Usually it's the money. After retirement, what goes out for insurance, medical care and a place to live can easily exceed what's coming in.

Retirement Security Inc. can help you design a retirement plan, whether you're planning your own or managing a parent's. We'll create a program to make sure the money's there when you need it.

Contrary to popular belief, your eyesight isn't the first thing to go.

And when that time comes, we'll help with every aspect. We help you purchase long-term care insurance, process your medical claims, and, if necessary, choose a new home. You can count on our referral services to help find a nursing home, create trusts and wills, plan your estate and arrange your finances. Just choose the services you need when you need them, then relax and enjoy your new life.

Call Retirement Security at 1-800-LT CARE5 (1-800-582-2735). We can show you how to keep your money from going before anything else.

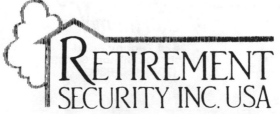

RETIREMENT SECURITY INC. USA

Serving individuals, families and corporations.
An MRM Group Company

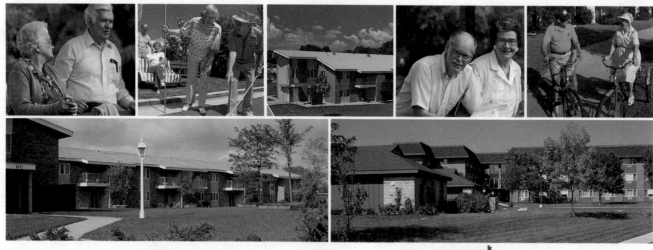

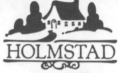

ORYX PRESS

ELDER SERVICES

1992 - 1993

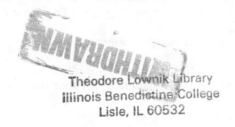
With the Cooperation of
Area Agency on Aging for the City of Chicago
Suburban Area Agency on Aging
And
Northeastern Illinois Area Agency on Aging

362.6025
E37
1992-93

Copyright © 1992 by
The Oryx Press
4041 North Central at Indian School Road
Phoenix, Arizona 85012-3397

Published simultaneously in Canada

Printed and Bound in the United States of America

∞ The paper used in this publication meets the minimum requirements of American National Standard for Information Science–Permanence of Paper for Printed Library Materials, ANSI Z39.48, 1984.

Library of Congress Cataloging-in-Publication Data

Elder services, 1992–1993 : the Greater Chicago area guide to
  eldercare.
      p.   cm.
   "With the cooperation of Area Agency on Aging for the City of
Chicago (Chicago Department on Aging and Disability), Suburban Area
Agency on Aging, Northeast Illinois Area Agency on Aging."
   Includes bibliographical references and indexes.
   ISBN 0-89774-664-3
   1. Aged–Services for–Illinois–Chicago Metropolitan Area–
–Directories. 2. Aged–Care–Illinois–Chicago Metropolitan Area–
–Directories. 3. Aged–Illinois–Chicago Metropolitan Area–
–Handbooks, manuals, etc. 4. Caregivers–Illinois–Chicago
Metropolitan Area–Handbooks, manuals, etc.   I. Oryx Press.
HV1471.C38E43 1992   92-3715
362.6'025'77311–dc20   CIP

✔ In order to support future editions of this publication would you please mention **Elder Services** each time you contact any advertiser, facility, or service.

Table of Contents

✔ In order to support future editions of this publication would you please mention **Elder Services** each time you contact any advertiser, facility, or service.

✔ In order to support future editions of this publication would you please mention **Elder Services** each time you contact any advertiser, facility, or service.

Help her now, and feel the warmth all winter.

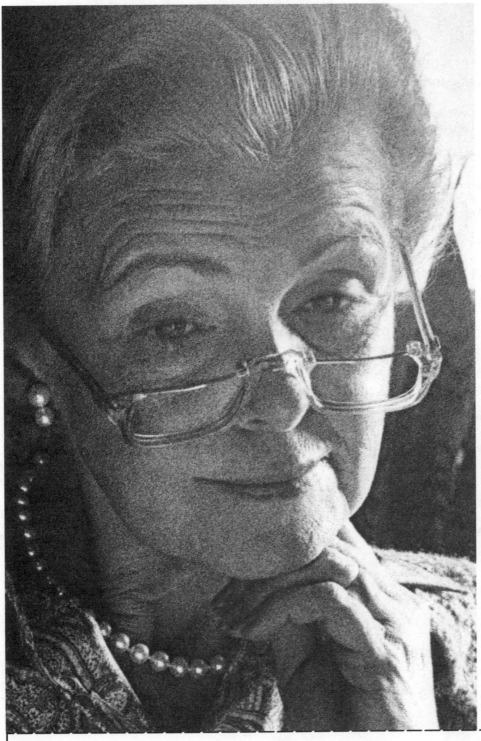

Protect loved ones with our Third Party plan. If you have friends or relatives who are ill, handicapped or elderly— this message is for you. In the unlikely event of a gas service interruption this winter, they might miss the notification from Peoples or North Shore Gas. But you can help them. You can volunteer to contact them through our Third Party plan. We urge you to fill out the form and have your friend or relative sign it. Just think how good that'll make you feel. Especially on the coldest nights. Return to Peoples Energy Corporation, Room 1159, 122 South Michigan Avenue, Chicago, Illinois 60603.

**Peoples Gas
North Shore Gas**
(312) 431-7004

DEPARTMENT OF HEALTH & HUMAN SERVICES

Office of the Secretary

Washington, D.C. 20201

Eldercare: Challenge for the 90's

Today, the nation's older population is healthier, better educated and living longer than ever before. At the same time, we have growing numbers of vulnerable older persons who are at risk of losing their independence. Our nation has a rich history of concern and action on behalf of its older citizens. Caring for our older relatives and friends who are at risk is an American tradition that should be preserved. Our goal is to help older persons remain active and independent in their own homes and communities for as long as possible. Eldercare is the response to this challenge. This word conveys the concept of caregiving and symbolizes the "culture of caring" which is needed to make our communities better places for all of us to mature today and into the 21st century.

Joyce T. Berry, Ph.D.

U.S. Commissioner on Aging

NATIONAL
ASSOCIATION
OF STATE UNITS
ON AGING

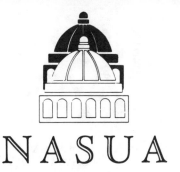

NASUA

2033 K Street, NW
Suite 304
Washington, DC 20006
(202) 785-0707

Independence and freedom of choice, without regard to age, sex, social or economic circumstance, are basic tenets of our democratic society. As these rights are preserved so is our sense of dignity and worth. Over the past 25 years, extending this guarantee to our elder citizens has become one of our nation's highest priorities. Reflective of this commitment, the leadership of our country has established policies and programs intended to preserve the autonomy and self-determination of older Americans.

One of the pivotal social structures charged with safeguarding the rights and advancing the interests of older people across the nation are the State Agencies on Aging. As a result of the passage of the Older Americans Act in 1965, there are 57 state and territorial government agencies established to further the social and economic agendas for older people in their respective states. The specific title of the State Agencies on Aging vary from state to state. It may be called a Department, Commission, Board, Office, or Bureau on Aging. In a few states, it carries the title Aging and Adult Services Administration.

The Older Americans Act, the cornerstone upon which all State Agency on Aging actions are based, sets forth ambitious, global goals for the nation's elderly. The strategies used by State Aging Agencies to achieve these goals are twofold. First, they operate a complex service system designed to complement and complete other human service systems in meeting the needs of the elderly. Simultaneously, they serve as effective and visible advocates for the elderly, working with both the public and the private sectors to ensure their responsiveness to the needs of older citizens. A few of the most challenging tasks they face today include: long term care, older worker employment, support to families, income maintenance, quality of care, housing development, nutrition, intergenerational programs and the targeting of services to persons in greatest need.

One of the highest objectives of State Agencies on Aging, together with their Association (NASUA), is to maximize the ability of older Americans to remain independent in their homes and communities as long as possible. Critical to achieving this goal is the role of the caregiver who provides support to the older person. It is essential, therefore, that both older people and caregivers be informed and knowledgeable about how to access available community and in-home services when they are needed.

A publication program such as <u>Elder Services</u> is designed to meet the evolving needs of older persons and caregivers. This publication supports our efforts to educate older people and caregivers about service options designed to support the independence of our nation's older citizens.

Daniel A. Quirk
Executive Director

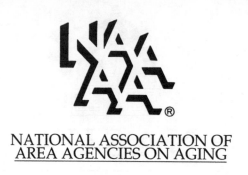

NATIONAL ASSOCIATION OF
AREA AGENCIES ON AGING

The first step for most people in dealing with personal or family issues relating to growing older is to locate sources of help. In fact, accessing information about community resources for older people is a growing concern among our nation's elderly and their caregivers. It is also a concern of the nation's Area Agencies on Aging.

Together with the U.S. Administration on Aging and 57 State Agencies on Aging, the 670 Area Agencies on Aging and their 20,000 + service contractors are part of what has been called America's Aging Network. Created under federal law to administer programs for all citizens over 60, the Aging Network is charged with advocating, designing, funding, and brokering public and private funds for a wide array of community services. Covering the entire nation, they are the vital link concerned with the creation of a comprehensive system of public and private services for older Americans.

Through contracts with over 20,000 local organizations, Area Agencies on Aging spend nearly $3 Billion annually to provide meals, transportation, senior centers, home care, and a wide variety of other services. Over 10 million Americans receive some form of assistance through the nationwide system of Area Agencies on Aging every year. Area Agencies are also strong advocates for seniors - often officially monitoring nursing homes and other institutions and participating in such activities as local land use decisions to ensure the housing needs of the seniors are being met. Finally, they are the source of information and referral for over 11 million requests annually.

Unfortunately, in many communities such services are not widely available. The lack of adequate community services has become a major family issue, an economic issue, and a healthcare issue. These resources are critical to help our nation's elderly maintain their health and independence in their homes and communities. Responding to the need among the nation's seniors has already begun to tax the resources of public service providers. However, increased demand for products and services can also lead to new opportunities for the private sector and force organizations to work together to be more creative and responsive in developing new products and services.

The aging of America will affect every part of our future - whether it's business trying to understand the new needs and attitudes of this age group, or employers struggling with how to help their employees care for their loved ones without affecting productivity. This is a problem the private sector and public sector can and should solve together.

Elder Services is an excellent resource for older Americans and their caregivers. NAAAA applauds this cooperative effort to provide a comprehensive, community-wide directory of services.

Jonathan D. Linkous
Executive Director

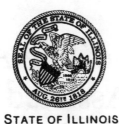

DEPARTMENT ON AGING

421 EAST CAPITOL AVENUE
SPRINGFIELD **62701**

Dear Readers,

The Illinois Department on Aging was established in 1973 by the State Legislature and charged with a mission to improve the quality of life for Illinois' older citizens. The Department is the only agency in the State authorized to receive and disburse Federal Older Americans Act funds, as well as State funds to Illinois' thirteen Area Agencies on Aging. These regional agencies re-allocate funding to community-based service providers who directly assist older adults, allowing them to remain in their own homes while avoiding nursing home placement as their only long term care option. We call this service delivery system, the Illinois Aging Network.

In addition to funding the agencies which serve adults, age 60 and older, the Department on Aging also plans, coordinates and evaluates the programs provided through the Aging Network. High priority is given to serving older individuals with greatest economic and social need.

Services provided through the Aging Network include: access services, such as transportation, case management and outreach; community services, like nutrition and employment programs, housing assistance and multipurpose senior centers; in-homes services, such as homemaker, chore housekeeping, residential repair and renovation and home-delivered meals; plus, many others. The Aging Network also coordinates elder abuse and neglect intervention services, a long term care ombudsman program and many separate initiatives to help special populations, like family caregivers and Alzheimer's victims.

The Illinois Department on Aging operates a nationwide toll-free information and referral number, **1-800-252-8966.** This number can be reached from 8:30 a.m. to 5 p.m., Monday through Friday. Older persons, their family members and anyone who is interested in learning more about services available through the Illinois Department on Aging and the State's Aging Network are welcome to call. This number is also an excellent access point for long-distance caregivers who need to find out about services available in other states.

The Department's mission and the Aging Network's goal is to help older people and their families. If this excellent resource directory does not answer all of your questions, please call **1-800-252-8966.** We care and we're here to help.

Yours truly,

Nancy S. Nelson

Nancy S. Nelson, Deputy Director
Illinois Department on Aging

Seniors Live The Active Life Through Assisted Living At ActiveLife Rental Retirement Communities

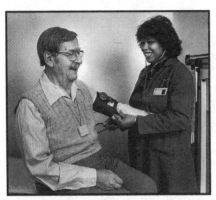

Blood pressure checks are just one of the many services offered to residents like Sam Naso at the Oak Park Arms and Hawthorn Lakes Retirement Communities.

He's known to the staff of the Oak Park Arms as "the man with the twinkling eyes," and you know exactly what they mean when you meet 81-year old Sam Naso.

This native Chicagoan talks easily about himself, his days as a bookkeeper at Ryan Insurance and his retirement at the Oak Park Arms. "I love my life here at the Oak Park Arms!" he relates enthusiastically.

Sam, a life-long bachelor, has Parkinson's Disease. His condition requires careful monitoring, which is available to him at the Oak Park Arms. That assistance allowed Sam to be a finalist for king of the Oak Park Arms' Senior Prom and a prize winner in the annual talent contest. Without the specialized care he receives, Sam would have to live in a nursing home.

Sam's alternative to life in a nursing home is an active life at the Oak Park Arms with his day-to-day care provided by First Choice Home Health and Family Support Services. First Choice maintains an on-site office staffed 24-hours a day.

Experienced staff members at ActiveLife Retirement Communities understand the special needs of their residents. From the Oak Park Arms in the western suburbs to Hawthorn Lakes in Vernon Hills, assisted living is top priority.

Both rental communities provide "more care" allowing residents to be "more carefree." Residents may choose from many assistance programs designed to meet specific needs. A resident may simply need to be accompanied to the dining room or reminded when a medication should be taken—or in some instances require 24-hour nursing service. Care services can be purchased on a monthly basis in packages which carefully profile the physical needs of the individual resident.

At the Oak Park Arms, First Choice Home Health and Family Support Services is the care provider. At Hawthorn Lakes, residents can choose health care services from LifeStyle Options, Inc. and Condell Medical Center.

With health needs secured, residents of the Oak Park Arms and Hawthorn Lakes Retirement Communities can enjoy a full range of activities including trips to concerts, plays and shopping. Both communities feature delicious restaurant dining, maid service and 24-hour security.

Give us a call and we'll show you how your patient can live a fuller more carefree life at Hawthorn Lakes or The Oak Park Arms Retirement Communities.

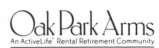

Oak Park Arms
An ActiveLife® Rental Retirement Community

408 S. Oak Park Avenue
Oak Park
(708) 386-4040

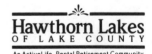

Hawthorn Lakes
OF LAKE COUNTY
An ActiveLife Rental Retirement Community

10 E. Hawthorn Parkway
Vernon Hills
(708) 367-0166

Preface
and How to Use This Book

The aging of the nation has created a new awareness of the needs of the elderly. Better health care and demographics have made elderly people among the fastest growing segments of the population, but with this growth has come an increased demand for quality eldercare. In response, a "culture of caring" has developed involving caregivers, professionals, and older people themselves. The goal of this culture is to provide the best care possible, while at the same time preserving the independence and dignity of the elderly and the well-being of the caregivers. In keeping with this goal, this book, *Elder Services 1992: The Greater Chicago Area Guide to Eldercare*, provides useful advice, practical information, and detailed descriptions of over 280 service-providing agencies, organizations, and associations in the greater Chicago metropolitan area. In addition, the lengthy "Directory of Facilities" in *Elder Services* gives information on 1,319 adult day care centers, home health care services, nursing homes, retirement facilities, Alzheimer's treatment centers, and medical rehabilitation facilities in the Chicago metropolitan area.

In an area as large and diverse as greater Chicago, the choices may seem overwhelming, but by providing so much information about the eldercare network in a single source, this *Guide* allows caregivers, professionals, and older people to find the long-term care arrangements that best meet their needs.

HOW TO USE THIS BOOK

A good approach, or point of entry, to *Elder Services* is for the reader to consult the "Glossary of Commonly Used Terms in Caregiving" in order to clarify any concepts or vocabulary with which he or she is unfamiliar.

Practical Advice and Information

Balancing the needs of elderly and those of caregivers is not an easy task. Many decisions have to be made about insurance, type of care needed, where the care should be provided, legal affairs, finances, and personal relations between caregivers and older people. The "Practical Advice and Information" section of this *Guide* provides useful insights into these topics in articles written by local experts.

- **Older Americans Act–Network on Aging** discusses the network created by the pas-

✓ In order to support future editions of this publication would you please mention **Elder Services** each time you contact any advertiser, facility, or service.

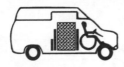
sage of The Older Americans Act (OAA) in 1965. The network consists of federal, state, and local agencies dedicated to implementing the objectives of OAA, which are listed. A chart clearly details their structure and the services they provide.

- **What Is Long-Term Care?** describes long-term care as a continuum of care ranging from those who are home and well to those who are institutionalized and immobile. The advancement along this continuum is determined by health and mental status and not by age. The article discusses what types of services make up long-term care and where these services are provided, noting that 80 percent of such care is provided by nonprofessionals.
- **Ethnicity and Aging** deals with the unique concerns of the aging members of over 100 different nationalities who reside in the Chicago metropolitan area. In particular, the isolation caused by linguistic and cultural barriers is discussed, and the need for personnel to work with these seniors is stressed. Organizations that may be available to provide assistance are listed.
- **Housing Alternatives for Seniors** is a source of comprehensive information concerning the option of "aging-in-place," or when that choice is not feasible, the many other opportunities that exist along the continuum from independent living to an institutional setting. The advantages and services generally available with each of these options are explored, and financial considerations and available programs are considered.

- **Accessing and Using the Home Care System** is an in-depth discussion of home care, including insurance benefits. The article differentiates between skilled care, covered by Medicare and many long-term policies, and personal care, which must be funded for the most part by the client or family. The team approach in a home health program, where the paraprofessional carries out the plan of the professionals, is explained.
- **Added Security through Caller ID** describes a new telephone service to be provided in the Chicago area that allows the customer to determine who is calling before answering the phone, thereby avoiding annoying calls from unknown callers. This service provides security and protection for older people, many of whom are exploited by harassing callers.
- **Independence at Home: Creative Opportunities** is an explanation of when it is appropriate for the family to step in and provide or hire the assistance that is needed by an aging individual. The author provides many ideas of services that make it possible for a person to age-in-place.
- **Caregiving: Managing the Responsibility** is an analysis of the responsibilities of the caregiver and the dilemma that this person faces when she or he must juggle the new role of caregiver with other commitments to family and employer. A helpful list, headed "What You Can Do," offers some solutions.
- **Support in the Workplace: Corporate Eldercare** is a discussion of corporate eldercare options that exist to meet the needs of a company and its employees. Program possibilities range from simply providing information and seminars to consultation and referral, flexible time, and financial assistance.
- **Volunteer Opportunities** discusses the many services provided for the aging population through volunteer programs. Also

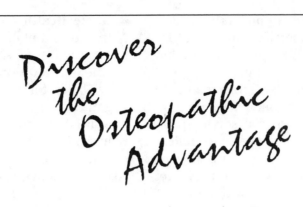

presented is the other side of the coin: the older person as a volunteer.

- **Preparing for Incompetence: Legal Considerations** focuses on those legal tools that do not require court intervention. Also explained are the concepts of power of attorney, the living will, the health care surrogate act, and the living trust.
- **Dealing with Costs of Long-Term Care** notes that eight out of ten families are directly affected by the long-term care (LTC) crisis. LTC is costly because it combines so many elements of care; federal programs do not provide enough money, and private insurance is inadequate in most cases. Home care is cheaper, and patients generally do better in a home-care situation, but costs of home care are rarely covered by insurance or federal funds. The author believes the solution to this problem may be adult day care because it is cheaper than institutionalization and provides the caregiver with more freedom and time to work. A list of key consumer LTC resources is also provided.

- **Long-Term Care Insurance** explains the profile of the perfect candidate for long-term care insurance and how the subscriber can find the best buy. Ratings for insurance companies are explained, and group plans are compared with individual plans. Most important is the language of the policy and making sure that definitions of eligibility standards are understood.
- **Veteran Benefits, Chicago Metropolitan Area** describes the benefits, which include pensions and medical care, available to millions of people in this country. This article includes the range of services, eligibility requirements, and Chicago-area service locations in detail.

Basic Resources for the Caregiver

This section of *Elder Services* includes checklists, a bibliography, helpline numbers to call, a glossary of often-used terms, and a list of and index to helpful organizations. All contain basic, useful resources for the caregiver or concerned family of an older adult.

✔ In order to support future editions of this publication would you please mention **Elder Services** each time you contact any advertiser, facility, or service.

- **Service Options and Opportunities** describes community services available in the Chicago area and the work of the local Area Agencies on Aging.
- **Helpful Organizations** lists more than 280 greater Chicago area agencies ranging from senior centers to social service providers to government services. An **Index** to this list helps users locate just the organizations they need, whether they are looking for senior centers with congregate dining or agencies that provide legal services.
- **Checklists** help caregivers evaluate the many aspects of these topics: whether a relative should live alone, needs for home care, questions to ask about care for a relative within your home, questions to ask about a day care center, and questions to ask when selecting a nursing home.
- **Helpline Numbers** lists 40 of the most important phone contacts a caregiver needs.
- **Helpful Materials for Caregivers** provides listings for helpful materials dealing with eldercare.

Directory of Facilities

In addition to narrative advice and basic resources, *Elder Services* provides a Directory of Facilities section.

Entries in this section were obtained from six databases, created and updated by the Oryx Press through continual mailings of questionnaires. All entries are for the greater Chicago area. Facilities are arranged according to the type of caregiving offered: Adult Day Care Centers, Home Health Care Services, Nursing Homes, Retirement Facilities, Alzheimer's Treatment Centers and Programs, and Medical Rehabilitation Facilities. Within each separate directory, facilities are arranged alphabetically by city and by facility name. Each entry contains core information–name, address, telephone number, and may include further description as follows:

- **Adult Day Care Centers**. Entries may detail number of clients, hours of operation, meals, and services offered.

- **Home Health Care Services**. Profiles may include number of clients; financial plans accepted; and services offered, including whether equipment and supplies are available for sale or rent, and if pickup and delivery is available.
- **Nursing Homes**. Entries may detail information on licensing, the number of beds and type of care, certification, admissions requirements, and full- and part-time staff. Languages spoken other than English are listed. Charts at the end of this section allow quick comparison of the facilities' features and the activities available at each nursing home.
- **Retirement Facilities**. For the first time in this edition, facilities are divided into "Sheltered and Congregate Care" and "Independent Living" sections. These descriptions may include the nature of the housing type and accommodations provided. Number of residents is often given, as are entrance age requirements and a list of services provided, such as medical care, nursing, therapy and rehabilitation, housekeeping, spiritual, social, recreational, security, shopping, central dining, and personal. Some facility profiles include average monthly and/or entrance fees.
- **Alzheimer's Treatment Centers and Programs**. Individual listings may describe the full-time, part-time, and consulting staff; the type of facility as determined by care programs provided; accreditations given; name of the parent institution or system and any affiliations; referral policy; insurance plans accepted; client services; and any age restrictions. Charts allow quick reference to compare facilities, programs, and services.
- **Medical Rehabilitation Facilities**. Profiles may include the full-time, part-time, and consulting staff; the type of facility; and accreditations given. The program profile may include referral methods, diagnostic services provided, financial coverages accepted, client services provided, and any additional information. Charts allow quick comparison of programs and services from center to center.

✔ In order to support future editions of this publication would you please mention **Elder Services** each time you contact any advertiser, facility, or service.

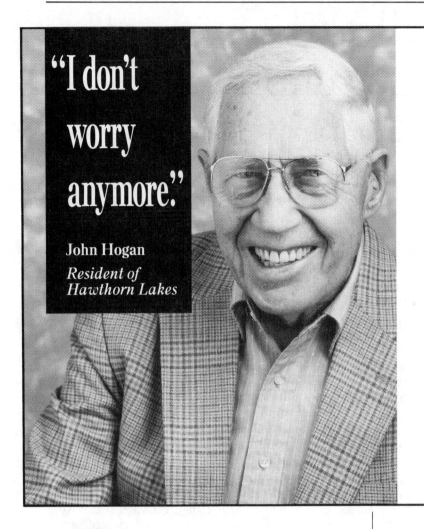
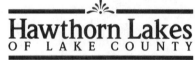

Indexes

The organizations and facilities listed in the directory section are also listed in the Indexes–first, alphabetically, for easy reference to facilities being considered, and, second, geographically, for those selecting facilities nearest their homes.

ACKNOWLEDGMENTS

A unique publication such as this would be impossible to produce without dedication and hard work. The editors acknowledge the tireless work and expertise of Magon Kinzie, Nancy Brim, Sam Mongeau, Barbara Flaxman, and Sandi Bourelle.

It is especially important to acknowledge Siri Nimitz-Nelson for her hard work and dedication.

This is the last edition of *Elder Services* to be published by The Oryx Press. Future editions in this series will be published by HCIA, 300 East Lombard Street, Baltimore, MD 21202. If, as you use this guide, you become aware of additional information or changes that should be made, please write HCIA, c/o Miss Mary Betch, or call toll free at 1-800-568-3282 and ask for the publications department. Every effort will be made to include such contributions in succeeding editions. In the event of a publication error, the sole responsibility of the publisher will be to enter corrected information in succeeding editions. Please also direct any such information to the editors at HCIA at the address given above.

A listing in the directory section of this *Guide* is by no means an endorsement of that facility by The Oryx Press or by HCIA and should not take the place of in-person visits to the centers, extensive personal evaluation, and consultation with local government and aging advocacy groups.

✔ In order to support future editions of this publication would you please mention **Elder Services** each time you contact any advertiser, facility, or service.

Glossary of Commonly Used Terms

AAA *See* Area Agency on Aging.

Accessory Apartment A separate living unit built within the basic frame of an existing single family home. Also known as an in-law apartment.

Activities Coordinator An individual who creates programs that provide recreation and entertainment for residents of a nursing home, retirement facility, or clients in a day care facility or senior center.

Activities of Daily Living (ADLs) These include getting out of bed, getting dressed and groomed, toileting and bathing, getting around the house, preparing meals, taking medications, communicating needs, handling finances, and household chores.

Acute Illness A sudden illness such as a heart attack or stroke. The cause is known and the condition curable.

Adult Home Sheltered housing or a group home. A facility designed with personal attention and a lifestyle closer to normal than that in a nursing home. Services are limited and may not include nursing care.

Advocacy Acting on behalf of others, in this case older people; i.e., when representatives for older persons collectively seek full service benefits and entitlement, including the expansion of benefits, which will assist all older people with these needs.

Ages Common terms for the elderly are: young old, 60-75 years; old, 76-84 years; very old, 85 years, and over.

Area Agency on Aging (AAA or Triple A) A nonprofit agency or unit of local government that plans and coordinates services for the elderly in a given geographic area.

Assessment *See* Geriatric Assessment.

Assisted Living Termed "Sheltered Care" in our facility directory section, these facilities provide residents some assistance with the activities of daily living. Although staff members may supervise the self-administration of medication, they may not administer medication or provide nursing care.

Board and Care Facility A small group living arrangement providing room, meals, housekeeping, and personal care services. *See also* Domiciliary Care Home.

Caregiver The person helping the elderly with everyday living.

Caregiver Support Self-help, support groups, and formal services which will assist and enable the caregiver to continue the helping relationship. *See also* Respite Care.

Carrier Watch A program where postal clerks watch for regular mail pickup by older persons who are registered with the Post Office. If mail is not picked up, an emergency contact is notified.

Case Coordination Units Agencies of the Area Agency on Aging which provide case management services.

Case (Care) Management Assessment, coordination, and monitoring of services by skilled social worker provided to an older person and his or her family. This service develops a care plan, information and assistance for needs, and regular follow-up to enable the older person to function as independently as possible. Some private geriatric care managers may also provide direct services such as counseling and home care.

Chore Housekeeping *See* Housekeeper.

Chronic Illness A physical or mental disability marked by long duration and/or frequent recurrence. It may be long-term and incurable but may be manageable with medical treatment.

Circuit Breaker A program where Illinois homeowners or renters aged 65 or older may annually apply for a rebate on property taxes or rent. Participants may also elect to use a portion of the rebate to enroll in the pharmaceutical assistance program and receive free medications for heart, blood pressure, diabetes, and/or arthritis.

Companion A person who assists with daily living activities of the elderly person. The companion has no nursing responsibilities. *See also* Housekeeper.

Congregate Dining A feature of a residential facility which provides hot or appropriate prepared meals in a social atmosphere.

Congregate Housing Individual apartments or single rooms in a multi-unit building planned and designed for older persons. Supportive services such as meals, transportation, housekeeping, and social and recreational activities are usually provided. Also referred to as shared housing.

Congregate Meals Programs that serve balanced nutritional meals in a social group setting.

Continuing Care Agreements Assignment of assets to a facility in exchange for care. Financial arrangements may include significant entrance and/or endowment fees in addition to monthly charges. Generally, some portion of principal is refunded to the resident's estate.

Continuing Care Communities Housing planned and operated to provide a continuum of services and accommodations for older adults including, but not limited to, independent living, congregate housing, assisted living, and nursing home care. Services are provided depending on the level of care required. *See also* Continuing Care Agreements.

Cooperative Apartments Independent apartment buildings where the residents are part-owners of the building. Owners have a part in the decision-making process of managing the building.

Counseling Services provided by trained therapists and social workers for individuals who require help in understanding and managing their needs and future directions.

Crisis Intervention Services that intervene at time of emotional and/or physical trauma.

Custodial Care Care that provides a safe environment for those who do not need a nursing home but are frail and can no longer live on their own. This service monitors health and provides meals and social activities.

Day Care Week-day structured programs in a communal setting, providing activities in addition to health-related and rehab services. Designed for the elderly who are physically or emotionally disabled and need protective environments. The program provides meals, activities, and personal care and health services. Because it secures the care of clients during the day, it provides respite for caregivers.

Dementia A group of brain disorders that disrupt normal thinking, cognitive abilities, memory, judgement, mood, and social functioning. It is not necessarily a part of the normal effects of aging.

Diagnostic Related Groups (DRGs) A group of illnesses for which the federal government has set a reimbursement cap under Medicare; this amount may or may not equal the cost of treatment or the cost billed to the consumer.

Discharge Planner A staff member of a hospital or nursing home who helps plan the future care of a patient when released into the community.

Domiciliary Care Home A group living arrangement that provides supervised meals, housekeeping, and personal care. *See also* Board and Care Facility.

Durable Power of Attorney *See* Power of Attorney.

Echo Housing A self-contained, free-standing, and temporary living unit which is occupied by a relative on the property of an adjacent single family dwelling. It is used for an aging relative and then removed when the need for proximity to the family is ended. Also referred to as a granny flat or mother-in-law suite.

Education for Older Persons A variety of enriching formal and informal classroom and field studies offered for a continuation of life-long learning.

Elder Abuse Emotional, physical, and/or financial mistreatment of older persons by those involved in their lives. Cases of abuse should be reported to an agency that will respond to reports by investigating, helping to relieve the problems, and arranging for services needed. *See* Emotional Abuse, Financial Exploitation, and Physical Abuse.

Emergency Response System A service where the older person is connected to a dispatch unit and/or medical facility via a remote transmitter and the telephone. If the remote transmitter is activated, efforts are made to contact the older person, his/her emergency contact, or paramedics.

Emotional Abuse The verbal threatening, harassment, or insulting of a person.

Employment Counseling Assistance in locating work and or training for gainful employment.

Escort A service that takes older persons to and from medical appointments and/or shopping.

Ethnic Services and Activities Programs that offer services of special interest to people from various ethnic groups.

Federally Subsidized Housing Rental housing built and operated with financial assistance from the US Department of Housing and Urban Development (HUD). Low- and moderate-income residents pay 30 percent of their income for rent and HUD pays the difference.

Financial Exploitation A situation where one's money and funds are misused or withheld.

Financial Services Programs where trained consultants help plan the monetary resources of older persons so they may be self-sufficient and have financial security.

Friendly Visitor One who regularly visits an isolated or institutionalized older person. These visits provide companionship and are usually made by a volunteer.

Gatekeeper Program A service where utility meter readers and other personnel are trained to recognize signs of possible illness or injury in order to link the older person with appropriate agencies in the community.

Geriatric Assessment Evaluation of the person's physical, psychological, and social condition by a professional team specializing in gerontology, usually a physi-

cian, nurse, and a social worker. The team then makes recommendations for future care.

Granny Flats *See* Echo Housing.

Guardianship A protective service for one who needs help making important decisions about paying bills, going to the doctor, and finding safe housing. The court appoints a responsible adult acting in a parental way to provide this protective service. May be limited to certain tasks and/or temporary.

Home Delivered Meals Nutritionally balanced meals delivered to the older person on a regular basis. Most programs can accommodate special diets and may provide additional snacks and/or weekend meals.

Home Equity Conversion Reverse annuity mortgages or sale leasebacks which allow an older person to turn up to 80 percent of his/her accumulated equity in a home into a monthly income plus guaranteed residence, either for a fixed period of time or for life. In reverse annuity mortgages, the home usually reverts to the lender (most often a bank), while in the sale leaseback the home is sold, usually to a relative, and then rented back to the older person. *See also* Reverse Mortgage Loan.

Home Health Aide A trained person who assists with personal care needs, such as bathing, dressing, walking, and monitoring oral medication.

Home Health Nurse A professional nurse who makes home visits with doctor's orders to evaluate the patient's condition, provide medical services, and possibly train the individual or family members in home health care.

Home Maintenance and Repair Services Programs designed to assist older persons to remain in their own homes or apartments by making repairs to the home at little or no cost to the residents. Can include yard work, painting, electrical or plumbing repairs, cement repairs, repairs to steps or porches, and/or the addition of adaptive devices for persons with disabilities.

Home Matching Programs A service where two or three persons are matched, typically with the assistance of an agency, to share an existing home or apartment of one of the older persons. This program should result in lower overall housing costs for the residents and also offer companionship. The residents have their own sleeping areas and share the common areas of the home. Frequently, service agreements are made by residents to assist with activities of daily living.

Homemaker *See* Housekeeper.

Homes for the Elderly Accommodations for people with health limitations. They range from private homes, which may only offer custodial care, to skilled nursing facilities.

Homestead Exemption In Illinois, a tax provision that reduces the equalized assessed valuation, therefore the real estate taxes, of a residential property owned and occupied by an Illinois resident aged 65 or older.

Hospice A range of services that combine personal and medical care designed to help those terminally ill and their families live as comfortably as possible. The emphases of these programs are to ease pain and offer dignified choices in the last stages of life.

Housekeeper A trained worker, hired privately or supervised by an agency, who provides assistance with cleaning, meal preparation, laundry, transportation, and shopping, and possibly personal care. Nursing care is not included.

Housing Assistance A service to help find suitable housing for an older person.

In-Home Services A program where trained personnel provide medical and/or nonmedical support to assist persons in their homes. These service providers may include homemakers, housekeepers, home health aides, or other workers who perform tasks for older people to enable them to remain in their own homes.

Independent Senior Apartments Self-contained living units for older adults who are able to care for themselves. Management may facilitate minimal access to community services and provide recreational services for voluntary use by residents. No medical services are provided.

Information and Assistance A program provided by many agencies and companies that finds and refers information and services for clients. Also called information and referral, or I & R.

Intake Personnel The first people usually encountered when contacting a service agency. This person will clarify the request and then refer the client to the proper department and/or service.

Intergenerational Programs Programs designed to blend the young, the old, and middle aged, or combinations thereof, offering opportunities for all to appreciate an enriching multigenerational environment.

Intermediate Care Assistance for those who are unable to dress, feed, bathe, or get around by themselves. It is usually provided in a nursing home and focuses on personal care and social work.

Legal Services Assistance and guidance on legal issues and legal representation, including advocacy, conservatorship, and power of attorney.

Life Care Communities *See* Continuing Care Communities.

Living Trust A legal, revocable document that names a person, known as a grantor, to manage property of the grantee according to the terms of the trust agreement.

Living Will A declaration of an individual's wishes regarding health care should the individual become incapacitated. Only applicable to terminal illnesses and is subject to the judgement of the individual's physician.

Long-Term Care The provision of services to persons of any age who suffer from chronic health impairment.

Long-Term Care Insurance An insurance policy issued by a private insurance company that covers the costs of nursing home care or home healthcare. This type of insurance policy is recommended for persons who have over $50,000 in assets, not including one's home or personal items, and an annual income over $15,000. Premiums and coverage vary depending on many factors.

Meal Sites Places where meals are prepared and served, such as senior centers and/or community locations.

Meals on Wheels *See* Home Delivered Meals.

Medicaid Insurance The part of the Medicare program that pays for nursing home care when the person cannot afford to pay these costs. The person must have spent nearly all of his or her assets and be a resident in a nursing home that participates in this program. There are many varying requirements in this program and current information should be researched when considering Medicaid.

Medical Director The physician appointed to help ensure the adequacy and appropriateness of the medical services provided to nursing home residents.

Medical Evaluation *See* Geriatric Assessment.

Medicare Insurance Federal government health insurance. Part A is for hospital and skilled nursing care. Part B covers physician services, home health services, therapies, and some other services.

Medigap Insurance An insurance policy purchased by the consumer, issued by a private insurance company, which covers health care costs above those covered by Medicare Part A or Part B. These policies do not cover most long-term care expenses.

Mother-in-Law Suites *See* Echo Housing.

Municipally Owned/Subsidized Housing A municipally funded building or program funded through bonds, taxes, and other pools of public money, which guarantees that the market rent will be paid to the management, although the tenant only pays a portion of the amount. *See also* Federally Subsidized Housing.

Neglect The failure to receive basic requirements for living such as food, medical care, clothing, shelter, or social contact.

Occupational Therapist A licensed therapist who helps a person relearn activities of daily living and may make adaptations in the home to enable the person to live more independently.

"Old" *See* Ages.

Ombudsman A program to advocate and protect the rights of residents in long-term care facilities by investigating complaints, mediating and resolving disputes, and initiating corrective action.

Pharmaceutical Assistance Program *See* Circuit Breaker.

Physical Abuse The mistreatment of a person, which includes rough handling, slapping, or hitting.

Physical Therapist A licensed therapist who provides individualized programs of exercise to improve physical mobility.

Power of Attorney A legal procedure that enables a person to give another person the authority to act on his or her behalf. Can be inclusive or exclusive and relate to money and/or health matters.

Property Tax Deferral A provision where property taxes on a residence owned and occupied by a person age 65 or older are deferred until the property is sold or the taxpayer no longer resides there, whereupon the taxes must be paid with minimal interest charges. May be continued by a surviving spouse aged 55 or older.

Protective Services Services that support an adult who may be abused, neglected, or exploited. Available from social services agencies and state agencies.

Recreation Activities of interest and fun.

Rehabilitation Therapeutic care for those who need intensive physical, occupational, or speech therapy to reach their full potential.

Residential Energy Assistance Partnership Program An Illinois program to provide financial assistance to income qualifying persons with high utility bills.

Respite Care Temporary care of the frail elderly to relieve caregivers of the stress of their time-consuming responsibilities. May be care in or out of the home and can range in duration from a few hours to several days. *See also* Caregiver Support.

Reverse Mortgage Loan A loan that involves payment *to*, rather than *from*, the homeowner. These monthly cash advances, available in Illinois to homeowners 62 or older, do not require repayment until the homeowners sell, move away, or die. The amount of the loan is based on the age of the youngest homeowner, the value of the home, and the interest rate.

Self-Care Bathing, dressing, toileting, and feeding of oneself.

Self-Help Group *See* Support Group.

Senior Centers Neighborhood centers offering a variety of social, health, nutritional, educational, and recreational programs.

Sewer Charge Exemption A provision where homeowners aged 65 or older can be excused from paying a sewer service charge.

Shared Housing *See* Congregate Housing.

Sheltered Care Care provided in a facility that should be licensed with a state regulating agency. Provides assistance with daily living but does not provide nursing care. Our directory section includes "Assisted Living" and "Board and Care Facilities" in this category.

Single Room Occupancy Hotels Properties primarily providing single furnished rooms for rent on a daily, weekly, or monthly basis with no lease. Usually occupied by low-income individuals. Also known as Transient Hotels or SRO's.

Skilled Level Care *See* Skilled Nursing Facility.

Skilled Nursing Facility (SNF) A facility that provides 24-hour medical nursing care by registered nurses, licensed practical nurses, and/or nurses aides. This is care for the seriously ill or severely disabled.

Social Worker A licensed counselor who assists the elderly and their families in understanding and coping with the practical, emotional, and psychological aspects of aging. The social worker may also monitor in-home services.

Supplemental Insurance See Medigap Insurance.

Support Group A group where individuals in similar situations meet to provide mutual support with the help of a trained leader.

Telephone Reassurance A service, usually provided by volunteers, which makes daily phone calls to elderly persons living alone. Provides social contact and can act in the event that the elderly person does not answer the telephone.

Transportation Services Free or low-cost transportation for people with special needs. Can be arranged on a regular basis or by appointment.

"Very Old" *See* Ages.

Veteran An individual who has been in active military service, discharged under conditions other than dishonorable, and has served the required time specified for VA eligibility.

Volunteer Services Opportunities for both those wanting to work without payment and those who use the various services provided by volunteers.

Weatherization Repairs Program A service similar to home maintenance and repair, but repairs focus on storm windows and doors, insulation, heating units, and weatherstripping.

Will Program A public service program of the Chicago Bar Association. This program offers eligible citizens a free, will-related consultation and the preparation of a will at a reduced cost.

"Young Old" *See* Ages.

WHY BE BOTHERED?

Wrong numbers. Unsolicited solicitations. Pranksters. Nosy neighbors. How do you separate these little annoyances from the phone calls you really care about? Like calls from your favorite friends and family?

The solution is Caller ID, new from Illinois Bell. Caller ID clearly shows the caller's number on a display screen that's attached to your phone. It's incredibly easy to use. And affordable, too.

When the phone rings and you're not sure how to answer, the answer is Caller ID.

CALLER ID.
For information and availability, call
1-800-428-2111
Dept. 89.

During its introduction, Caller ID will give you numbers of calls placed within your local Illinois Bell calling area. Both you and the caller must be in specially-equipped calling areas for numbers to appear on your display screen. Display equipment is purchased separately. If you want to block the appearance of your number when you place a call, dial *67 on your touchtone phone, or 1167 on rotary dials. The activation of your blocking is confirmed with a stutter, followed by a dial tone.

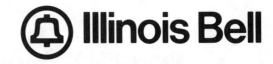

 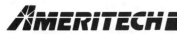

PRACTICAL ADVICE AND INFORMATION

Show this page to your family and friends. You could save a life.

Someone you care about probably has diabetes and doesn't know it.

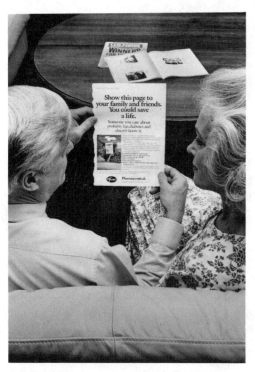

It's estimated that eleven million Americans have diabetes, yet less than half of them know it. Patients with diabetes run a risk of high blood pressure, heart attacks, kidney disease, or blindness.

And yet today's physicians know more about the disease and how to manage it than ever before. Treatment has become increasingly simple and effective, making it possible for a great many diabetics to live normal lives.

That means there's more reason than ever to know the warning signs of diabetes:

- **A history of diabetes in the family**
- **Overtiredness for no apparent reason**
- **Overweight and age over 40**
- **Excessive thirst**
- **More frequent urination**
- **Bruises, cuts, or infections that take longer than normal to heal**

If some of these warning signs seem to apply to you, or to one of your family or friends, it's time for a visit to the doctor.

For reprints of this message, write to: Pharmaceuticals Group, Pfizer Inc, Save A Life, P.O. Box 3852D, Grand Central Station, New York, NY 10163.

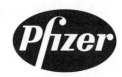

Pharmaceuticals
A PARTNER IN HEALTHCARE™

Older Americans Act–
Network on Aging

The National Association of State Units on Aging (NASUA) is the agency overseeing 57 state and territorial government agencies established to further the social and economic agendas for older people. The Older Americans Act, described here, is the cornerstone on which all state agency on aging actions are based.

THE OLDER AMERICANS ACT–THE FOUNDATION

The passage of the Older Americans Act in 1965 by the U.S. Congress affirmed our nation's high sense of commitment to the well-being of older citizens. The goal of the Older Americans Act (OAA) is to remove barriers to economic and personal independence and to ensure the availability of appropriate services for those older individuals who need them.

More specifically, the OAA embraces the following objectives for assuring older Americans–

- Adequate income
- Best possible physical and mental health
- Suitable housing
- Full restorative services for those who require institutional care and a comprehensive array of community-based long-term care services to sustain older people at home
- Opportunity for employment
- Retirement in health, honor, and dignity
- Civic, cultural, educational, and recreational opportunities
- Community services that provide a continuum of care for the vulnerable elderly
- Benefits from research
- Freedom to plan and manage their lives

IMPLEMENTING THE OAA

To implement these objectives, the Older Americans Act created structures at the federal, state, and local levels. Taken together they are often referred to as the Network on Aging. The aging network has as its common goal to provide maximum opportunities for older people to live independent, meaningful, and dignified lives in their own homes and communities as long as possible and to protect the rights of older people who need to live in care-providing facilities.

Today, the OAA Network on Aging includes the U.S. Administration on Aging, a part of the Department of Health and Human Services; 57 State Agencies on Aging–one in each state and territory; 670 Area Agencies on Aging–local agencies designated by the state–covering all geographic areas of the country; and 27,000 local service-provider organizations,

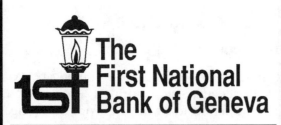

which offer supportive and nutritional services to approximately 9 million older Americans each year.

Since 1965 a broad range of programs and services has evolved from the efforts of the aging network. Although services vary, based on local needs, commonly available services include the following:

In-Home Services encompass a wide array of supportive services for older people who are homebound due to illness, disability, or other reasons. These services allow older people to stay in their own homes or with family members as long as possible. In-home services may include home health care, personal care, homemaking, chore services, home delivered meals, friendly visiting, telephone reassurance, and respite services to assist family caregivers.

Services in the Community are available at various locations in the community. These services may include adult day care, senior center programs, legal assistance, congregate meals, health/fitness programs, elder abuse/protective services, housing services, home repair, employment services, and volunteer opportunities.

Access Services ensure that an older person or family member is linked with appropriate services as needed. Access services may include information and referral, transportation, escort services, and case management.

Services to Residents of Care-Providing Facilities are designed to protect and improve the quality of life of older people living in nursing homes, board and care homes, or residential care facilities. The Long Term Care Ombudsman Program serves as a patients' rights advocate; investigates complaints; negotiates resolutions to problems; and educates the community on how to select a quality facility, and on financial, legal, and regulatory issues related to the residents and facilities.

NETWORK ON AGING

Each community offers a range of supportive services based on the priority needs of residents 60 years of age or over. Not all the above listed services are available in all communities. Your State Agency on Aging or Area Agency on Aging can assist you in locating the services you or a family member may need.

✔ In order to support future editions of this publication would you please mention **Elder Services** each time you contact any advertiser, facility, or service.

What Is Long-Term Care?

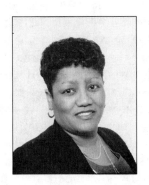

EDNA F. BRIGGS

Edna F. Briggs holds a doctorate in Public Administration from the University of Southern California, with an emphasis in health services administration and gerontology. She has more than 22 years of experience with Los Angeles County in positions such as hospital dietician at Los Angeles County/USC Medical Center and Harbor General/UCLA Medical Center; as health facilities consultant in dietetics and food service with the Department of Health Services, Health Facilities Division; as planning and contracts management supervisor and long-term care coordinator with the Los Angeles County Area Agency on Aging; and as intergovernmental relations staff in the Executive Office of the Department of Community and Senior Services. Dr. Briggs is currently a division chief with the Los Angeles County Department of Health Services, Public Health Programs and Services.

Many families, agencies, and communities at-large are faced with a major problem–how to provide needed and effective care to older persons. This concern may be focused on a parent or on another close family member, a friend, a co-worker, or a client. Obtaining services in a timely manner is a major issue.

Some older persons are well and mobile, while others may have severe disabilities and numerous health problems. Many older persons are concerned with safety, freedom, independence, and maintaining themselves in the community for as long as possible. The preferred community residential setting is their own homes rather than confinement to an institution. Families and friends (caregivers) form an important support network. They share older persons' concerns and assist in identifying and accessing needed services and in making other important decisions.

The type of care typically needed by older persons has historically been referred to as "long-term care." It is important that we clearly understand what long-term care entails, who may require it and why, and what settings and services may be needed and/or available.

DEFINING LONG-TERM CARE

Traditional long-term care has been used as a catch-all term that, until recently, has been synonymous with care of the aged in nursing homes. Many changes occur with aging, and older individuals often have multiple, complex needs, which can be met in settings other than institutions. More important, while the need for institutionaliza-

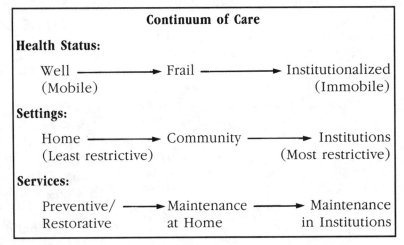

Continuum of Care

Health Status:

Well ⟶ Frail ⟶ Institutionalized
(Mobile)   (Immobile)

Settings:

Home ⟶ Community ⟶ Institutions
(Least restrictive)   (Most restrictive)

Services:

Preventive/ ⟶ Maintenance ⟶ Maintenance
Restorative   at Home   in Institutions

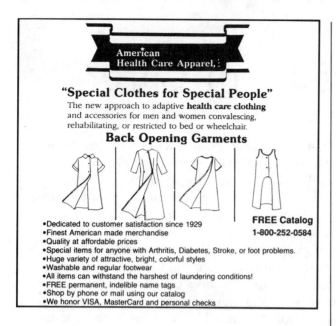
tion may increase dramatically with age, studies have shown that most older individuals prefer to remain in their own homes for as long as possible.

Viewing long-term care along a continuum, as illustrated on the previous page, allows for an expanded definition that ranges from the home and community to an institution. It is important to note that (1) advancement along the continuum may be determined more by health status and level of physical or mental impairment, rather than age; (2) movement along the continuum may be bidirectional (both ways), rather than unidirectional (one-way); (3) a mix of health and social services may be needed either as a single service and/or in combination in different situations; and (4) the continuum is basically near-infinite, that is, for some persons it can extend from home to the grave.

Consider the following cases. Two people may retire at age 60, both obtaining information and referral, congregate meals, and socialization services from the local senior center. At some point, case one encounters an accident that requires admission to an acute care hospital for treatment and care. Home is the preferred discharge setting, where caregivers provide assistance. Initially and for a short period, services are provided by a home health nurse. The family caregiver works; therefore, the older person receives home delivered meals daily and is transported to the adult day health care center two days per week for rehabilitation services. This person's condition eventually improves and he/she returns to the senior center to resume activities.

In case two, hospitalization occurs due to a progressive ailment that reduces mobility, and eventually requires home care for a long period of time. Transportation to and from medical visits, home delivered meals, and homemaker services are provided by public and private agencies, as this person lives alone and there are no family members or friends to help. The individual eventually suffers an episode that requires hospitalization, followed by the need for specialized nursing care and special medical equipment for an indefinite period. Clearly this person's home care options may be extremely limited and may require that some time, or the rest of his/her life, be spent in a nursing home or other institutional setting.

Long-term care is best defined as a continuum consisting of an array of health (preventive, diagnostic, therapeutic, rehabilitative), social (supportive, maintenance), and personal care services that address the needs of persons who require assistance. Services may be formal (provided by health care professionals) or informal (provided by caregivers–family and friends), and may be provided intermittently or continuously over time. Consequently, multiple options are available to allow older persons and their caregivers the freedom to select the preferred or least-restrictive option.

WHO NEEDS LONG-TERM CARE?

The need for long-term care is not necessarily identified with particular diagnoses, but rather with physical, mental, or social disabilities that impair functioning necessary for daily living and protecting oneself against abuse, neglect, and exploitation. It is important to note that, although the need for long-term care increases with age, conditions which require these services can affect individuals of all ages. Victims of accidents and other mishaps, persons born with mental and developmental disabilities, also require assistance with activities of daily living and basic protection.

Although age is not the sole indicator of need for long-term care services, the greatest number of persons within the total population requiring this care will be older persons. Health and mobility do decline with advancing age. Although acute conditions are common in the elderly, chronic conditions are most frequently reported by persons residing in their own homes. These include arthritis, hypertension, hearing impairment, heart disease, arteriosclerosis, visual impairment, and diabetes. By the seventh and eighth decades of life, chances of being impaired in some way, and of being in need of health and supportive services, are great. Most persons over the age of 75 tend to have one or more disabilities. Persons age 85 and over, the extreme aged or old-old, have been the fastest growing segment of the aged population. These persons are generally described as (1) being vulnerable, frail, or functionally impaired; (2) being at-risk of institutionalization; (3) most likely to live alone in their own homes; (4) requiring assistance with activities of daily living (walking, bathing, eating); and (5) being in need of assistance in maintaining maximum independence and dignity in a home environment.

Caregivers are central to the long-term care process because they are key providers of supervision and organization of services. Of the total care that is provided, approximately 20 percent comes from professionals, while 80 percent or more is provided by family and friends. Spouses are a particularly high-risk group of caregivers as they are more prone to be aged themselves and likely to have health problems that may be exacerbated by the caregiver burden (physical labor, emotional strain, disruption in family relationships). Despite the problems associated with caregiving, caregivers continue to provide assistance. Therefore, it is important that, when identifying those who require services, caregivers must be included both as *providers* and *users* of long-term care services, especially respite care.

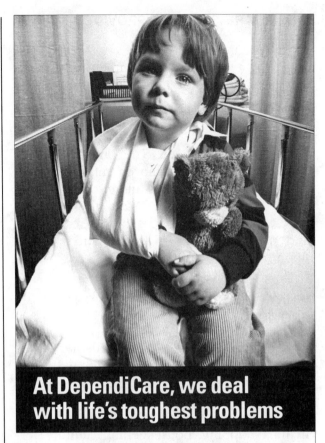

At DependiCare, we deal with life's toughest problems

✔ In order to support future editions of this publication would you please mention **Elder Services** each time you contact any advertiser, facility, or service.

WHERE ARE SERVICES PROVIDED?

The continuum of care exists and operates in a complex environment which includes a range of interacting factors. These factors include a continuum of least and most restrictive settings–home, community, or institution–and services based upon health status and need. The cases discussed above illustrate that movement along the continuum is dynamic, rather than static. There are no restrictive boundaries between the settings, and services may be required and used singly or in combination, based upon need.

WHAT SERVICES ARE NEEDED OR PROVIDED

An array of services are available within the continuum, such as home delivered meals, homemaker/chore services, and home health care for persons who need assistance with instrumental activities of daily living (shopping, housekeeping, laundry) either in their homes or in the homes of relatives and friends. Others, such as adult day health care, rehabilitation, or day treatment hospitals are designed for persons with functional impairments who require assistance with activities of daily living (eating, dressing, bathing) for extended periods of time.

Acute care and mental hospitals provide emergency and critical care, while skilled nursing homes are designed to serve both the relatively short-term needs of post-hospital discharge patients as well as the needs of those with severe or chronic disabilities. Other examples of types of services are listed as follows:

Home:
    Visiting Nurse
    Home Health Aide
    Meals
    Transportation
    Housing
    Life Management
    Financial Assistance
    Protective Services
    Health Education

    Telephone Reassurance
    Counseling
    Legal Services
    Support Groups
    Senior Companions
    Information and Referral
    Emergency Assistance

Home/Community:
    Hospice
    Adult Day Care
    Caregiver Respite
    Senior Center
    Alzheimer Day Care

Community:
    Adult Day Health Care
    Rehabilitation Hospital
    Geriatric Medical Services
    Community Mental Health
    Shared Housing
    Hospital Outpatient Clinics
    Ambulatory Care Centers
    Other Outpatient Clinics

Community/Institutions:
    Retirement Homes
    Board and Care Homes
    Domiciliary Care
    Independent Living Centers
    Health Maintenance Organizations

Institutions:
    Acute Care Hospitals
    Mental Hospitals
    Rehabilitation Hospitals
    Skilled Nursing Homes
    Intermediate Care Facilities

SUSTAINING THE CONTINUUM

The goal of long-term care should be to postpone advancement along the continuum, by the linking of services, in an attempt to address the needs of the older person in the least restrictive manner. Making the continuum work for those who need it, when they need it, is another challenge. Sustaining the continuum often requires that users be able to negotiate a complex maze of agencies and service systems which form a network within the community. Further, the network must be sustained through mutual relationships that rely on coordination and collaboration, rather than competition, in order to ensure system maintenance.

While the total long-term care environment described here consists of multiple types of services and programs, all services are not available in all communities where needed. Functionally impaired persons and their caregivers often are unable to travel the course through the existing system and identify or access needed services.

Case management is a service designed to navigate the system on behalf of those who need assistance. This service consists of a set of activities that results in: (1) the provision of information to those who request it; (2) an exchange of program and client information between service providers; (3) an assessment of needs and development of a plan of care; (4) coordination and monitoring of services delivered in accordance with the plan of care; and (5) evaluation of service delivery and periodic client reassessment of needs.

In summary, defining long-term care encompasses more than nursing home care. A better definition includes elements of health status, varied settings for which services are provided, and offers multiple services based upon need. This concept is supportive of the preferences expressed most by older persons–to remain in their homes in the community–and allows for institutionalization when needed and/or desired by individuals and their caregivers.

Ethnicity and Aging

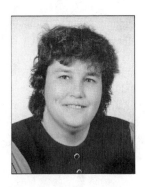

JANET M. LOGAN

Janet M. Logan is the former director of planning for the Chicago Department on Aging and former assistant director of public policy for the Alzheimer's Association, having spent more than ten years as a gerontology professional. Ms. Logan completed coursework toward a Ph.D. in Social Policy from the Florence Heller School in Advanced Studies in Social Welfare and is currently working on her dissertation.

The greater Chicago metropolitan area is a mosaic of ethnic and linguistic diversity. It is estimated that representatives of over 105 different nationalities are represented in the city of Chicago's population alone. Recent changes in patterns of immigration have increasingly brought the needs of the limited English-speaking elderly to the attention of the three local area agencies on aging (Chicago Department of Aging, Suburban Area Agency on Aging, and the Northeastern Illinois Area Agency on Aging): entities that are responsible for planning and coordinating services to persons aged 60 and over.

The isolation created by language and cultural barriers is often an overwhelming problem for an older person. For example, imagine that you are a recent transplant to the Chicago area from a nation that is largely agricultural in origin. While your children may have been acculturated through education to a modern urban lifestyle, you may find coping with urban congestion extremely stressful. In some cases, traditional social roles affording the elderly special levels of respect in their homeland may be absent from westernized life.

Often cultural and linguistic barriers encountered by various ethnic groups are determined by circumstances of immigration. Individuals who have voluntarily emigrated may have had more time to prepare for adjustment to a different society and culture. Many ethnic elderly have moved to the United States to join their adult children and to provide additional support in raising grandchildren.

Others may have come to the United States to escape political, economic, or religious persecution. Many recent refugees have fled their homelands in the aftermath of war and economic dislocation and thus had little time to prepare for such a major move.

In 1987, the Chicago Department on Aging, in conjunction with the Retirement Research Foundation, McArthur Foundation, and the Chicago Community Trust, commissioned the Pacific/Asian American Mental Health Research Center of the University of Illinois at Chicago to perform an Ethnic Elderly Needs Assessment. Organizations from various ethnic groups participated in data collection, including Asian Human Services of Chicago, ASI, Cambodian Association of Illinois, Chinese American

Service League, Greek-American Community Services, Japanese American Service Committee, Korean American Senior Center, Lithuanian Human Services Council of the USA, National Association for Hispanic Elderly, Polish Welfare Association, and South-East Asia Center. Major findings of the study indicate a need for service providers to make available more materials and personnel to work with non-English-speaking elderly. Recent immigrants also appear to suffer more than American-born elderly from mental health problems, especially depression. It was also noted that some groups may be aware of available service programs but are hesitant to use them. This may be due to traditional reliance on informal support networks, such as the family.

Ethnic ties are important to those persons concerned about transmitting a sense of history and culture to future generations. Society is enriched through maintenance of these connections.

The Area Agencies on Aging of Metropolitan Chicago are very interested in working with seniors from all ethnic groups in the community. In addition, there are many ethnic organizations providing hands-on assistance to senior citizens. These ethnic or-

ganizations are included in the "Helpful Organizations" section of this book.

Housing Alternatives for Seniors

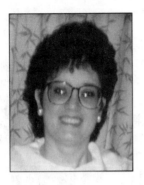

TAMARA L. ANDREW

Ms. Andrew joined the Suburban Area Agency on Aging in June, 1988. In February, 1989, she became a suburban senior housing specialist for the Area Agency as a part of what was formerly the Illinios Housing Leadership Network (IHLN). The IHLN was a two-year demonstration project funded by the federal Administration on Aging Discretionary Grant Program. Ms. Andrew is currently involved with the Suburban Senior Housing Alternatives Program funded by the Retirement Research Foundation, which is a two-year program designed to continue and enhance the initiatives established by the IHLN.

Ms. Andrew holds a Master's of Science in rural sociology, with emphasis in demography and aging issues, from the University of Missouri and Bachelor's of Science degrees from Southwest Missouri State University in urban and regional planning and in sociology.

Although most seniors prefer to "age-in-place," it makes good planning sense to consider housing that *could* serve as an alternative. When a crisis arises, seniors and their families can avoid making ill-informed decisions about alternative housing and possible changes in lifestyle by becoming familiar with different housing options in their area.

The American Association for Retired Persons' Housing Options for Older Americans provides a guide that seniors and their families can use in making decisions about housing alternatives. One suggestion is to make two lists: (1) "reasons for staying" and (2) "reasons for moving." It is important to choose a housing alternative that is appropriate in terms of need and financial capabilities.

STAYING AT HOME–SUPPORTIVE OPTIONS

In-Home Services

When a senior chooses to stay in his/her own home/apartment, in-home services can be accessed to make that stay an appropriate and safe decision. These services can be tailored to the specific needs of the individual(s) needing the service(s). In-home services can include:

- Case management and coordination
- Home delivered meals
- Transportation
- Chore help/housekeeping
- Friendly visiting
- Telephone reassurance
- Outreach
- Legal assistance
- Respite services

Individuals interested in obtaining information on senior services available in their areas should refer to the "Helpful Organizations" section of this book.

Home Repair/Maintenance

Most seniors own their residences. A number of elderly homeowners have limited cash incomes and find

HOUSING ALTERNATIVES FOR SENIORS 13

We take the effort out of moving.

- ❤ Moving company selection and coordination
- ❤ Packing and unpacking
- ❤ Sorting and sale of belongings
- ❤ Organization of closets, cupboards and cabinets
- ❤ Change-of-address services

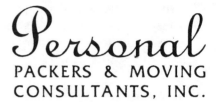

Personal
PACKERS & MOVING
CONSULTANTS, INC.

Get your move off to a smooth start. . .call Bob Copeland for our free *Moving Assessment Booklet* at (312) 248-5638

B O N D E D   I N S U R E D

themselves in a "house rich/cash poor" situation. These homeowners may find it increasingly difficult to afford needed home repair/maintenance, taxes, and utility costs. One important factor that can keep home repair costs to a minimum is to perform systematic, preventative home maintenance. Many experts suggest conducting spring or fall inspections. Additionally, it is a good practice to conduct outside structural inspections after severe weather. The earlier a problem is detected, the earlier the repair can take place. A number of villages/municipalities throughout the Chicago area provide financial assistance to qualifying homeowners for single family rehabilitation with funding from the Community Development Block Grant program (CDBG). (See "Home Equity Conversion" and "Tax Assistance Programs" below.)

Home Equity Conversion

A few programs are now available in Illinois to assist senior homeowners in converting home equity into usable dollars. Home equity conversion can include reverse mortgage plans, deferred payment loans, sale-leaseback, and life estate plans. The most common programs are reverse mortgage loans and deferred payment loans.

A reverse mortgage (RM) is exactly what its name implies: a mortgage that involves payments *to,* rather than *from,* the homeowner. This special type of loan guarantees to homeowning seniors monthly cash advances, or occasional lump sums, that do not require repayment until the homeowners sell the home, move away, or die. Unlike normal home mortgages or home equity loans, RMs require no employment income, clean consumer credit, or repayment for as long as the senior citizen or couple live in their home. The specific amounts available are a function of the age of the youngest homeowner, the appraised home value, and the interest rate. Potential borrowers should know that there are several different types of RM loans and are urged to discuss these with their lending institutions. Reverse mortgage loans are now available in Illinois to homeowners 62 years or older.

Real estate property tax deferral is the most common use of deferred payment loans. In Illinois the Senior Citizens Real Estate Tax Deferral Program allows qualified senior citizens to defer part or all of the property taxes on their personal residences. It is a form of low-interest loan that is to be repaid after the taxpayer's death or at the time the property is sold. For information on how to apply, interested property owners should contact their local county collector's office.

✔ In order to support future editions of this publication would you please mention **Elder Services** each time you contact any advertiser, facility, or service.

Tax Assistance Programs

Programs that offer additional assistance to homeowners and renters include:

- The Circuit Breaker, which reduces the burden of taxes on qualifying seniors and disabled individuals through an annual direct payment to participants.
- Senior Homestead Exemption, which provides a tax break for homeowners 65 years and older. It reduces the equalized assessed valuation of an eligible residence.
- Homeowners Exemption, which eliminates up to $3,500 of the increase in a home's taxable value over what is was in 1977. There is no age requirement, only proof of ownership.
- Sewer Tax Rebate, which provides a rebate to senior citizens within the legal boundaries of a respective village/municipality. Township Assessor and County Collection offices can provide interested individuals with information on tax assistance programs.

Adaptation or Design Modification

As an individual ages in place, the physical design and structure of a home or apartment may be adapted to meet his or her physical needs. For example, ramps and chair lifts or other assistive devices may be installed to make a home more accessible. Senior homeowners may even consider renovating homes to accommodate other persons, such as caregivers or housemates. (See "Accessory Apartments" and "Homesharing" below.)

Accessory Apartments

Sometimes referred to as an "in-law apartment," an accessory apartment is a private living unit within a single family dwelling. This type of housing may be appropriate for an older homeowner wishing to remain in a home because it offers added income from the rental of the apartment or the rest of the house and better utilization of space. However, major structural changes are often required to produce a separate living unit, and local zoning restrictions may impede the development of this option.

HOUSING OPTIONS AWAY FROM HOME

When a senior makes the decision to move from his/her home, several options may be available depending upon his/her financial status. The following is a brief description of options that may be available in the greater Chicago area. Some options may be multiresident, others multiunit, and some may be limited because of local zoning restrictions.

Assisted Living and Sheltered Care

This is an option for older persons who have some functional impairment restricting them to a less independent lifestyle. While not uniformly defined or regulated by the State of Illinois, these housing situations, sometimes referred to as board and care, are for those who need short- or long-term care but do not require skilled nursing care or continuous medical/personal care. The distinction between assisted living and sheltered care is that sheltered care is regulated by the state.

Congregate Care Facilities

Congregate care (or congregate housing) applies to a multiunit house specifically designed to provide supportive services to its residents, who typically reside in self-contained apartments or single rooms and are provided supportive services, which may include meals, housekeeping, transportation, and social and recreational activities. In Chicago and the older "ring" suburbs, congregate facilities are sometimes called retirement hotels.

Continuing Care Retirement Communities/Life Care Communities (CCRC/LCC)

CCRC's/LCC's are designed to provide a continuum of care for older adults ranging from independent living to long-term care.

The level of assistance or care varies according to the individual's level of functional impairment. Services are often bundled or packaged, giving residents an array from which to choose. These services may be included in monthly fees or may be separate charges depending on service levels and need.

The majority of CCRC's/LCC's may (1) require a refundable deposit (within limitations); (2) require a nonrefundable application fee; (3) require a substantial endowment or entrance fee; (4) charge higher than average monthly fees; and (5) require the provision of instructions for health care (e.g., the use of a durable power of attorney). Many CCRC's/LCC's include long-term care insurance in monthly fees and service packaging.

Often used interchangably, there are subtle differences between CCRC's and LCC's. The primary difference between them is in the financial packaging.

ECHO Housing

Elder Cottage Housing Opportunity is a self-contained, free-standing temporary housing unit. Generally, ECHO units are installed adjacent to an existing family home by adult children for use by their aging parent(s) or relatives. This is an option that is not frequently used in the greater Chicago area because of zoning restrictions and high land costs.

Homesharing

This housing situation allows for unrelated persons to reside together in one household. Homesharing usually involves a home-provider, a home-seeker, and sometimes an agency to screen applications and suggest potential matches. Homesharing participants may choose to share living expenses and housekeeping duties. Sometimes the home-seeker provides services to the home-provider in lieu of rent. While some people want or need help with expenses or tasks of daily living, others are primarily interested in companionship and/or security. There are

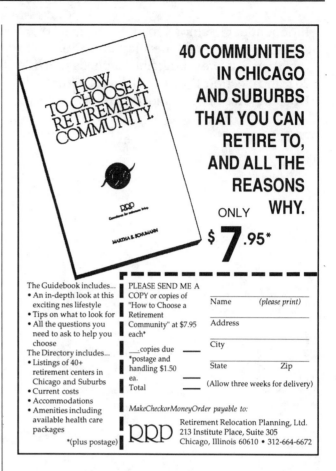

several agencies throughout the greater Chicago area that provide homesharing or matching services.

Shared Group Living

This option involves a limited number of unrelated people living cooperatively in a single household or dwelling. Services provided in this setting often include cooking, laundering, housekeeping, and maintenance. This situation is not often available because of local zoning that restricts the number of unrelated persons living in one household (usually three or less).

Independent Senior Apartments

Independent senior apartments are structures with self-contained living units for older adults who are able to care for themselves. Management may provide limited social/recreational programming services but does not provide congregate meal service.

✔ In order to support future editions of this publication would you please mention **Elder Services** each time you contact any advertiser, facility, or service.

Independent senior apartments are often subsidized through development loans or rental assistance programs such as Section 202 and Section 8 of the National Affordable Housing Act. Local and/or county housing authorities have information on how to apply for rental subsidies.

For further information on housing, please refer to the sections of this publication entitled "Helpful Organizations" and "Helpful Materials for Caregivers."

Accessing and Using the Home Care System

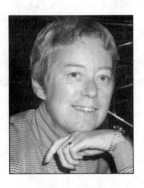

DORIS DREYER HIRN

Since 1985, Doris Dreyer Hirn has been executive director/administrator of Chicago Home Health Services and has served on its board since 1972. This agency has been presented the Governors Award for Excellence and Innovation in Home Care by the Illinois Department of Public Health. From 1975-1985 Hirn established and operated Suburban Home Health Services in Des Plaines.

Chair of the HCFA Region V Reimbursement Committee, Ms. Hirn represented Illinois on the Regional Intermediary Transition Team. She served on the Board of the Illinois Home Care Council and on the National Association for Home Care's Federal Regulatory Affairs Committee. She is active in the Long Term Care Task Force, the Illinois Financial Managers Forum, and the National Financial Managers Forum.

Ms. Hirn conducts seminars for national and state healthcare associations, serves as a consultant to governmental and private organizations, and has published articles on many healthcare and administrative issues.

Ms. Hirn attended Colby Junior College, Hofstra University, and Northwestern University.

Arranging for care received in the home is often confusing because it is divided into two distinctly separate systems. The first is professional skilled healthcare, which follows fairly rigid eligibility requirements and is billed to an insurance program. The other segment is paraprofessional support and personal care, available under funded programs or through individual payment. Which system is chosen is based upon the individual's immediate needs, medical condition, physical status, and living environment. Today's shorter hospital stays, limited family caregiving, outpatient surgeries, and longer lifespans have clearly created the need for both home care systems in the healthcare planning process.

The basic differences between skilled home healthcare and home care (personal care) are the professional levels of the personnel involved, the time spent with the patient, the services provided, and the methods of payment.

SKILLED HOME HEALTH CARE

Home healthcare is ordered by the physician or can be requested from the social service worker or discharge planner before the patient is discharged from the hospital. The home health agency arranges for a registered nurse, working with orders, to visit the patient at home to develop a plan of care for the medical condition and discuss the recovery expectations. The physician, patient, family, and home health agency team all participate in planning the care, treatment, and goal setting throughout the rehabilitation process. Examples of providers of this care are nurses, therapists, nutritionists, medical social workers, or certified home health aides who provide skilled care under the orders of a doctor and come and go on a regular basis to treat medical problems. These skilled practitioners also teach the caregivers and patient how to manage an illness or disability and confer regularly with the physician, reporting on the patient's condition, making changes in the care as needed, and accessing the other team services as they are needed.

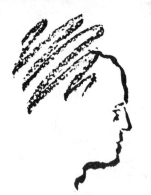

Skilled home healthcare is a team concept, with the nurse or therapist as the care coordinator. The office staff of the agency, however, also participates in the team approach. The billing department, familiar with all public and private insurance programs, can resolve insurance problems. The staff nutritionist can provide advice, special diets, and meal preparation suggestions to patient and caregivers, even making a home visit to resolve eating problems.

The nursing supervisors, on call 24 hours a day, are available for advice or problem solving in between staff visits. They can also arrange for supply and equipment deliveries and laboratory tests ordered by the doctor. The agency social worker can access community resources for transportation, Meals on Wheels, financial assistance, self-help programs, and can visit the home to provide planning assistance when discharge from agency services approaches.

The agency field staff, including the nurses, therapists, social workers, and home health aides, must all meet the requirements set by federal and state laws for education, experience, and ongoing training. They are employed by the home health agency and are covered by agency professional liability insurance, as are the office staff. They drive their own cars, and will see four to six patients each day, sharing on-call weekend duty.

Home health aides provide only personal care related to the medical condition; for example, keeping the patient clean and comfortable and implementing exercise programs developed by the therapist. They are usually in the home for two to four hours per visit and follow the care instructions developed by the nurse as well as by the therapist.

Case management is a widely used benefit for the client which enables the agency to monitor the patient's progress and recovery as skilled services are withdrawn. Caregivers instructions can be altered as the recovering patient's needs change. Case management provides access to all other agency and community services should they be needed–serving as an ongoing resource to the patient and family. All of the skilled services discussed can be billed to Medicare, Medicaid, or health insurance companies.

HOME CARE (PERSONAL CARE)

Home care personnel are registered and practical nurses, homemakers, home health aides, and companions who stay with the patient for extended periods, providing personal care, housekeeping, cooking, and assisting with their ordinary daily activities. They are paid by the patient, private insurance policies, or locally funded social service agencies.

This care is generally arranged by the patient and family, perhaps through referrals by the hospital, social service worker, or physician. Typically, a nurse visits the home with the prospective employee to establish the schedule, plan the care program, and discuss responsibilities and financial arrangements.

FINANCING SHORT-TERM AND LONG-TERM CARE

The costs of home care can be evaluated only when separated into categories of (1) long- and short-term duration and (2) into skilled or personal care. Because the nature of long-term care is ongoing, it is often dif-ficult to find a single source of stable reimbursement for an entire illness. Short-term care often is paid by insurers because it is specific to a current medical episode and has a projected duration. Planning and payment approval are usually arranged in 30- and 60-day segments.

The cost of skilled home healthcare is higher than personal homecare because it is a state and federally regulated industry demanding a sophisticated administrative structure. The homemaker-home health aide agencies are usually regulated under the same laws as employment agencies and are able to keep their costs in a more affordable range. Almost all home healthcare is paid for by insurers: Medicare, Medicaid, or health insurance companies. In contrast, the majority of personal homecare is fully or partially paid for by the user, unless the patient meets the financial criteria for community services or has long-term care insurance policies that include personal care.

Home healthcare is a rehabilitation program, designed to help the patient regain the maximum independence possible, promote recovery from an acute episode, and teach coping skills for lifestyle changes. Combined with the ongoing personal homecare support component, the patient today has the choice to recover at home, and remain in that home by utilizing the growing resources now available.

Added Security through Caller ID

BARRY CALPINO

Barry Calpino is the manager of Consumer and Small Business Market Communications for Ameritech in Chicago. He has served in several marketing posts at the company, including product management, market research, and advertising. Mr. Calpino is a graduate of Marquette University in Milwaukee and Northwestern University's Kellogg Graduate School of Business. He is a member of Alpha Sigma Nu, the Jesuit National Honor Society.

The telephone, an older person's link to his or her community and a potentially life-saving device, can, in many instances, also be the source of harassment and exploitation. A response to this problem is a new technology that has been compared with a "peephole" on one's telephone. As protection against harassing and exploitive calls, the technology allows subscribers to identify the telephone number of the incoming call before answering.

Introduced in the Chicago area in January 1992, this new technology promises to have a marked impact on solving the problem of unwanted and frightening calls. The service was approved by the Illinois Commerce Commission and introduced by Illinois Bell. A special device, connected to the subscriber's telephone, will display the telephone number of the incoming call as it is ringing.

In studies of geographic areas in which this service has already been introduced, law enforcement officials have reported a major drop in cases of harassing and obscene telephone calls. This technology becomes a *deterrent* to the criminal by taking off the "mask" that protects the unwanted caller. The intruder will have to deal with the new reality that s/he can no longer hide under anonymity.

Although this program provides a new form of home security that has never been seen before, and brings a fairly dramatic change in the way that we live, it has been met with a high level of controversy. Many were concerned that, while protecting the privacy of the callee, it eliminated too much privacy/anonymity for the caller. The Commerce Commission settled this dispute by requiring that all callers be offered the free option of having their numbers blocked from the callee on a per-call basis. This solution will maintain the caller's anonymity, while clearly sending the signal to the callee that the incoming call is blocked. The callee will have the option of not answering the call, thereby providing home security.

In a world of changing technologies, the ways we communicate with one another are changing also. The communications industry continues to pioneer and contribute greatly to the independence and dignity of older people. This exciting new service will help families feel more secure about older residents living independently. As with all new technology and change, it will take time, but with time will come real benefits.

Independence at Home: Creative Opportunities

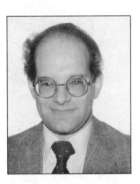

ROBERT N. MAYER

Rob Mayer is the founder and chief executive officer of HomeCorps, which helps older adults and people with disabilities achieve an independent living environment at home through a comprehensive program of home delivered services throughout the greater Chicago area. Prior to founding HomeCorps, he spent 17 years in human resource management and executive development. He also has been an active member of the older adult community for the past seven years as president of the Hulda B. and Maurice L. Rothschild Foundation, a private philanthropy that works to improve the quality of life for older adults in the Chicago area. Rob Mayer holds a Ph.D. from Northwestern University and an M.B.A. from the University of Chicago.

Over time, you have noticed that your grandmother, who is living alone, has exhibited a decline in her hearing. You sometimes have to repeat things or speak slowly. Occasionally, it takes Grandma a bit longer to remember once familiar names and telephone numbers. She misplaces frequently used objects such as her house keys and her reading glasses. You recently came across a stack of overdue medical bills in one of her desk drawers.

Grandma's house was her pride and joy. The little flower garden was always perfectly trimmed. It seemed that the floors were waxed daily and the furniture dusted on the hour. In the past year, however, you have noticed that dust is beginning to accumulate. The garden is sporting a growth of weeds amongst the roses and, though it is mid-May, the storm windows have not yet been removed. Upon closer inspection, you also notice that the gutters are clogged.

Grandma's physician is prescribing a number of medications to deal with some problems, such as hypertension, but you suspect that she isn't always taking her pills when she is supposed to. Her reaction speed is slower, which has caused at least two minor traffic accidents over the past year, yet she insists on driving herself.

One day, you get a telephone call. Grandma tells you that she doesn't want to be any trouble, but she thinks she may have hurt herself. In a frenzy, you drop everything, run over to her house, and discover her sitting on the floor by the telephone. An X-ray reveals that she fractured her leg when she tripped over the door threshold to the kitchen.

Grandma insists that she is just fine and doesn't need any help at home. She is not willing to give up either her house or her independence. She won't move in with you and won't have someone live with her. You and your family are all she really needs, she has told you. However, because of your career and family obligations you can't spend as much time with Grandma as she expects and probably needs. You are concerned that she is no longer able to fully care for herself alone in her house. You feel emotionally torn, guilty, and frustrated.

SERVICE OPTIONS

This scenario is being played and replayed across the country, with infinite variations as families increasingly are called upon to deal with caregiving complexities that accompany an aging population. Fortunately, services and products are now available in response to the growing need for creative options. Any number of these services and products can be packaged together to provide a comprehensive support program–a program that will afford the family the peace of mind and respite they need and, at the same time, allow the older individual the independence she or he wants and deserves.

Companion Service

Companion services, available for a a few hours a day or 24-hour live-ins, can perform a multitude of tasks ranging from cleaning, laundry, and shopping, to meal preparation. Properly trained companions can also handle personal hygiene needs, dressing, and exercise requirements. The number of hours of companion support is a function of a client's ability to handle the normal tasks of daily living and the willingness to accept a nonfamily caregiver in the home.

A family may choose to directly employ a companion, or to engage the services of an organization which will provide, supervise, and be responsible for the quality and performance of their companions. While the first option is less expensive, it places responsibilities on family caregivers for employment issues that they may not be prepared to undertake. For example, they must be in compliance with the relevant tax laws regarding social security, unemployment, and income tax withholding. The family must also arrange for scheduling, bonding, replacement coverage, etc. Should the companion leave suddenly for any reason, there may be no ready replacement.

The selection of a good companion/caregiver makes an important difference in the quality of life for an older person. A thorough on-site assessment of the required skills and personality must be made before selecting a caregiver. The caregiver needs to be someone with whom the family feels comfortable. Most important, the client is going to be spending time alone with this person. She or he and the caregiver need to be able to develop a mutual understanding and a positive relationship.

Strong skills and references alone are not sufficient to ensure quality care. In the scenario presented, the family should look for someone who will make it her job to support the client's independence and at the same time maximize the quality of life by motivating and stimulating, not just maintaining. The companion should also be capable of acting promptly in an emergency and be able to clearly communicate with Grandma's other caregivers.

In selecting a companion service, ask these questions about the companions on the staff: Are they given physicals and screened for drugs? Are their backgrounds checked for felony convictions? If they drive, do they have clean motor vehicle records? Are they bonded? How often will the service make a supervisory visit to check on the companion, and will you be charged for that visit? Will the service conduct an initial site assessment and introduce a back-up companion so that a familiar face is available if the primary companion becomes ill or requires time off for any reason? Most important, how strong is their guarantee if you are not satisfied?

For older individuals, independence is of paramount importance. Therefore, find out if services will be available to the family as required, rather than per the agency's schedule. The family should be a partner in the development of a schedule and plan of activity, as well as in the selection of a caregiver. This is a very different relationship from the traditional nurse-patient dynamic which emphasizes nurse control and patient/family compliance.

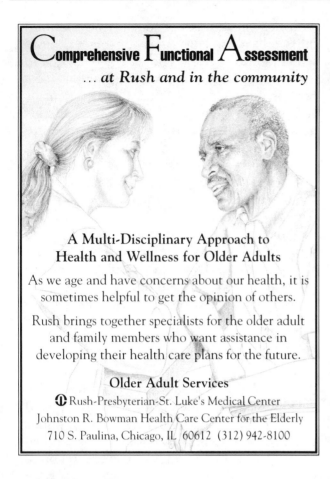

Comprehensive Functional Assessment
... at Rush and in the community

A Multi-Disciplinary Approach to Health and Wellness for Older Adults

As we age and have concerns about our health, it is sometimes helpful to get the opinion of others.

Rush brings together specialists for the older adult and family members who want assistance in developing their health care plans for the future.

Older Adult Services

Rush-Presbyterian-St. Luke's Medical Center
Johnston R. Bowman Health Care Center for the Elderly
710 S. Paulina, Chicago, IL 60612 (312) 942-8100

Medication Management

A major cause of disability in older adults is medication abuse. We are not talking about the conscious over- or under-consumption of medication, but rather the confusion caused by the need for older adults to take different prescriptions at different times and in different dosages. If Grandma doesn't remember which medications she has taken from the six bottles by her bedside, there is no way to be certain, short of counting the remaining pills, whether she has consumed the correct quantities. It is, however, neither cost effective nor convenient for someone to visit Grandma daily for the sole purpose of laying out the day's medication.

Today there are many medication packaging programs available which can ease this confusion considerably. There are simple plastic drawers that can be labelled by the day or hour. There are more sophisticated dispensing machines that alert the client by sound and light when a medication is due to be taken and then dispenses the appropriate

dosages. There are also environmentally sound bubble packages that show, at a glance, medication taken and medication remaining. Another advantage of these bubble packages is that they are returnable for a refund if for any reason any of the prepackaged medications are not used.

Personal and Emergency Response Systems

"I've fallen and I can't get up." By now, we all recognize the parody of the emergency response industry. If one can get past the parodies and the scams that have unfortunately characterized this industry, there are some fine, cost-effective services available that provide prompt assistance and support for those living alone. However, it is first important to understand the difference between an emergency response system and a personal response system.

Emergency response systems have been around the longest. Typically, a system consists of a hand-held wireless call button, which the client can either wear or carry in a pocket. In an emergency, the client presses the button to summon help. The button transmits a signal to a remote device connected to the telephone line. This device automatically dials the number of a central monitoring station and sends a coded signal. The monitoring station personnel translate the signal into an address to which they then send assistance. Such assistance may range from a neighbor to the paramedics, depending on the instructions from the family. More sophisticated systems allow the client to converse directly with monitoring center personnel and tell them exactly the nature of the emergency so that the appropriate persons can be contacted to respond.

Personal response systems have socialization as their focus. They can be as simple as a daily telephone call to remind clients to take their medication and to ask about their day. Alternatively, clients may be encouraged to call whenever they feel lonely or scared. Of course, the system is also available at the touch of a button in case of an emergency. More sophisticated personal response sys-

✔ In order to support future editions of this publication would you please mention **Elder Services** each time you contact any advertiser, facility, or service.

tems have hand-held call buttons that put the client in two-way voice communication with a monitoring station.

How do you select a system without being taken? Don't buy. Rent or lease the equipment. That way, you can cancel the service at any time without being stuck with a lot of high-priced hardware. You also will not be left with an expensive piece of useless equipment if the manufacturer or monitoring center goes out of business. Does the unit contain a battery backup in case of power loss? What personal information is maintained in the monitor center files for reference in case of emergency? If you are considering a voice system, find out who the people are who monitor the calls. How are they trained? Are they supervised by registered nurses?

There are a number of systems with special features that may be of value. For example, some can be configured to include smoke or fire detectors. Some allow you to answer the telephone with the press of a button and converse without picking up the telephone receiver. There are also some systems that have designed optional accessories so that they may be used by people with physical disabilities.

Home Adaptation

Changes in mobility, sensory activity, and lifestyle that accompany the aging process demand a slightly different living environment. Some common home adaptations include lever door latches, large cabinet pulls, bathroom grab bars, and rocker light switches, just to name a few. There is also now a whole array of creative products available which make the tasks of daily living easier. For example, there are "helping hands" to assist with reaching; hooks to assist with clothing buttons and zippers; oversized handles for eating utensils and writing instruments; raised bath and toilet seats; and large numbered telephones and playing cards.

To ensure that a home is configured to support an older person's physical needs, a family member should spend some time with the person, carefully observing how he or she handles everyday activities at home. What activities or tasks appear to be difficult? Are there tasks she or he tends to avoid altogether? Another option is to consider home environment assessment by a consultant. Most home adaptations are relatively simple and inexpensive and can be made by a competent home repair service.

Home Maintenance

According to the U.S. Department of Health and Human Services, falls are the leading cause of death from injury for people over age 65. Therefore, special attention needs to be paid to safety hazards. Loose stairs, uneven floorboards, and inadequate handholds can all contribute to an unsafe home environment.

Fire hazards are another safety concern. The U.S. Consumer Product Safety Commission estimates that home heating equipment is associated with approximately 30 percent of all residential fires. Flammable upholstery and volatile liquids are next highest. Attention is also required for a number of other potential fire hazards such as frayed electrical wires or overloaded outlets. Also needed are smoke detectors placed in key areas.

Because home safety is so important, periodic safety surveys are strongly recommended. Local fire prevention bureaus often will conduct these kinds of inspections for their community. Otherwise, such inspections are available through private agencies.

When family and neighbors are no longer able to keep up with the ongoing maintenance requirements of the home, a good home maintenance service can be engaged to handle such routine seasonal chores as gutter cleaning. A little assistance in restoring the flower garden would also probably be appreciated. Community volunteers can sometimes be found for this type of work as well. Regardless of who does the work, be certain that it carries a guarantee if the client is not satisfied.

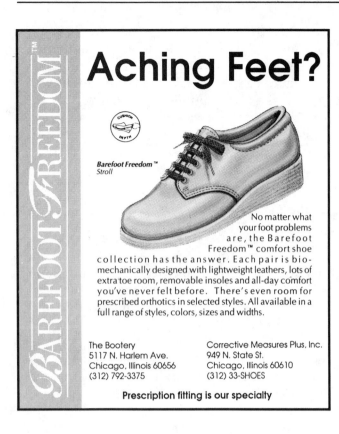
Medical Claims Assistance

Older adults are often faced with a confusing array of medical bills, insurance policies, and the maintenance of appropriate health care expense records. A single brief hospitalization may generate up to a half-dozen or more different invoices and insurance claim notices. Overlooked insurance premium notices can cause important policies to be cancelled, leaving the client without key coverage.

Some communities have retired accountants available who volunteer to assist with the necessary bookkeeping and records maintenance. There are independent services that will help families interpret insurance benefits and ensure that the maximum benefit is gained from available insurance coverages. A good service will follow all claims from initial filing to final reconciliation. They will evaluate claims paid and will communicate directly with the insurance carrier to resolve any disagreements over coverage or claims disputes.

Transportation

The family's concern over an older person's driving is an emotionally charged issue. Driving represents a symbol of independence which is not easily eliminated. Furthermore, there are a multitude of activities important to an older person's lifestyle which require transportation. Depriving him or her of the ability to get around will likely result in feelings of isolation, depression, and increased dependence on the family to meet transportation needs.

In response to this concern, many areas have developed transportation systems especially for the older population, providing convenient pickup and drop-off locations and frequent service. For example, there may be shuttle buses that run from the local senior center to shopping malls or professional office buildings where physicians' offices are located.

Community-sponsored transportation using specially designed vans for the physically challenged is available in many areas. Use of this service, however, is often limited to clients who can obtain a letter from a physician which certifies medical necessity. Furthermore, to utilize these services, the client must be able to self-propel a wheelchair or be accompanied by a caregiver.

There are many medicar and ambulance services available which also use specially designed transportation equipment. However, the cost of these services can be prohibitive, unless covered by insurance. Discretionary travel, such as shopping, the hairdresser, or dinner with the family, which is not related to medical necessity, is not a covered expense.

Some home service organizations have developed programs which couple transportation with the services of a professional caregiver. A trained caregiver transports the client in the client's vehicle of choice (often the client's own car) to the destination; accompanies him or her to the appointment or errand; then brings him or her safely home. This allows for the safe and convenient transport of the client, while supporting continuing care needs. The cost of this service is frequently less than one-half of the cost of traditional ambulance services.

Nutrition

An appropriate nutritional intake is also important for the physical well-being of older adults. Nutritional requirements change, and often diets may require modification as part of a comprehensive treatment plan for any number of ailments such as heart disease, hypertension, or adult onset diabetes. To assist people at home with diet and meal preparation, many communities have developed "Meals on Wheels" programs. They vary somewhat from area to area, but typically, they employ a cadre of community volunteers to prepare the food at a local senior center and deliver one or two meals a day directly to each client's home. The meals are delivered completely prepared and ready to eat, including disposable utensils. One meal is usually delivered hot. All meals are specially prepared to meet specific dietary requirements under the supervision of a staff dietician.

Financing Options

Neither Medicare, the federal health care plan for people aged 65 and older, nor private Medigap supplemental insurance will cover most of these expenses, which are unrelated to an acute illness. Fortunately, there are now a number of good long-term care insurance programs available that will cover these kinds of services. In addition, there are organizations that will offer to purchase a life insurance policy for immediate funds, which can then be used to increase comfort and offset expenses incurred during the older person's lifetime. If his or her mortgage is paid off, the older person's home equity is another source of funds.

Summary

We have discussed just a few of the community-sponsored and private services available to assure older citizens like Grandma independence and high quality of

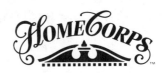
life while living in the comfort of their own homes.

Most areas have resources to help locate these services. Some areas have published directories of older adult services and have created senior activity centers. Others have community information and referral centers, which maintain information on local support services. Most medical centers have created older adult affinity groups and offer special medical and support programs to this population. Note, however, that institutionally affiliated programs often only provide referrals to their own services.

Few directories or information and referral centers have the resources to monitor the quality of the providers on their lists. Families should carefully review the practices, quality assurance programs, and guarantees of any service they are considering in addition to price. In any event, there is no reason why our story can't have a happy ending. Grandma's family has put in place a creative and comprehensive program of products and services, comfortable for the family and responsive to her needs, so that she can continue to enjoy the quality of life and independence both she and the family desire.

Caregiving: Managing the Responsibility

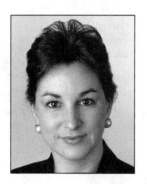

GERALDINE GALLAGHER

Geraldine Gallagher earned a master's degree in education, with a focus on aging, from Northwestern University in Evanston, Illinois, as well as a bachelor's degree from Northwestern's Medill School of Journalism. She has served as public information officer for the State of Illinois Department on Aging in Chicago. She was the editor of *Access Chicago* magazine, a monthly consumer publication for people 50 and older, and she was an assistant editor for *Mature Outlook*, a national magazine for older adults. She is also a freelance writer who specializes in the areas of aging, health, and education.

American families are faced with a rather startling fact: a midlife woman today can expect to spend more years caring for an aging parent than she does for her own child. Frequently, these years of care overlap, creating what sociologists have called "women in the middle," "the sandwich generation," "kin keepers," "the super woman squeeze," and "the daughter track."

But these clever catch phrases do not do justice to the work of caregivers–people who try to balance the needs of their spouses, their children, their parents, and frequently their jobs–not to mention their own needs.

Nancy Hooyman is just one example of the millions of caregivers around the country who busily juggles conflicting physical and emotional demands on her time and attention. Hooyman lives with her husband and two children in Seattle, and a few years ago spent several months commuting to Ohio to help her father, then 85, find a nursing home for his second wife. At the time, her ten-year-old son had come down with a severe case of mononucleosis, and her husband was facing serious job-related stress. Meanwhile, friends from Norway had settled into the family's home for a visit, and, as if this all weren't enough, the plumbing in the Hooyman house blew.

"I felt like a rubber band stretched between Seattle and Ohio," says Hooyman, who is co-author of *Taking Care: Supporting Older People and Their Families* (New York: Free Press, 1985) and dean of the University of Washington's School of Social Work. After her father's wife died, Hooyman again returned to Ohio. "I tried to explain to (my son) Kevin why I had to go. He was still sick, and he was in tears. It did create a lot of guilt," she says quietly.

Hooyman's split responsibilities are familiar to many in their 40s, 50s, 60s, and even 70s, experts say. The American Association of Retired Persons estimates that there are at least 7 million caregivers, more than three-quarters of whom are women, and more than half of whom are also employed outside the home. The bulk of care for vulnerable elderly–more than 80 percent–is provided by informal caregivers, usually daughters or wives.

CAREGIVING: BEHIND THE NUMBERS

Surviving America has a long tradition of families caring for their own. As far back as the 1700s, surviving historical documents show that adult children were legally and morally charged with caring for their aging parents. So, though caregiving is talked about a lot today, it's hardly a new topic. Nevertheless, the Census Bureau paints the picture of a series of demographic shifts which have conspired to make it a crucial issue for the 1990s.

- The American population is aging at an unprecedented rate. During the past decade the number of people 65 and older has increased by 23 percent. And the 85-plus age segment, the group that requires the most care, has risen by 44 percent.
- Life expectancy has soared to 72 for men and 79 for women born in 1989. These numbers are up from 65 for males born about four decades ago and 71 for females born then. Contrast these numbers with turn-of-the-century figures of mid-40s for people born then.
- The steady increase in divorce over the past several decades has implications for tomorrow's caregivers. Divorced older adults who do not remarry won't be able to count on support from a spouse. And the 25-percent rise in the number of single elderly women expected by the year 2000 means that the responsibility of caring for them will likely lie with their children.
- Young people today are delaying marriage and childbearing, effectively prolonging their emotional and (sometimes) financial ties to their parents. Compounding this is the growing number of adult children returning to the parental nest as single parents or after a divorce or job loss.

And ironically, research shows that many of these people do not even realize they are caregivers. "It's like the old saying: If it looks like a duck, walks like a duck, and quacks like a duck, well, it's probably a duck," says Victor L. Wirth, former director of the Illinois Department on Aging, which launched its caregiving initiative in 1986 and provides support services to thousands of Illinois residents who might otherwise have to opt for nursing home care. "These individuals have all the characteristics of caregivers and are performing all the duties: handling financial, medical or legal paperwork; accompanying their parent to medical appointments; preparing meals; or helping with housekeeping, home repair or personal grooming. Though they may not call themselves caregivers, they are doing the job—and from an emotional and physical perspective, they may be paying the price."

Mirca Liberti of Levittown, Pennsylvania, who 15 years ago founded the nonprofit support group, Children of Aging Parents (CAPS), after caring for her blind, terminally ill father while working full-time, knows how dear that price can be. "I watched my dad deteriorate right before my eyes. I almost wished my dad were dead. It wasn't that I didn't love him—it was really out of love and compassion that I felt this. I resented what was happening to my life and to him."

However, caregivers and experts alike point out that there is also often a positive side, offering families the opportunity to bolster intergenerational bonds. "This has definitely brought my daughters closer to their grandparents," says Elaine Shocket, a north suburban Chicago woman who helps her father care for her 87-year-old mother who has suffered from Alzheimer's disease for the past 12 years. "They are very close to their grandfather. And there are times they have to be there for him. He has always been there for them in the past. And if I am at the office and am not available, he will call them instead."

"People are living longer, and there are greater opportunities (for them) to deal with grandchildren as adults—and grandchildren can also begin to take over caregiving responsibilities," says Victoria Bumagin, MSSW, ACSW, BCD, a Wilmette-based gerontology consultant and co-author of *Helping the Aging Family* (Glenview, IL: Scott, Foresman, 1990) and *Aging Is a Family Affair* (New York: T.Y. Crowell, 1979). Grandparents and grandchildren often develop close relationships, she adds with a smile, because as the old saying goes, "They have an enemy in common."

But family relationships can also begin to suffer, especially if a spouse or children feel that they are getting the short end of the bargain. "Spouses have come to (support group) meetings and admitted their marriages were on the rocks because of their new roles as caregivers," Liberti explains.

Whether the effect on family relationships is positive or not-so-positive is usually determined by the state of these relationships before the adult child becomes a caregiver to an older parent, says Bumagin, who consults with caregivers, older adults and their families. "Often, too," she adds, "caregivers can feel overwhelmed by their responsibilities" and find that they don't have enough time to spend with children and spouses.

The stress of caregiving, whether in the caregiver's home or the parent's home, can take its toll physically and emotionally. "You feel frustration and agony," says Shocket, whose mother's Alzheimer's disease makes her disoriented–sometimes not recognizing family members, forgetting what stage she is at in life or losing all sense of time's passing. "I have not had a complete night's sleep without some kind of nightmare–that she'll get lost, which she has three or four times in the past. My other fear is of abuse–that someone will hurt her or take advantage of her. I've learned not to panic in front of my mother when things upset me–I can't show fear, sadness or anger on my face because it just upsets her. I have found that the best medicine is free: kindness and a smile." But sometimes it's all just too much. "Inwardly, I break down and cry. In a way, I'm treating her like a child. But she's my mom, I haven't really had a mom for about 12 years," says Shocket, who has taken over many hands-on care responsibilities. And, Shocket in turn, serves as the sounding board and confidant for her father who can no longer rely on his wife in that role. "We talk at least twice a day, sometimes more often. He misses that communication. He's really quite lonely. He misses his wife–and yet she is there."

The stresses of caregiving can be as difficult whether the older relative lives nearby or in another state, as Steve Cohn of suburban Chicago has discovered. Cohn's father, now 90 and suffering from dementia, lived on his own, with five-day-a-week home help, in the southwestern United States after his wife passed away several years ago. The combination of a stroke and progressive dementia forced Cohn to bring his father to Chicago to live and be cared for. In the interim years, Cohn moved his father down south again, at the older gentleman's insistence, but had to again bring him to this area for care. "Sometimes it is harder being far way," explains Cohn, who has taken over his father's financial affairs and care management, "but overall, it is much more difficult to have him here."

Because the dementia has caused his father to lash out at the family, especially Cohn, the day-to-day stress can become overwhelming. "The most difficult thing for me is getting on with my life," says Cohn, whose home and office are just minutes from his father's long-term care facility. "There is continuous, overshadowing guilt. He does not enjoy life; he asks me to help him kill himself. When parenting a parent, you do the best you can within the parameters of not ruining your own life. You see the parent who raised and nurtured you being destroyed–by frailty and loss of control, and nothing is going to turn that process around." Cohn and his wife are faced with what he calls a "double-whammy" because her mother, too, is becoming more frail and needs assistance.

Men and women often take on caregiving roles differently, Bumagin adds. "Traditionally, men participate in their own way. Even when it is the husband's mother, usually the daughter-in-law assumes some of the responsibilities. They will take over the financial duties and management of care. Men are more likely to hire help than women, who feel it is their responsibility. Women find it harder to turn those caregiving tasks over to someone else."

Adding a job to the balance of personal and family relationship issues can complicate the situation for caregivers. "More than half of all caregivers are also holding down jobs outside the home," Wirth says. "So when a caregiver leaves the office at 5 or 6 p.m. every day, he or she is returning home to yet another full-time job. Though more employers are beginning to respond to the needs of caregivers–with flex time, elder care referral, caregiver support groups, group long-term care insurance and informational seminars–the workplace still has a long way to go."

Caregiving is "really a Catch-22," Hooyman says. "If you don't do it, you feel guilty. If you do it, but haven't enough time to do it well, you (still) end up feeling guilty and may be penalized in the workforce. When you try to do it all, you wind up exhausted and not doing a good job in anything."

The key, says Wirth, former director of the Illinois Department on Aging, is to help older adults and their families access the intricate network of support services available in their communities. "By simply bringing services into the home, we can frequently relieve the stress on caregivers and many times help an older person to 'age in place'–to maintain independence and remain in his or her own home as long as possible."

Bumagin agrees. "If we're dealing with caregivers who are giving too much, I ask what they are *really* able to do and determine to what extent they can relinquish some of the responsibility. What are they willing and able to do? What is reasonable to do without jeopardizing other parts of

their life? We take stock and set limits," she explains. "Caregivers often need permission to do something for themselves. Here we're dealing with emotional costs. The love and affection of the family is the most important thing they can give. And it doesn't cost them very much if they are not already overwhelmed with caregiving responsibilities. There are services that can be purchased at a variety of levels and costs. The need to bring in services does not reflect inadequacy on the part of the caregiver–rather, they are saving that part of themselves, (the love and affection), that is most important to the older person."

WHAT YOU CAN DO

There are no easy answers for caregivers, but experts in the fields of aging and family relations offer the following tips:

• *Ask for help.* Don't fall into the super woman (or man) squeeze if other family members are available to help out. Enlist the support of your spouse, children, siblings–even close friends and neighbors. Sometimes people are not aware of the stresses that face caregivers or how much they welcome a helping hand. And by spreading caregiving duties among the spouse and children, they are less likely to feel alienated or left out. If help is offered, don't be too proud to accept.

• *Don't assume that a widowed or elderly parent needs assistance* or should be moved out of his or her own home. Older people cherish their autonomy and often are quite capable of living on their own–sometimes with help from family, volunteers, or social services. They may resent being moved, having responsibility yanked away from them unneccessarily, or having decisions made for them without their input.

• *Consider bringing a companion or home care professional* into your home or your parent's home if he or she cannot be left alone. Social service agencies sometimes work on a sliding fee scale and volunteer caregiver networks operate through many churches, synagogues, and community groups to provide low-cost help to tired caregivers. Even if you can afford to hire home care just a couple of evenings a month, the time for yourself will be worth it. A burned-out caregiver cannot provide good quality care.

- *Contact your Area Agency on Aging or the Illinois Department on Aging* for information about the support services available to you and your parent–they may include transportation, home-delivered meals, homemaker assistance, chore housekeeping, a companion, personal grooming, respite or adult day care, legal and housing information, and more (in Chicago, call 312-744-4016; in the suburbs, call 708-383-0258; elsewhere in Illinois, call 1-800-252-8966).

- *Look into adult day care and respite care,* which provides day, overnight, and weeklong care for older adults, giving the caregiver a well-deserved break. These programs are frequently offered by local hospitals, nursing homes, or senior centers.

- *Be realistic about the care you can provide.* If a parent requires around-the-clock medical attention, for example, a long-term care facility may be the only answer.

- *Talk with friends.* Caregivers require an emotional outlet when the stress becomes too overwhelming. Friends sometimes can be more objective sounding boards than family members because they aren't as close to the situation.

- *Contact support groups,* many of which are offered by area hospitals, religious groups, senior centers, and community organizations and can serve as an outlet for caregivers.

- *Consider seeking professional help* if the pressure becomes more than discussions with friends or peers can relieve. Contact a clergy member, a counselor, or a doctor.

- *Be honest about your situation with colleagues.* The workplace has adjusted to

provide more flexibility for mothers, but it hasn't yet caught up with the need for caregiver resources. Though more and more companies are beginning to address caregiver concerns, a little open discussion could raise consciousness at your office and make your boss and co-workers more aware of the situation you are facing at home.

- *Read the popular literature* for suggestions. You will find dozens of titles in the self-help, family, relationship, and psychology shelves of your local library or bookstore. Sometimes it helps to know that millions of people face the same pressures–and you might benefit from their experiences.

- *Discuss finances, living arrangements and health care preferences* with parents before they actually need assistance, if possible. This will ease your mind when you have to take over responsibilities.

- *Finally, realize that you can't do it all,* and no one should expect that you do. Take on as much responsibility as you can, but don't feel guilty for what you are unable to handle.

Support in the Workplace: Corporate Eldercare

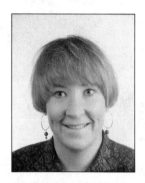

CHRISTI LENNOX

Christi Lennox is the director of Aging and the Workplace, a program of the Illinois Alliance for Aging, a not-for-profit membership organization providing leadership throughout Illinois to create and improve services for older people and their families. She received her M.A. in gerontology from Roosevelt University.

Eldercare benefits. They're being called the employee benefit of the '90s and with good reason. Trends affecting the American workforce include an increasing number of older individuals, a decreasing pool of workers from which to draw, and an increasing average workforce age. Companies cannot avoid feeling the impact of an older America. To soften the effects of these realities, companies must learn which elder care programs and options are available and which best fit their business and employee needs.

THE STAGE IS SET

"Hello, Susan? I'll be in late this morning. I have to take my father to the Doctor."

"My mother is being discharged from the hospital tomorrow–I'll need to take the day off."

"Another organization with whom I am interviewing offers family care benefits. Do you?"

Around the Chicago area and across the country employers are beginning to hear the concerned voices of their employees and feel the impact of an increasingly aging society. It is a society in which families desire to remain involved in the care of their older relatives and organizations strive for a competitive edge only achieved by attracting and retaining the best and brightest workers. Successfully recruiting the elite of this diminishing labor pool is not always easy. It requires responding to the increasing demands of workers to provide a work environment that is supportive of their family roles.

Indeed, the voices of employed elder caregivers will get louder. Society is poised at the threshold of a major demographic revolution with significant implications for employers, employees, and the families of which they are a part. Experts believe that the business consequences of elder caregiving by employees will far surpass those yet confronted in the realm of child care.

Increase in Size of Population

In the Chicago area alone the population of those over the age of 65 has increased by 32.5 percent since 1970 and is projected to increase an additional 50 percent in the next 30 years. Moreover, the group of individuals over the age of 85 has increased its numbers by 83 percent since 1970 and is expected to repeat that feat in the next 30 years. As the number of older people increases, there is a greater likelihood that a significant number of individuals in the workplace (as many as 30 percent) will be involved in elder care.

Anticipated Labor Shortage

Added to this demographic scenario is the anticipated shortage of workers that have the skills and talents to meet the needs of companies facing global economic competition. A recent Illinois report released by the Governor's Task Force on Human Resource Development points to a significant decrease in the anticipated number of skilled individuals entering the workforce over the next decade.

Increase in Average Age of Workforce

By the year 2000, the average age of the workforce will reach nearly 40 years, an age at which elder caregiving begins to peak. These caregivers are likely to be among the most experienced and loyal of a company's employees.

Providing care to an older relative involves an extensive range of physical, emotional, and financial needs and a complicated network of in-home and community services. It is also of indefinite and unpredictable duration. Caregiving introduces demands on individuals which spill over in their work environment. Absenteeism, late arrivals, excessive personal phone use, and lowered productivity are common among these employees.

If employers are to obtain optimum productivity from their caregiving employees they will need to provide the kind of work environment that allows balance between work and the caregiving role. Companies that ignore the connection between their end-of-quarter earnings and family-supportive work environments will suffer the consequences: higher turnover, increased training costs, and lower productivity.

EMPLOYER-SPONSORED ELDERCARE PROGRAMS

Employers have begun to conduct employee surveys and form task forces to explore and investigate options for addressing eldercare concerns. They know that their bottom line depends on it. But what kinds of programs and services are available?

There is a broad range of activities and services that will support employees in their caregiving roles while minimizing the impact these roles have on workplace performance. Offering some kind of program places companies in the "family-friendly" circle of corporate America–a guideline being used with increasing frequency by individuals considering employment moves. Contrary to common perception, these activities need not be costly or difficult to administer.

Information. Surveys have shown time and again that what employed caregivers request most is information–information about the range of available community services, about procedures for obtaining services, about Medicare and Medicaid. Information can be conveyed in a number of ways. A regular column or section in an employee newsletter devoted to caregiving concerns is easy to produce and reaches a wide number of employees. Creating a library that includes caregiving manuals, aging services directories, and handy checklists is a helpful alternative. Holding a "caregiver's fair," where a host of service-to-the-aging providers are available to offer general information and answer employees' questions, is another option.

Educational seminars. Educational seminars for employees on topics such as the aging process, Medicare and other health payment systems, legal issues, and housing options for the elderly are among the most efficient and productive ways to support and inform employed caregivers. Typically held over the lunch hour, seminars can reach a large number of employees and provide much-needed basic information.

Consultation and referral. More and more companies are beginning to recognize the effectiveness of providing individualized eldercare expertise to their employees. Offered either in person or through access to a telephone helpline, this option provides employees with information that is specific to their situation. Counselors help the employees articulate their concerns, clarify their options, and guide them to community resources that will assist them in their caregiving roles. The counselors are able to quickly assess the employee's situation and appropriately target the search for solutions.

Easing time constraints. The average caregiver spends six to ten hours a week in caregiving responsibilities. A somewhat smaller yet significant percentage of caregivers provide as much as 35 hours a week of assistance. While employers cannot create more time in a worker's day, they can help their employees manage their time by allowing flexible work hours, part-time hours, job sharing, or telecommuting. While not feasible in every organization, easing time constraints is one of the most effective ways to help employees maintain a balance between work and family.

Financial assistance. Companies can alleviate the financial crunch by providing vouchers to subsidize the aging services that employees use and by offering dependent care assistance programs, and long-term care insurance.

Research Is Important

Determining which of the many options will best meet the needs of a company and its employees will take some work. Employee surveys allow a company to learn the extent of caregiving among its employees as well as which programs will best assist them. Developing employee focus groups can be an effective method for determining the desirability and potential utilization of particular programs. Many professional benefits and human resource associations include work and family committees that can serve as resources. Finally, consulting the increasing number of publications that address this issue provides information on selecting options and on what other companies are doing. (See "Resources," below.)

Several of the program alternatives described are likely to involve contracting with an outside vendor. This outside provider may be a private consultant or consulting firm, a private, not-for-profit organization, or a public entity. References from other companies who have previously used a particular provider of eldercare programs is an important factor in making a final selection.

In Summary

Employers will be facing with increasing frequency the issues related to elder caregiving by their employees. However, by addressing the needs and concerns of these workers, and implementing eldercare benefits programs, companies can reduce the business impact of eldercare responsibilities. The bottom line–companies attract and *keep* valued and skilled workers.

RESOURCES

Bureau of National Affairs. 1989. *Special Survey Report: Eldercare and the Workplace.* Washington, DC: Bureau of National Affairs.

Creedon, Michael. 1987. *Issues for an Aging America: Employees and Eldercare.* Bridgeport, CT: University of Bridgeport, Center for the Study of Aging.

Families and Work Institute. 1991. *The Corporate Reference Guide to Work-Family Programs.* New York: Family and Work Institute.

Morgan, Hal and Kerry Tucker. 1991. *Companies that Care.* New York: Simon and Schuster.

New York Business Group on Health. 1986. *Employer Support for Employee Caregivers.* New York: New York Business Group on Health.

Scharlach, Andrew E., Ph.D., Beverly F. Lowe, Ph.D., and Edward L. Schneider, M.D. 1991. *Elder Care and the Work Force: Blueprint for Action.* Lexington, MA: Lexington Books.

Volunteer Opportunities

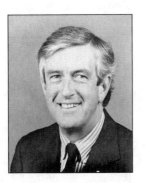

DONALD R. SMITH

Donald R. Smith is the commissioner of the Chicago Department on Aging, the Area Agency on Aging for the City of Chicago. A veteran of city government with 27 years of service, he has developed innovative urban programs in the areas of education, employment, day care, aging, disability, and community development. Mr. Smith founded the Raymond Hilliard Adult Education Center of Chicago and also served as a former deputy director for the Office of the Mayor, Chicago Model Cities Program.

ALEXANDRA LYONS

Alexandra Lyons is director of volunteer services at the Chicago Department on Aging. She manages the Department's "Light Up Chicago–Volunteer One-to-One" program, which links government, corporations and the public to provide volunteer services to seniors residing in Chicago. She holds a Master's Degree in Public Health from the University of Illinois at Chicago with a concentration in gerontology and health resource management.

"Ask not what your country can do for you, but what you can do for your country." –*John F. Kennedy*

Volunteering is a time-honored tradition that is as American as apple pie, the flag, and motherhood. Giving service by one's free will is a wonderful precept that has helped strengthen and improve our communities, while also enriching the lives of others. Based on a "self-help" concept, volunteerism is people helping themselves while helping others.

Nationally, people of all ages are volunteering their time for many types of organizations and human causes. Over 80 million people across America volunteer an average of five hours per week, devoting time to infants, children, young adults, and senior citizens. The only criterion for a volunteer is a genuine spirit of caring.

As America comes of age, assistance is on the rise for the elderly through volunteer organizations. In the Chicago area, several programs use volunteers to provide much-needed assistance with errands, shopping, household chores, and transportation for the elderly. The burdens of isolation and loneliness that are often experienced by homebound elderly are eased with the comfort of friendly visits by volunteers.

Our greatest volunteer resources are older adults who spend their retirement years giving to others. Surveys report that almost 45 percent of adults over age 55 and 29 percent over 75 years of age are active volunteers for various community and human service organizations. The commitment and energies of older volunteer adults both provide means for enriching their lives and make them the backbone of many volunteer organizations.

Many of the older volunteers are retired professionals, returning to their areas of expertise, for example, a retired electrician who helps to rehabilitate inner-city housing or a lawyer who donates time to a free legal clinic. The compensation for volunteering is most rewarding–the development of new skills, meeting new people, and the sensation of helping someone in need.

In response to increasing volunteer opportunities and program needs, metropolitan Chicago has launched the nation's first comprehensive, computerized volunteer

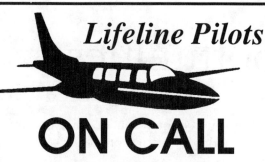
network program–The Volunteer Referral Service. This service is a collaborative venture of seven volunteer service providers in Chicago, which includes the City of Chicago's Light Up Chicago One-to-One volunteer program. It is sponsored by the Volunteer Network (formerly Community and Management Assistance Program), an organization with excellent experience in the recruitment and training of volunteers for the public and private sectors.

The service screens and registers organizations that need volunteers–social service agencies, schools, hospitals, nursing homes, cultural groups–and links volunteers according to interest and experience. Volunteers are trained if needed, then linked to organizations throughout Chicago's six-county area and Northwest Indiana. The Volunteer Referral Service projects that over 10,000 volunteers are expected to be placed with hundreds of registered agencies.

The Volunteer Referral Service will offer opportunities for older persons who are willing to give of themselves through volunteering as well as provide volunteers to work with the elderly.

Interested volunteers are encouraged to contact one of the volunteer referral sites or other volunteer organizations listed in the "Helpful Organizations" section of this book.

Preparing for Incompetence: Legal Considerations

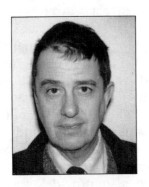

THOMAS GRIPPANDO

Thomas Grippando has been practicing law for 25 years. He is an attorney with United Charities Legal Aid Bureau and specializes in public benefits. He is also co-director of the John Marshall Law Program for Community Developers and Social Workers, offering a 12-week training program for social service providers, which (a) informs the providers about laws that protect their clients; (b) identifies appropriate referrals; and (c) prepares the service provided to advocate for the client.

Most of us are capable of conceiving of our own death. To prepare for that eventuality, we may prepare a will or place property in joint tenancy or in a trust. These steps ensure that our loved ones will receive our assets after we pass away.

In contrast, we rarely consider the possibility of losing our mental ability to manage our property or to make decisions about our medical treatment. While death is viewed as inevitable, the state of incompetency is considered to be totally improbable. Yet, we know of families who have experienced needless suffering while a loved one remained in a permanent comatose state. We know of elderly persons with diminished faculties who were financially exploited. This article discusses some of the protections available under Illinois law and focuses on those legal tools that do not require court intervention.

Each of the protections described here is available without having to file an action in court to declare that a person is disabled to the point of incompetency. They do not, however, eliminate the need for guardianship proceedings in all cases. For example, Joe can no longer manage his property or make decisions about medical treatment. He has not created a living trust, nor has he signed a power of attorney. In order to protect that property from exploitation, and in order to ensure that proper decisions are made about his health care, a guardianship may well be necessary. The services of a lawyer are required. Court costs and attorneys have to be paid. If Joe's estate includes substantial liquid assets, the guardian will have to post a bond and the fees for that bond will come from Joe's estate. A judge, who does not know the disabled person, will make important decisions as to the person's care and financial affairs.

There are advantages in a guardianship. The guardian's decisions are reviewed by the court. If the guardian embezzles the ward's funds, the bond covers any losses. Bonds are not required for the legal tools listed below and there is no judicial monitoring. In the case of embezzlement, one's only recourse is to sue the wrongdoer.

POWER OF ATTORNEY

If "A" is competent, "A" can authorize "B" to make decisions about "A"'s property (for example, bank accounts, rental units, etc.) and about "A"'s health. "B," the person who has this authority, is referred to as an agent. This authority is known as "power of attorney."

A power of attorney will continue even after the person who grants the authority becomes incompetent. However, the person granting the power must be competent at the time the power of attorney authorization is signed. This authority continues even after that individual has been declared incompetent by a court, and a guardian is appointed. In a certain sense, a power of attorney could continue after death, in that the individual could give the agent authority to decide how the body is to be disposed of or if it is to be used for medical research. For example, if "A" later becomes incompetent or is in a comatose state, "B" can still make these decisions. Even if "A" has been declared incompetent and a guardian appointed, "B" would retain this authority unless the court strips him or her of that authority.

This is an awesome power and should not be given lightly. In the past, power of attorney was of limited use because third parties would be at risk in relying upon the agent's authority. For example, if John authorized Tom to withdraw some money from a bank but later withdrew that authorization, the bank would be liable if it honored that authorization and gave the money to Tom. However, under a recent amendment to Illinois law, third parties are entitled to rely upon the authorization unless they have actual knowledge of fraud or knowledge that the authorization has been revoked.

Authorization could empower the agent to engage in real estate transactions; financial institution transactions; stock and bond transactions; tangible personal property transactions; safe deposit box transactions; insurance and annuity transactions; retirement plan transactions; Social Security, unemployment, and military benefits transactions; tax matters; claims and litigation; estate transactions; and virtually every other type of transaction.

The statute also provides for power of attorney to make health care decisions. "A" can give "B" the authority to be informed about, to consent to, or to refuse or to withdraw any type of health care for "A" and all powers that "A" as a parent may have to control or consent to health care for a minor child. Thus, you can give authority to make decisions about your own health care and the health care provided to your child. With respect to your own health care, you can give the agent legal right to make decisions about withholding or withdrawing life-sustaining or death-delaying procedures.

One can revoke authorization by burning, tearing, or destroying the power of attorney document, by written revocation, or by any oral or any other expression of intent to revoke the agency in the presence of a witness 18 years or older who signs and dates a writing confirming that such expression of intent was made. Neither the attending physician nor any other health provider may act as a health care agent.

The Illinois state legislature observed that the right of an individual to decide about personal care overrides the obligation of the physician and other health care providers to render care or to preserve life and health. The statute now provides that: (1) an individual has a right to control all aspects of his/her personal care and medical treatment including the right to decline medical treatment or to direct that it be withdrawn, even if death ensues, and (2) the individual can delegate this responsibility to the agent. Medical providers are immune from liability for following those instructions.

On the other hand, the doctor need not do anything that would violate his/her conscience and may refuse to comply. The agent is then responsible to make the necessary arrangements for the transfer of the patient to another provider.

This tool is not restricted to the elderly. With this power of attorney, families with mentally ill adult children can monitor the medication the adult child receives in a mental health facility.

Forms for power of attorney can be obtained at stationery stores. This is a serious matter and anyone signing this form should be fully informed of its consequences.

LIVING WILL

A living will is a set of instructions to health providers explaining that the person making the will does not wish extraordinary means to be used to keep the person alive when there is no reasonable expectation that the individual will recover. It must use certain wording and be witnessed by two persons. The living will would be used where the individual, at the time of the illness, is not able to express his/her intent. These forms are also available at stationery stores.

HEALTH CARE SURROGATE ACT

The Health Care Surrogate Act permits your family and friends to make health care decisions (including the decision to forego life-sustaining treatment) when you are mentally unable to make a decision. Those who make the decision are referred to as surrogate decison-makers. The Act would apply where an individual has not signed a power of attorney or a living will, or where the terms of power of attorney or living will are not applicable to the patient's situation.

Family or friends can make the decision without having to go to court. No court proceedings are required. The doctors would only request the "surrogate decison-makers" determine which services should be provided and which ones should be stopped, including tube feeding. The law only comes into effect where the patient lacks the capacity to make a decision as to medical services and one of the three conditions listed below exists:

(1) terminal condition (no reasonable prospect of cure or recovery, death is imminent and the application of life-sustaining treatment would only prolong the dying process);

(2) permanent unconsciousness;

(3) an incurable or irreversible condition.

In selecting the surrogate decision-maker, the following priorities apply:

(a) the patient's guardian;

(b) the patient's spouse;

(c) any adult son or daughter of the patient;

(d) either parent of the patient;

(e) any adult brother or sister of the patient;

(f) any adult grandchild of the patient;

(g) a close friend of the patient;

(h) the patient's guardian of the estate.

For example, Joe does not have a guardian and his wife died five years ago. His only children are two adult daughters. The daughters would be the surrogate decision-makers.

APPOINTMENT OF REPRESENTATIVE PAYEE

If a Social Security or Supplemental Security Income (SSI) beneficiary is unable to manage his/her benefits, one who is concerned about the beneficiary's welfare can request that he/she be named as the representative payee by the Social Security Ad-

---

ministration (SSA). One must complete the appropriate SSA forms, which are available at local offices. The representative payee must complete an annual report explaining how the benefits were spent. SSA has the obligation to investigate reports of the representative payee's misuse of funds.

LIVING TRUST

A trust is simply an arrangement whereby "A" transfers property to "B" for the benefit of "A" or another party. For example, Joe could enter into an agreement with Frank whereby Frank will receive $50,000; but those monies can only be used to meet Joe's needs. The trust agreement could provide that upon Joe's death the remainder of the money would be distributed to those persons designated by Joe as his beneficiaries. If, after creating the trust, Joe's condition deteriorated to the point that he could no longer manage his money, the trust would still be valid. Frank would dole out the monies pursuant to the terms of the trust. Joe would still have the benefit of the monies in the trust, but would be protected from exploitation. Obviously, Joe would have to have a great deal of confidence in Frank.

Dealing with Costs of Long-Term Care

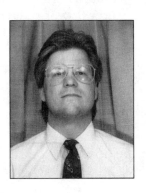

JOHN F. WASIK

John F. Wasik is editor and publisher of "The Conscious Consumer", a newsletter based in Wauconda, Illinois. He has also written for *The New York Times*, *Parade*, *The Saturday Evening Post*, and *Consumer Digest*.

Jim Spiro, 69, a retired Army Brigadier General, didn't know what to do when his wife contracted Alzheimer's disease. Until she succumbed to the disease a few years ago, his wife required custodial care for the last eight years of her life. Since he couldn't qualify for federal aid because he was drawing a modest pension and social security, Spiro says he's now starting a new career just to pay the bills of his wife's care, which cost him about $1,000 to $1,500 a *week* when *he* was hospitalized and unable to take care of her.

"I found somebody to take care of my wife (at home); most people don't 'luck out' that way," Spiro noted. "Friends and relatives don't know how to deal with the situation, so they fade away."

Fortunately, there is an abundance of public and private resources that are available specifically to caregivers struggling with the high cost of long-term care (LTC)–costs that threaten families with financial ruin.

The LTC crisis directly affects eight out of ten American families, and more than half of those families must pay for the care out of pocket. At an average cost of more than $25,000 a year, LTC facilities can often cost up to $60,000 a year. The most painful part of the LTC problem is that it's estimated the high costs of LTC will force nearly one million Americans this year into poverty. For example, few are prepared for nursing home costs, one of the largest components of LTC. A 1985 Harvard/Blue Cross study found that 63 percent of the elderly who entered nursing homes exhausted their life savings in 13 weeks; nearly half of those surveyed would be impoverished within only three months of entering the facility. With the cost of nursing homes ranging from $20,000 to $60,000 a year, the result of long-term care can be devastating to a family's lifetime savings.

Why is the cost of these conditions so oppressive in an age of "safety net" programs such as Medicare, Medicaid, and Social Security Disability Income? Because federal laws, like private health insurance programs, are filled with bureaucratic curbs that make it difficult to receive financial help–especially for middle-class Americans.

Who pays for most of these costs? For the most part, families and individuals, and to a lesser extent, private insurance. Keep in mind that some 37 million Americans have no insurance at all, and a difficult-to-estimate but larger group is underinsured.

While the government is squeezed by the need to cut back social programs because of budget deficits, the costs of LTC will grow dramatically because of an aging US population. At present, it costs $40 billion to care for Alzheimer's disease patients alone. Add those costs to the expenses of an expanding elderly nursing home population (although the vast majority of those needing LTC don't live there), which will grow from 1.6 million to 4.6 million from 1989 to 2040, and you have an explosion in LTC costs over the next generation.

Despite what many Americans believe, the Medicare program only pays for some 2 percent of LTC costs. Because Medicare only pays for 150 days of nursing care (following hospitalization), it was never meant to take care of LTC needs. That leaves the medical program of last resort–Medicaid–to pick up some 42 percent of LTC costs. But in order to qualify for Medicaid, a recipient must meet federal "poverty-level" income standards. That means a person must be impoverished in order to qualify for Medicaid. Ironically, the steep costs of LTC do indeed impoverish Americans. That's why families need to plan carefully to finance the often overwhelming costs of LTC.

WHY LONG-TERM CARE COSTS SO MUCH

Whenever 24-hour care is provided, the recipient is paying for a premium service. LTC services are expensive because they generally combine three types: (1) Skilled care, involving licensed health professionals such as doctors and registered nurses; (2) Intermediate care, which combines some medical personnel and specialists with lesser training; and (3) Custodial care, which covers the basic necessities such as meals, cleaning, and other daily activities. LTC facilities may either specialize in one type of care or offer the different levels in one setting.

For example, there are facilities that offer nothing but custodial care and others that combine a condominium-like setting with a health insurance plan. In full-service facilities, a person is paying for skilled and semi-skilled medical assistance; custodial and housekeeping services; activities; and social directors, and other personnel; food service; and administrative and other management expenses. Even in a lower-cost home-care setting, while saving money on administrative and some custodial expenses, medical, food, and housekeeping specialists are still needed.

In the most service-oriented facilities, costs escalate because of full resident medical staff and support facilities, private rooms, outside transportation services, and a full range of therapy and social activities.

LTC is costly in general because it combines so *many* services. As one might expect, the more service is needed the more it will cost. To wit: Skilled services are the most expensive and custodial the least expensive. How much should these facilities charge? It varies greatly on the quality of care available, the institution, and how the service is paid for.

HOW TO PAY FOR LONG-TERM CARE: A BRIEF LOOK

Home Care

Of all the LTC solutions being explored, care provided in the home has the greatest amount of support because it's less expensive than institutions and is a preferred care environment. According to the National Association for Home Care (NAHC), daily home care costs an average of $15,000 a year, versus as much as $60,000 a year for a high-quality nursing home. Although the home care average is still expensive, consider that NAHC research has found that home care postpones institutionalization, costs a fraction as much as hospitalization, keeps families together, and allows the maximum amount of freedom for the individual.

Home care is perhaps the best LTC option for the patient because research (from the NAHC and other leading groups) has shown that children and adults recover faster and with a lessened risk of infection at home than in an institution. Some 85 percent of home care is provided by volunteer "caregivers," typically spouses, relatives, and community workers. But about 5.5 million people who could benefit from outside assistance aren't receiving the help they need.

The most nagging drawback in paying for home care is that it's rarely covered by health insurers, barely covered by federal programs, and may not be available or of a high quality in many areas. Again, Medicaid doesn't consistently provide home health benefits, but a person can qualify who meets certain state/federal poverty-level guidelines or obtains a "waiver" of state Medicaid rules. Since Medicaid is a federal program administered by the states, the state agency responsible for the program should be queried. Medicare also provides some home care help, but that's also limited.

Private insurance for home care is available, but most policies contain several exclusions that diminish the coverage. And, at present, there are only 20 companies that sell separate home care policies. Again, like private LTC insurance (many policies offer home care "riders" at extra cost), this coverage becomes more expensive as the policy holder grows older.

For millions at home, though, home care is still the best alternative. Home care is provided by nearly 11,000 home care agencies. Of those groups, slightly more than half are "Medicare-certified," which means some Medicare reimbursement is available. They are also checked out by Medicare officials from time to time. That may not be a critical point since only 1.5 million out of 4 million people receive Medicare support. For more information, contact the nearest area agency on aging or write to the NAHC. (See "Getting Help: Key Consumer LTC Resources," at the end of this article.)

Adult Day Care

As its name implies, this is a basic service providing care for disabled adults who can be dropped off at a day care center in

the morning and picked up in the evening. Although it's in a nascent stage, this service will grow by leaps and bounds–especially because it's a lower-cost alternative to a nursing home. According to Dorothy Howe of the National Council on Aging, Inc., there are about 2,000 adult day care centers operating throughout 50 states, up from just 12 in 1970. She estimates that they range in cost from $27 to $31 a day. Angela Heath of the American Association of Retired Persons, however, estimates the range from free to $50 a day, depending upon the program. The more extensive programs naturally cost more, although public and private funding helps defray the costs, but the remainder of the charges are paid out-of-pocket by the person being cared for or by the caregiver.

Providing transportation, medical care, counseling, social activities, therapies, and nutrition, adult day care may be one of the most promising alternatives for adult LTC. Companies such as Holiday Inn are even exploring the concept. When choosing a day care center, make sure it complies with state regulations and can provide the necessary services (medical, proper nutrition, etc.). Also visit the center to make a visual inspection. For more information, see "Getting Help: Key Consumer LTC Resources," below.

Continuing-Care Retirement Communities

This is an option that costs the most but offers a large selection of services for the elderly. Continuing-care communities (formerly called "Life Care" communities) are essentially residential complexes that provide LTC services. The better facilities are accredited by the American Association of Homes for the Aging (AAHA) and provide everything from transportation, housekeeping, and medical care to recreation. This comprehensive approach has a price, though. "Members" of these communities pay one-time "entry" fees ranging from $30,000 to $100,000 and monthly charges ranging from $600 to $2,000. An "All-inclusive" facility, for example, covers nearly every LTC expense, but costs an average $63,328 for the entry fee and $940 a month, according to Deborah Cloud of the AAHA.

After a lump-sum payment up front and a monthly assessment thereafter, the communities also include a health insurance policy as part of the package. Variations on continuing care offer "shared" or "congregate" housing, which is usually less expensive but offers fewer services.

Estate Planning

While this isn't necessarily a way to pay for LTC, it can help prepare a family legally for circumstances that develop in an LTC situation. For example, Peter Strauss, a New York estate planning attorney, recommends looking into establishing "Durable Power of Attorney." This gives a family member or friend power to make financial decisions in the case of mental incapacity (like Alzheimer's disease). It also can help loved ones make the best possible decisions for their dependents. Joel Dobris, a law professor at the University of California at Davis, notes: "My mom's 84, and she told me she wants all of her money spent keeping her *out* of a nursing home." The best advice in this area is to seek out a quality estate-planning attorney.

Private LTC Insurance

Although one of the emerging "solutions" to the problem of how to pay for long-term care, it isn't for everyone; it's a complex product that needs to be studied carefully. Millions may be needlessly buying worthless or exorbitantly priced policies. LTC insurance is primarily bought to cover nursing home, home care, or skilled custodial care expenses and to preserve a family's assets from the ravages of nursing home bills.

The policies, issued by over 130 insurers at present, are becoming popular because of the soaring cost of nursing homes and the likelihood of facing such confinement in later years. The Health Insurance Association of America (HIAA), an industry trade group, has found that an "estimated 40 percent of elderly Americans will spend some time in a nursing home in their life."

Premiums on individual LTC policies range from $250 a year to $2,500 a year, according to HIAA. The average policy pays about $60 a day in benefits and $30 for home care, if that additional coverage is chosen. Most companies won't insure policyholders in their 70s or 80s. In fact, a 1988 Brookings Institution study showed that fewer than one-half of all older people could even afford a decent policy–especially dangerous for those who needed it the most and couldn't afford it due to their health or age.

The quality and utility of private LTC insurance varies greatly. Public service professionals who work with the elderly candidly agree that no one policy is ideal; many are riddled with clauses that lower the chances of a payout. A 1988 survey by the United Seniors Health Co-operative (USHC) in Washington, DC, found that beneficiaries of leading LTC policies had little chance of getting reimbursed for a claim. Their findings confirmed earlier research done by the General Accounting Office that revealed "nearly all policies contained restrictive clauses that attempt to establish medical necessity . . . these clauses, however, tend to reduce the likelihood that the policies will pay benefits . . . ."

These restrictions typically excluded those with "pre-existing conditions" such as Alzheimer's disease, or wouldn't pay unless the policyholder received "prior hospitalization," again an unlikely occurrence with Alzheimer's patients. Be on the lookout for these phrases when buying coverage.

Responding to that criticism, insurers have improved these policies dramatically because of better consumer awareness and tougher state laws. There are industry guidelines for LTC policies, but they're largely suggestions for state regulators. Although the trade group representing state insurance regulators–The National Association of Insurance Commissioners (NAIC)–recently issued "model legislation" that recommends LTC policy standards, insurers are not legally obliged to use the model. To date, though, 23 states have adopted laws similar to the NAIC model and nine more states are considering it. But consumer advocates have also criticized the NAIC rules for not going far enough to protect policyholders.

Who should buy a private LTC plan? Most financial planners recommend you buy LTC insurance if you have savings of $50,000 and under.

"If you're very wealthy and have retirement income (in excess of) $100,000, you don't need it (insurance)," advises Robert Bingham, a Cleveland-based estate planning attorney. "Those with retirement incomes of $30,000 to $50,000 should consider it." Better rates are available for those who are younger and in good health, but those in their late 70s or early 80s are unlikely to qualify.

It's also possible to buy "living benefit" life insurance policies that carry "riders" that will pay for LTC expenses, but only about 20 companies offer the complex plans, and they provide life insurance first and coverage second. Most of the policies pay a percentage (from 25 to 100 percent) of their accumulated cash value for LTC expenses, according to the American Council of Life Insurance. The benefits are actually prepayments of what the policy would pay out in "death benefits." Like all of the LTC policies, they are complicated, often expensive (depending upon age and health), and have many coverage restrictions. Although a promis-

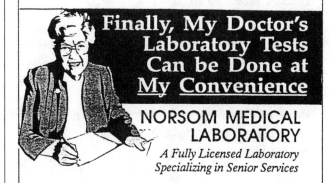

✔ In order to support future editions of this publication would you please mention **Elder Services** each time you contact any advertiser, facility, or service.

ing private insurance development, they should be eyed with extreme caution because they will be refined and made more flexible as the market for them grows. Home care is also available through a "rider," but it, too, is available at additional cost.

Several employers, such as General Foods, Proctor & Gamble, and American Express, are beginning to offer LTC insurance in a group plan to their employees (also see information about group plans on page 50, "Long-Term Care Insurance"). Check your personnel office to see if your company is offering this fringe benefit, which is usually significantly less expensive than the individual policies.

GETTING HELP: KEY CONSUMER LTC RESOURCES

Good Places to Start

The state, county, or local area agency on aging is a primary resource and may be the best place to start when it is not clear what kind of help is needed. The telephone numbers are listed in the "Helpful Organizations" section of this book. Another good resource is the local American Association of Retired Persons chapter.

Another course to follow when a course of action has not yet been determined is to employ a "geriatric care manager." He or she will locate the resources and facilities that will suit your needs and your budget. Contact Aging Network Services, 4400 East-West Highway, Bethesda, MD 20814; 301-657-4329.

To locate an attorney well-versed in LTC and estate planning, send a stamped, self-addressed envelope to the National Academy of Elder Law Attorneys, 655 North Alvernon, Suite 108, Tucson, AZ 85711.

Home Care

The National Association on Home Care, 519 C Street, NE, Stanton Park, Washington, DC 20002 is a group that represents home-care agencies and professionals. Although they have several publications, ask for their booklet *How to Choose a Home Care Agency.* The publication outlines the process, standards, and rights in dealing with a home-care agency.

Adult Day Care

The National Institute on Adult Day Care, c/o The National Council on Aging, Inc., 600 Maryland Avenue, SW, Wing 100, Washington, DC 20024, not only represents the adult day care industry, but can provide extensive information on the subject.

Continuing Care Communities

The best resource on this subject is the American Association of Homes for the Aging, 1129 20th Street, NW, Suite 412, Washington, DC 20036. Send them a self-addressed, stamped envelope to receive a list of accredited facilities and consumer brochures on Continuing Care Retirement Communities.

Insurance

The best booklet ($6.95) on the subject is published by the United Seniors Health Cooperative, located at 1334 G Street, NW, Suite 500, Washington, DC 20005. They publish *Long-Term Care: A Dollars and Sense Guide,* which details how to buy the policies, the pitfalls involved, and questions to ask an insurance agent.

Berkeley Planning Associates, a health insurance consulting firm in Oakland, California, has prepared a booklet designed to evaluate a person's need and financial ability to pay for LTC insurance. Called *How Do I Pay for My Long-Term Health Care,* it answers a host of questions on LTC. It's available by sending $7.95 (add 7% for sales tax if you live in California) to BPA Guidebook, 440 Grand Avenue, Oakland, CA 94610.

Long-Term Care Insurance

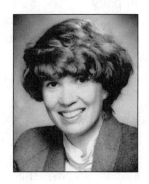

PEGGY PANNKE

Peggy Pannke, president of the National Consumer Oriented Agency, is a nationally recognized author and lecturer on the subject of long-term care insurance. As a consumer advocate, she was invited to Capitol Hill to address the Health Insurance Association of America. Improvements in long-term care insurance recommended by Ms. Pannke have been adopted verbatim by several major insurance companies. Interviewed on radio and television, she has also been featured in *The New York Times, Crain's Chicago Business,* and *Financial Planning* magazine. Pannke is best known for her dynamic seminars on long-term care insurance and her free presentations.

THE "GOOD NEWS" ABOUT LONG-TERM CARE INSURANCE

Six years ago, after watching my grandmother lose her savings and assets during her nursing home confinement, I decided to specialize in long-term care insurance. The changes in the industry during those years have proven that there really are insurance companies with "hearts."

Six years ago, the nursing home insurance that was available was full of restrictions (three-day hospital stays, skilled care only, and no home care). Today, even the average policies require no prior hospital stays, cover custodial (personal) care, and offer home care benefits.

Close to 2,000,000 people now have long-term care insurance, according to Carl Schramm, president of the Health Insurance Association of America; 425,000 LTC policies were sold in 1990 alone, and the numbers are increasing dramatically.

With average nursing home stays approaching four years, according to the *New England Journal of Medicine* (February 28, 1991), costs exceeding $150,000–$300,000 per person are no longer uncommon. The much-publicized Brandeis University study, showing that one out of two women will need to enter a nursing home at some time in her life, is added impetus to look at long-term care insurance.

Most people know they can't count on Medicare. Medicare still does not cover any custodial care (the kind of care needed by 95 percent of those needing care). Fewer than 2 percent of people who need skilled care ever get coverage from Medicare.

How Can You Find Excellent Long-Term Care Insurance?

Long-term care insurance is offered today by 134 insurance companies, but 75 percent of all LTC policies were sold by 12 insurers. The following are suggestions for finding the best buy.

Ratings

Look for insurance companies that have earned high ratings from at least one of the major rating companies: A.M. Best (the biggest rating company with a long track record), Standard & Poor's, Moody's, and Duff & Phelps. This is a good first step in finding the right LTC policy.

Track Record

Be sure that the highly rated insurance company has had its long-term care insurance on the market for at least two years! Past experience has shown that a certain percentage of the new LTC plans will pull out of the market after 12 or 18 months. A minimum of two years also allows for checking on their premium stability and claims payments. Plans that have been on the market for 5 years, 10 years, or 15 years, with no rate increases and good claims payment histories, have proven their commitment to long-term care insurance.

Group Plans or Individual Plans

Limited-enrollment group long-term care insurance often arrives by mail. You can recognize these plans by looking for a deadline or a day by which you must enroll. They come in many forms: retirement community groups, attorneys' groups, association groups, mail order plans, etc. Insurance companies using limited enrollments reserve the right to close the group at any time, leaving you in a group with only a few other people. This protects the insurance companies, but is not necessarily consumer-oriented. Why? Look in the certificate language (group plans refer to "certificates" whereas individual plans provide "policies"). According to the language, the insurance company reserves the right to increase premiums by group. If your group were very small, any claims would lead to rate increases. In some cases, the insurance company reserves the right to cancel by group! You may want more security.

Seventy-five percent of all LTC insurance policies were sold to individuals and only 16 percent were sold to groups, according to the recent HIAA survey. Most people who purchase long-term care insurance feel more secure with an individual policy. Individual policies are open to everyone in your state. There may be 10,000 people in the same policy form with you, and, if one of those 10,000 people had a large claim, it would be diluted and would not affect your premiums.

Individual LTC policies marked "Guaranteed Renewable" can never be cancelled.

The Importance of "Clean" Policy Language

Here's where you might need some expert advice. Hidden deep in some long-term care insurance plans is what I call a "weasel clause"–a clause allowing the insurance company to weasel out of paying your claim.

Many legitimate long-term care plans base benefit eligibility on Activities of Daily Living (ADLs) such as eating, continence, bathing, transferring, etc. It sounds logical that if you need assistance in your ADLs, you should get some benefit from your long-term care insurance policy. However, one insurance company requires "continual one-on-one assistance" in 2 out of 5 ADLs. The problem is that insurance companies use their own definitions of the ADLs, e.g.:

Eating

"A person is considered able to feed himself . . . even if he is being tube fed"

Continence

"A person is considered continent . . . even if he is catheterized"

Contrast this with "clean" policy language found in recommended LTC plans which allow a person who needs assistance (of any kind) with activities of daily living to receive benefits.

Attained Age or Level Premiums

Some policies seem less expensive than others, but make sure the reason isn't because the premiums are based on attained age. These policies cost more every year. By the time the policy is really necessary it probably would be unaffordable.

Much better are the level premiums found in approved policies. With those policies you lock in your premium at the age you are when you purchase it. For example, if you purchase a lifetime LTC policy offering you lifetime nursing home care starting at a $100 per day benefit, which increases by 5 percent compounded annually for life, and lifetime at-home care (in your home) starting at $50 per day and also increasing for life, and first-day benefit, you will lock in an annual premium of $495 if you are a healthy 59 year old. You will always pay the rate of a 59-year-old person, even when you are 94. The plan used in this example would pay the person approximately $90,000 per year for life when it was needed.

You are always better off locking in a premium at your age today rather than waiting until next year. The younger you are, the lower the level premium you lock in. Waiting until you are older will not save you money! If your health deteriorates, you may not even qualify for long-term care insurance.

Good Home Care Plans

Like many people, you may prefer a long-term care plan that offers home care benefits, or a stand-alone home care plan. When you think of home care, you are probably thinking of care for personal needs, help with bathing, eating, etc. Some of the less advanced home care plans only pay a full benefit for professional services provided by a nurse, physician, or licensed therapist, or services provided exclusively by professional medical personnel, as if you were a hospital patient. Much better are the many approved home care plans that pay the full benefit for personal care services and pay benefits for home health aides and adult day care.

Policies that let your doctor, or your nurse certify that you need help are best. What kind of help? Not only continual one-on-one assistance. Much better are those approved plans that allow active hands-on help, supervisory stand-by help, and/or directional, reminding help because many people require help as a consequence of loss of short- or long-term memory, reasoning powers, or recognition of whereabouts or time. Whether caused by Alzheimer's, senility, or anything else, look for clearly stated coverage for cognitive impairments.

All approved LTC plans contain a waiver of premium. This means that when you spend a certain number of days in a nursing home (specified in the policy), you stop paying for the insurance. Several insurance companies now offer the waiver for home care, too.

Be a Savvy Shopper

You are safest if you contact a specialist in long-term care insurance who is not employed by any insurance companies and who has many years of experience. Expect to be shown several different companies' plans and to compare their rates and benefits. There is no need to pay an annual premium when you apply. Most companies will accept a quarterly deposit–we know of two companies that require no deposit at time of application. But DO SOMETHING NOW! Many very intelligent seniors who have investigated every long-term care plan on the market, still end up with "analysis paralysis." For that reason, National Consumer Oriented Agency has prepared a simple checklist that is available to help sort through all these variables. Write to National Consumer Oriented Agency at 2200 East Devon, Des Plaines, IL 60018 for your free checklist.

✔ In order to support future editions of this publication would you please mention **Elder Services** each time you contact any advertiser, facility, or service.

Veteran Benefits, Chicago Metropolitan Area

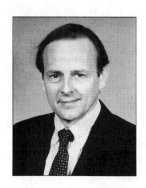

DAVID K. SULLIVAN

David K. Sullivan is the medical center planner for the VA Lakeside Medical Center in Chicago. Dr. Sullivan, whose experience includes six years with the City of Chicago Health Systems Agency, earned an M.B.A. in finance from Northwestern University and a Ph.D. from Georgetown University.

The Department of Veterans Affairs (VA) provides a wide variety of benefits to the nation's 27,000,000 veterans and their families. A veteran is an individual who has been in active military service and discharged under conditions other than dishonorable and has served the required time specified for VA eligibility. About one of three US citizens is a potential VA beneficiary. In the Chicago metropolitan area, there are approximately 900,000 veterans; of those, 240,000, or 27 percent, are 65 years of age and older.

VA benefits include pensions for wartime veterans (especially those 65 years of age and older); compensation for a military service injury; education and training; home mortgage loans; specially adapted homes, clothing, and autos for disabled veterans; life and mortgage insurance; burial fees; survivors' financial assistance; various forms of employment assistance; and medical care. Nonmedical VA benefits are handled through the VA regional office at 536 South Clark Street, Chicago 60680, (312) 663-5510.

Medical care for veterans is available in the Chicago area at four medical centers and two satellite outpatient clinics. Five community-based facilities provide readjustment counseling for Vietnam veterans and their families. The addresses and telephone numbers of the four medical centers are:

Edward Hines, Jr. VA Hospital
Roosevelt Rd and 5th Ave
Hines, IL 60141
(708) 343-7200

VA Lakeside Medical Center
333 E Huron St
Chicago, IL 60611
(312) 943-6600

VA Medical Center North
  Chicago
3001 Green Bay Rd
North Chicago, IL 60064
(708) 688-1900

VA West Side Medical Center
820 S Damen Ave
Chicago, IL 60612
(312) 666-6500

The outpatient clinics are:

Adam Benjamin, Jr.
  Outpatient Clinic
  (affiliated with VA
  Lakeside Medical Center)
9330 Broadway
Crown Point, IN 46307
(219) 662-0001

VA Medical Center
  North Chicago
  Outpatient Clinic
1601 Parkview Ave
Rockford, IL 61107
(815) 395-5576

✔ In order to support future editions of this publication would you please mention **Elder Services** each time you contact any advertiser, facility, or service.

The Illinois Department of Veterans Affairs (IDVA) also operates a 300-bed nursing home in Manteno, Illinois, 50 miles south of downtown Chicago, (815) 468-6581; a 626-bed nursing home and 150-bed domiciliary in Quincy, Illinois, 280 miles south of Chicago, (217) 222-8641; and a 120-bed nursing home in LaSalle, Illinois, 75 miles southwest of Chicago, (815) 223-0303. The IDVA Chicago office is located in Suite 4-650, State of Illinois Building, 100 West Randolph Street, Chicago 60601, (312) 814-2460. The City of Chicago's Commission on Human Relations has a veteran liaison, Suite 6A, 500 North Peshtigo Court, Chicago 60611, (312) 744-7582. Many counties in the Chicago metropolitan area have veterans' assistance offices.

The four Chicago-area VA medical centers provide virtually every type of medical care from basic outpatient services to high-technology programs such as cardiac surgery and radiation therapy. The centers offer acute medical, surgical, and psychiatric hospital care; dialysis treatment; dental and vision care; and long-term (extended) care in nursing homes, domiciliaries, adult day health care centers, community residences, and hospital-based home care programs. Specialty programs include rehabilitation of the blind, drug and alcohol abuse treatment, post traumatic stress disorder (PTSD) treatment, and spinal cord injury treatment. Many services are specially tailored to geriatric patients.

In recent years the VA has made special efforts to customize medical services for the nation's 1,200,000 women veterans. VA medical centers now have women veterans' coordinators for the 35,000 women veterans who reside in the Chicago area. The coordinators for the four Chicago area hospitals are:

Barbara Savage, Social Work Service
    Hines, (708) 216-2051

Anne McDermott, RN, Utilization Review
    Lakeside, (312) 943-6600, Ext 575

Claire Cafaro, Social Work Service
    North Chicago, (708) 688-1900, Ext 4111

Audrey Winfrey, RN, Nursing Service
    West Side, (312) 665-6500, Ext 2750/ 2752

Donna Charles, RN, Voluntary Service
    West Side, (312) 665-6500, Ext 2334

VA medical facilities have social work departments which provide counseling services, including individual and group psycho-social therapy, to patients and their families and assistance with posthospital care including resource management and referral to other VA and community services.

Eligibility for VA medical care varies according to the particular medical treatment (for example, inpatient or outpatient care) as well as the individual veteran's income and other factors. There are two principal eligibility categories:

Mandatory: Eligible for hospital care without co-payment. This group includes veterans with incomes below $18,200 annually ($21,800 if married), veterans with a certified service–connected medical condition (an injury or disability incurred or aggravated while in military service), former POWs, and others.

Discretionary: Eligible for hospital care with co-payment if space and other resources are available. This eligibility category includes all those not in the mandatory category; for example, a veteran with no dependents and income above $18,200 annually. The hospital co-payment is equal to the Medicare deductible ($628 in 1991) for the first 90 days of care during any 365-day period.

To obtain additional information on VA programs, eligibility requirements, and financial considerations, contact a VA office in your area. (See "United States Government" in the blue pages of your telephone directory.) In the Chicago area, the best source for general inquiries is the Chicago VA regional office, 536 South Clark Street, (312) 663-5510 or toll-free 1-800-972-5327. Veteran service organizations, which have offices at 536 South Clark Street, are excellent sources of information and guidance on VA eligibility, benefits, and system access.

If a veteran's medical condition is not an emergency, he/she should make an appointment with the VA medical center before arriving for treatment. Better yet, veterans should consult a VA or veterans service organization counselor before actually needing care to review eligibility status and required documentation so that when the time comes for medical care, treatment can begin with minimum delay.

Publications with more detailed information on VA benefits include:

Department of Veterans Affairs, *Federal Benefits for Veterans and Dependents*, published annually in March. About 100 pages.

Department of Veterans Affairs, *A Summary of VA Benefits*, published biannually (even numbered years) in September. About 40 pages.

These publications can be obtained from the Chicago VA regional office at 536 South Clark Street, Chicago 60680, (312) 663-5510. The four Chicago area VA medical centers also have brochures describing their services and related information.

✔ In order to support future editions of this publication would you please mention **Elder Services** each time you contact any advertiser, facility, or service.

BASIC RESOURCES FOR THE CAREGIVER

You might not be able to give your parents good health, but you can give them good health care.

As your parents grow older, their healthcare requirements will also change. And that is the benefit of having a system of healthcare services working for you. Whether you have concerns about where your parents will reside in the future, or whether you have already identified a need for more comprehensive medical care, Central DuPage Health System has a continuum of services to respond to their needs:

A Life-care Retirement Community Wyndemere provides a gracious living environment and comprehensive services to its residents. We will be opening our retirement community in 1993. Please call for additional information.

Alzheimer's Assessment Program Central DuPage Hospital, in conjunction with Community Convalescent Center of Naperville and the Alzheimer's Disease Center of Rush-Presbyterian-St. Luke's Hospital, offers professional and personal resources for the evaluation and management of this disease.

Home Healthcare Services and Home IV Therapy
Community Nursing Service of DuPage brings a full range of healthcare services into the home, including skilled nursing care; therapies; social service; home health aide, homemaker, and Hospice services.

Intermediate/Skilled Care Facility Community Convalescent Center of Naperville is committed to meeting the distinct needs of older adults, including short-term care for convalescence or rehabilitation, long-term care and Alzheimer's care.

For more information on how Central DuPage Health System can make health care work for you and your parents, please call our Information and Referral Service at **708-260-2685**.

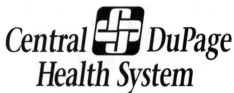

Central ✚ DuPage Health System

1151 E. Warrenville Road
Naperville, Illinois 60563

M a k i n g   H e a l t h   C a r e   W o r k   F o r   Y o u .

Service Options and Opportunities

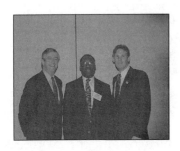

JONATHAN LAVIN

Jonathan Lavin is executive director of the Suburban Area Agency on Aging. He is the legislative chairman of the Illinois Association of Area Agencies on Aging and Illinois Coalition on Aging. He recently served on the Board of Directors of the National Association of Area Agencies on Aging, and was the State of Illinois Coordinator for the National Long-Term Care Campaign. He was a division director and project coordinator with the City of Chicago's Office on Aging for five years before joining the Area Agency in 1978.

DONALD R. SMITH

Donald R. Smith is the commissioner of the Chicago Department on Aging, the Area Agency on Aging for the City of Chicago. A veteran of city government with 27 years of service, he has developed innovative urban programs in the areas of education, employment, day care, aging, disability, and community development. Mr. Smith founded the Raymond Hilliard Adult Education Center of Chicago and also served as a former deputy director for the Office of the Mayor, Chicago Model Cities Program.

CHARLES JOHNSON

Charles Johnson has been executive director of the Northeastern Illinois Area Agency on Aging since 1974. Before that, he served as deputy director and director of neighborhood centers at the Kankakee County Community Action Agency. Mr. Johnson recently served as president of the Illinois Association of Area Agencies on Aging. He has been instrumental in the development of aging services in Illinois and is considered an advocate for aging services.

The senior population aged 60 and over in metropolitan Chicago numbers 1,148,649 and makes up 15.5 percent of the total population. The number of older persons in northeastern Illinois represents 59.6 percent of the total Illinois senior population. Within this nine-county region resides a rich blend of different ethnic, racial, economic, and social groups. Eighty-eight percent of the senior minority population in Illinois and 91 percent of the Hispanic elderly live in this region.

Diversity in lifestyles, foods, politics, religion, and language makes the Chicago area one of the most exciting in the world. In developing plans for serving the older segment of this population the goal must be to provide professional and quality services that emphasize each person's right to choose from as many options as possible to promote his or her maximum control and self-determination.

The aging service organizations described and listed in the "Helpful Organizations" section of this book reflect the enthusiasm and complexion of the communities they serve. Local citizens serve as staff, boards of directors, elected officers, and a tremendous volunteer corps. Programs are designed to meet high standards of service in many different types of settings. Service planners and advocates for the aging are concerned that services range from vigorous senior activity programs to the most intensive but caring long-term residential facilities.

As we look at aging services in this region, we appreciate the many opportunities and options provided to our senior populations. Older job hunters have access to outstanding employment preparedness and placement services. New eldercare programs are designed to provide the children or spouses of older persons with needed information and support to help meet their caregiving requirements while still meeting expectations of employers. There are many educational, social, health, nutrition, and leisure services and programs provided by the outstanding multipurpose senior centers throughout the region. A full range of volunteer opportunities exist in the number of settings serving all generations, especially the elderly.

Federal, state, and local governments serve older persons with benefit and service programs, including the Older Americans Act and the Illinois Act on Aging (and the City of Chicago Ordinance on Aging), which authorize support to the area agencies on aging programs.

We look for new opportunities to ensure that there are housing options and improved use of existing housing to help the older person live in a supportive and comfortable environment. We appreciate the health care, nutrition, and support services that help the older person with chronic health conditions to recuperate from illness, to overcome barriers to independence, and to spend the last months of life with comfort and dignity. We are pleased by the emergence of outstanding adult day care services and innovative group and personal care services.

Life is full of circumstances that often reduce options and decisions that provide future directions. As Robert Frost illustrated in the "Road Not Taken," we decide which road we will follow and probably will never have a chance to discover what it would have been like had we chosen the other. The goal of service providers for the aging is to allow older persons a chance to choose roads leading to new opportunities and challenges. Over time, choices may be limited by changes in health and reductions in functional ability. Social support may be lost through the death of friends and relatives or the moving of friends to others areas of the country. Service programs for the aging strive to assist our citizens even when the choices are not quite so wide, to help them proactively choose the roads they will take, and to make every trip as rewarding and positive as possible.

Robert Frost says he chose the road less traveled and that made all the difference. We know that the programs, benefits, and services identified within this volume make a difference to over 350,000 older persons in metropolitan Chicago. These citizens have been served through the outstanding community-based senior service programs of the City of Chicago Department on Aging, Suburban Area Agency on Aging for Cook County outside of Chicago, and the Northeastern Illinois Area Agency on Aging serving Du Page, Lake, Will, Kankakee, McHenry, Grundy, Kane, and Kendall counties. All three area agencies on aging are pleased that this resource is available. We ask that you use the services and benefits, volunteer to assist in the described programs, and offer support through contributions to not-for-profit service agencies or encouragement of your community to recognize and provide resources for strong senior service programs.

In the following articles all of the above will be explained and suggestions will be offered on how to reach an appropriate service source.

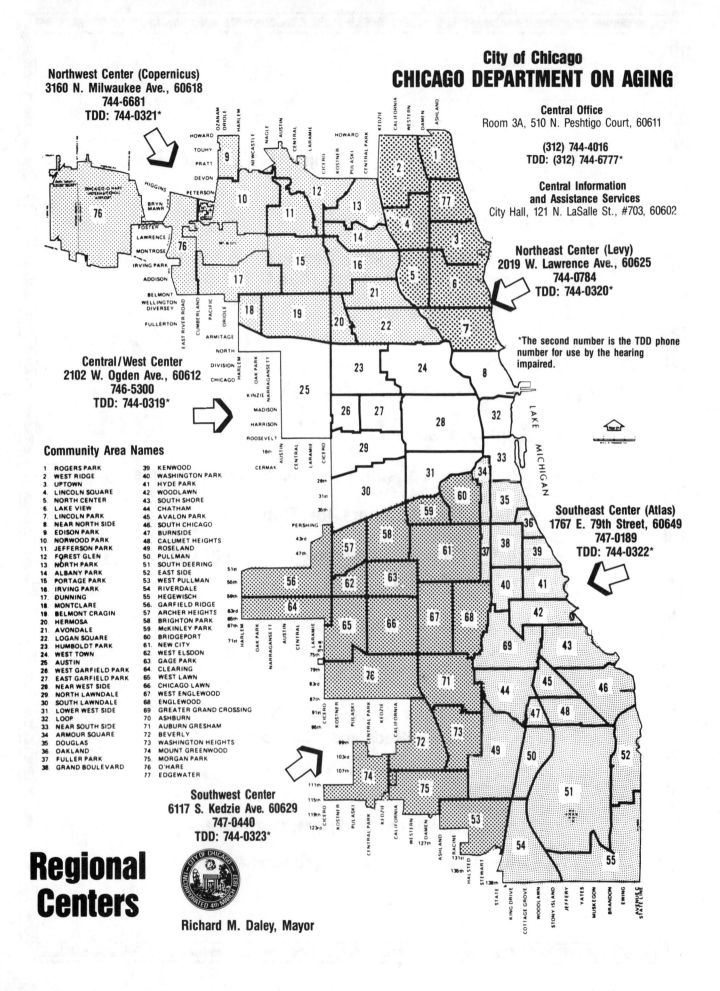

City of Chicago
CHICAGO DEPARTMENT ON AGING

Northwest Center (Copernicus)
3160 N. Milwaukee Ave., 60618
744-6681
TDD: 744-0321*

Central Office
Room 3A, 510 N. Peshtigo Court, 60611

(312) 744-4016
TDD: (312) 744-6777*

**Central Information
and Assistance Services**
City Hall, 121 N. LaSalle St., #703, 60602

Northeast Center (Levy)
2019 W. Lawrence Ave., 60625
744-0784
TDD: 744-0320*

*The second number is the TDD phone
number for use by the hearing
impaired.

Central/West Center
2102 W. Ogden Ave., 60612
746-5300
TDD: 744-0319*

Southeast Center (Atlas)
1767 E. 79th Street, 60649
747-0189
TDD: 744-0322*

Community Area Names

1 ROGERS PARK
2 WEST RIDGE
3 UPTOWN
4 LINCOLN SQUARE
5 NORTH CENTER
6 LAKE VIEW
7 LINCOLN PARK
8 NEAR NORTH SIDE
9 EDISON PARK
10 NORWOOD PARK
11 JEFFERSON PARK
12 FOREST GLEN
13 NORTH PARK
14 ALBANY PARK
15 PORTAGE PARK
16 IRVING PARK
17 DUNNING
18 MONTCLARE
19 BELMONT CRAGIN
20 HERMOSA
21 AVONDALE
22 LOGAN SQUARE
23 HUMBOLDT PARK
24 WEST TOWN
25 AUSTIN
26 WEST GARFIELD PARK
27 EAST GARFIELD PARK
28 NEAR WEST SIDE
29 NORTH LAWNDALE
30 SOUTH LAWNDALE
31 LOWER WEST SIDE
32 LOOP
33 NEAR SOUTH SIDE
34 ARMOUR SQUARE
35 DOUGLAS
36 OAKLAND
37 FULLER PARK
38 GRAND BOULEVARD
39 KENWOOD
40 WASHINGTON PARK
41 HYDE PARK
42 WOODLAWN
43 SOUTH SHORE
44 CHATHAM
45 AVALON PARK
46 SOUTH CHICAGO
47 BURNSIDE
48 CALUMET HEIGHTS
49 ROSELAND
50 PULLMAN
51 SOUTH DEERING
52 EAST SIDE
53 WEST PULLMAN
54 RIVERDALE
55 HEGEWISCH
56 GARFIELD RIDGE
57 ARCHER HEIGHTS
58 BRIGHTON PARK
59 McKINLEY PARK
60 BRIDGEPORT
61 NEW CITY
62 WEST ELSDON
63 GAGE PARK
64 CLEARING
65 WEST LAWN
66 CHICAGO LAWN
67 WEST ENGLEWOOD
68 ENGLEWOOD
69 GREATER GRAND CROSSING
70 ASHBURN
71 AUBURN GRESHAM
72 BEVERLY
73 WASHINGTON HEIGHTS
74 MOUNT GREENWOOD
75 MORGAN PARK
76 O'HARE
77 EDGEWATER

Southwest Center
6117 S. Kedzie Ave. 60629
747-0440
TDD: 744-0323*

Regional
Centers

Richard M. Daley, Mayor

Options for Our Aging Society Right in Your Community

Understanding the needs of older persons and searching for resources to meet their needs can be both time-consuming and frustrating. With over thirty years experience in service to older adults, the **Chicago Department on Aging** creates service options and makes them available right in your community.

Our staff of caring professionals provides a wide spectrum of programs for older adults. Our major goal is to keep seniors independent, healthy and active.

Programs and Services for Older Adults

- INFORMATION AND ASSISTANCE
- CASE MANAGEMENT
- CHICAGO FUND ON AGING AND DISABILITY
- CHORE/HOUSEKEEPING
- ELDERCARE/Chicago *sm
- EMPLOYMENT SERVICES
- FOSTER GRANDPARENTS
- HOME DELIVERED MEALS

- LIFE ENRICHMENT PROGRAMS
- LIGHT-UP CHICAGO (VOLUNTEER PROGRAM)
- RESPITE
- PROTECTIVE SERVICES
- REGIONAL CENTERS
- GOLDEN DINERS
- TRANSPORTATION

Northeast Center (Levy)
2019 W. Lawrence Ave., 60625
744-0784
TDD: 744-0320 *

Southwest Center
6117 S. Kedzie Ave., 60629
747-0440
TDD: 744-0323 *

Central/West Center
2102 W. Ogden Ave., 60612
746-5300
TDD: 744-0319 *

Southeast Center (Atlas)
1767 E. 79th Street, 60649
747-0189
TDD: 744-0322 *

Northwest Center (Copernicus)
3160 N. Milwaukee Ave., 60618
744-6681
TDD: 744-0321 *

* The second number is the TDD phone number for use by the hearing impaired.

The **Chicago Department on Aging** is the **Area Agency on Aging for Chicago,** designated to address the needs and concerns of our aging society.

Call us for more information, (312) 744-4016
or TDD: (312) 744-6777.

City of Chicago
Richard M. Daley
Mayor

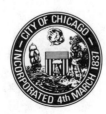

Chicago Department
on Aging
Donald R. Smith
Commissioner

*service mark

NORTHEASTERN ILLINOIS AREA AGENCY ON AGING

Serving the eight (8) northeastern Illinois counties since 1974. Services funded or coordinated by Northeastern Illinois meet the diverse needs of the most rapidly growing population in Illinois.

Contact the **Case Coordination Unit** in your area for information and assistance on services and programs for older persons:

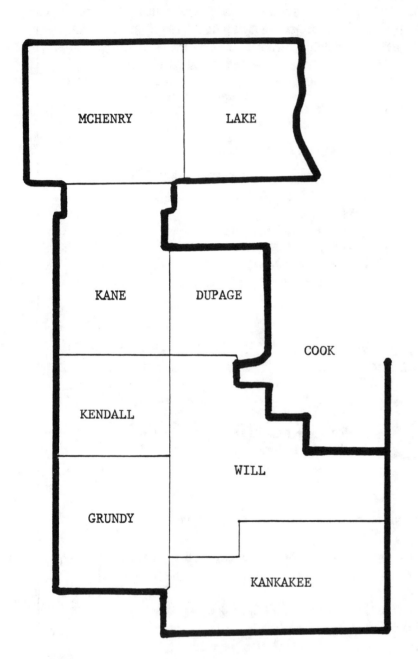

DUPAGE
DuPage Co Dept of Human Services
(708) 682-7990

GRUNDY
Grundy Co Senior Citizens Council
(815) 634-2254

KENDALL
Senior Service Associates, Inc
(708) 741-0404

MCHENRY
Senior Service Associates, Inc.
(815) 344-3555

KANE
Senior Service Associates, Inc
(708) 741-0404

KANKAKEE
Catholic Charities
Senior Outreach & Referral
(815) 932-1921

LAKE
Catholic Charities
(815) 546-5733

WILL
Senior Services of Will County
(815) 723-9713

"WORKING HARDER TO MAKE AGING EASIER"

West Chicago Office: (708) 293-5990

Kankakee Office: (815) 939-0727
                                   (800) 528-2000

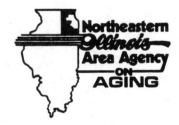

YOU'RE A PHONE CALL AWAY!
FROM SERVICES FOR OLDER PERSONS IN YOUR COMMUNITY

Northeastern Illinois Area Agency on Aging plans and coordinates services for older persons in eight northern Illinois counties.

➡Are you living in or do you have an elderly loved one living in **DuPage, Grundy, Kane, Kendall, Kankakee, Lake, McHenry or Will** county?

➡Do you need **information and assistance** to find out more about the following services or programs available to older adults?

- case management
- home delivered meals
- outreach
- transportation
- protective services
- employment services
- recreational/social opportunities

- volunteer opportunities
- congregate dining centers
- community care program
- legal services
- respite care
- senior centers
- and more ....

The agencies listed are there to answer your questions.

DUPAGE
DuPage County Department of Human Services
(708) 682-7990

KANE
Senior Services Associates, Inc.
(708) 741-0404

GRUNDY
Grundy County Senior Citizens Council
(815) 634-2254

KANKAKEE
Catholic Charities
Senior Outreach & Referral
(815) 932-1921

KENDALL
Senior Service Associates, Inc
(708) 741-0404

LAKE
Catholic Charities
(815) 546-5733

MCHENRY
Senior Service Associates, Inc
(815) 344-3555

WILL
Senior Services of Will County
(815) 723-9713

Northeastern Illinois Area Agency on Aging's mission, not unlike a family caregiver, health care professional, etc, is to enable older persons to remain independent, active and in their own home for as long as possible.

The Area Agency on Aging is your resource for information, training, and advocacy on every aspect on aging. Please call us for more information:

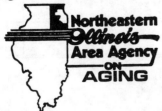

West Chicago Office
(708) 293-5990

Kankakee Office
(815) 929-0727
(800) 528-2000

"Working Harder to Make Aging Easier"

Suburban Aging Network
Service Providers

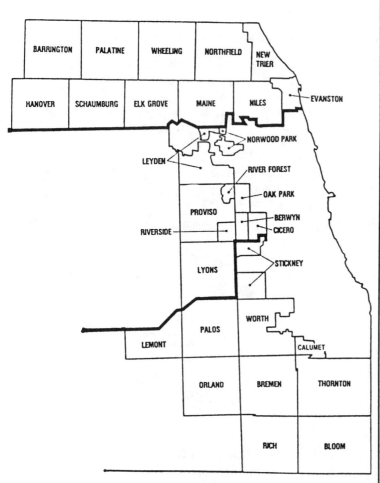

Serving the Suburbs
of Cook County, Illinois

SERVICE PROVIDERS	TELE-PHONE (708)	TOWNSHIP(S) SERVED
Lutheran Social Services of Illinois/Home Helps for Seniors	596-6690	Municipalities of Dolton, Thornton, Burnham, Calumet City, Lansing, Phoenix, East Hazel Crest, Riverdale, and South Holland
PLOWS Council on Aging	422-6722	Palos, Lemont, Orland and Worth
South Suburban Senior Services/Catholic Charities	596-2222	Bloom, Bremen, Calumet, Rich and the municipalities of Blue Island, Harvey, Dixmoor, Homewood, and Markham of Thornton Township
Stickney Public Health District	424-9200	Stickney
Berwyn Cicero Council on Aging	863-3552	Berwyn and Cicero
Leyden Family Service Senior Citizens	455-3929	Leyden
Oak Park Township Senior Services	383-8060	Oak Park and River Forest
Proviso Council on Aging	547-5600	Proviso Township with the exceptions of Brookfield and LaGrange Park Villages
Seniors Assistance Center	456-7979	Norwood Park
Southwest Suburban Center on Aging	354-1323	Lyons, Riverside and the Villages of Brookfield and LaGrange Park
Family Counseling Service of Evanston & Skokie Valley	328-2404	Evanston and Niles
Kenneth W. Young Centers: Center for Senior Services - West	885-1631	Elk Grove and Schaumburg
Center for Senior Services - North	253-5500	Barrington, Hanover, Palatine and Wheeling
North Shore Senior Center	446-8750	Maine, New Trier and Northfield

Suburban Area Agency on Aging

The Suburban Area Agency on Aging serves the suburbs of Cook County through a network of funded service providers. The Area Agency is responsible for developing local systems of social and nutritional support services to assist elderly persons to remain independent in their homes and communities.

"One-stop shopping" is available to older persons and caregivers through comprehensive community-based, long term care services provided through the suburban aging network.

Area Agency Funded Services

Access Services
- Information & Referral
- Case Management/Coordination
- Transportation
- Outreach
- Gatekeeper Program

Community Services
- Housing Assistance
- Legal Assistance
- Multi-Purpose Senior Centers
- Senior Employment Program
- Senior Lunch Program

In-Home Services
- Home Delivered Meals
- Telephone Reassurance
- Chore Housekeeping
- Friendly Visiting
- Respite Services

Protective Services
- Nursing Home Ombudsman
- Elder Abuse Intervention

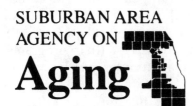

SUBURBAN AREA AGENCY ON **Aging**

Suburban Area Agency on Aging
1146 Westgate, Suite LL 112
Oak Park, IL 60301-1054
708-383-0258 (Voice and TDD)

All Participants Will Be Afforded Equal Admission To Programs/Activities

Where to Turn for Help

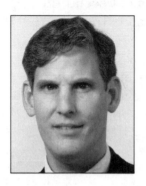

JONATHAN LAVIN

Jonathan Lavin is the executive director of the Suburban Area Agency on Aging. He is the legislative chairman of the Illinois Association of Area Agencies on Aging and Illinois Coalition on Aging. He recently served on the Board of Directors of the National Association of Area Agencies on Aging and was the State of Illinois Coordinator for the National Long-Term Care Campaign. Under his leadership, the Area Agency has developed major case management, advocacy, elder abuse interventions, nutrition, and communication programs. Mr. Lavin was a division director and project coordinator with the City of Chicago's Office on Aging for five years before joining the Area Agency in 1978.

The following is a listing of organizations that provide services to older persons who reside in the metropolitan Chicago area. The section is organized by city and name of the agency. Some organizations are centered in one location but serve the entire region. Others have out-station offices throughout the region. Very few service agencies specialize in only one type of service activity. The index to this section lists entries by service classification.

Note those agencies that are listed as providing multiple services. Most community-based senior service organizations are listed in this category. Some of the varied services these agencies provide may not be listed. It is recommended that the community-based service program be considered first when searching for appropriate assistance to meet the older person's needs.

In the city of Chicago, the central information and assistance number, (312) 744-4016, is the key to all aging services. In suburban Cook County and the collar counties, the Case Coordination Unit is the key for most service contacts. In northwestern Indiana, the Lake County Economic Opportunity Council is the central location to call, (219) 937-3500 (or for Indiana residents (800) 826-7871).

The agencies identified in this section provide older persons, caregivers, and professionals in the field of aging, a selection of services or benefits. Services should be provided in the least restrictive environment–meaning that the agency personnel must make the older person's self-determination and dignity their driving motivation in providing services. Most of the agencies listed are responsible to a code or set of standards for service delivery.

The services listed are classified by common characteristics in meeting the need(s) of the older person, family, or friends. Senior service agencies are creative and attempt to understand and adapt their programs to meet the needs of various communities and of various ethnic, religious, or individual conditions. This means the following service definitions are not represented as the actual service offered by each and every agency. Ask the provider agency for a full description of the attributes and limitations of their service provision.

✔ In order to support future editions of this publication would you please mention **Elder Services** each time you contact any advertiser, facility, or service.

A major source of service funding in the metropolitan area is the Older Americans Act. There are no fees for services provided under the Older Americans Act, but voluntary contributions are encouraged. Eligibility is determined by age (over 60) and by the need for the service. There are no income eligibility requirements for Older Americans Act services. Other services are provided through the Illinois Community Care Program, which is directed to older persons with demonstrated needs for service and who qualify for assistance based on income or asset levels. Both Older Americans Act and Community Care Program services are accessed through the same case management agencies, allowing for all older persons to apply for an appropriate service from the same case managers.

Your community may have other services available through the park district, local government, private agencies, and other not-for-profit agencies. The information and referral (I&R) office or case manager can give you information on these services, their eligibility requirements, and any costs.

Comprehensive Care for Older Adults

Northwestern Memorial Hospital's Department of Geriatric Services provides a comprehensive range of readily available medical, psychiatric and health education services for older adults. Our staff of geriatricians, geriatric nurse specialists, geriatric clinical social workers and other health care professionals will assist you and your patients in a variety of ways.

Northwestern's Geriatric Services include:

"Healthy Transitions" membership program: keeps you informed about health-related topics and services

Geriatric Evaluation Service: comprehensive evaluations which assess and treat total medical, functional and psychosocial needs, with the goal of maintaining independence

Older Adult Program, Institute of Psychiatry: outpatient and inpatient treatment

Geriatric Health Ministry: geriatric nurses work with churches and synagogues to promote health and wellness

Communi-Call: an in-home emergency response communication system

Northwestern Memorial Home Health Care/ Services, Inc.: comprehensive home care services throughout the Chicago metropolitan area

The Hospice Program: home and hospital care for the terminally ill

For more information, or to refer a patient,
call the Healthy Transitions coordinator at
(312) 908-4335

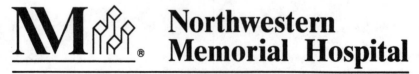

Northwestern
Memorial Hospital

Organizations

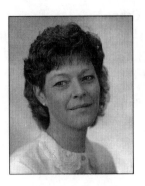

SIRI L. NIMITZ-NELSON

Siri Nimitz-Nelson has recently completed a course of study in gerontology at Montay College and is now pursuing a degree in geriatric social work at Northeastern Illinois University. She participated in a GSA Fellowship survey on implementation of fees for services presented at the 1989 Illinois Governor's Conference for the Aging. She also is a personal financial manager, and has been for seventeen years, in the Chicago area. For this edition of *Elder Services* she has compiled the "Organizations" section as well as "Helpful Materials for Caregivers," "Helpline Numbers," "Checklists," and "Glossary," and edited the section of "Practical Advice and Information."

The Abbey Leisure Center
407 W St Charles Rd, Elmhurst, IL 60126
(708) 833-9766
FUNCTIONS: Senior center; Congregate dining

Access Wisdom Inc
288 N Addison, Elmhurst, IL 60126
(708) 530-2847, 832-3071 FAX
FUNCTIONS: Information & referral; Counseling

Addison Park District
120 E Oak, Addison, IL 60101
(708) 833-0100
FUNCTIONS: Congregate dining

Alcoholics Anonymous
205 W Wacker Dr Ste 422, Chicago, IL 606 06
(312) 346-1475
FUNCTIONS: Support groups; Counseling

Alexian Brothers Medical Centers
800 Biesterfield Rd, Elk Grove Village, IL 60007
(708) 437-5500
FUNCTIONS: Medical health services

ALJO Medical Transport
3333 W Peterson Ste 10, Chicago, IL 60659
(312) 583-2800
OTHER SERVICES: Medical & nonmedical transport for handicapped persons
See ad page xvi

Alliance for the Mentally Ill
833 N Orleans St, Chicago, IL 60610
(312) 642-3338
FUNCTIONS: Information & referral; Support groups

Alzheimer's Disease Association—Chicago Area Chapter
4709 Golf Rd Ste 1015, Skokie, IL 60076
(708) 933-2413, Helpline (708) 933-1000
FUNCTIONS: Information & referral; Caregiver support; Counseling; Educational programs

Alzheimer's Family Care Center
5522 N Milwaukee Ave, Chicago, IL 60630
(312) 283-6502
FUNCTIONS: Information & referral; Caregiver support; Day care; Counseling

Alzheimer's Family Care Hospice
1725 West Harrison Ste 1030, Chicago, IL 60612
(312) 942-4463
FUNCTIONS: Hospice

✓ In order to support future editions of this publication would you please mention *Elder Services* each time you contact any advertiser, facility, or service.

American Academy of Ophthalmology
PO Box 6988, San Francisco, CA 94011
(800) 222-3937
FUNCTIONS: Information & referral; Educational programs; Publications

American Academy of Physical Medicine & Rehabilitation
122 S Michigan Ave Ste 1300, Chicago, IL 60603
(312) 922-9366
FUNCTIONS: Information & referral; Educational programs; Publications

American Association of Retired Persons (AARP)—Chicago Area
2720 Des Plaines Ave Ste 113, Des Plaines, IL 60018
(708) 298-2852
FUNCTIONS: Information & referral; Educational programs; Publications
OTHER SERVICES: Pre- & postretirement counseling

American Cancer Society—Illinois Division
77 E Monroe Ste 1300, Chicago, IL 60603
(312) 641-6150
FUNCTIONS: Information & referral; Educational programs

American Diabetes Association
6 N Michigan Ave Ste 1202, Chicago, IL 60602
(312) 346-1805
FUNCTIONS: Information & referral; Educational programs

American Foundation for the Blind
20 N Wacker Dr, Chicago, IL 60606
(800) 232-5463
FUNCTIONS: Information & referral; Educational programs; Publications; Counseling

American GI Forum
217 W Washington St, Waukegan, IL 60085
(708) 336-1298
FUNCTIONS: Ethnic services & activities

American GI Forum—Women's Auxiliary
431 Franklin St, Waukegan, IL 60085
(708) 623-4906
FUNCTIONS: Ethnic services & activities

American Health Care Apparel
334 Church St, Easton, PA 18042
(800) 252-0584
OTHER SERVICES: Specialized apparel and footwear for people with special needs. Adaptations and alterations available. Free catalog available.
See ad page 6

American Heart Association of Metropolitan Chicago
20 N Wacker Dr, Chicago, IL 60606
(312) 346-4675

FUNCTIONS: Information & referral; Educational programs

American Indian Center
1630 W Wilson, Chicago, IL 60640
(312) 275-5871
FUNCTIONS: Ethnic services & activities

American Red Cross
43 E Ohio, Chicago, IL 60611
(312) 440-2000
FUNCTIONS: Social services
OTHER SERVICES: Disaster services

American Spanish Institute
2619 W Armitage, Chicago, IL 60647
(312) 278-5130
FUNCTIONS: Ethnic services & activities; In-home services

Antioch Senior Center
817 Holbek Dr, Antioch, IL 60002
(708) 395-7120
FUNCTIONS: Senior center; Congregate dining

Apostolic Assembly
922 Washington St, Waukegan, IL 60085
(708) 336-0150
FUNCTIONS: Ethnic services & activities

Area 1 Agency on Aging
5518 Calumet Ave, Hammond, IN 46320
(219) 937-3500, (800) 826-7871
FUNCTIONS: Information & referral; Advocacy; Congregate dining; Ombudsman services
OTHER SERVICES: Pre-nursing home admission screening; addresses of congregate dining sites available from this office

Argo-Summit Senior Nutrition Site
7438 W 62nd Pl, Summit IL 60501
(708) 458-9380
FUNCTIONS: Home delivered meals; Congregate dining

The Ark
2341 W Devon, Chicago, IL 60659
(312) 973-1000
FUNCTIONS: Information & referral; Case management; In-home services; Home delivered meals
OTHER SERVICES: Kosher meals available

Arlington Heights Library
500 N Dunton, Arlington Heights, IL 60004
(708) 392-0100
FUNCTIONS: Energy assistance program; Educational programs

Arthritis Foundation—Illinois Chapter
79 W Monroe St Ste 510, Chicago, IL 60603
(800) 572-2397
FUNCTIONS: Information & referral; Educational programs; Support groups

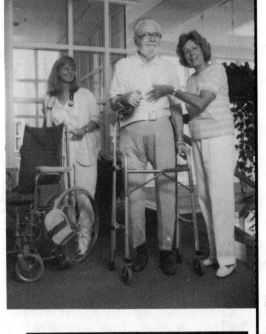

Arts Unlimited
55 E Washington St Ste 1934, Chicago, IL 60602
(312) 332-0093
OTHER SERVICES: Entertainment & arts workshops

ASI
2619 W Armitage, Chicago, IL 60647
(312) 278-5130
FUNCTIONS: Ethnic services & activities

Asian Human Services of Chicago
4753 N Broadway Ste 818, Chicago, IL 60640
(312) 728-2235
FUNCTIONS: Ethnic services & activities

Asociacion Latina de Servicios Educacionales Inc
3616 Elm St, East Chicago, IN 46312
(219) 398-1337
FUNCTIONS: Information & referral; Counseling

Association House of Chicago
2150 W North Ave, Chicago, IL 60647
(312) 276-0084
FUNCTIONS: Information & referral; Support groups; Counseling; In-home services; Ethnic services & activities

Association of Indians in America
211 W 79th St, Burr Ridge, IL 60521
(312) 996-0041

FUNCTIONS: Ethnic services & activities

Aurora Township Senior Center
33 S Stolp, Aurora, IL 60506
(708) 897-4035
FUNCTIONS: Senior center; Congregate dining

Austin Peoples Action Center
5931 W Corcoran, Chicago, IL 60644
(312) 921-2121
FUNCTIONS: Ethnic services & activities

Autumn Country Club
627 N LaGrange Rd, Frankfort, IL 60423
(708) 469-0060
FUNCTIONS: Senior center

Warren Barr Pavilion of Illinois Masonic Medical Center
66 W Oak St, Chicago, IL 60610
(312) 337-5400
FUNCTIONS: Day care; Social services; Recreation; Volunteer opportunities; Educational programs; Publications

Barrington Area Senior Citizens Center Inc
235 Lions Dr, Barrington, IL 60010
(708) 381-0687
FUNCTIONS: Senior center; Congregate dining

✔ In order to support future editions of this publication would you please mention *Elder Services* each time you contact any advertiser, facility, or service.

Beacon Neighborhood House
1422 S Ashland Ave, Chicago, IL 60608
FUNCTIONS: Ethnic services & activities

Beecher Community Center
908 Game Farm Rd, Yorkville, IL 60560
(708) 553-5777
FUNCTIONS: Senior center

Bensenville Home Society—Castle Towers
325 S York Rd, Bensenville, IL 60106
(708) 766-5800
FUNCTIONS: Congregate dining

Berwyn/Cicero Council on Aging
5817 W Cermak Rd, Cicero, IL 60650
(708) 863-3552
FUNCTIONS: Information & referral; Educational programs; Case management; In-home services; Friendly visits; Home delivered meals; Home repairs; Senior center; Recreation; Congregate dining; Transportation; Energy assistance program; Case coordination unit; Protective services; Volunteer opportunities; Legal assistance; Medical assessments; Multiple services

Bethel New Life Inc
367 N Karlov, Chicago, IL 60624
(312) 342-6550
FUNCTIONS: Information & referral; Day care; In-home services; Home repairs; Housing assistance; Energy assistance program

Bloom Township Senior Citizens Services
425 S Halsted St, Chicago, IL 60401
(708) 754-9400 Ext 45
FUNCTIONS: Information & referral; Transportation; Case management; Multiple services

Bloomingdale Township Senior Center
6 N 050 Rosedale Rd, Bloomingdale, IL 60108
(708) 529-7794
FUNCTIONS: Senior center; Congregate dining

Blue Island Senior Citizens Project
13051 S Greenwood, Blue Island, IL 60406
(708) 597-8608
FUNCTIONS: Information & referral; Multiple services

Bolingbrook Senior Center
230 E Briarcliff, Bolingbrook, IL 60439
(708) 739-4590
FUNCTIONS: Congregate dining; Senior center

The Bootery
5117 N Harlem Ave, Chicago, IL 60656
(312) 792-3375
OTHER SERVICES: Specialize in corrective, orthopedic, and comfort footwear. Nursing home and retirement center visits available.
See ad page 26

Bradley Bourbannais Senior Citizens
700 W North St, Bradley, IL 60915
(815) 937-3743
FUNCTIONS: Senior center

Bremen Township Senior Services
16361 S Kedzie Ave, Markham, IL 60426
(708) 596-6880
FUNCTIONS: Multiple services

Buehler Center on Aging—Northwestern University
750 N Lake Shore Dr Ste 521, Chicago, IL 60611
(312) 503-3087
FUNCTIONS: Educational programs

Burbank-Stickney Senior Lunch Center
7730 S LeClaire Ave, Burbank, IL 60459
(708) 636-8850
FUNCTIONS: Home delivered meals; Congregate dining

Burmese American Association of Chicago
6830 N Lincoln Ave, Chicago, IL 60646
(312) 478-6800
FUNCTIONS: Ethnic services & activities

Calumet City Youth & Family Services
145 167th St, Calumet City, IL 60409
(708) 891-8743
FUNCTIONS: Volunteer opportunities

Calumet Township Senior Citizens Service Center
12633 S Ashland Ave, Calumet Park, IL 60643
(708) 597-1075
FUNCTIONS: Multiple services; Home delivered meals; Congregate dining

Cambodian Assistance Project
1105 W Lawrence Ave Ste 214, Chicago, IL 60640
(312) 878-7090
FUNCTIONS: Ethnic services & activities

Cary Grove Senior Center
441 W Main St, Cary, IL 60013
(708) 639-8118
FUNCTIONS: Senior center; Congregate dining

Casa Central
1041 N California, Chicago, IL 60622
(312) 276-1902
FUNCTIONS: Ethnic services & activities; Day care; Congregate dining

Catholic Charities—Chicago
126 N Des Plaines Ave, Chicago, IL 60606
(312) 236-5172
FUNCTIONS: Information & referral; Educational programs; Case management; Counseling; In-home services; Friendly visits; Senior center; Recreation; Support groups; Legal assistance; Multiple locations

Catholic Charities of Chicago
5801-C N Pulaski Rd, Chicago, IL 60646
(312) 583-9224
FUNCTIONS: Case coordination unit; Multiple services

Catholic Charities—Joliet
411 Scott St, Joliet, IL 60432
(815) 723-3405
FUNCTIONS: Ethnic services & activities

Catholic Charities—Round Lake
116 N Lincoln Ave, Round Lake, IL 60073
(708) 546-5733
FUNCTIONS: Case coordination unit; Multiple services

Catholic Family Services—Crown Point
109 E Joliet St, Crown Point, IN 46307
(219) 769-2165
FUNCTIONS: Information & referral; Counseling
OTHER SERVICES: Emergency assistance available

Catholic Family Services—East Chicago
4012 Elm St, East Chicago, IN 46312
(219) 397-5803
FUNCTIONS: Information & referral; Counseling
OTHER SERVICES: Emergency assistance available

Catholic Family Services—Gary
509 W Ridge Rd, Gary, IN 46408
(219) 980-1318
FUNCTIONS: Information & referral; Counseling
OTHER SERVICES: Emergency assistance available

Catholic Family Services—Michigan City
524 C Franklin Square, Michigan City, IN 46360
(219) 879-9312
FUNCTIONS: Information & referral; Counseling
OTHER SERVICES: Emergency assistance available

Catholic Family Services—Portage
3147 Willowcreek Rd, Portage, IN 46368
(219) 762-1177
FUNCTIONS: Information & referral; Counseling
OTHER SERVICES: Emergency assistance available

Catholic Family Services—Whiting
6919 Indianapolis Blvd, Whiting, IN 46394
(219) 844-4883
FUNCTIONS: Information & referral; Counseling
OTHER SERVICES: Emergency assistance available

Caza Aztlan
1401 S Racine Ave, Chicago, IL 60608
(312) 666-5508
FUNCTIONS: Ethnic services & activities

The Center of Concern
1580 N Northwest Hwy Ste 223, Park Ridge, IL 60068
(708) 823-0453
FUNCTIONS: Multiple services; Will services

Central DuPage Hospital
25 N Winfield Rd, Winfield, IL 60190
(708) 682-1600
FUNCTIONS: Information & referral; Caregiver support; Case management; Educational programs; Exercise; Home health services; In-home services; Hospice; Medical assessments; Medical health services; Mental health services; Publications; Respite services; Social services; Support groups; Volunteer opportunities
OTHER SERVICES: Medicare forms assistance
See ad page 138

Central Park Towers
120 S State St, Elgin, IL 60120
(708) 742-6037
FUNCTIONS: Congregate dining

Centro Cristo Ray
315 N Root St, Aurora, IL 60505
(708) 851-1890
FUNCTIONS: Ethnic services & activities

Centro de Informacion y Progreso
62 Fountain Square Plaza, Elgin, IL 60120
(708) 695-9050
FUNCTIONS: Ethnic services & activities

Channahon Park District
PO Box 227, Channahon, IL 60410
(815) 467-5361
FUNCTIONS: Senior center

Charter Hospital of Northwest Indiana
101 W 61st Ave, Hobart, IN 46342
(800) 722-4555
FUNCTIONS: Mental health services

Cheney Company
3186 MacArthur, Northbrook, IL 60062
(800) 568-1222, (708) 498-2366
OTHER SERVICES: Handicap accessibility products
See ad page 172

Chicago Dept on Aging
510 N Peshtigo Ct 3A, Chicago, IL 60615
(312) 744-4016, 744-6777 TDD
FUNCTIONS: Information & referral; Advocacy; Caregiver support; Case management; Congregate dining; Counseling; Educational programs; Employment; Ethnic services & activities; Exercise; Friendly visits; Home delivered meals; Home repairs; In-home services; Legal assistance; Medicare & supplemental security income assistance; Ombudsman services; Recreation; Respite services; Senior center; Social services; Transportation; Volunteer opportunities; Multiple locations; Multiple services
See ad page 77

✔ In order to support future editions of this publication would you please mention *Elder Services* each time you contact any advertiser, facility, or service.

Chicago Dept on Aging Central/West Region Senior Center

2102 W Ogden Ave, Chicago, IL 60612
(312) 746-5300, 746-0319 TDD
FUNCTIONS: Information & referral; Senior center; Congregate dining; Educational programs; Recreation
OTHER SERVICES: Life enrichment programs. Call for reservations and meal times for the following dining sites: Casa Central, 1335 N California Ave; Central/West Senior Center, 2102 W Ogden Ave; Chinese Community Center, 250 W 22nd Pl; Division-LaSalle Apartments, 116 W Elm St; Fifth City, 3350 W Jackson Blvd; Greater Union Baptist Church, 1956 W Warren Blvd; Greenview Apartments, 847 N Greenview Ave; Hilliard Senior Center, 54 W Cermak Rd; Las Americas, 1611 S Racine Ave; Millard Congregational Church, 2301 S Central Park Ave; Parkview Apartments, 3916 W Washington Blvd; Prime Food Caterers, 5643 W North Ave; St Elizabeth's Hospital, 1431 N Claremont Ave; St Pius Church, 1909 S Ashland Ave; Sullivan Senior Center, 1633 W Madison St; Ukrainian Social Service Bureau, 2355 W Chicago Ave; Wicker Park Apartments, 1414 N Damen Ave.
See ad page 77

Chicago Dept on Aging Northeast Region—Levy Senior Center

2019 W Lawrence Ave, Chicago, IL 60625
(312) 744-0784, 744-0320 TDD
FUNCTIONS: Information & referral; Educational programs; Recreation; Congregate dining; Senior center
OTHER SERVICES: Life enrichment programs. Call for reservations and meal times for the following dining sites: Clark Irving Apartments, 3920 N Clark St; Colin Kelley Amvet Hall, 2051 W Belmont Ave; Dickens-Burling Apartments, 2111 N Halsted Ave; Filipino American Council, 1332 W Irving Park Rd; Fisher Apartments, 5821 N Broadway; Japanese American Service Center, 4427 N Clark St; Levy Center, 2019 W Lawrence Ave; Lakeview Presbyterian Church, 716 W Addison St; Larrabee Senior Apartments, 1845 N Larrabee Ave; Lincoln-Sheffield Apartments, 2640 N Sheffield Ave; Luther Memorial Church, 2500 W Wilson Ave; North Shore Baptist Church, 5244 N Lakewood Ave; Queen of Angels Church, 2330 W Sunnyside Ave; Schneider Apartments, 1750 W Peterson Ave; Sheridan-Argyle Apartments, 4945 N Sheridan Rd; Sheridan-Leland Apartments, 4645 N Sheridan Rd; South East Asia Center, 1124 W Ainslie St; St Ignatius Church, 6559 N Glenwood Ave; St Alphonsus Church, 2936 N Southport Ave; St Peter's Episcopal Church, 621 W Belmont Ave.
See ad page 77

Chicago Dept on Aging Northwest Region—Copernicus Senior Center

3160 N Milwaukee Ave, Chicago, IL 60618
(312) 744-6681, 744-0321 TDD
FUNCTIONS: Information & referral; Senior center; Congregate dining; Educational programs; Recreation

OTHER SERVICES: Life enrichment programs. Call for reservations and meal times for the following dining sites: Copernicus Center, 3160 N Milwaukee Ave; Golden Flame Restaurant, 6417 W Higgins Ave; Samil United Church of Christ, 4201 N Troy St; Mayfair Lutheran Church, 4335 W Lawrence Ave; Montrose Baptist Church, 4411 N Melvina Ave; Korean American Community Services, 3839 W Harding Ave; Palmer Square Golden Diners Club, 3228 W Palmer St; St Andrew's Lutheran Church, 5447 W Addison St; St Cyprian's Church, 6501 W Belmont Ave; St Luke's Church, 2649 N Francisco Ave; St Stephen's Church, 4348 W Parker Ave; Westtown Baptist Church, 1909 N Fairfield Ave.
See ad page 77

Chicago Dept on Aging Southeast Region—Atlas Senior Center

1767 E 79th St, Chicago, IL 60649
(312) 747-0189, 744-0322 TDD
FUNCTIONS: Information & referral; Senior center; Congregate dining; Educational programs; Recreation
OTHER SERVICES: Life enrichment programs. Call for reservations and meal times for the following dining sites: 111th Street YMCA, 4 E 111th St; 91st & South Chicago Apartments, 9177 S South Chicago Ave; Altgeld Gardens, 951 E 132nd Pl; Armour Square Senior Center, 3150 S Wentworth Ave; Church of the Good Shepherd, 5700 S Prairie; De Sales Senior Center, 10160 S Avenue "J"; Francis Atlas Center, 1767 E 79th St; Hegewisch Methodist Church, 13501 S Burley Ave; Hyde Park Neighborhood Club, 5480 S Kenwood Ave; Judge Green Apartments, 4030 S Lake Park Ave; Kenneth Campbell Apartments, 6360 S Minerva Ave; Langley Apartments, 4930 S Langley Ave; Lincoln Perry Apartments, 3245 S Prairie Ave; Park Manor Congregational Church, 7000 S King Dr; Paul Stewart Building, 400 E 41st St; Princeton Apartments, 4250 S Princeton Ave; Shields Senior Center, 344 W 28th Pl; Slater Senior Center, 4218 S Cottage Grove Ave; South Chicago Neighborhood House, 8458 S Mackinaw Ave; South Chicago Apartments, 661 E 69th St; South Chicago YMCA, 3039 E 91st St; Sutherland Hotel, 4647 S Drexel; St James AME Church, 9256 S Lafayette Ave; Tabernacle-Willa Rawls Manor, 4120 S Indiana Ave; Trumbull Park Community Center, 10530 S Oglesby Ave; Zion Lutheran Church, 8455 S Stoney Island Ave.
See ad page 77

Chicago Dept on Aging Southwest Region Senior Center

6117 S Kedzie Ave, Chicago, IL 60629
(312) 747-0440, 744-0323 TDD
FUNCTIONS: Information & referral; Senior center; Congregate dining; Educational programs; Recreation
OTHER SERVICES: Life enrichment programs. Call for reservations and meal times for the following dining sites: Ada Niles Senior Center, 6414 S Halsted; Ada Park, 11250 S Ada Ave; Benton Community Settlement, 3052 S Gratten Ave; Bethany Union Church, 1750 W 103rd St; Bethel Terrace, 900 W

63rd Pkwy; Brainard Center, 8700 S Laflin St; Five Holy Martyrs Church, 4327 S Richmond Ave; Immaculate Heart—Back of the Yards, 4501 S Ashland Ave; Major Robert Lawrence Apartments, 655 W 65th St; Mt Greenwood Salvation Army, 11355 S Central Park Ave; Our Lady of Good Counsel Church, 3528 S Hermitage Ave; Southwest Senior Center, 6117 S Kedzie Ave; St Daniel the Prophet Church, 5330 S Nashville Ave; St Nicholas of Tolentine Church, 3721 W 62nd St; St Gall's Church, 5511 S Sawyer Ave; Yale Apartments, 6401 S Yale Ave; Vincennes Senior Center, 7316 S Yale Ave.

See ad page 77

Chicago Hearing Society
332 S Michigan Ave, Chicago, IL 60604
(312) 939-6888
FUNCTIONS: Medical health services
OTHER SERVICES: Audiological services & screening; Hearing aid loan program

Chicago Heights Senior Sunshine Club
1203 W End Ave, Chicago Heights, IL 60411
(708) 754-4575
FUNCTIONS: Home delivered meals; Congregate dining

Chicago Housing Authority
22 W Madison St, Chicago, IL 60602
(312) 567-6013
FUNCTIONS: Housing assistance

Chicago Lighthouse for the Blind
1850 W Roosevelt Rd, Chicago, IL 60608
(312) 666-1331
FUNCTIONS: Information & referral; Educational programs
OTHER SERVICES: Orientation services for the blind

Chicago Lung Association
1440 W Washington Blvd, Chicago, IL 60607
(312) 243-2000
FUNCTIONS: Information & referral; Educational programs

Chicago Medical Society
512 N Dearborn St, Chicago, IL 60610
(312) 670-2550
OTHER SERVICES: Physician referral

Chicago Roseland Coalition
43 E 110th St, Chicago, IL 60628
(312) 261-2252
FUNCTIONS: Ethnic services & activities

Chicago Transit Authority (CTA)—Special Services
(312) 664-7200 Ext 3394
OTHER SERVICES: Information regarding routes & special services on the CTA

✓ In order to support future editions of this publication would you please mention *Elder Services* each time you contact any advertiser, facility, or service.

Chicago Volunteer Legal Services
203 N Wabash Ave Ste 2300, Chicago, IL 60601
(312) 332-1624
FUNCTIONS: Legal assistance
OTHER SERVICES: Assistance & referral for free or low-
cost legal services

Children of Aging Parents
2761 Trenton Rd, Levittown, PA 19056
(215) 945-6900
FUNCTIONS: Information & referral
OTHER SERVICES: Service resources throughout the country for caregivers

Chinese American Civic Council
2249 S Wentworth, Chicago, IL 60616
(312) 225-0234
FUNCTIONS: Ethnic services & activities

Chinese American Service League
310 W 24th Pl, Chicago, IL 60616
(312) 791-0418
FUNCTIONS: Ethnic services & activities; Energy assistance program

Chinese Consolidated Benevolent Association
250 W 22nd Pl, Chicago, IL 60616
(312) 225-6198
FUNCTIONS: Congregate dining; Ethnic services & activities

Chinese Mutual Aid Association
1100 W Argyle St, Chicago, IL 60640
(312) 784-2900
FUNCTIONS: Ethnic services & activities

Church of the Brethren
155 Boulder Hill, Montgomery, IL 60538
(708) 896-0247
FUNCTIONS: Congregate dining

Citizens Information Service of Illinois
332 S Michigan Ave Ste 1142, Chicago, IL 60604
(312) 939-4636
FUNCTIONS: Information & referral; Educational programs; Publications
OTHER SERVICES: Furnishes nonpartisan information regarding government and politics through a telephone information service.

Claim Cure
4611 W Davis, Skokie, IL 60076
(708) 674-8016
FUNCTIONS: Medical claims & billing assistance

Peter Claver Center
172 S Chicago, Joliet, IL 60432
(815) 722-6361
FUNCTIONS: Ethnic services & activities

Coal City Senior Citizens
580 S Broadway, Coal City, IL 60416
(815) 634-2254
FUNCTIONS: Senior center; Congregate dining

Coalition of Limited English-Speaking Elderly Inc
327 S LaSalle St Ste 920, Chicago, IL 60604
(312) 922-5890
FUNCTIONS: Ethnic services & activities

Colony Park
550 E Thornhill, Carol Stream, IL 60188
(708) 682-9000
FUNCTIONS: Congregate dining

Community & Economic Development Association (CEDA)
224 N Des Plaines St, Chicago, IL 60606
(312) 207-5444
FUNCTIONS: Information & referral; Day care; Counseling; In-home services; Friendly visits; Home delivered meals; Home repairs; Recreation; Congregate
dining; Transportation; Energy assistance program;
Medical assessments; Housing assistance; Multiple
locations; Multiple services

Community Contracts
1035 E State St, Geneva, IL 60134
(708) 232-9100
FUNCTIONS: Information & referral; In-home services;
Home health services; Energy assistance program

Community Day Care
1005 Grant, Downers Grove, IL 60515
(708) 968-1060
FUNCTIONS: Congregate dining

Community House
8th and Madison, Hinsdale, IL 60521
(708) 323-7500
FUNCTIONS: Information & referral; Educational programs; Employment

Community House of Hinsdale Senior Center
415 W 8th St, Hinsdale, IL 60521
(708) 323-7500
FUNCTIONS: Senior center

Community Nursing Service West Hospice
330 Eastern Ave, Bellwood, IL 60104
(708) 547-5480
FUNCTIONS: Hospice

Community Nutrition Network Inc
274 N Des Plaines St, Chicago, IL 60606
(312) 207-5290
FUNCTIONS: Home delivered meals; Congregate dining

Community Senior Center
130 E Cook Ave, Libertyville, IL 60048
(708) 367-8210
FUNCTIONS: Senior center; Congregate dining

Concerned Citizens of Little Village
2553 S Millard, Chicago, IL 60618
(312) 521-1097
FUNCTIONS: Ethnic services & activities

Concerned Relatives of Nursing Home Patients
3130 Mayfield Rd, Cleveland, OH 44118
(216) 321-0403
FUNCTIONS: Information & referral

Cook County Office of the Public Guardian
221 N LaSalle St Ste 1555, Chicago, IL 60601
(312) 609-5300
FUNCTIONS: Protective services
OTHER SERVICES: Acts as guardian for individuals who are mentally or physically disabled

Cook County Senior Citizen's Legal Services
1146 Westgate St Ste 200, Oak Park, IL 60301
(708) 524-2600
FUNCTIONS: Information & referral; Legal assistance
OTHER SERVICES: Free legal services offered for emergency cases. Referrals for other cases.

Corrective Measures Plus
949 N State St, Chicago, IL 60610
(312) 33-SHOES
OTHER SERVICES: Specialize in corrective, orthopedic, and comfort footwear. Nursing home and retirement center visits available.
See ad page 26

Council for Jewish Elderly
3003 W Touhy Ave, Chicago, IL 60645
(312) 508-1000
FUNCTIONS: Information & referral; Educational programs; Caregiver support; Day care; Respite services; Support groups; Case management; Counseling; Home health services; In-home services; Friendly visits; Home delivered meals; Senior center; Congregate dining; Ethnic services & activities; Respite services; Medical assessments; Legal assistance; Multiple services

Council for Jewish Elderly Adult Day Care Center
1015 Howard St, Evanston, IL 60202
(708) 492-1400
FUNCTIONS: Day care; Support groups; Caregiver support

Counseling Center of Lakeview
3225 N Sheffield, Chicago, IL 60657
(312) 549-5886
FUNCTIONS: In-home services; Counseling

Deatherage-Drdak Senior Center
230 E Briarcliff, Bolingbrook, IL 60440
(708) 739-1300
FUNCTIONS: Senior center

Deerfield Senior Center
835 Hazel, Deerfield, IL 60015
(708) 945-0650
FUNCTIONS: Senior center

DeKalb County Hospice
615 N First Ste 204, DeKalb, IL 60115
(815) 756-3000
FUNCTIONS: Hospice

Des Plaines Community Senior Center
1040 Thacker St, Des Plaines, IL 60016
(708) 298-0111
FUNCTIONS: Senior center

Des Plaines Municipal Offices
1420 Miner St, Des Plaines, IL 60016
(708) 391-5492
FUNCTIONS: Multiple services; Will services

Des Plaines Senior Nutrition Site—Des Plaines Mall
700 Pearson Space T-103, Des Plaines, IL 60016
(708) 390-0755
FUNCTIONS: Home delivered meals; Congregate dining

Des Plaines Valley Health Center
6138 S Archer Rd, Summit, IL 60501
(708) 458-0831
FUNCTIONS: Medical health services

Downers Grove Park District Senior Center
935 Maple Ave, Downers Grove, IL 60515
(708) 963-1314
FUNCTIONS: Senior center; Congregate dining

Dundee Township Park District
2 Pine, Carpentersville, IL 60110
(708) 426-5339
FUNCTIONS: Senior center; Congregate dining

DuPage County Dept of Human Resources
421 N County Farm Rd, Wheaton, IL 60187
(708) 682-7990
FUNCTIONS: Case coordination unit; Volunteer opportunities; Multiple services

DuPage County Health Dept
111 N County Farm Rd, Wheaton, IL 60187
(708) 682-7400
FUNCTIONS: Information & referral

DuPage Senior Citizens Council
837 S Westmore Bldg A-6, Lombard, IL 60148
(708) 620-0804
FUNCTIONS: Information & referral; Home delivered meals; Recreation; Congregate dining; Volunteer opportunities

✔ In order to support future editions of this publication would you please mention *Elder Services* each time you contact any advertiser, facility, or service.

East Chicago Operation Hope
1819 Broadway, East Chicago, IN 46312
(219) 398-9526
FUNCTIONS: Information & referral; Case management;
    Congregate dining; Educational programs; Employ-
    ment; Energy assistance program; Home delivered
    meals; In-home services; Recreation; Senior center;
    Transportation
OTHER SERVICES: Addresses of congregate dining sites
    available from this office

Eastern Will County Senior Services
PO Box 579, 25864 S Chestnut, Monee, IL 60449
(708) 534-2323
FUNCTIONS: Senior center; Congregate dining

El Centro Pan Americano
325 E Galena, Aurora, IL 60505
(708) 892-2224
FUNCTIONS: Ethnic services & activities

El Primer Paso
325 E Galena Blvd, Aurora, IL 60505
(708) 892-7600
FUNCTIONS: Ethnic services & activities

El Valor Corporation
1850 W 21st St, Chicago, IL 60618
(312) 666-4511
FUNCTIONS: Ethnic services & activities

**Ela Township Senior Center—Harry Knigge Senior
Civic Center**
95 E Main St, Lake Zurich, IL 60047
(708) 438-0303
FUNCTIONS: Senior center; Congregate dining

Elder Link Inc
2000 N Racine Ste 2182, Chicago, IL 60614
(312) 929-4514
FUNCTIONS: Information & referral; Case management;
    Financial services; Educational programs; Medicare
    & supplemental security income assistance; Mul-
    tiple services
OTHER SERVICES: Assistance with Medicare, Medicaid,
    and insurance benefits. Help with financial plan-
    ning for long-term care services.
See ad page 45

Eldercare America
PO Box 1533, Rockville, MD 20849
(301) 340-6511
FUNCTIONS: Information & referral; Advocacy; Educa-
    tional programs; Publications
OTHER SERVICES: A membership organization which pro-
    motes the well being, dignity, and independence
    of older persons and their families. Workshops and
    videotapes available.

Elderly in Distress
6233 N Pulaski Ste 303, Chicago, IL 60646
(312) 202-1569

FUNCTIONS: In-home services
OTHER SERVICES: Physician home visits

Elder-Med at Our Lady of Mercy Hospital
24 Joliet Rd, Dyer, IN 46311
(219) 322-6839
FUNCTIONS: Information & referral; Counseling

Elk Grove Senior Center
225 E Elk Grove Blvd, Elk Grove, IL 60007
(708) 364-7224
FUNCTIONS: Senior center; Congregate dining

Englewood Community Health Organization
938 W 69th St, Chicago, IL 60621
(312) 962-5600
FUNCTIONS: Ethnic services & activities

Epilepsy Foundation of Greater Chicago
20 E Jackson Blvd, Chicago, IL 60604
(312) 939-8622
FUNCTIONS: Information & referral; Educational pro-
    grams; Counseling; Support groups

Erie Family Health Center
1656 W Chicago Ave, Chicago, IL 60622
(312) 666-3488
FUNCTIONS: Case management; Counseling; Home
    health services; In-home services; Home delivered
    meals; Recreation; Support groups; Financial ser-
    vices; Energy assistance program

Erie Neighborhood House
1347 W Erie, Chicago, IL 60622
(312) 666-3430
FUNCTIONS: Counseling; Friendly visits; Home deliv-
    ered meals

ESSE
41 Park Blvd, Glen Ellyn, IL 60137
(708) 853-1005
FUNCTIONS: Congregate dining; Day care

Evanston Commission on Aging
2100 Ridge Ave, Evanston, IL 60204
(708) 866-2919
FUNCTIONS: Ombudsman services; Multiple services;
    Will services

**Evanston Senior Nutrition Center—Fleetwood-
Jourdain Center**
1655 Foster St, Evanston, IL 60201
(708) 864-2850
FUNCTIONS: Home delivered meals; Congregate dining

Evergreen Park Senior Center
3450 West 97th St, Evergreen Park, IL 60642
(708) 422-8776
FUNCTIONS: Multiple services

Fairview Baptist Home
7 S 241 Fairview Ave, Downers Grove, IL 60516
(708) 852-4350
FUNCTIONS: Information & referral; Educational programs; Support groups; Respite services; Counseling; Friendly visits; Recreation; Housing assistance

Family Care Service of Metropolitan Chicago
234 S Wabash Ave, Chicago, IL 60604
(312) 427-8790
FUNCTIONS: Caregiver support; Respite services; Home health services; Case management; In-home services; Friendly visits

Family Counseling Service of Evanston & Skokie Valley—Evanston
1114 Church St, Evanston, IL 60201
(708) 327-2404
FUNCTIONS: Information & referral; Case coordination unit; Case management; Counseling; Mental health services; Protective services

Family Counseling Service of Evanston & Skokie Valley—Skokie
5210 Main St, Skokie, IL 60076
(708) 328-2404
FUNCTIONS: Information & referral; Case coordination unit; Case management; Counseling; Mental health services; Protective services

Family Services Association of Greater Elgin Area
22 S Spring St, Elgin, IL 60120
(708) 695-3680
FUNCTIONS: Information & referral; Case management; Counseling; Caregiver support; Support groups

Federal Information Center
PO Box 600, Cumberland, MD 21501-0600
(800) 366-2998
OTHER SERVICES: Information & referral related to functions of federal government agencies

Filipino American Council of Chicago
1332 W Irving Park Rd, Chicago, IL 60613
(312) 281-1210
FUNCTIONS: Congregate dining; Ethnic services & activities

Filipino Association of America
PO Box 121, Waukegan, IL 60085
FUNCTIONS: Ethnic services & activities

First Baptist Church
401 N Genesee, Waukegan, IL 60085
(708) 623-2821
FUNCTIONS: Ethnic services & activities

First National Bank of Geneva
21 N 3rd St, Geneva, IL 60134
(708) 232-6700
FUNCTIONS: Financial services; Retirement benefits; Multiple locations
OTHER SERVICES: Trust services; Asset management accounts; "Senior Citizen Now" accounts
See ad page 4

Five Hospital Homebound Elderly Program
600 W Diversey Pkwy Ste 200, Chicago, IL 60614
(312) 549-5822
FUNCTIONS: Information & referral; Educational programs; Case management; Counseling; Home health services; In-home services; Friendly visits; Medical assessments
See ad page 158

Ford Heights Community Service Senior Center
1647 S Cottage Grove Ave, Ford Heights, IL 60411
(708) 758-2510
FUNCTIONS: Senior center; Home delivered meals; Congregate dining

Fox Lake Senior Center
57 Martin Dr, Fox Lake, IL 60020
(708) 587-2046
FUNCTIONS: Senior center

Fox River Grove Senior Center
402 Northwest Highway, Fox River Grove, IL 60021
(708) 639-9751
FUNCTIONS: Senior center

Fox Valley Hospice
113 E Wilson, Batavia, IL 60510
(708) 879-6064
FUNCTIONS: Hospice

Fox Valley Park District
150 W Illinois Ave, Aurora, IL 60506
(708) 859-8606
FUNCTIONS: Senior center

Franklin Park Senior Nutrition Site—Centre Place
10040 Addison Ave, Franklin Park, IL 60131
(708) 678-8777
FUNCTIONS: Home delivered meals; Congregate dining

Gary Community Mental Health Center
1100 W 6th Ave, Gary, IN 46402
(219) 885-4264
FUNCTIONS: Mental health services

Gary Neighborhood Services Inc
21st & Adams St, Gary, IN 46407
(219) 883-0431
FUNCTIONS: Information & referral; Counseling

Geneva Park District
710 Western Ave, Geneva, IL 60134
(708) 232-4542
FUNCTIONS: Senior center

✔ In order to support future editions of this publication would you please mention *Elder Services* each time you contact any advertiser, facility, or service.

Geriatric Resource Consultants Inc
160 Cary Ave, Highland Park, IL 60035
(708) 432-3490
OTHER SERVICES: Care management
See ad page 32

Gideon Baptist Church
1000 Yeoman, Waukegan, IL 60085
(708) 662-7672
FUNCTIONS: Ethnic services & activities

Glen Ellyn Drop-In Center
535 Duane, Glen Ellyn, IL 60137
(708) 469-5000
FUNCTIONS: Senior center

Glen Ellyn Park District Senior Adult Program
501 Hill St, Glen Ellyn, IL 60137
(708) 858-2462
FUNCTIONS: Senior center

Glen Ellyn Senior Service Center
493 Forest Ave, Glen Ellyn, IL 60137
(708) 858-6325
FUNCTIONS: Senior center

Glenview Senior Center Rugen Community Center
901 Shermer Rd, Glenview, IL 60025
(708) 724-4793
FUNCTIONS: Multiple services

Golden Agers Service Foundation
6355 S Cottage Grove, Chicago, IL 60637
(312) 667-1000
FUNCTIONS: Ethnic services & activities

Golden Diners Senior Center
3510 Bay Rd, Crystal Lake, IL 60012
(708) 459-4261
FUNCTIONS: Senior center; Congregate dining

Gottlieb Memorial Hospital
701 W North Ave, Melrose Park, IL 60160
(708) 450-4526
FUNCTIONS: Information & referral; Exercise; Home health services; In-home services; Medical assessments; Medical health services; Mental health services; Respite services; Recreation; Social services; Support groups
OTHER SERVICES: Emergency response system; Educize (arthritis exercise) program; Social club; Gottlieb Gold Seniors membership program
See ad page 127

Governor's Office of Citizens Assistance—Senior Action Center
100 W Randolph St Ste 9-100, Chicago, IL 60601
(312) 917-2754
OTHER SERVICES: Information & referral related to state government, consumer information, and complaints

Grace Lutheran Church
493 Forest View, Glen Ellyn, IL 60137
(708) 858-6325
FUNCTIONS: Congregate dining

Grant Hospital of Chicago—Prime Life
550 W Webster Ave, Chicago, IL 60614
(312) 883-3775
FUNCTIONS: Information & referral; Educational programs; Medical assessments; Medical health services; Recreation

Greater Elgin Senior Center
101 S Grove Ave, Elgin, IL 60120
(708) 741-0404
FUNCTIONS: Senior center; Congregate dining

Greater Faith Baptist Church
565 Powell, Waukegan, IL 60085
(708) 244-4400
FUNCTIONS: Ethnic services & activities

Greater Hammond Community Services
119 State St, Hammond, IN 46320
(219) 932-4800
FUNCTIONS: Information & referral; Case management; Congregate dining; Educational programs; Employment; Energy assistance program; Home delivered meals; In-home services; Recreation; Senior center; Transportation
OTHER SERVICES: Addresses of congregate dining sites available from this office

Greek American Community Services
3940 N Pulaski Rd, Chicago, IL 60641
(312) 545-0303
FUNCTIONS: Ethnic services & activities; Friendly visits

Grundy Community Hospice
201 Liberty St Ste 253, Morris, IL 60450
(815) 942-8252
FUNCTIONS: Hospice

Grundy County Health Dept
111 E Illinois Ave, Morris, IL 60450
(815) 941-3111
FUNCTIONS: Case coordination unit; Multiple services

H P Medical Claim Consultants
5010 W Bonner Dr, McHenry, IL 60050
(815) 385-2739
FUNCTIONS: Medical claims & billing assistance
See ad page 83

Hammond Community Center
5550 Sohl Ave, Hammond, IN 46320
(219) 833-7377
FUNCTIONS: Information & referral; Counseling; Day care
OTHER SERVICES: Emergency food

Hanover Township
8 N 180 Route 59, Bartlett, IL 60103
(708) 837-0301
FUNCTIONS: Multiple services

Harris Bank
111 W Monroe, Chicago, IL 60603
(312) 461-BANK
FUNCTIONS: Financial services; Retirement benefits
OTHER SERVICES: Trust, asset management, & banking
    services
See ad on back cover

Hartman Center
Irving and Collins St, Joliet, IL 60433
(815) 741-7279
FUNCTIONS: Senior center; Congregate dining

Harvard Senior Center
12 N Ayer St, Harvard, IL 60033
(708) 943-6844
FUNCTIONS: Senior center; Congregate dining

Harvey High Rise
15306 S Robey, Harvey, IL 60426
(708) 596-6530
FUNCTIONS: Home delivered meals

Health Insurance Planners
500 N Skokie Blvd Ste 625, Northbrook, IL 60062
(708) 291-3061
OTHER SERVICES: Consultants for personal and group
    health and long-term care insurance

Heartland Luxury Bath Systems Inc
374 Balm Ct, Wood Dale, IL 60191
(708) 595-9555
OTHER SERVICES: Slip resistant bath tubs & showers
See ad page 154

Hebron Senior Center
9908 St Albans St, Hebron, IL 60034
(708) 648-4072
FUNCTIONS: Senior center; Congregate dining

Hellenic Foundation
5700 N Sheridan Rd, Chicago, IL 60660
(312) 728-2603
FUNCTIONS: Ethnic services & activities

Help at Home
7429 N Western, Chicago, IL 60645
(312) 508-0000
FUNCTIONS: Caregiver support; Respite services; In-
    home services

Hemlock of Illinois
PO Box A3883, Chicago, IL 60690
(312) 477-7228
FUNCTIONS: Advocacy; Educational programs; Publica-
    tions

OTHER SERVICES: Supports the option of voluntary eu-
    thanasia for the terminally ill.

Highland Park Senior Center
54 Laurel, Highland Park, IL 60035
(708) 432-4110
FUNCTIONS: Senior center

Hill Memorial Center
416 Ontario St, Joliet, IL 60435
(815) 723-0942
FUNCTIONS: Ethnic services & activities

Hinsdale Hospital—ConfiCare
120 N Oak, Hinsdale, IL 60521
(708) 887-4141
FUNCTIONS: Information & referral; Caregiver support;
    Case management; Counseling; Day care; Educa-
    tional programs; Employment; Exercise; Friendly
    visits; Home delivered meals; Home health ser-
    vices; Hospice; In-home services; Medical assess-
    ments; Medical health services; Mental health ser-
    vices; Respite services; Social services; Support
    groups; Volunteer opportunities
See ad page 73

Hobart Township Community Services
275 29th Ave, Lake Station, IN 46405
(219) 962-7080
FUNCTIONS: Information & referral; Case management;
    Congregate dining; Educational programs; Employ-
    ment; Energy assistance program; Home delivered
    meals; In-home services; Recreation; Senior center;
    Transportation
OTHER SERVICES: Addresses of congregate dining sites
    available from this office

Holiday Inn Hotel
345 W Rand Rd, Elgin, IL 60120
(708) 695-5000
FUNCTIONS: Congregate dining

✔ In order to support future editions of this publication would you please mention *Elder Services* each time you contact
any advertiser, facility, or service.

Holy Ghost Church
254 N Wood Dale Rd, Wood Dale, IL 60191
(708) 860-2975
FUNCTIONS: Ethnic services & activities

Home Companion Services
38 North Austin, Oak Park, IL 60302
(708) 386-1324
FUNCTIONS: In-home services

Home Hospice—Visiting Nurse Association North
2008 Dempster St, Evanston, IL 60202
(708) 328-1900
FUNCTIONS: Hospice

HomeCorps
550 W Jackson Blvd Ste 430, Chicago, IL 60661-5716
(800) 745-HOME
FUNCTIONS: Information & referral; Caregiver support;
   Case management; Counseling; Educational pro-
   grams; Friendly visits; Home health services; Home
   repairs; In-home services; Medical assessments;
   Respite services; Social services; Transportation;
   Medical claims & billing assistance
OTHER SERVICES: Medication management; Personal re-
   assurance & emergency response systems
See ads pages 27, 159

Honduran Association of Waukegan
2935 N Butrick, Waukegan, IL 60085
(708) 623-5715
FUNCTIONS: Ethnic services & activities

Horizon Hospice
2800 N Sheridan Rd Ste 108, Chicago, IL 60657
(312) 871-3658
FUNCTIONS: Hospice

Hospice Care Chicagoland
200 W 22nd St, Lombard, IL 60148
(708) 495-8484
FUNCTIONS: Hospice

Hospice Care Chicagoland North
4433 W Touhy Ste 270, Lincolnwood, IL 60646
(708) 679-9400
FUNCTIONS: Hospice

Hospice of DuPage Inc
22 W 600 Butterfield Rd, Glen Ellyn, IL 60137
(708) 469-5556
FUNCTIONS: Hospice

Hospice of Highland Park Hospital
718 Glenview Ave, Highland Park, IL 60035
(708) 480-3858
FUNCTIONS: Hospice

Hospice of Illinois Medical Center
836 W Wellington, Chicago, IL 60657
(312) 883-7048
FUNCTIONS: Hospice

Hospice of Little Company of Mary Hospital
2800 W 95th St, Evergreen Park, IL 60642
(708) 422-2600 ext 5367
FUNCTIONS: Hospice

Hospice of Northeastern Illinois Inc
450 W Highway 22, Barrington, IL 60010
(708) 381-5599
FUNCTIONS: Hospice

Hospice of the North Shore
2821 Central St, Evanston, IL 60642
(708) 866-4601
FUNCTIONS: Hospice

Hospice of West Suburban Hospital
12 W Lake St, Oak Park, IL 60302
(708) 383-4663
FUNCTIONS: Hospice

Hospice Suburban South
PO Box 258, 2609 Flossmoor Rd, Flossmoor, IL 60422
(708) 957-7177
FUNCTIONS: Hospice

Hotel Baker Living Center
100 W Main St, St Charles, IL 60174
(708) 584-2100
FUNCTIONS: Congregate dining
See ad page 296

Howard Area Community Center
7648 N Paulina St, Chicago, IL 60626
(312) 262-6622
FUNCTIONS: Information & referral; Case management;
   Housing assistance; Support groups; Educational
   programs; Medicare & supplemental security income assistance; Volunteer opportunities; Social
   services

Hull House Association
118 Clinton St Ste 200, Chicago, IL 60606
(312) 726-1526
FUNCTIONS: Information & referral; Educational programs; Caregiver support; Support groups; Case
   management; Home delivered meals; Friendly visits; Congregate dining; Senior center; Legal assistance

Humana Michael Reese Hospital
2929 S Ellis, Chicago, IL 60616
(312) 791-2748
FUNCTIONS: Counseling; Medical assessments

Hyde Park Neighborhood Association
5480 S Kenwood Ave, Chicago, IL 60615
(312) 643-4062
FUNCTIONS: Educational programs; Home delivered
   meals; Senior center; Recreation; Congregate dining; Day care; Transportation

Illinois Alliance for Aging

327 S LaSalle St Ste 920, Chicago, IL 60604
(312) 922-5890
FUNCTIONS: Information & referral; Advocacy; Employment; Housing assistance; Protective services; Volunteer opportunities
See ad page 61

Illinois Association of Homes for the Aging

911 N Elm St Ste 228, Hinsdale, IL 60521
(708) 325-6170
FUNCTIONS: Educational programs; Day care; Respite services; Support groups; Home health services; Hospice; Housing assistance

Illinois Attorney General's Office

100 W Randolph St, Chicago, IL 60601
(312) 814-3000
FUNCTIONS: Information & referral; Educational programs; Energy assistance program
OTHER SERVICES: Consumer protection; Advocacy for seniors through the state's legal system

Illinois Chinese American Residence (I-Care)

501 Cass, Westmont, IL 60559
(708) 963-9631
FUNCTIONS: Ethnic services & activities; Congregate dining

Illinois Citizens for Better Care

220 S State St Ste 800, Chicago, IL 60604
(312) 663-5120
FUNCTIONS: Information & referral; Medicare & supplemental security income assistance
OTHER SERVICES: Advocacy group for nursing home residences & their families concerned with the quality of care & life in nursing homes

Illinois Dept of Rehab Services—Services for the Visually Handicapped

100 W Randolph St Ste 8-100, Chicago, IL 60601
(312) 917-3377
FUNCTIONS: Information & referral
OTHER SERVICES: Training & adaptation services for the visually impaired

Illinois Dept on Aging—Chicago

100 W Randolph, Chicago, IL 60601
(312) 814-2636
FUNCTIONS: Information & referral

Illinois Dept on Aging—Springfield

421 E Capitol Ave, Springfield, IL 62701
(800) 252-8966
FUNCTIONS: Information & referral

Illinois Home Care Council

222 W Ontario Ste 430, Chicago, IL 60610
(312) 335-9922
OTHER SERVICES: Information & referral regarding agencies that provide in-home services

Illinois Masonic Medical Center

836 W Wellington Ave, Chicago, IL 60657
(312) 883-7027
FUNCTIONS: Information & referral; Educational programs; Caregiver support; Day care; Respite services; Support groups; Case management; Counseling; Medical assessments; Home health services; Hospice; Friendly visits; Recreation; Transportation; Legal assistance

Illinois Migrant Council—Aurora

818 E New York St, Aurora, IL 60505
(708) 820-7088
FUNCTIONS: Ethnic services & activities

Illinois Migrant Council—Momence

120 E Washington St, Momence, IL 60954
(815) 472-3914
FUNCTIONS: Ethnic services & activities

Illinois Migrant Council—Mundelein

105 N Seymour Ave, Mundelein, IL 60060
(708) 566-0420
FUNCTIONS: Ethnic services & activities

Illinois State Medical Society

20 N Michigan Ave, Chicago, IL 60602
(312) 782-1654
OTHER SERVICES: Physician referral; Speakers bureau

Immanuel Residence

1122 Gilbert, Downers Grove, IL 60515
(708) 832-1310
FUNCTIONS: Congregate dining

Indiana Dept of Human Services

PO Box 7983, Indianapolis, IN 46207
(800) 622-4972
FUNCTIONS: Information & referral; Ombudsman services

Ingalls Hospital—Senior Life Program

One Ingalls Dr, Harvey, IL 60426
(708) 333-3331
FUNCTIONS: Medical health services; Educational programs

Institute of Medicine of Chicago

332 S Michigan Ave Ste 1558, Chicago, IL 60604
(312) 663-0040
FUNCTIONS: Educational programs

Interfaith Housing Center of the Northern Suburbs

620 Lincoln Ave, Winnetka, IL 60093
(708) 256-4780
FUNCTIONS: Housing assistance

Marie Irwin Community Center

18120 Highland Ave, Homewood, IL 60430
(708) 957-7275
FUNCTIONS: Senior center

Japanese American Citizens League
5415 N Clark, Chicago, IL 60640
(312) 728-7171
FUNCTIONS: Ethnic services & activities

Japanese American Service Committee
4427 N Clark St, Chicago, IL 60640
(312) 275-7212
FUNCTIONS: Information & referral; Educational programs; Caregiver support; Day care; Counseling; In-home services; Home delivered meals; Senior center; Recreation; Congregate dining; Support groups; Medical assessments; Housing assistance; Legal assistance; Ethnic services & activities

Jewish Family & Community Service Central & South Chicago
205 W Randolph St Ste 1100, Chicago, IL 60606
(312) 263-5523
FUNCTIONS: Information & referral; Educational programs; Caregiver support; Day care; Support groups; Case management; Counseling; Medical health services; In-home services; Home delivered meals; Senior center; Financial services; Legal assistance

Jewish Family & Community Service North Chicago
2710 W Devon, Chicago, IL 60645
(312) 274-1324
FUNCTIONS: Information & referral; Educational programs; Caregiver support; Day care; Support groups; Case management; Counseling; Medical health services; In-home services; Home delivered meals; Senior center; Financial services; Legal assistance

Jewish Federation of Metro Chicago
One S Franklin St 6th Fl, Chicago, IL 60606
(312) 346-6700
FUNCTIONS: Ethnic services & activities

Joliet Area Community Hospice Inc
337 W Jefferson St, Joliet, IL 60435
(815) 744-4104
FUNCTIONS: Hospice

Jones Memorial Community Center
229 E 15th St, Chicago Heights, IL 60411
(708) 757-5395
FUNCTIONS: Multiple services

Kankakee County Senior Citizens Center
657 E Court St, Kankakee, IL 60901
(815) 937-5600
FUNCTIONS: Senior center

Meyer Kaplan JCC Senior Program
5050 Church St, Skokie, IL 60076
(708) 675-2200
FUNCTIONS: Educational programs; Recreation; Exercise

Kennedy Senior Citizens Building
2200 Oneida, Joliet, IL 60435
(815) 729-9273
FUNCTIONS: Congregate dining

Kenwood-Oakland Community Organization
1236-48 E 46th St, Chicago, IL 60653
(312) 548-7500
FUNCTIONS: Ethnic services & activities

Kin Care
3318 N Lincoln Ave, Chicago, IL 60657
(312) 975-7777
FUNCTIONS: Information & referral; Case management; Respite services
OTHER SERVICES: Convalescent & respite care for those in need of temporary care in private homes.

Kingwood Hospital
3714 S Franklin, Michigan City, IN 46360
(219) 873-1616
FUNCTIONS: Mental health services

Korean American Association of Chicago
5491 N Lincoln Ave, Chicago, IL 60659
(312) 878-1900
FUNCTIONS: Ethnic services & activities

Korean American Community Service
4300 N California Ave, Chicago, IL 60618
(312) 583-5501
FUNCTIONS: Educational programs; Support groups; Counseling; Medical assessments; In-home services; Friendly visits; Housing assistance; Senior center; Recreation; Congregate dining; Financial services; Legal assistance; Energy assistance program

Korean American Senior Association of Chicagoland
4750 N Sheridan Rd Ste 415, Chicago, IL 60640
(312) 878-8617
FUNCTIONS: Energy assistance program; In-home services; Friendly visits; Recreation; Financial services; Legal assistance; Housing assistance; Ethnic services & activities

Korean American Senior Center
4750 N Sheridan Rd Ste 280, Chicago, IL 60640
(312) 878-7272
FUNCTIONS: Energy assistance program; In-home services; Friendly visits; Recreation; Financial services; Legal assistance; Housing assistance; Ethnic services & activities

Korean Self-Help Community Center
4934 N Pulaski, Chicago, IL 60630
(312) 545-8348
FUNCTIONS: Ethnic services & activities

LaGrange Memorial Hospice
6406 Joliet Rd, Countryside, IL 60525
(708) 352-6696
FUNCTIONS: Hospice

Lake County Community Civic Organization
1030 Judge Ave, Waukegan, IL 60085
(708) 662-1943
FUNCTIONS: Ethnic services & activities

Lake County Prosecutor's Office Adult Protective Services
2293 N Main St, Crown Point, IN 46307
(219) 755-3720
FUNCTIONS: Legal assistance

Lake County Urban League
122 W Madison St, Waukegan, IL 60085
(708) 249-3770
FUNCTIONS: Ethnic services & activities

Lake Forest Hospital Hospice
660 N Westmoreland Rd, Lake Forest, IL 60045
(708) 234-5600 ext 6446
FUNCTIONS: Hospice

Lake Forest—Lake Bluff Gorton Senior Center
400 E Illinois Rd, Lake Forest, IL 60045
(708) 234-2209
FUNCTIONS: Senior center

Laotian Service Center
4740 N Sheridan Rd Ste 320, Chicago, IL 60640
(312) 271-0004
FUNCTIONS: Ethnic services & activities

LaSalle Senior Center
300 W Hill St, Chicago, IL 60610
(312) 787-3756
FUNCTIONS: Information & referral; Counseling; In-home services; Friendly visits; Home repairs; Housing assistance; Senior center; Recreation; Congregate dining; Transportation

Latino Institute
228 S Wabash 6th Fl, Chicago, IL 60604
(312) 663-3603
FUNCTIONS: Ethnic services & activities

League of United Latin American Citizens (LULAC)
117 N Genesee St, Waukegan, IL 60085
(708) 336-1004
FUNCTIONS: Ethnic services & activities

Legal Aid Society of Greater Hammond
232 Russell St, Hammond, IN 46320
(219) 932-2787
FUNCTIONS: Legal assistance

Legal Assistance Foundation of Chicago
343 S Dearborn St Ste 700, Chicago, IL 60604
(312) 651-3100
FUNCTIONS: Legal assistance
OTHER SERVICES: Free or low-cost legal services for low-income elderly

Legal Services Program of Greater Gary
530 Broadway, Gary, IN 46402
(219) 886-3161
FUNCTIONS: Legal assistance

Levy Center
1700 Maple, Evanston, IL 60201
(708) 869-0727
FUNCTIONS: Senior center

Leyden Family Service
10009-A W Grand Ave, Franklin Park, IL 60131
(708) 455-3929
FUNCTIONS: Information & referral; In-home services; Case management; Protective services; Transportation; Multiple services

Leyden Township Senior Citizens Program
10200 W Grand Ave, Franklin Park, IL 60131
(708) 455-8616
FUNCTIONS: Information & referral; Case management; Protective services; Multiple services

Lifeline Pilots
913 Harrington, Champaign, IL 61821
(217) 373-4195
OTHER SERVICES: Volunteer organization of pilots with planes providing free air transportation for disaster relief and assisting agencies, organizations, and people with special medical needs. Limits: No stretchers or life support equipment can be accepted.
See ad page 38

Lifeline—Rest Haven
16250 Prince Dr, South Holland, IL 60473
(708) 877-4800
OTHER SERVICES: Personal response system monitored 24 hours a day by trained personnel who immediately respond & send help for user's needs
See ad on page i

Lifelink Corporation
331 S York Rd, Bensenville, IL 60106
(708) 766-3570
FUNCTIONS: Counseling; Home delivered meals; Housing assistance; Support groups

Lincoln West Hospital—Golden Years Program
2544 W Montrose, Chicago, IL 60618
(312) 267-2200
FUNCTIONS: Medical assessments; Medical health services; Social services; Educational programs; Support groups; Transportation; Information & referral

✔ In order to support future editions of this publication would you please mention *Elder Services* each time you contact any advertiser, facility, or service.

OTHER SERVICES: Program providing free health screening and transportation for their other clinic services, including physician visits, counseling, and educational programs. Lunch and socialization provided on day of visit.
See ads pages xv, 88

Lincolnwood Senior Services
6918 N Keeler, Lincolnwood, IL 60646
(708) 673-1540
FUNCTIONS: Multiple services

Lisle Park District
5801 Westview, Lisle, IL 60532
(708) 969-0992
FUNCTIONS: Senior center; Congregate dining

Lithuanian Community Services
7218 S Whipple, Chicago, IL 60629
(312) 434-0935
FUNCTIONS: Ethnic services & activities

Lithuanian Human Services
2711 W 71st St, Chicago, IL 60629
(312) 476-2655
FUNCTIONS: Information & referral; Educational programs; Counseling; Medical assessments; In-home services; Friendly visits; Home delivered meals; Housing assistance; Senior center; Recreation; Congregate dining; Transportation; Energy assistance program; Ethnic services & activities

Little Brothers—Friends of the Elderly
1658 W Belmont Ave, Chicago, IL 60657
(312) 477-7702
FUNCTIONS: Information & referral; In-home services; Friendly visits; Home delivered meals; Housing assistance; Senior center; Transportation

Little Company of Mary Hospital Senior Services
2800 W 95th St, Evergreen Park, IL 60642
(708) 422-0360
FUNCTIONS: Medical health services

Living-at-Home Program
1015 W Howard St, Evanston, IL 60202
(708) 492-9400
FUNCTIONS: Information & referral; Caregiver support; Day care; Case management; Counseling; In-home services; Home delivered meals; Social services; Support groups; Educational programs
OTHER SERVICES: Consulting; Assessments

Lockport Congregational Church
700 E 9th St, Lockport, IL 60441
(815) 838-5885
FUNCTIONS: Senior center; Congregate dining

Lombard Community Senior Center
205 W Maple, Lombard, IL 60148
(708) 629-9707
FUNCTIONS: Senior center

Lord & Taylor Learning Together Center of Northbrook Court
1455 Lake Cook Rd, Northbrook, IL 60062
(708) 489-2500 Ext 377
FUNCTIONS: Educational programs

Loyola University Medical Center
2160 S First Ave, Maywood, IL 60153
(708) 216-9000
FUNCTIONS: Medical health services

Lutheran Community Services for the Aged
800 W Oakton St, Arlington Heights, IL 60004
(708) 253-3710
FUNCTIONS: Information & referral; Respite services; Support groups; Counseling; Medical health services; Publications; Case management; In-home services; Home delivered meals; Volunteer opportunities; Hospice; Educational programs
OTHER SERVICES: Short-term admissions for respite & hospice care
See ads pages 69, 202

Lutheran Social Services of Illinois—Chicago
8704 S Constance, Chicago, IL 60617
(312) 935-1100
FUNCTIONS: Case coordination unit

Lutheran Social Services of Illinois—Des Plaines
1001 E Touhy Ave Ste 50, Des Plaines, IL 60018
(708) 635-4600
FUNCTIONS: Information & referral; Educational programs; Caregiver support; Day care; Case management; Counseling; Medical assessments; In-home services; Home delivered meals; Senior center; Protective services; Volunteer opportunities

Lutheran Social Services of Illinois—Elmhurst
590 Spring Rd, Elmhurst, IL 60126
(708) 279-6074

FUNCTIONS: Ethnic services & activities; Multiple services

Lutheran Social Services of Illinois—Home Helps for Seniors
640 E 168th Pl, South Holland, IL 60473
(708) 596-6690
FUNCTIONS: Information & referral; Case management; In-home services; Transportation; Protective services

MacNeal Hospital
3249 S Oak Park Ave, Berwyn, IL 60402
(708) 795-9100
FUNCTIONS: Medical health services; Mental health services; Medical assessments; Caregiver support; Support groups; Social services; Home health services; In-home services; Home delivered meals; Educational programs; Publications; Multiple locations

MAGA Ltd Group
701 Lee St Ste 730, Des Plaines, IL 60016
(708) 699-4072
OTHER SERVICES: Long-term care insurance, counseling, & education

Maine Township Senior Services
1700 Ballard Rd, Park Ridge, IL 60068
(708) 297-2510
FUNCTIONS: Information & referral; Multiple services

Maple Terrace Apartments
905 2nd Ave, Aurora, IL 60506
(708) 851-1491
FUNCTIONS: Congregate dining

Martin Manor
310 W Martin Ave, Naperville, IL 60540
(708) 355-7551
FUNCTIONS: Congregate dining

Mayslake Village Senior Center
1801 35th St, Oak Brook, IL 60521
(708) 654-3242
FUNCTIONS: Senior center

Maywood Senior Nutrition Site
1108 W Madison St, Maywood, IL 60153
(708) 450-3500
FUNCTIONS: Home delivered meals; Congregate dining

Ada S McKinley Community Services
725 S Wells, Chicago, IL 60612
(312) 554-0600
FUNCTIONS: Ethnic services & activities

Medical Claim Services Inc
669 Graceland Ave, Des Plaines, IL 60016
(708) 298-9380
FUNCTIONS: Medicare & supplemental security income assistance; Medical claims & billing assistance

OTHER SERVICES: Insurance coverage review; Co-insurance claims filed
See ad page 33

Medical Personnel Pool—Oak Lawn
10735 S Cicero Ste 200, Oak Lawn, IL 60453
(708) 422-2934
FUNCTIONS: In-home services; Medical health services; Respite services; Hospice; Multiple locations; Multiple services
OTHER SERVICES: Services available 24 hours a day, 7 days a week

Medical Personnel Pool—Oak Park
1515 N Harlem Ste 101, Oak Park, IL 60302
(708) 383-7320
FUNCTIONS: In-home services; Medical health services; Respite services; Hospice; Multiple locations; Multiple services
OTHER SERVICES: Services available 24 hours a day, 7 days a week

Medicare Claims (Part B)
Walk-in office: 233 N Michigan Ave; Claims: PO Box 4422, Marine, IL 62959
(800) 642-6930
FUNCTIONS: Medical claims & billing assistance
OTHER SERVICES: Information & service regarding Medicare insurance claims

Mental Health Association in Lake County
2450 169th St, Hammond, IN 46323
(219) 845-2720
FUNCTIONS: Mental health services

Mental Health Association of Greater Chicago
104 S Michigan Ave, Chicago, IL 60603
(312) 781-7780
FUNCTIONS: Information & referral; Educational programs; Publications

Mercy Center for Health Care Services
1325 N Highland, Aurora, IL 60506
(708) 859-2222 ext 3740
FUNCTIONS: Information & referral; Medical health services; Medical assessments; Mental health services; Congregate dining; Home delivered meals; Social services; Counseling; Case management; Support groups; Caregiver support; Educational programs; Publications; Volunteer opportunities; Multiple locations
OTHER SERVICES: ADVANTAGE Senior Program
See ad page 90

Mercy Hospital & Medical Center—Eldercare
Stevenson Expressway at King Dr (26th St), Chicago, IL 60616
(312) 567-5678
FUNCTIONS: Information & referral; Educational programs; Home health services; Support groups; Publications; Recreation; Medical claims & billing assistance

✓ In order to support future editions of this publication would you please mention *Elder Services* each time you contact any advertiser, facility, or service.

OLDER ADULT
Psychiatric Program

Mercy Center's Older Adult Psychiatric Program is a psychiatric inpatient unit for adults over 50 who suffer from depression, anxiety or other psychological problems. The program offers two specialized treatment tracks:

The Acute Care Program
A holistic, short-term program for older adults who are having difficulty coping with everyday living as a result of an acute or chronic psychiatric disorder.

Care for the Cognitively-Impaired
An intensive, highly structured, short-term program that includes diagnostic testing to determine if symptoms are the result of normal aging or an irreversible brain pathology.

In both tracks, comprehensive medical care under the direction of a psychiatrist is combined with specialized programming in a multi-disciplinary setting. Special emphasis is placed on the unique social, psychological, spiritual, and physical needs of each individual.

For more information about the program, call (708) 859-2222, extension 3740.

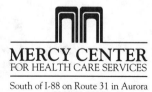

MERCY CENTER
FOR HEALTH CARE SERVICES
South of I-88 on Route 31 in Aurora
708/859-2222

OTHER SERVICES: Housecalls program; Alzheimer's disease center; Home safety assessments
See ads pages 116, 161, 351

Meridian Hospice
1525 East 53rd St Ste 1107, Chicago, IL 60615
(312) 955-5529
FUNCTIONS: Hospice

Methodist Hospital
5025 N Paulina St, Chicago, IL 60640
(312) 271-9040
FUNCTIONS: Information & referral; Medical assessments; Home health services; Medical health services; In-home services; Home delivered meals

Metro Corps of Gary Inc
1100 Massachusetts, Gary, IN 46402
(219) 886-3155
FUNCTIONS: Information & referral; Case management; Congregate dining; Educational programs; Employment; Energy assistance program; Home delivered meals; In-home services; Recreation; Senior center; Transportation
OTHER SERVICES: Addresses of congregate dining sites available from this office

Metropolitan YMCA Third Age Program
2100 S Indiana, Chicago, IL 60616
(312) 850-6550
FUNCTIONS: Ethnic services & activities

Mexican Society
1149 Lincoln, North Chicago, IL 60064
FUNCTIONS: Ethnic services & activities

Mile Square Health Center Inc
2040 W Washington Blvd, Chicago, IL 60612
(312) 421-3266
FUNCTIONS: Educational programs; Support groups; Case management; Counseling; Medical assessments; Home health services; Transportation

Howard Mohr Community Center Senior Citizen Program
7640 Jackson Blvd, Forest Park, IL 60130
(708) 771-7737
FUNCTIONS: Multiple services

Morris Senior Center
913 Pine St, Morris, IL 60450
(815) 942-9565
FUNCTIONS: Senior center

Morton Grove Senior Center
6101 Capulina Ave, Morton Grove, IL 60053
(708) 965-4100
FUNCTIONS: Multiple services

Mt Prospect Senior Citizens Center
50 S Emerson St, Mt Prospect, IL 60056
(708) 870-5680
FUNCTIONS: Senior center

Mt Sinai Baptist Church
2401 Argonne, North Chicago, IL 60064
(708) 689-4422
FUNCTIONS: Ethnic services & activities

Mujeres Latinas en Accion
1823 W 17th St, Chicago, IL 60608
(312) 226-1544
FUNCTIONS: Ethnic services & activities

Mundelein Senior Center
1200 Regent Dr, Mundelein, IL 60060
(708) 566-4790
FUNCTIONS: Senior center; Congregate dining

NAACP
2335 Meadow Lane, North Chicago, IL 60064
(708) 623-5839
FUNCTIONS: Ethnic services & activities

Naperville Park District
18 W Jefferson, Naperville, IL 60540
(708) 420-4210
FUNCTIONS: Congregate dining; Senior center

National Association for Home Care
519 C St NE, Washington, DC 20002
(202) 547-7424
FUNCTIONS: Information & referral

National Association of Claims Assistance Professionals Inc
4724 Florence Ave, Downers Grove, IL 60515
(708) 963-3500
FUNCTIONS: Information & referral; Educational programs
OTHER SERVICES: Nationwide referral for assistance with Medicare & health insurance claims
See ad page 91

National Association of Hispanic Elderly
2600 W Touhy, Chicago, IL 60645
(312) 262-5300
FUNCTIONS: Ethnic services & activities

National Association of Private Geriatric Care Managers
1315 Talbott Tower, Dayton, OH 45402
(513) 222-2621
FUNCTIONS: Information & referral

National Caucus & Center on Black Aged
2100 S Indiana Ste 122, Chicago, IL 60616
(312) 225-2500
FUNCTIONS: Ethnic services & activities; Employment

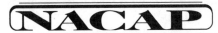
National Caucus & Center on Black Aged—Membership Chapter
PO Box 64846, Chicago, IL 60664
(312) 814-2919
FUNCTIONS: Advocacy; Educational programs
OTHER SERVICES: Organization concerned with the quality of life for minority elderly

National Consumer Oriented Agency
2200 E Devon, Des Plaines, IL 60018
(708) 299-1996
FUNCTIONS: Medicare & supplemental security income assistance
OTHER SERVICES: Seminars; Review of insurance needs; Sales of long-term care insurance policies
See ad page 50

National Council of Jewish Women
53 W Jackson Blvd Ste 835, Chicago, IL 60604
(312) 987-1927
FUNCTIONS: Ethnic services & activities

National Council on the Aging Inc
409 3rd St SW, Washington, DC 20024
(202) 479-1200
FUNCTIONS: Publications

National Health Information Clearinghouse
PO Box 1133, Washington, DC 20013
(800) 336-4797
FUNCTIONS: Information & referral

✔ In order to support future editions of this publication would you please mention *Elder Services* each time you contact any advertiser, facility, or service.

National Hospice Foundation & Home Care
519 C St NE, Washington, DC 20002
(202) 547-6586
OTHER SERVICES: National hospice information & referrals

National Resource Center on Health Promotion & Aging
601 "E" St NW Ste 5B, Washington, DC 20049
(202) 434-2200
FUNCTIONS: Information & referral; Publications; Educational programs

Native American Education Services
2838 W Peterson, Chicago, IL 60659
(312) 761-5000
FUNCTIONS: Ethnic services & activities

Native American Outpost
4740 N Clark, Chicago, IL 60640
(312) 769-0205
FUNCTIONS: Ethnic services & activities

New Horizon Community Center
305 W Jackson, Naperville, IL 60540
(708) 420-4210
FUNCTIONS: Senior center

New Lennox Community Park District
1 Manor Dr, New Lennox, IL 60451
(815) 485-7187
FUNCTIONS: Congregate dining

Ada S Niles Senior Center
6414 S Halsted St, Chicago, IL 60621
(312) 874-2400
FUNCTIONS: Information & referral; Counseling; Housing assistance; Congregate dining

Niles Senior Citizens Services
8060 Oakton, Niles, IL 60648
(708) 967-6100
FUNCTIONS: Multiple services; Will services

Niles Township Sheltered Workshop
8050 Monticello Ave, Skokie, IL 60076
(708) 679-5610
FUNCTIONS: Employment; Day care

Norsom Medical Laboratory—Chicago
4600 N Ravenswood Ave, Chicago, IL 60647
(708) 867-8831
OTHER SERVICES: Lab services 7 days a week
See ad page 47

Norsom Medical Laboratory—Harwood
7343 W Wilson Ave, Harwood Heights, IL 60656
(708) 867-8831
OTHER SERVICES: Lab services 7 days a week
See ad page 47

North Chicago Senior Center
1919 Sherman Ave, North Chicago, IL 60064
(708) 473-4898
FUNCTIONS: Senior center; Congregate dining

North Shore Senior Center
7 Happ Rd, Northfield, IL 60093
(708) 446-8750
FUNCTIONS: Information & referral; Educational programs; Caregiver support; Day care; Respite services; Support groups; Case management; Counseling; Medical assessments; Home health services; In-home services; Friendly visits; Housing assistance; Senior center; Recreation; Transportation; Financial services; Energy assistance program; Protective services; Volunteer opportunities; Case coordination unit; Multiple services
See ad page 144

North Stickney Senior Lunch Center
6721 W 40th St, Stickney, IL 60402
(708) 788-9100
FUNCTIONS: Congregate dining; Home delivered meals

North Suburban Self-Help Center
233 Briar Lane, Highland Park, IL 60035
(708) 433-4130
FUNCTIONS: Ethnic services & activities

Northbrook Senior Center
1810 Walters, Northbrook, IL 60062
(708) 291-2988
FUNCTIONS: Multiple services

Northeastern Illinois Area Agency on Aging—Kankakee
KCC W Campus Bldg 5 River Rd PO Box 809, Kankakee, IL 60901
(815) 929-0727, (800) 528-2000
FUNCTIONS: Information & referral; Caregiver support; Educational programs; Employment; Publications; Advocacy; Multiple locations; Multiple services
OTHER SERVICES: Gatekeeper program; Speakers bureau; Corporate Caring program
See ad page 93

Northeastern Illinois Area Agency on Aging—West Chicago
245 W Roosevelt Rd Bldg 6, West Chicago, IL 60185
(708) 293-5990
FUNCTIONS: Information & referral; Caregiver support; Educational programs; Employment; Publications; Advocacy; Multiple locations; Multiple services
OTHER SERVICES: Gatekeeper program; Speakers bureau; Corporate Caring program
See ad page 93

Northeastern Illinois University Student Volunteer Corps
5500 N St Louis C-311, Chicago, IL 60625
(312) 794-6115
FUNCTIONS: Volunteer opportunities

Northshore Eldercare Management
1019 South Blvd, Evanston, IL 60202
(708) 866-7466
FUNCTIONS: Information & referral; Case management; Counseling; Educational programs

Northwest Community Hospital Home Hospice
800 W Central, Arlington Heights, IL 60005
(708) 259-1000 Ext 5194
FUNCTIONS: Hospice

Northwest Counseling Center
6229 N Northwest Hwy, Chicago, IL 60631
(312) 774-7555
FUNCTIONS: Information & referral; Counseling

Northwestern Memorial Hospital Dept of Geriatric Services
750 N Lake Shore Dr Ste 601, Chicago, IL 60611
(312) 908-4335
FUNCTIONS: Information & referral; Medical health services; Mental health services; Medical assessments; Educational programs; Home health services; In-home services; Hospice
OTHER SERVICES: Emergency response system; Geriatric health ministry; Senior membership program
See ad page 70

Northwestern Memorial Hospital Hospice Program
303 Superior St, Chicago, IL 60611
(312) 908-7476
FUNCTIONS: Hospice

Nursefinders
4415 W Harrison Ste 437, Hillside, IL 60126
(708) 449-3850
FUNCTIONS: Day care; Respite services; Home health services; In-home services

Oak Lawn Senior Center
5330 W 95th St, Oak Lawn, IL 60453
(708) 499-0240
FUNCTIONS: Senior center

Oak Lawn Senior Nutrition—Pilgrim Faith Church
9420 S 52nd Ave, Oak Lawn, IL 60453
(708) 422-5180
FUNCTIONS: Home delivered meals; Congregate dining

Oak Park Senior Center
500 S Maple, Oak Park, IL 60304
(708) 848-7050
FUNCTIONS: Senior center; Home delivered meals; Congregate dining; Recreation; Educational programs; Employment

Oak Park Senior Nutrition Center
1108 W Madison St, Maywood, IL 60153
(708) 450-7080
FUNCTIONS: Congregate dining

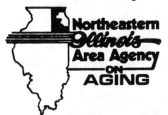
✔ In order to support future editions of this publication would you please mention *Elder Services* each time you contact any advertiser, facility, or service.

Oak Park Township Senior Services
105 S Oak Park Ave, Oak Park, IL 60302
(709) 383-8060
FUNCTIONS: Information & referral; In-home services; Case management; Senior center; Case coordination unit; Protective services

Older Adult Rehabilitation Service (OARS)
5817 W Cermak Rd, Cicero, IL 60650
(708) 656-3722
FUNCTIONS: Caregiver support; Senior center; Congregate dining; Transportation

Older Women's League (OWL)
734 Noyes, Evanston, IL 60201
(708) 869-1831
FUNCTIONS: Information & referral; Advocacy
OTHER SERVICES: Advocacy of economic and health issues for mid-life and older women

Operation Able
180 N Wabash Ave 8th Fl, Chicago, IL 60601
(312) 782-3335
FUNCTIONS: Information & referral; Educational programs; Employment

Operation Push—Mt Zion Baptist Church
McKinley and Erie, Joliet, IL 60436
(815) 723-9445
FUNCTIONS: Congregate dining; Ethnic services & activities

Orland Park Senior Nutrition Center
255 Orland Park Dr, Orland Park, IL 60426
(708) 460-1850
FUNCTIONS: Congregate dining

Orland Township Senior Services
15100 S 94th Ave, Orland Park, IL 60462
(708) 403-4222
FUNCTIONS: Transportation

Osteopathic Hospitals & Medical Centers
20201 S Crawford Ave, Olympia Fields, IL 60461
(708) 747-4000
FUNCTIONS: Information & referral; Home health services; Medical health services; Medical assessments; Mental health services; Publications; Volunteer opportunities; Multiple locations
OTHER SERVICES: Golden VIP Club; Physician referral
See ad page xvii

PACE
550 W Algonquin Rd, Arlington Heights, IL 60005
(708) 364-7223
FUNCTIONS: Information & referral; Transportation

Palatine Township Senior Citizens Council
721 S Quentin Rd, Palatine, IL 60067
(708) 991-1112

FUNCTIONS: Congregate dining; Home delivered meals; Friendly visits; Senior center; Volunteer opportunities; Educational programs; Social services; Respite services; Caregiver support; Support groups; Recreation; Exercise
OTHER SERVICES: Free income tax assistance

Palos Area Transportation Services for the Elderly
8455 W 103rd St, Palos Hills, IL 60465
(708) 430-4500
FUNCTIONS: Transportation

Park Forest Nurses PLUS Home Health Care
200 Forest Blvd, Park Forest, IL 60466
(708) 748-1112
FUNCTIONS: Medical health services

Park Place Senior Center
306 W Park St, Arlington Heights, IL 60005
(708) 253-5500
FUNCTIONS: Information & referral; Case management; Home delivered meals; Case coordination unit; Protective services; Volunteer opportunities; Support groups; Senior center; Congregate dining; Multiple services

Park Ridge Senior Center
100 South Western Ave, Park Ridge, IL 60068
(708) 692-3597
FUNCTIONS: Multiple services; Will services

Parkside Senior Services—Lutheran General Health Care
1775 Dempster St 1S, Park Ridge, IL 60068
(708) 696-7770
FUNCTIONS: Information & referral; Counseling; In-home services; Home delivered meals; Day care; Senior center; Medical health services; Support groups; Educational programs; Volunteer opportunities
OTHER SERVICES: Geriatric assessments; Emergency response system; Intergenerational programs
See ads pages 140, 202, 301

Pathways Consultants for Senior Living Inc
PO Box 14363, Chicago, IL 60614
(312) 935-9038
FUNCTIONS: Housing assistance; Case management; Social services
OTHER SERVICES: Consulting & referrals of housing options
See ad page 95

Pavilion Senior Center
199 N First St, Wheeling, IL 60090
(708) 459-2670
FUNCTIONS: Multiple services; Senior center

Peace Memorial Manor
3737 Highland, Downers Grove, IL 60515
(708) 963-3780
FUNCTIONS: Congregate dining

Pembroke Senior Citizens Center
PO Box 488, Hopkins Park, IL 60944
(815) 944-5283
FUNCTIONS: Senior center; Congregate dining

Peoples Gas
122 S Michigan Ave, Chicago, IL 60602
(312) 431-7004
OTHER SERVICES: Special arrangements may be made for notification to a third party of nonpayment to avoid gas shut-off.
See ad on page ix

Peoples Resource Center
107 W Indiana, Wheaton, IL 60187
(708) 682-3844
FUNCTIONS: Ethnic services & activities

Personal Packers & Moving Consultants Inc
3020 N Clybourn, Chicago, IL 60618
(312) 248-5638
FUNCTIONS: Housing assistance
OTHER SERVICES: Complete moving services; On-site and phone consultation for residence search, locating and coordinating moving company, real estate agent, home repair and design services; Estate shrinkage and liquidation; Change-of-address services; Full packing, unpacking, and closet organization services.
See ad page 13

Phoenix Senior Nutrition Center
650 E Phoenix Dr, Phoenix, IL 60426
(708) 331-2408
FUNCTIONS: Congregate dining; Home delivered meals

Plainfield Park District
100 W Ottawa St, Plainfield, IL 60544
(815) 436-6699
FUNCTIONS: Congregate dining

PLOWS Council on Aging
4700 W 95th St Ste 106, Oak Lawn, IL 60453
(708) 422-6722
FUNCTIONS: Information & referral; Educational programs; Caregiver support; Case management; Medical assessments; In-home services; Friendly visits; Home delivered meals; Housing assistance; Transportation; Legal assistance; Energy assistance program; Protective services; Case coordination unit; Multiple services; Will services

Polish National Alliance
1200 N Ashland, Chicago, IL 60622
(312) 286-0500
FUNCTIONS: Ethnic services & activities

Polish Welfare Association
3834 N Cicero Ave, Chicago, IL 60641
(312) 282-8206
FUNCTIONS: Information & referral; Advocacy; Ethnic services & activities

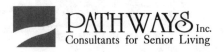

Porter County Council on Aging
1005 Campbell, Valparaiso, IN 46383
(219) 464-9736
FUNCTIONS: Information & referral; Case management; Congregate dining; Educational programs; Employment; Energy assistance program; Home delivered meals; In-home services; Recreation; Senior center; Transportation
OTHER SERVICES: Addresses of congregate dining sites available from this office

Porter-Starke Services Inc
2535 Portage Mall, Portage, IN 46368
(219) 762-9556
FUNCTIONS: Mental health services

PRC Paratransit Services Inc
1700 Ballard Rd, Park Ridge, IL 60068
(708) 297-5067
FUNCTIONS: Transportation

Presbyterian Home
3200 Grant St, Evanston, IL 60201
(708) 492-2900
FUNCTIONS: Educational programs; Day care; Respite services; Support groups; Counseling; Medical assessments; Friendly visits; Housing assistance; Recreation; Congregate dining; Transportation

Prisoner Release Ministry Inc
203 N Ottawa, Joliet, IL 60431
(815) 723-8998
FUNCTIONS: Ethnic services & activities

Prospect Heights Senior Center
110 W Camp McDonald Rd, Prospect Heights, IL 60070
(708) 394-2848
FUNCTIONS: Senior center

✔ In order to support future editions of this publication would you please mention *Elder Services* each time you contact any advertiser, facility, or service.

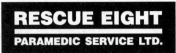
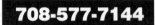
Proviso Council on Aging

439 Bohland Ave, Bellwood, IL 60104
(708) 547-5600
FUNCTIONS: Information & referral; Case management; Case coordination unit; Protective services; Senior center; Volunteer opportunities; Day care; Transportation; In-home services; Friendly visits; Home delivered meals; Congregate dining

Puerta Albierta

25975 N Diamond Lake Rd, Mundelein, IL 60060
(708) 566-0066
FUNCTIONS: Ethnic services & activities

Puerto Rican Society

150 S Sheridan Rd, Waukegan, IL 60085
(708) 662-1437
FUNCTIONS: Ethnic services & activities

Quad County Urban League

305 E Benton, Aurora, IL 60505
(708) 897-5335
FUNCTIONS: Ethnic services & activities

Rainbow Hospice Inc

460 S Northwest Hwy Ste 103, Park Ridge, IL 60068
(708) 292-0050
FUNCTIONS: Hospice

Referral & Emergency Service

824 Broadway, Gary, IN 46402
(219) 886-1586
FUNCTIONS: Information & referral; Counseling
OTHER SERVICES: Emergency assistance available

Regional Transit Authority (RTA)

Chicago (312) 836-7000, Suburbs (800) 972-7000
OTHER SERVICES: Information regarding routes & special services on the RTA

Rehabilitation Institute of Chicago

345 E Superior St, Chicago, IL 60611
(312) 908-6000
FUNCTIONS: Medical health services
OTHER SERVICES: In- & out-patient services for physical, social, & vocational services; Arthritis therapy

Rescue Eight Paramedic Service

208 W University, Arlington Heights, IL 60004
(708) 577-7144
OTHER SERVICES: Advance life support, basic life support, & wheelchair livery service
See ad page 96

Resource Center for the Elderly

306 W Park St, Arlington Heights, IL 60005
(708) 577-7070
OTHER SERVICES: Information & referral regarding shared housing

Respitecare

2008 Dempster St, Evanston, IL 60202
(708) 328-1900
FUNCTIONS: Information & referral; Respite services; Caregiver support; In-home services; Support groups
OTHER SERVICES: Assessments done for daily & nursing needs

Retirement Relocation Planning Inc

213 Institute Pl Ste 305, Chicago, IL 60610
(312) 664-6672
FUNCTIONS: Housing assistance
OTHER SERVICES: Through consulting, seminars, and media, helps seniors and their families select the best retirement community to meet their needs.
See ad on page 15

Retirement Security Inc—An MRM Group

820 N Orleans Ste 320, Chicago, IL 60610
(312) 664-5252
FUNCTIONS: Financial services; Retirement benefits; Information & referral
OTHER SERVICES: Programs for individuals & corporations wishing to purchase long-term care insurance
See ad page iii

Rich Township Senior Center

22013 Governors Hwy, Richton Park, IL 60471
(708) 748-5454
FUNCTIONS: Transportation; Multiple services

Rich Township Senior Nutrition Program

480 Lakewood, Park Forest, IL 60466
(708) 747-2700
FUNCTIONS: Congregate dining

River Forest Community Center Senior Program

412 Thatcher, River Forest, IL 60305
(708) 771-6159
FUNCTIONS: Recreation

Riverain Point
200 N Island Ave, Batavia, IL 60510
(708) 879-1790
FUNCTIONS: Congregate dining

Robbins Senior Center
3518 W 139th St, Robbins, IL 60472
(708) 389-1910
FUNCTIONS: Senior center; Home delivered meals; Congregate dining

Rolling Meadows Senior Center
3705 Pheasant Dr, Rolling Meadows, IL 60008
(708) 818-3205
FUNCTIONS: Senior center

Roosevelt University
430 S Michigan Ave, Chicago, IL 60605
(312) 341-3860
FUNCTIONS: Educational programs

Round Lake Area Senior Center
814 Hart Rd, Round Lake, IL 60073
(708) 546-8558
FUNCTIONS: Senior center; Congregate dining

Rush-Presbyterian-St Lukes Medical Center—Bowman Center
710 S Paulina, Chicago, IL 60612
(312) 942-7161
FUNCTIONS: Medical health services; Caregiver support; Educational programs; Medical assessments; Support groups; Information & referral
OTHER SERVICES: Rehabilitation & geropsychiatric services
See ad page 24

Rush-Presbyterian-St Luke's Medical Center—Older Adult Services
1653 W Congress, Chicago, IL 60612
(312) 942-8100
FUNCTIONS: Information & referral; Support groups; Medical assessments; Medical health services; Caregiver support; Educational programs; Publications
OTHER SERVICES: Comprehensive geriatric assessment
See ad page 24

St Alexis Church
400 W Wood St, Bensenville, IL 60106
(708) 350-7656
FUNCTIONS: Ethnic services & activities

St Anthony Medical Center
Main and Franciscan Rd, Crown Point, IN 46307
(217) 663-8120
FUNCTIONS: Caregiver support; Educational programs; Home delivered meals; Home health services; Medical health services; Mental health services; Social services; Volunteer opportunities
See ad page 245

St Augustine's Center for American Indians
4512 N Sheridan Rd, Chicago, IL 60640
(312) 784-1050
FUNCTIONS: Ethnic services & activities

St Catherine Hospital
4321 Fir St, Hammond, IN 46312
(219) 392-7600
FUNCTIONS: Respite services; In-home services

St Charles Pastoral Center
401 S Independence Blvd, Romeoville, IL 60441
(815) 838-8100
FUNCTIONS: Ethnic services & activities

St Francis Hospice
1000 Skokie Blvd Ste 325, Wilmette, IL 60091
(708) 256-7882
FUNCTIONS: Hospice

St James Hospice
610 E Water St, Pontiac, IL 61764
(815) 842-2828 Ext 3329
FUNCTIONS: Hospice

St Joseph Church
509 S Utica, Waukegan, IL 60085
(708) 623-2655
FUNCTIONS: Ethnic services & activities

St Joseph Hospital & Health Care Center—Center for Healthy Aging
2900 N Lake Shore Dr, Chicago, IL 60657
(312) 975-3155
FUNCTIONS: Information & referral; Educational programs; Publications; Multiple services; Medical claims & billing assistance
OTHER SERVICES: Physician referral; Senior membership program; Discounts
See ad page 11

St Joseph Hospital of Elgin
77 N Airlite St, Elgin, IL 60123-4912
(708) 695-3200
FUNCTIONS: Information & referral; Case management; Counseling; Day care; Educational programs; Exercise; Home delivered meals; Home health services; In-home services; Medical assessments; Mental health services; Publications; Respite services; Social services; Support groups; Volunteer opportunities; Multiple locations
OTHER SERVICES: Senior Spirit Program
See ads pages 18, 168

St Mary of Nazareth Hospital Center
2233 W Division, Chicago, IL 60622
(312) 770-2000
FUNCTIONS: Medical health services; Mental health services; Home health services; Social services; Volunteer opportunities
OTHER SERVICES: No-cost Medicare program; Heart Club; Diabetic program
See ad page 162

✔ In order to support future editions of this publication would you please mention *Elder Services* each time you contact any advertiser, facility, or service.

St Mary's Church—Spanish Center
140 N Oakwood, West Chicago, IL 60185
(708) 231-7156
FUNCTIONS: Ethnic services & activities

St Petronille Catholic Church
420 Glenwood Ave, Glen Ellyn, IL 60137
(708) 469-0404
FUNCTIONS: Ethnic services & activities

St Thomas Hospice
7 Salt Creek Lane Ste 101, Hinsdale, IL 60521
(708) 920-8300
FUNCTIONS: Hospice

Salem Towers
1315 Rowell Ave, Joliet, IL 60433
(815) 726-3194
FUNCTIONS: Congregate dining

Salvation Army
300 3rd Ave, Joliet, IL 60433
(815) 726-4834
FUNCTIONS: Ethnic services & activities

Salvation Army—Family Services
4800 N Marine Dr, Chicago, IL 60640
(312) 275-6233
FUNCTIONS: Respite services; Support groups; Counseling; In-home services

Salvation Army Golden Diners
132 E Prairie St, Marengo, IL 60152
(708) 568-7176
FUNCTIONS: Senior center; Congregate dining

Salvation Army of Elgin
316 Douglas, Elgin, IL 60120
(708) 695-4951
FUNCTIONS: Congregate dining

Salvation Army—Second Horizon Senior Center
437 E Galena, Aurora, IL 60505
(708) 897-7299
FUNCTIONS: Senior center; Congregate dining

Salvation Army Senior Services & Center
148 N Harrison, Kankakee, IL 60901
(815) 933-1603
FUNCTIONS: Senior center

Schaumburg Health & Human Services
101 Schaumburg Ct, Schaumburg, IL 60193
(708) 894-4500
FUNCTIONS: Counseling; Medical assessments; Home health services; Friendly visits; Senior center; Congregate dining; Medical health services

Schaumburg Senior Center
505 N Springinsguth Rd, Schaumburg, IL 60193
(708) 490-7026
FUNCTIONS: Senior center

Schaumburg Senior Nutrition Site—The Barn
231 Civic Dr, Schaumburg, IL 60193
(708) 529-7496
FUNCTIONS: Home delivered meals; Congregate dining

SCR Medical Transportation Service
1900 S Wabash, Chicago, IL 60616
(312) 791-0800
OTHER SERVICES: Medical & nonmedical special services carrier

Self-Help Center
1600 Dodge Ste S-122, Evanston, IL 60201
(708) 328-0470
FUNCTIONS: Information & referral; Support groups
OTHER SERVICES: Referrals to over 300 self-help groups

Senior Adult Center—Leaning Tower YMCA
6300 W Touhy, Niles, IL 60648
(708) 647-8222
FUNCTIONS: Senior center

Senior Care Consultants
2700 W Touhy Ave, Chicago, IL 60645
(708) 780-5403
FUNCTIONS: Information & referral; Case management; Counseling
OTHER SERVICES: Comprehensive geriatric care management service; Support group facilitators; Assessments of special needs

Senior Centers of Metropolitan Chicago
501 W Surf St, Chicago, IL 60657
(312) 525-3480
FUNCTIONS: Information & referral; Educational programs; Support groups; Case management; In-home services; Friendly visits; Home delivered meals; Senior center; Recreation; Legal assistance

Senior Citizens Center Golden Age Chateau
15652 S Homan Ave, Markham, IL 60426
(708) 596-6680
FUNCTIONS: Senior center; Home delivered meals; Congregate dining

Senior Citizens of Schaumburg Township Inc
25 Illinois Blvd, Hoffman Estates, IL 60196
(708) 882-1929
FUNCTIONS: Transportation; Multiple services; Will services

Senior Club of Lake County
905 Muirfield, Waukegan, IL 60085
FUNCTIONS: Ethnic services & activities

Senior Outreach & Referral
657 E Court St Ste 200, Kankakee, IL 60901
FUNCTIONS: Case coordination unit; Multiple services

Senior Service Association of McHenry County
3519 N Route 31, McHenry, IL 60050
(815) 344-3555
FUNCTIONS: Senior center; Congregate dining

Senior Service Center
310 N Joliet St, Joliet, IL 60432
(815) 723-9713
FUNCTIONS: Congregate dining

Senior Services Associates Inc—Beecher Community Building
908 Game Farm Rd, Yorkville, IL 60560
(708) 553-5777
FUNCTIONS: Case coordination unit; Congregate dining; Multiple services

Senior Services Associates Inc—Elgin
101 S Grove St, Elgin, IL 60120
(708) 741-0404
FUNCTIONS: Case coordination unit; Multiple services

Senior Services Associates Inc—McHenry
3519 N State Rte 31, McHenry, IL 60050
(708) 344-3555
FUNCTIONS: Case coordination unit; Multiple services

Senior Services Center of Will County
310 N Joliet St, Joliet, IL 60431
(708) 723-9713
FUNCTIONS: Case coordination unit; Multiple services; Senior center

Seniors Assistance Center
7500 W Montrose, Norridge, IL 60634
(708) 456-7979
FUNCTIONS: Information & referral; Case management; Protective services; Home delivered meals; Friendly visits; Transportation; Will services

SER—Jobs for Progress Inc
117 N Genesee St, Waukegan, IL 60085
(708) 336-1004
FUNCTIONS: Ethnic services & activities

Share Health Plan of Illinois
One Pierce Pl Ste 600, Itasca, IL 60143
(708) 250-3250
OTHER SERVICES: Health care coverage for groups & individuals on Medicare, including specialized health care coverage for nursing home residents.
See ad page 125

Shawsau Temple
401 Baldwin, Waukegan, IL 60085
FUNCTIONS: Ethnic services & activities

Shiloh Baptist Church
800 S Genesee, Waukegan, IL 60085
(708) 662-9361
FUNCTIONS: Ethnic services & activities

Silver Harvest Senior Delight
341 N St Joseph Ave, Kankakee, IL 60901
(815) 933-7883
FUNCTIONS: Congregate dining

Simon Foundation for Continence
PO Box 815, Wilmette, IL 60091
(800) 23SIMON, (708) 864-3913
FUNCTIONS: Information & referral; Support groups; Educational programs; Publications
OTHER SERVICES: Information & self-help for people, and their families, who suffer with incontinence

Albert J Smith Activities Center
5120 Galitz, Skokie, IL 60077
(708) 673-0500
FUNCTIONS: Senior center; Home delivered meals; Multiple services

Social Security & Medicare (Part A)
105 W Adams St, Chicago, IL 60603
(800) 772-1213
OTHER SERVICES: Information & referral regarding financial assistance, disability benefits, and retirement insurance

South Lake County Community Services
7000 W 137th Pl, Cedar Lake, IN 46303
(219) 374-5476
FUNCTIONS: Information & referral; Case management; Congregate dining; Educational programs; Employment; Energy assistance program; Home delivered meals; In-home services; Recreation; Senior center; Transportation
OTHER SERVICES: Addresses of congregate dining sites available from this office

South Suburban Senior Services—Catholic Charities
15300 S Lexington Ave, Harvey, IL 60426
(708) 596-2222
FUNCTIONS: Information & referral; Case management; Case coordination unit; Counseling; Protective services; In-home services; Transportation; Home delivered meals; Respite services; Advocacy; Senior center; Congregate dining

Southeast Asia Center
1124 W Ainslie, Chicago, IL 60640
(312) 989-6927
FUNCTIONS: Congregate dining; Energy assistance program

Southeastern Grundy Senior Citizens
207 Liberty, Gardner, IL 60424
(815) 237-2727
FUNCTIONS: Senior center; Congregate dining

✔ In order to support future editions of this publication would you please mention *Elder Services* each time you contact any advertiser, facility, or service.

Southlake Center for Mental Health—Hobart
1348 S Lake Park Ave, Hobart, IN 46342
(219) 842-4040
FUNCTIONS: Mental health services

Southlake Center for Mental Health—Merrillville
8555 Taft St, Merrillville, IN 46410
(219) 769-4005
FUNCTIONS: Mental health services

Southlake Center for Mental Health—Merrillville
290 A E 90th Dr, Merrillville, IN 46410
(219) 736-9115
FUNCTIONS: Mental health services

Southlake Center for Mental Health—Schererville
2001 U S 41, Schererville, IN 46375
(219) 322-6622
FUNCTIONS: Mental health services

Southwest Suburban Center on Aging
111 W Harris, LaGrange, IL 60525
(708) 354-1323
FUNCTIONS: Information & referral; Educational programs; Support groups; Case management; Counseling; Medical assessments; In-home services; Friendly visits; Home delivered meals; Senior center; Recreation; Congregate dining; Transportation; Financial services; Legal assistance; Energy assistance program; Case coordination unit; Protective services; Senior center; Case management; Multiple services

Spanish Center
309 N Eastern Ave, Joliet, IL 60432
(815) 727-3683
FUNCTIONS: Ethnic services & activities

STAR Hospice—St Therese Medical Center
2615 Washington St, Waukegan, IL 60085
(708) 360-2220
FUNCTIONS: Hospice

Stickney Public Health District
5635 State Rd, Burbank, IL 60459
(708) 424-9200 ext 18
FUNCTIONS: Information & referral; Case coordination unit; Case management; Protective services; Multiple services

Stickney Township Office on Aging
5635 State Rd, Burbank, IL 60459
(708) 424-9200
FUNCTIONS: Information & referral; Congregate dining; Home delivered meals; Multiple services

Anita Stone Jewish Community Center
18600 Governors Hwy, Flossmoor, IL 60422
(708) 799-7650
FUNCTIONS: Support groups

Stryker Building
102 Stryker, Joliet, IL 60436
(815) 725-9119
FUNCTIONS: Congregate dining

Suburban Area Agency on Aging
1146 Westgate Ste LL112, Oak Park, IL 60301
(708) 383-0258
FUNCTIONS: Information & referral; Caregiver support; Employment; Housing assistance; Publications; Protective services; Volunteer opportunities; Multiple services
OTHER SERVICES: Gatekeeper program; Services for abused & neglected elderly; Speakers bureau
See ad page 101

Terra Nova Films Inc
9848 S Winchester Ave, Chicago, IL 60643
(312) 881-8491
FUNCTIONS: Educational programs
OTHER SERVICES: Consulting and production of videos. Film festivals and seminars may be arranged. Over 70 topics related to aging available for rent or purchase.

Thornton Township Senior Services
333 E 162nd St, South Holland, IL 60473
FUNCTIONS: Congregate dining; Transportation; Multiple services

Travelers & Immigrants Aid
327 S LaSalle Ste 1500, Chicago, IL 60604
(312) 435-4500
FUNCTIONS: Ethnic services & activities

Tri-City Comprehensive Community Mental Health Center Inc—East Chicago
3901 Indianapolis Blvd, East Chicago, IN 46312
(219) 398-7050
FUNCTIONS: Mental health services

Tri-City Comprehensive Community Mental Health Center Inc—Hammond
229 Ogden Ave, Hammond, IN 46320
(219) 932-7234
FUNCTIONS: Mental health services

TriCity Family Services
321 Hamilton St, Geneva, IL 60134
(708) 232-1070
FUNCTIONS: Counseling

Trinity Adults
405 S Rush, Roselle, IL 60172
(708) 894-3263
FUNCTIONS: Congregate dining

Trinity AME Church
210 South Ave, Waukegan, IL 60085
(708) 623-8529
FUNCTIONS: Ethnic services & activities

Troy Township Senior Citizens Center
25448 Beith Rd, Joliet, IL 60436
(815) 467-5777
FUNCTIONS: Senior center; Congregate dining

Twin Cities Community Services
3550 Pennsylvania Ave, East Chicago, IN 46312
(219) 397-7924
FUNCTIONS: Information & referral; Counseling; Educational programs; Recreation; Medical health services

Ukrainian Social Service
2355 W Chicago Ave, Chicago, IL 60622
(312) 235-2895
FUNCTIONS: Congregate dining; Energy assistance program

United Charities North Center
3445 N Central Ave, Chicago, IL 60634
(312) 282-9535
FUNCTIONS: Information & referral; Case management; Support groups; Caregiver support; Counseling; Advocacy; Financial services

United Charities of Chicago
3214 W 63rd, Chicago, IL 60629
(312) 776-1900
FUNCTIONS: Case coordination unit

United Charities of Chicago Senior Services
14 E Jackson Blvd, Chicago, IL 60604
(312) 986-4000
FUNCTIONS: Information & referral; Educational programs; Caregiver support; Respite services; Support groups; Case management; Medical assessments; In-home services; Financial services; Legal assistance; Case coordination unit; Multiple services

United Methodist Church
East Kahler Rd, Wilmington, IL 60481
(815) 476-7555
FUNCTIONS: Congregate dining

United Parkinson Foundation
360 W Superior St, Chicago, IL 60610
(312) 664-2344
FUNCTIONS: Information & referral; Publications; Educational programs

United Way of Chicago—Crusade of Mercy
221 N LaSalle St, Chicago, IL 60603
(312) 580-2800
FUNCTIONS: Multiple locations; Multiple services

United Way of Will County Volunteer Services
54 N Ottawa, Joliet, IL 60431
(815) 723-8510
FUNCTIONS: Volunteer opportunities

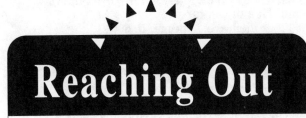
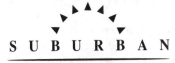
✔ In order to support future editions of this publication would you please mention *Elder Services* each time you contact any advertiser, facility, or service.

University of Chicago Hospital—Windemere Senior Health Center
5549 S Cornell Ave, Chicago, IL 60637
(312) 702 8840
FUNCTIONS: Medical health services; Social services; In-home services; Case management; Counseling; Educational programs

The University of Illinois Hospital & Clinics Geriatric Assessment Center
901 S Wolcott, Chicago, IL 60612
(312) 996-3039, (800) 488-3628
FUNCTIONS: Information & referral; Counseling; Medical assessments; Medical health services
OTHER SERVICES: Incontinence control
See ad page 56

Valley View Community Center
Rte 30 and Wolfe Rd, Frankfort, IL 60423
(815) 469-1499
FUNCTIONS: Senior center; Congregate dining

Vernon Hills Senior Citizens
290 Evergreen Dr, Vernon Hills, IL 60061
(708) 362-3893
FUNCTIONS: Senior center

Veterans Benefits Administration
536 S Clark St (Mail: Box 8136), Chicago, IL 60680
(312) 663-5510, (800) 827-0466
FUNCTIONS: Information & referral; Educational programs; Caregiver support; Support groups; Medical assessments; Medical health services; Recreation

Victory Memorial Hospital & Health Services
1324 N Sheridan Rd, Waukegan, IL 60085
(708) 360-4246
FUNCTIONS: Information & referral; Home health services; Medical assessments; Educational programs; Respite services; Medical health services; Mental health services; Housing assistance; Support groups; Caregiver support; Social services; Day care; Volunteer opportunities; Medical claims & billing assistance
OTHER SERVICES: Out-patient bathing & hygiene assistance; Speakers bureau; Physician referral; Better Breathers Club; Stroke rehabilitation; Chemical dependency program; Senior Passport (assistance with Medicare & insurance claims)

Vietnamese Community Service Center
4833 N Broadway 2nd Fl, Chicago, IL 60640
(312) 728-3700
FUNCTIONS: Ethnic services & activities

Visiting Nurse Association Hospice of Chicago
322 S Green St 3rd Fl, Chicago, IL 60607-3599
(312) 738-8622
FUNCTIONS: Hospice

Visiting Nurse Association of Chicago
322 S Green St, Chicago, IL 60607
(312) 738-0299
FUNCTIONS: Respite services; Case management; Home health services; Hospice; In-home services; Friendly visits

Volunteer Network
300 W Washington Ste 1414, Chicago, IL 60606
(312) 201-3550
FUNCTIONS: Volunteer opportunities

Vriangato Association
819 S Jackson, Waukegan, IL 60085
FUNCTIONS: Ethnic services & activities

Warren Township Senior Center
17801 W Washington St, Gurnee, IL 60031
(708) 244-1101
FUNCTIONS: Senior center

Waukegan Park District Older Adult Program—Lilac Cottage Senior Center
1917 N Sheridan Rd, Waukegan, IL 60087
(708) 360-4770
FUNCTIONS: Senior center

Waukegan Senior Center
1 N Genesee, Waukegan, IL 60085
(708) 249-3500
FUNCTIONS: Senior center; Congregate dining

Wayne Township Seniors
29 W 777 Hahndorf Rd, West Chicago, IL 60185
(708) 231-7140
FUNCTIONS: Senior center

Weinstein Brothers Memorial Chapels
111 Skokie Blvd, Wilmette, IL 60091
(709) 256-5700
FUNCTIONS: Educational programs; Support groups
OTHER SERVICES: Seminars

Wellspring Gerontological Service
179 W Washington Ste 360, Chicago, IL 60602
(312) 201-9696
FUNCTIONS: Day care; Financial services; Home health services; In-home services; Respite services; Support groups

West Chicago Community Center of Winfield Township
306 Main St, West Chicago, IL 60185
(708) 293-0022
FUNCTIONS: Congregate dining

West Suburban Hospital Medical Center
Erie at Austin Blvd, Oak Park, IL 60304
(708) 383-6200

FUNCTIONS: Information & referral; Medical health services; Medical assessments; Educational programs; Publications; Home health services; Hospice; Social services; Support groups; Multiple locations; Medical claims & billing assistance

OTHER SERVICES: AdvantAge program (discounts & claim assistance)

West Towns Hospice
1441 South Harlem Ave, Berwyn, IL 60402
(708) 749-7171
FUNCTIONS: Hospice

Westmont Park District Senior Citizens Center
75 E Richmond, Westmont, IL 60559
(708) 963-5150
FUNCTIONS: Senior center; Congregate dining

Wheaton Center
2 Wheaton Center, Wheaton, IL 60187
(708) 462-7082
FUNCTIONS: Congregate dining

Wheaton Park District Senior Center
666 S Main St, Wheaton, IL 60187
(708) 665-4710
FUNCTIONS: Senior center

Wheeling Township Services
1616 N Arlington Heights Rd, Arlington Heights, IL 60004
(708) 259-7730
FUNCTIONS: Information & referral; Home delivered meals; Educational programs; Social services; Exercise; Transportation

Willowbrook/Burr Ridge/Pleasant Dale Senior Center
10 S 474 Madison St, Burr Ridge, IL 60521
(708) 920-1969
FUNCTIONS: Senior center

Woodstock Nutrition Center
1155 Walden Oaks Dr, Woodstock, IL 60098
(815) 338-7772
FUNCTIONS: Congregate dining

World Relief Corporation
1028 College Ave, Wheaton, IL 60187
(708) 665-0235
FUNCTIONS: Ethnic services & activities

John C Wunsch
77 W Washington St Ste 1420, Chicago, IL 60602
(312) 855-0705
FUNCTIONS: Legal assistance
OTHER SERVICES: Firm concentrates in civil litigation
See ad page 40

YMCA of Metropolitan Chicago
2100 S Indiana Ave, Chicago, IL 60616
(312) 808-3505
FUNCTIONS: In-home services; Housing assistance; Senior center; Recreation; Congregate dining

YMCA of Metropolitan Chicago
4251 W Irving Park Rd, Chicago, IL 60641
(312) 777-7500
FUNCTIONS: In-home services; Housing assistance; Senior center; Recreation; Congregate dining

York Township Senior Center
1502 S Meyers Rd, Lombard, IL 60148
(708) 620-2424
FUNCTIONS: Senior center; Congregate dining

Kenneth W Young Center for Senior Citizens—Arlington Heights
306 W Park St, Arlington Heights, IL 60005
(708) 253-5500
FUNCTIONS: Information & referral; Educational programs; Day care; Case management; Counseling; Medical assessments; In-home services; Friendly visits; Home delivered meals; Housing assistance; Transportation; Financial services; Legal assistance; Case coordination unit; Protective services; Volunteer opportunities; Senior center; Support groups; Multiple services; Will services

Kenneth W Young Center for Senior Citizens—Hoffman Estates
2500 W Higgins Rd Ste 655, Hoffman Estates, IL 60195
(708) 885-1631
FUNCTIONS: Information & referral; Educational programs; Case management; Counseling; Medical assessments; In-home services; Friendly visits; Home delivered meals; Housing assistance; Transportation; Financial services; Legal assistance; Case coordination unit; Protective services; Volunteer opportunities; Support groups; Multiple services; Will services

YWCA
220 E Chicago St, Elgin, IL 60120
(708) 742-7930
FUNCTIONS: Ethnic services & activities

Zion Senior Center—Zion Park District
2600 Emmaus Ave, Zion, IL 60099
(708) 746-2330
FUNCTIONS: Senior center; Congregate dining

✔ In order to support future editions of this publication would you please mention *Elder Services* each time you contact any advertiser, facility, or service.

Index to Organizations

Advocacy

Area 1 Agency on Aging
Chicago Dept on Aging
Eldercare America
Hemlock of Illinois
Illinois Alliance for Aging
National Caucus & Center on Black Aged—Membership Chapter
Northeastern Illinois Area Agency on Aging—Kankakee
Northeastern Illinois Area Agency on Aging—West Chicago
Older Women's League (OWL)
Polish Welfare Association
South Suburban Senior Services—Catholic Charities
United Charities North Center

Caregiver support

Alzheimer's Disease Association—Chicago Area Chapter
Alzheimer's Family Care Center
Central DuPage Hospital
Chicago Dept on Aging
Council for Jewish Elderly
Council for Jewish Elderly Adult Day Care Center
Family Care Service of Metropolitan Chicago
Family Services Association of Greater Elgin Area
Help at Home
Hinsdale Hospital—ConfiCare
HomeCorps
Hull House Association
Illinois Masonic Medical Center
Japanese American Service Committee
Jewish Family & Community Service Central & South Chicago
Jewish Family & Community Service North Chicago
Living-at-Home Program
Lutheran Social Services of Illinois—Des Plaines
MacNeal Hospital
Mercy Center for Health Care Services
North Shore Senior Center
Northeastern Illinois Area Agency on Aging—Kankakee
Northeastern Illinois Area Agency on Aging—West Chicago
Older Adult Rehabilitation Service (OARS)
Palatine Township Senior Citizens Council
PLOWS Council on Aging
Respitecare
Rush-Presbyterian-St Lukes Medical Center—Bowman Center

Rush-Presbyterian-St Luke's Medical Center—Older Adult Services
St Anthony Medical Center
Suburban Area Agency on Aging
United Charities North Center
United Charities of Chicago Senior Services
Veterans Benefits Administration
Victory Memorial Hospital & Health Services

Case coordination unit

Berwyn/Cicero Council on Aging
Catholic Charities of Chicago
Catholic Charities—Round Lake
DuPage County Dept of Human Resources
Family Counseling Service of Evanston & Skokie Valley—Evanston
Family Counseling Service of Evanston & Skokie Valley—Skokie
Grundy County Health Dept
Lutheran Social Services of Illinois—Chicago
North Shore Senior Center
Oak Park Township Senior Services
Park Place Senior Center
PLOWS Council on Aging
Proviso Council on Aging
Senior Outreach & Referral
Senior Services Associates Inc—Beecher Community Building
Senior Services Associates Inc—Elgin
Senior Services Associates Inc—McHenry
Senior Services Center of Will County
South Suburban Senior Services—Catholic Charities
Southwest Suburban Center on Aging
Stickney Public Health District
United Charities of Chicago
United Charities of Chicago Senior Services
Kenneth W Young Center for Senior Citizens—Arlington Heights
Kenneth W Young Center for Senior Citizens—Hoffman Estates

Case management

The Ark
Berwyn/Cicero Council on Aging
Bloom Township Senior Citizens Services
Catholic Charities—Chicago
Central DuPage Hospital
Chicago Dept on Aging
Council for Jewish Elderly
East Chicago Operation Hope
Elder Link Inc

Erie Family Health Center
Family Care Service of Metropolitan Chicago
Family Counseling Service of Evanston & Skokie Valley—Evanston
Family Counseling Service of Evanston & Skokie Valley—Skokie
Family Services Association of Greater Elgin Area
Five Hospital Homebound Elderly Program
Greater Hammond Community Services
Hinsdale Hospital—ConfiCare
Hobart Township Community Services
HomeCorps
Howard Area Community Center
Hull House Association
Illinois Masonic Medical Center
Jewish Family & Community Service Central & South Chicago
Jewish Family & Community Service North Chicago
Kin Care
Leyden Family Service
Leyden Township Senior Citizens Program
Living-at-Home Program
Lutheran Community Services for the Aged
Lutheran Social Services of Illinois—Des Plaines
Lutheran Social Services of Illinois—Home Helps for Seniors
Mercy Center for Health Care Services
Metro Corps of Gary Inc
Mile Square Health Center Inc
North Shore Senior Center
Northshore Eldercare Management
Oak Park Township Senior Services
Park Place Senior Center
Pathways Consultants for Senior Living Inc
PLOWS Council on Aging
Porter County Council on Aging
Proviso Council on Aging
St Joseph Hospital of Elgin
Senior Care Consultants
Senior Centers of Metropolitan Chicago
Seniors Assistance Center
South Lake County Community Services
South Suburban Senior Services—Catholic Charities
Southwest Suburban Center on Aging
Stickney Public Health District
United Charities North Center
United Charities of Chicago Senior Services

University of Chicago Hospital—Windemere Senior Health Center
Visiting Nurse Association of Chicago
Kenneth W Young Center for Senior Citizens—Arlington Heights
Kenneth W Young Center for Senior Citizens—Hoffman Estates

Congregate dining

The Abbey Leisure Center
Addison Park District
Antioch Senior Center
Area 1 Agency on Aging
Argo-Summit Senior Nutrition Site
Aurora Township Senior Center
Barrington Area Senior Citizens Center Inc
Bensenville Home Society—Castle Towers
Berwyn/Cicero Council on Aging
Bloomingdale Township Senior Center
Bolingbrook Senior Center
Burbank-Stickney Senior Lunch Center
Calumet Township Senior Citizens Service Center
Cary Grove Senior Center
Casa Central
Central Park Towers
Chicago Dept on Aging
Chicago Dept on Aging Central/West Region Senior Center
Chicago Dept on Aging Northeast Region—Levy Senior Center
Chicago Dept on Aging Northwest Region—Copernicus Senior Center
Chicago Dept on Aging Southeast Region—Atlas Senior Center
Chicago Dept on Aging Southwest Region Senior Center
Chicago Heights Senior Sunshine Club
Chinese Consolidated Benevolent Association
Church of the Brethren
Coal City Senior Citizens
Colony Park
Community & Economic Development Association (CEDA)
Community Day Care
Community Nutrition Network Inc
Community Senior Center
Council for Jewish Elderly
Des Plaines Senior Nutrition Site—Des Plaines Mall
Downers Grove Park District Senior Center
Dundee Township Park District
DuPage Senior Citizens Council
East Chicago Operation Hope
Eastern Will County Senior Services
Ela Township Senior Center—Harry Knigge Senior Civic Center
Elk Grove Senior Center
ESSE
Evanston Senior Nutrition Center—Fleetwood-Jourdain Center
Filipino American Council of Chicago

Ford Heights Community Service Senior Center
Franklin Park Senior Nutrition Site—Centre Place
Golden Diners Senior Center
Grace Lutheran Church
Greater Elgin Senior Center
Greater Hammond Community Services
Hartman Center
Harvard Senior Center
Hebron Senior Center
Hobart Township Community Services
Holiday Inn Hotel
Hotel Baker Living Center
Hull House Association
Hyde Park Neighborhood Association
Illinois Chinese American Residence (I-Care)
Immanuel Residence
Japanese American Service Committee
Kennedy Senior Citizens Building
Korean American Community Service
LaSalle Senior Center
Lisle Park District
Lithuanian Human Services
Lockport Congregational Church
Maple Terrace Apartments
Martin Manor
Maywood Senior Nutrition Site
Mercy Center for Health Care Services
Metro Corps of Gary Inc
Mundelein Senior Center
Naperville Park District
New Lennox Community Park District
Ada S Niles Senior Center
North Chicago Senior Center
North Stickney Senior Lunch Center
Oak Lawn Senior Nutrition—Pilgrim Faith Church
Oak Park Senior Center
Oak Park Senior Nutrition Center
Older Adult Rehabilitation Service (OARS)
Operation Push—Mt Zion Baptist Church
Orland Park Senior Nutrition Center
Palatine Township Senior Citizens Council
Park Place Senior Center
Peace Memorial Manor
Pembroke Senior Citizens Center
Phoenix Senior Nutrition Center
Plainfield Park District
Porter County Council on Aging
Presbyterian Home
Proviso Council on Aging
Rich Township Senior Nutrition Program
Riverain Point
Robbins Senior Center
Round Lake Area Senior Center
Salem Towers
Salvation Army Golden Diners
Salvation Army of Elgin
Salvation Army—Second Horizon Senior Center
Schaumburg Health & Human Services

Schaumburg Senior Nutrition Site—The Barn
Senior Citizens Center Golden Age Chateau
Senior Service Association of McHenry County
Senior Service Center
Senior Services Associates Inc—Beecher Community Building
Silver Harvest Senior Delight
South Lake County Community Services
South Suburban Senior Services—Catholic Charities
Southeast Asia Center
Southeastern Grundy Senior Citizens
Southwest Suburban Center on Aging
Stickney Township Office on Aging
Stryker Building
Thornton Township Senior Services
Trinity Adults
Troy Township Senior Citizens Center
Ukrainian Social Service
United Methodist Church
Valley View Community Center
Waukegan Senior Center
West Chicago Community Center of Winfield Township
Westmont Park District Senior Citizens Center
Wheaton Center
Woodstock Nutrition Center
YMCA of Metropolitan Chicago
York Township Senior Center
Zion Senior Center—Zion Park District

Counseling

Access Wisdom Inc
Alcoholics Anonymous
Alzheimer's Disease Association—Chicago Area Chapter
Alzheimer's Family Care Center
American Foundation for the Blind
Asociacion Latina de Servicios Educacionales Inc
Association House of Chicago
Catholic Charities—Chicago
Catholic Family Services—Crown Point
Catholic Family Services—East Chicago
Catholic Family Services—Gary
Catholic Family Services—Michigan City
Catholic Family Services—Portage
Catholic Family Services—Whiting
Chicago Dept on Aging
Community & Economic Development Association (CEDA)
Council for Jewish Elderly
Counseling Center of Lakeview
Elder-Med at Our Lady of Mercy Hospital
Epilepsy Foundation of Greater Chicago
Erie Family Health Center
Erie Neighborhood House
Fairview Baptist Home
Family Counseling Service of Evanston & Skokie Valley—Evanston

✔ In order to support future editions of this publication would you please mention *Elder Services* each time you contact any advertiser, facility, or service.

Family Counseling Service of Evanston
    & Skokie Valley—Skokie
Family Services Association of Greater
    Elgin Area
Five Hospital Homebound Elderly
    Program
Gary Neighborhood Services Inc
Hammond Community Center
Hinsdale Hospital—ConfiCare
HomeCorps
Humana Michael Reese Hospital
Illinois Masonic Medical Center
Japanese American Service Committee
Jewish Family & Community Service
    Central & South Chicago
Jewish Family & Community Service
    North Chicago
Korean American Community Service
LaSalle Senior Center
Lifelink Corporation
Lithuanian Human Services
Living-at-Home Program
Lutheran Community Services for the
    Aged
Lutheran Social Services of
    Illinois—Des Plaines
Mercy Center for Health Care Services
Mile Square Health Center Inc
Ada S Niles Senior Center
North Shore Senior Center
Northshore Eldercare Management
Northwest Counseling Center
Parkside Senior Services—Lutheran
    General Health Care
Presbyterian Home
Referral & Emergency Service
St Joseph Hospital of Elgin
Salvation Army—Family Services
Schaumburg Health & Human Services
Senior Care Consultants
South Suburban Senior
    Services—Catholic Charities
Southwest Suburban Center on Aging
TriCity Family Services
Twin Cities Community Services
United Charities North Center
University of Chicago
    Hospital—Windemere Senior Health
    Center
The University of Illinois Hospital &
    Clinics Geriatric Assessment Center
Kenneth W Young Center for Senior
    Citizens—Arlington Heights
Kenneth W Young Center for Senior
    Citizens—Hoffman Estates

Day care

Alzheimer's Family Care Center
Warren Barr Pavilion of Illinois
    Masonic Medical Center
Bethel New Life Inc
Casa Central
Community & Economic Development
    Association (CEDA)
Council for Jewish Elderly
Council for Jewish Elderly Adult Day
    Care Center
ESSE

Hammond Community Center
Hinsdale Hospital—ConfiCare
Hyde Park Neighborhood Association
Illinois Association of Homes for the
    Aging
Illinois Masonic Medical Center
Japanese American Service Committee
Jewish Family & Community Service
    Central & South Chicago
Jewish Family & Community Service
    North Chicago
Living-at-Home Program
Lutheran Social Services of
    Illinois—Des Plaines
Niles Township Sheltered Workshop
North Shore Senior Center
Nursefinders
Parkside Senior Services—Lutheran
    General Health Care
Presbyterian Home
Proviso Council on Aging
St Joseph Hospital of Elgin
Victory Memorial Hospital & Health
    Services
Wellspring Gerontological Service
Kenneth W Young Center for Senior
    Citizens—Arlington Heights

Educational programs

Alzheimer's Disease
    Association—Chicago Area Chapter
American Academy of Ophthalmology
American Academy of Physical
    Medicine & Rehabilitation
American Association of Retired
    Persons (AARP)—Chicago Area
American Cancer Society—Illinois
    Division
American Diabetes Association
American Foundation for the Blind
American Heart Association of
    Metropolitan Chicago
Arlington Heights Library
Arthritis Foundation—Illinois Chapter
Warren Barr Pavilion of Illinois
    Masonic Medical Center
Berwyn/Cicero Council on Aging
Buehler Center on
    Aging—Northwestern University
Catholic Charities—Chicago
Central DuPage Hospital
Chicago Dept on Aging
Chicago Dept on Aging Central/West
    Region Senior Center
Chicago Dept on Aging Northeast
    Region—Levy Senior Center
Chicago Dept on Aging Northwest
    Region—Copernicus Senior Center
Chicago Dept on Aging Southeast
    Region—Atlas Senior Center
Chicago Dept on Aging Southwest
    Region Senior Center
Chicago Lighthouse for the Blind
Chicago Lung Association
Citizens Information Service of Illinois
Community House
Council for Jewish Elderly
East Chicago Operation Hope

Elder Link Inc
Eldercare America
Epilepsy Foundation of Greater
    Chicago
Fairview Baptist Home
Five Hospital Homebound Elderly
    Program
Grant Hospital of Chicago—Prime Life
Greater Hammond Community Services
Hemlock of Illinois
Hinsdale Hospital—ConfiCare
Hobart Township Community Services
HomeCorps
Howard Area Community Center
Hull House Association
Hyde Park Neighborhood Association
Illinois Association of Homes for the
    Aging
Illinois Attorney General's Office
Illinois Masonic Medical Center
Ingalls Hospital—Senior Life Program
Institute of Medicine of Chicago
Japanese American Service Committee
Jewish Family & Community Service
    Central & South Chicago
Jewish Family & Community Service
    North Chicago
Meyer Kaplan JCC Senior Program
Korean American Community Service
Lincoln West Hospital—Golden Years
    Program
Lithuanian Human Services
Living-at-Home Program
Lord & Taylor Learning Together
    Center of Northbrook Court
Lutheran Community Services for the
    Aged
Lutheran Social Services of
    Illinois—Des Plaines
MacNeal Hospital
Mental Health Association of Greater
    Chicago
Mercy Center for Health Care Services
Mercy Hospital & Medical
    Center—Eldercare
Metro Corps of Gary Inc
Mile Square Health Center Inc
National Association of Claims
    Assistance Professionals Inc
National Caucus & Center on Black
    Aged—Membership Chapter
National Resource Center on Health
    Promotion & Aging
North Shore Senior Center
Northeastern Illinois Area Agency on
    Aging—Kankakee
Northeastern Illinois Area Agency on
    Aging—West Chicago
Northshore Eldercare Management
Northwestern Memorial Hospital Dept
    of Geriatric Services
Oak Park Senior Center
Operation Able
Palatine Township Senior Citizens
    Council
Parkside Senior Services—Lutheran
    General Health Care
PLOWS Council on Aging

Porter County Council on Aging
Presbyterian Home
Roosevelt University
Rush-Presbyterian-St Lukes Medical
    Center—Bowman Center
Rush-Presbyterian-St Luke's Medical
    Center—Older Adult Services
St Anthony Medical Center
St Joseph Hospital & Health Care
    Center—Center for Healthy Aging
St Joseph Hospital of Elgin
Senior Centers of Metropolitan Chicago
Simon Foundation for Continence
South Lake County Community
    Services
Southwest Suburban Center on Aging
Terra Nova Films Inc
Twin Cities Community Services
United Charities of Chicago Senior
    Services
United Parkinson Foundation
University of Chicago
    Hospital—Windemere Senior Health
    Center
Veterans Benefits Administration
Victory Memorial Hospital & Health
    Services
Weinstein Brothers Memorial Chapels
West Suburban Hospital Medical
    Center
Wheeling Township Services
Kenneth W Young Center for Senior
    Citizens—Arlington Heights
Kenneth W Young Center for Senior
    Citizens—Hoffman Estates

Employment

Chicago Dept on Aging
Community House
East Chicago Operation Hope
Greater Hammond Community Services
Hinsdale Hospital—ConfiCare
Hobart Township Community Services
Illinois Alliance for Aging
Metro Corps of Gary Inc
National Caucus & Center on Black
    Aged
Niles Township Sheltered Workshop
Northeastern Illinois Area Agency on
    Aging—Kankakee
Northeastern Illinois Area Agency on
    Aging—West Chicago
Oak Park Senior Center
Operation Able
Porter County Council on Aging
South Lake County Community
    Services
Suburban Area Agency on Aging

Energy assistance program

Arlington Heights Library
Berwyn/Cicero Council on Aging
Bethel New Life Inc
Chinese American Service League
Community & Economic Development
    Association (CEDA)
Community Contracts
East Chicago Operation Hope

Erie Family Health Center
Greater Hammond Community Services
Hobart Township Community Services
Illinois Attorney General's Office
Korean American Community Service
Korean American Senior Association of
    Chicagoland
Korean American Senior Center
Lithuanian Human Services
Metro Corps of Gary Inc
North Shore Senior Center
PLOWS Council on Aging
Porter County Council on Aging
South Lake County Community
    Services
Southeast Asia Center
Southwest Suburban Center on Aging
Ukrainian Social Service

Ethnic services & activities

American GI Forum
American GI Forum—Women's
    Auxiliary
American Indian Center
American Spanish Institute
Apostolic Assembly
ASI
Asian Human Services of Chicago
Association House of Chicago
Association of Indians in America
Austin Peoples Action Center
Beacon Neighborhood House
Burmese American Association of
    Chicago
Cambodian Assistance Project
Casa Central
Catholic Charities—Joliet
Caza Aztlan
Centro Cristo Ray
Centro de Informacion y Progreso
Chicago Dept on Aging
Chicago Roseland Coalition
Chinese American Civic Council
Chinese American Service League
Chinese Consolidated Benevolent
    Association
Chinese Mutual Aid Association
Peter Claver Center
Coalition of Limited English-Speaking
    Elderly Inc
Concerned Citizens of Little Village
Council for Jewish Elderly
El Centro Pan Americano
El Primer Paso
El Valor Corporation
Englewood Community Health
    Organization
Filipino American Council of Chicago
Filipino Association of America
First Baptist Church
Gideon Baptist Church
Golden Agers Service Foundation
Greater Faith Baptist Church
Greek American Community Services
Hellenic Foundation
Hill Memorial Center
Holy Ghost Church
Honduran Association of Waukegan

Illinois Chinese American Residence
    (I-Care)
Illinois Migrant Council—Aurora
Illinois Migrant Council—Momence
Illinois Migrant Council—Mundelein
Japanese American Citizens League
Japanese American Service Committee
Jewish Federation of Metro Chicago
Kenwood-Oakland Community
    Organization
Korean American Association of
    Chicago
Korean American Senior Association of
    Chicagoland
Korean American Senior Center
Korean Self-Help Community Center
Lake County Community Civic
    Organization
Lake County Urban League
Laotian Service Center
Latino Institute
League of United Latin American
    Citizens (LULAC)
Lithuanian Community Services
Lithuanian Human Services
Lutheran Social Services of
    Illinois—Elmhurst
Ada S McKinley Community Services
Metropolitan YMCA Third Age Program
Mexican Society
Mt Sinai Baptist Church
Mujeres Latinas en Accion
NAACP
National Association of Hispanic
    Elderly
National Caucus & Center on Black
    Aged
National Council of Jewish Women
Native American Education Services
Native American Outpost
North Suburban Self-Help Center
Operation Push—Mt Zion Baptist
    Church
Peoples Resource Center
Polish National Alliance
Polish Welfare Association
Prisoner Release Ministry Inc
Puerta Albierta
Puerto Rican Society
Quad County Urban League
St Alexis Church
St Augustine's Center for American
    Indians
St Charles Pastoral Center
St Joseph Church
St Mary's Church—Spanish Center
St Petronille Catholic Church
Salvation Army
Senior Club of Lake County
SER—Jobs for Progress Inc
Shawsau Temple
Shiloh Baptist Church
Spanish Center
Travelers & Immigrants Aid
Trinity AME Church
Vietnamese Community Service Center
Vriangato Association
World Relief Corporation
YWCA

✔ In order to support future editions of this publication would you please mention *Elder Services* each time you contact
any advertiser, facility, or service.

Exercise

Central DuPage Hospital
Chicago Dept on Aging
Gottlieb Memorial Hospital
Hinsdale Hospital—ConfiCare
Meyer Kaplan JCC Senior Program
Palatine Township Senior Citizens
    Council
St Joseph Hospital of Elgin
Wheeling Township Services

Financial services

Elder Link Inc
Erie Family Health Center
First National Bank of Geneva
Harris Bank
Jewish Family & Community Service
    Central & South Chicago
Jewish Family & Community Service
    North Chicago
Korean American Community Service
Korean American Senior Association of
    Chicagoland
Korean American Senior Center
North Shore Senior Center
Retirement Security Inc—An MRM
    Group
Southwest Suburban Center on Aging
United Charities North Center
United Charities of Chicago Senior
    Services
Wellspring Gerontological Service
Kenneth W Young Center for Senior
    Citizens—Arlington Heights
Kenneth W Young Center for Senior
    Citizens—Hoffman Estates

Friendly visits

Berwyn/Cicero Council on Aging
Catholic Charities—Chicago
Chicago Dept on Aging
Community & Economic Development
    Association (CEDA)
Council for Jewish Elderly
Erie Neighborhood House
Fairview Baptist Home
Family Care Service of Metropolitan
    Chicago
Five Hospital Homebound Elderly
    Program
Greek American Community Services
Hinsdale Hospital—ConfiCare
HomeCorps
Hull House Association
Illinois Masonic Medical Center
Korean American Community Service
Korean American Senior Association of
    Chicagoland
Korean American Senior Center
LaSalle Senior Center
Lithuanian Human Services
Little Brothers—Friends of the Elderly
North Shore Senior Center
Palatine Township Senior Citizens
    Council
PLOWS Council on Aging

Presbyterian Home
Proviso Council on Aging
Schaumburg Health & Human Services
Senior Centers of Metropolitan Chicago
Seniors Assistance Center
Southwest Suburban Center on Aging
Visiting Nurse Association of Chicago
Kenneth W Young Center for Senior
    Citizens—Arlington Heights
Kenneth W Young Center for Senior
    Citizens—Hoffman Estates

Home delivered meals

Argo-Summit Senior Nutrition Site
The Ark
Berwyn/Cicero Council on Aging
Burbank-Stickney Senior Lunch Center
Calumet Township Senior Citizens
    Service Center
Chicago Dept on Aging
Chicago Heights Senior Sunshine Club
Community & Economic Development
    Association (CEDA)
Community Nutrition Network Inc
Council for Jewish Elderly
Des Plaines Senior Nutrition Site—Des
    Plaines Mall
DuPage Senior Citizens Council
East Chicago Operation Hope
Erie Family Health Center
Erie Neighborhood House
Evanston Senior Nutrition
    Center—Fleetwood-Jourdain Center
Ford Heights Community Service
    Senior Center
Franklin Park Senior Nutrition
    Site—Centre Place
Greater Hammond Community Services
Harvey High Rise
Hinsdale Hospital—ConfiCare
Hobart Township Community Services
Hull House Association
Hyde Park Neighborhood Association
Japanese American Service Committee
Jewish Family & Community Service
    Central & South Chicago
Jewish Family & Community Service
    North Chicago
Lifelink Corporation
Lithuanian Human Services
Little Brothers—Friends of the Elderly
Living-at-Home Program
Lutheran Community Services for the
    Aged
Lutheran Social Services of
    Illinois—Des Plaines
MacNeal Hospital
Maywood Senior Nutrition Site
Mercy Center for Health Care Services
Methodist Hospital
Metro Corps of Gary Inc
North Stickney Senior Lunch Center
Oak Lawn Senior Nutrition—Pilgrim
    Faith Church
Oak Park Senior Center
Palatine Township Senior Citizens
    Council
Park Place Senior Center

Parkside Senior Services—Lutheran
    General Health Care
Phoenix Senior Nutrition Center
PLOWS Council on Aging
Porter County Council on Aging
Proviso Council on Aging
Robbins Senior Center
St Anthony Medical Center
St Joseph Hospital of Elgin
Schaumburg Senior Nutrition Site—The
    Barn
Senior Centers of Metropolitan Chicago
Senior Citizens Center Golden Age
    Chateau
Seniors Assistance Center
Albert J Smith Activities Center
South Lake County Community
    Services
South Suburban Senior
    Services—Catholic Charities
Southwest Suburban Center on Aging
Stickney Township Office on Aging
Wheeling Township Services
Kenneth W Young Center for Senior
    Citizens—Arlington Heights
Kenneth W Young Center for Senior
    Citizens—Hoffman Estates

Home health services

Central DuPage Hospital
Community Contracts
Council for Jewish Elderly
Erie Family Health Center
Family Care Service of Metropolitan
    Chicago
Five Hospital Homebound Elderly
    Program
Gottlieb Memorial Hospital
Hinsdale Hospital—ConfiCare
HomeCorps
Illinois Association of Homes for the
    Aging
Illinois Masonic Medical Center
MacNeal Hospital
Mercy Hospital & Medical
    Center—Eldercare
Methodist Hospital
Mile Square Health Center Inc
North Shore Senior Center
Northwestern Memorial Hospital Dept
    of Geriatric Services
Nursefinders
Osteopathic Hospitals & Medical
    Centers
St Anthony Medical Center
St Joseph Hospital of Elgin
St Mary of Nazareth Hospital Center
Schaumburg Health & Human Services
Victory Memorial Hospital & Health
    Services
Visiting Nurse Association of Chicago
Wellspring Gerontological Service
West Suburban Hospital Medical
    Center

Home repairs

Berwyn/Cicero Council on Aging
Bethel New Life Inc
Chicago Dept on Aging
Community & Economic Development
  Association (CEDA)
HomeCorps
LaSalle Senior Center

Hospice

Alzheimer's Family Care Hospice
Central DuPage Hospital
Community Nursing Service West
  Hospice
DeKalb County Hospice
Fox Valley Hospice
Grundy Community Hospice
Hinsdale Hospital—ConfiCare
Home Hospice—Visiting Nurse
  Association North
Horizon Hospice
Hospice Care Chicagoland
Hospice Care Chicagoland North
Hospice of DuPage Inc
Hospice of Highland Park Hospital
Hospice of Illinois Medical Center
Hospice of Little Company of Mary
  Hospital
Hospice of Northeastern Illinois Inc
Hospice of the North Shore
Hospice of West Suburban Hospital
Hospice Suburban South
Illinois Association of Homes for the
  Aging
Illinois Masonic Medical Center
Joliet Area Community Hospice Inc
LaGrange Memorial Hospice
Lake Forest Hospital Hospice
Lutheran Community Services for the
  Aged
Medical Personnel Pool—Oak Lawn
Medical Personnel Pool—Oak Park
Meridian Hospice
Northwest Community Hospital Home
  Hospice
Northwestern Memorial Hospital Dept
  of Geriatric Services
Northwestern Memorial Hospital
  Hospice Program
Rainbow Hospice Inc
St Francis Hospice
St James Hospice
St Thomas Hospice
STAR Hospice—St Therese Medical
  Center
Visiting Nurse Association Hospice of
  Chicago
Visiting Nurse Association of Chicago
West Suburban Hospital Medical
  Center
West Towns Hospice

Housing assistance

Bethel New Life Inc
Chicago Housing Authority
Community & Economic Development
  Association (CEDA)
Fairview Baptist Home

Howard Area Community Center
Illinois Alliance for Aging
Illinois Association of Homes for the
  Aging
Interfaith Housing Center of the
  Northern Suburbs
Japanese American Service Committee
Korean American Community Service
Korean American Senior Association of
  Chicagoland
Korean American Senior Center
LaSalle Senior Center
Lifelink Corporation
Lithuanian Human Services
Little Brothers—Friends of the Elderly
Ada S Niles Senior Center
North Shore Senior Center
Pathways Consultants for Senior Living
  Inc
Personal Packers & Moving Consultants
  Inc
PLOWS Council on Aging
Presbyterian Home
Retirement Relocation Planning Inc
Suburban Area Agency on Aging
Victory Memorial Hospital & Health
  Services
YMCA of Metropolitan Chicago
Kenneth W Young Center for Senior
  Citizens—Arlington Heights
Kenneth W Young Center for Senior
  Citizens—Hoffman Estates

Information & referral

Access Wisdom Inc
Alliance for the Mentally Ill
Alzheimer's Disease
  Association—Chicago Area Chapter
Alzheimer's Family Care Center
American Academy of Ophthalmology
American Academy of Physical
  Medicine & Rehabilitation
American Association of Retired
  Persons (AARP)—Chicago Area
American Cancer Society—Illinois
  Division
American Diabetes Association
American Foundation for the Blind
American Heart Association of
  Metropolitan Chicago
Area 1 Agency on Aging
The Ark
Arthritis Foundation—Illinois Chapter
Asociacion Latina de Servicios
  Educacionales Inc
Association House of Chicago
Berwyn/Cicero Council on Aging
Bethel New Life Inc
Bloom Township Senior Citizens
  Services
Blue Island Senior Citizens Project
Catholic Charities—Chicago
Catholic Family Services—Crown Point
Catholic Family Services—East Chicago
Catholic Family Services—Gary
Catholic Family Services—Michigan
  City
Catholic Family Services—Portage

Catholic Family Services—Whiting
Central DuPage Hospital
Chicago Dept on Aging
Chicago Dept on Aging Central/West
  Region Senior Center
Chicago Dept on Aging Northeast
  Region—Levy Senior Center
Chicago Dept on Aging Northwest
  Region—Copernicus Senior Center
Chicago Dept on Aging Southeast
  Region—Atlas Senior Center
Chicago Dept on Aging Southwest
  Region Senior Center
Chicago Lighthouse for the Blind
Chicago Lung Association
Children of Aging Parents
Citizens Information Service of Illinois
Community & Economic Development
  Association (CEDA)
Community Contracts
Community House
Concerned Relatives of Nursing Home
  Patients
Cook County Senior Citizen's Legal
  Services
Council for Jewish Elderly
DuPage County Health Dept
DuPage Senior Citizens Council
East Chicago Operation Hope
Elder Link Inc
Eldercare America
Elder-Med at Our Lady of Mercy
  Hospital
Epilepsy Foundation of Greater
  Chicago
Fairview Baptist Home
Family Counseling Service of Evanston
  & Skokie Valley—Evanston
Family Counseling Service of Evanston
  & Skokie Valley—Skokie
Family Services Association of Greater
  Elgin Area
Five Hospital Homebound Elderly
  Program
Gary Neighborhood Services Inc
Gottlieb Memorial Hospital
Grant Hospital of Chicago—Prime Life
Greater Hammond Community Services
Hammond Community Center
Hinsdale Hospital—ConfiCare
Hobart Township Community Services
HomeCorps
Howard Area Community Center
Hull House Association
Illinois Alliance for Aging
Illinois Attorney General's Office
Illinois Citizens for Better Care
Illinois Dept of Rehab
  Services—Services for the Visually
  Handicapped
Illinois Dept on Aging—Chicago
Illinois Dept on Aging—Springfield
Illinois Masonic Medical Center
Indiana Dept of Human Services
Japanese American Service Committee
Jewish Family & Community Service
  Central & South Chicago

✔ In order to support future editions of this publication would you please mention *Elder Services* each time you contact
any advertiser, facility, or service.

Jewish Family & Community Service
   North Chicago
Kin Care
LaSalle Senior Center
Leyden Family Service
Leyden Township Senior Citizens
   Program
Lincoln West Hospital—Golden Years
   Program
Lithuanian Human Services
Little Brothers—Friends of the Elderly
Living-at-Home Program
Lutheran Community Services for the
   Aged
Lutheran Social Services of
   Illinois—Des Plaines
Lutheran Social Services of
   Illinois—Home Helps for Seniors
Maine Township Senior Services
Mental Health Association of Greater
   Chicago
Mercy Center for Health Care Services
Mercy Hospital & Medical
   Center—Eldercare
Methodist Hospital
Metro Corps of Gary Inc
National Association for Home Care
National Association of Claims
   Assistance Professionals Inc
National Association of Private
   Geriatric Care Managers
National Health Information
   Clearinghouse
National Resource Center on Health
   Promotion & Aging
Ada S Niles Senior Center
North Shore Senior Center
Northeastern Illinois Area Agency on
   Aging—Kankakee
Northeastern Illinois Area Agency on
   Aging—West Chicago
Northshore Eldercare Management
Northwest Counseling Center
Northwestern Memorial Hospital Dept
   of Geriatric Services
Oak Park Township Senior Services
Older Women's League (OWL)
Operation Able
Osteopathic Hospitals & Medical
   Centers
PACE
Park Place Senior Center
Parkside Senior Services—Lutheran
   General Health Care
PLOWS Council on Aging
Polish Welfare Association
Porter County Council on Aging
Proviso Council on Aging
Referral & Emergency Service
Respitecare
Retirement Security Inc—An MRM
   Group
Rush-Presbyterian-St Lukes Medical
   Center—Bowman Center
Rush-Presbyterian-St Luke's Medical
   Center—Older Adult Services
St Joseph Hospital & Health Care
   Center—Center for Healthy Aging

St Joseph Hospital of Elgin
Self-Help Center
Senior Care Consultants
Senior Centers of Metropolitan Chicago
Seniors Assistance Center
Simon Foundation for Continence
South Lake County Community
   Services
South Suburban Senior
   Services—Catholic Charities
Southwest Suburban Center on Aging
Stickney Public Health District
Stickney Township Office on Aging
Suburban Area Agency on Aging
Twin Cities Community Services
United Charities North Center
United Charities of Chicago Senior
   Services
United Parkinson Foundation
The University of Illinois Hospital &
   Clinics Geriatric Assessment Center
Veterans Benefits Administration
Victory Memorial Hospital & Health
   Services
West Suburban Hospital Medical
   Center
Wheeling Township Services
Kenneth W Young Center for Senior
   Citizens—Arlington Heights
Kenneth W Young Center for Senior
   Citizens—Hoffman Estates

In-home services

American Spanish Institute
The Ark
Association House of Chicago
Berwyn/Cicero Council on Aging
Bethel New Life Inc
Catholic Charities—Chicago
Central DuPage Hospital
Chicago Dept on Aging
Community & Economic Development
   Association (CEDA)
Community Contracts
Council for Jewish Elderly
Counseling Center of Lakeview
East Chicago Operation Hope
Elderly in Distress
Erie Family Health Center
Family Care Service of Metropolitan
   Chicago
Five Hospital Homebound Elderly
   Program
Gottlieb Memorial Hospital
Greater Hammond Community Services
Help at Home
Hinsdale Hospital—ConfiCare
Hobart Township Community Services
Home Companion Services
HomeCorps
Japanese American Service Committee
Jewish Family & Community Service
   Central & South Chicago
Jewish Family & Community Service
   North Chicago
Korean American Community Service
Korean American Senior Association of
   Chicagoland

Korean American Senior Center
LaSalle Senior Center
Leyden Family Service
Lithuanian Human Services
Little Brothers—Friends of the Elderly
Living-at-Home Program
Lutheran Community Services for the
   Aged
Lutheran Social Services of
   Illinois—Des Plaines
Lutheran Social Services of
   Illinois—Home Helps for Seniors
MacNeal Hospital
Medical Personnel Pool—Oak Lawn
Medical Personnel Pool—Oak Park
Methodist Hospital
Metro Corps of Gary Inc
North Shore Senior Center
Northwestern Memorial Hospital Dept
   of Geriatric Services
Nursefinders
Oak Park Township Senior Services
Parkside Senior Services—Lutheran
   General Health Care
PLOWS Council on Aging
Porter County Council on Aging
Proviso Council on Aging
Respitecare
St Catherine Hospital
St Joseph Hospital of Elgin
Salvation Army—Family Services
Senior Centers of Metropolitan Chicago
South Lake County Community
   Services
South Suburban Senior
   Services—Catholic Charities
Southwest Suburban Center on Aging
United Charities of Chicago Senior
   Services
University of Chicago
   Hospital—Windemere Senior Health
   Center
Visiting Nurse Association of Chicago
Wellspring Gerontological Service
YMCA of Metropolitan Chicago
Kenneth W Young Center for Senior
   Citizens—Arlington Heights
Kenneth W Young Center for Senior
   Citizens—Hoffman Estates

Legal assistance

Berwyn/Cicero Council on Aging
Catholic Charities—Chicago
Chicago Dept on Aging
Chicago Volunteer Legal Services
Cook County Senior Citizen's Legal
   Services
Council for Jewish Elderly
Hull House Association
Illinois Masonic Medical Center
Japanese American Service Committee
Jewish Family & Community Service
   Central & South Chicago
Jewish Family & Community Service
   North Chicago
Korean American Community Service
Korean American Senior Association of
   Chicagoland

Korean American Senior Center
Lake County Prosecutor's Office Adult
    Protective Services
Legal Aid Society of Greater Hammond
Legal Assistance Foundation of
    Chicago
Legal Services Program of Greater Gary
PLOWS Council on Aging
Senior Centers of Metropolitan Chicago
Southwest Suburban Center on Aging
United Charities of Chicago Senior
    Services
John C Wunsch
Kenneth W Young Center for Senior
    Citizens—Arlington Heights
Kenneth W Young Center for Senior
    Citizens—Hoffman Estates

Medical assessments

Berwyn/Cicero Council on Aging
Central DuPage Hospital
Community & Economic Development
    Association (CEDA)
Council for Jewish Elderly
Five Hospital Homebound Elderly
    Program
Gottlieb Memorial Hospital
Grant Hospital of Chicago—Prime Life
Hinsdale Hospital—ConfiCare
HomeCorps
Humana Michael Reese Hospital
Illinois Masonic Medical Center
Japanese American Service Committee
Korean American Community Service
Lincoln West Hospital—Golden Years
    Program
Lithuanian Human Services
Lutheran Social Services of
    Illinois—Des Plaines
MacNeal Hospital
Mercy Center for Health Care Services
Methodist Hospital
Mile Square Health Center Inc
North Shore Senior Center
Northwestern Memorial Hospital Dept
    of Geriatric Services
Osteopathic Hospitals & Medical
    Centers
PLOWS Council on Aging
Presbyterian Home
Rush-Presbyterian-St Lukes Medical
    Center—Bowman Center
Rush-Presbyterian-St Luke's Medical
    Center—Older Adult Services
St Joseph Hospital of Elgin
Schaumburg Health & Human Services
Southwest Suburban Center on Aging
United Charities of Chicago Senior
    Services
The University of Illinois Hospital &
    Clinics Geriatric Assessment Center
Veterans Benefits Administration
Victory Memorial Hospital & Health
    Services
West Suburban Hospital Medical
    Center
Kenneth W Young Center for Senior
    Citizens—Arlington Heights

Kenneth W Young Center for Senior
    Citizens—Hoffman Estates

Medical claims & billing assistance

Claim Cure
H P Medical Claim Consultants
HomeCorps
Medical Claim Services Inc
Medicare Claims (Part B)
Mercy Hospital & Medical
    Center—Eldercare
St Joseph Hospital & Health Care
    Center—Center for Healthy Aging
Victory Memorial Hospital & Health
    Services
West Suburban Hospital Medical
    Center

Medical health services

Alexian Brothers Medical Centers
Central DuPage Hospital
Chicago Hearing Society
Des Plaines Valley Health Center
Gottlieb Memorial Hospital
Grant Hospital of Chicago—Prime Life
Hinsdale Hospital—ConfiCare
Ingalls Hospital—Senior Life Program
Jewish Family & Community Service
    Central & South Chicago
Jewish Family & Community Service
    North Chicago
Lincoln West Hospital—Golden Years
    Program
Little Company of Mary Hospital Senior
    Services
Loyola University Medical Center
Lutheran Community Services for the
    Aged
MacNeal Hospital
Medical Personnel Pool—Oak Lawn
Medical Personnel Pool—Oak Park
Mercy Center for Health Care Services
Methodist Hospital
Northwestern Memorial Hospital Dept
    of Geriatric Services
Osteopathic Hospitals & Medical
    Centers
Park Forest Nurses PLUS Home Health
    Care
Parkside Senior Services—Lutheran
    General Health Care
Rehabilitation Institute of Chicago
Rush-Presbyterian-St Lukes Medical
    Center—Bowman Center
Rush-Presbyterian-St Luke's Medical
    Center—Older Adult Services
St Anthony Medical Center
St Mary of Nazareth Hospital Center
Schaumburg Health & Human Services
Twin Cities Community Services
University of Chicago
    Hospital—Windemere Senior Health
    Center
The University of Illinois Hospital &
    Clinics Geriatric Assessment Center
Veterans Benefits Administration
Victory Memorial Hospital & Health
    Services

West Suburban Hospital Medical
    Center

Medicare & supplemental security income assistance

Chicago Dept on Aging
Elder Link Inc
Howard Area Community Center
Illinois Citizens for Better Care
Medical Claim Services Inc
National Consumer Oriented Agency

Mental health services

Central DuPage Hospital
Charter Hospital of Northwest Indiana
Family Counseling Service of Evanston
    & Skokie Valley—Evanston
Family Counseling Service of Evanston
    & Skokie Valley—Skokie
Gary Community Mental Health Center
Gottlieb Memorial Hospital
Hinsdale Hospital—ConfiCare
Kingwood Hospital
MacNeal Hospital
Mental Health Association in Lake
    County
Mercy Center for Health Care Services
Northwestern Memorial Hospital Dept
    of Geriatric Services
Osteopathic Hospitals & Medical
    Centers
Porter-Starke Services Inc
St Anthony Medical Center
St Joseph Hospital of Elgin
St Mary of Nazareth Hospital Center
Southlake Center for Mental
    Health—Hobart
Southlake Center for Mental
    Health—Merrillville
Southlake Center for Mental
    Health—Schererville
Tri-City Comprehensive Community
    Mental Health Center Inc—East
    Chicago
Tri-City Comprehensive Community
    Mental Health Center
    Inc—Hammond
Victory Memorial Hospital & Health
    Services

Multiple locations

Catholic Charities—Chicago
Chicago Dept on Aging
Community & Economic Development
    Association (CEDA)
First National Bank of Geneva
MacNeal Hospital
Medical Personnel Pool—Oak Lawn
Medical Personnel Pool—Oak Park
Mercy Center for Health Care Services
Northeastern Illinois Area Agency on
    Aging—Kankakee
Northeastern Illinois Area Agency on
    Aging—West Chicago
Osteopathic Hospitals & Medical
    Centers
St Joseph Hospital of Elgin

✔ In order to support future editions of this publication would you please mention *Elder Services* each time you contact
any advertiser, facility, or service.

United Way of Chicago—Crusade of Mercy
West Suburban Hospital Medical Center

Multiple services

Berwyn/Cicero Council on Aging
Bloom Township Senior Citizens Services
Blue Island Senior Citizens Project
Bremen Township Senior Services
Calumet Township Senior Citizens Service Center
Catholic Charities of Chicago
Catholic Charities—Round Lake
The Center of Concern
Chicago Dept on Aging
Community & Economic Development Association (CEDA)
Council for Jewish Elderly
Des Plaines Municipal Offices
DuPage County Dept of Human Resources
Elder Link Inc
Evanston Commission on Aging
Evergreen Park Senior Center
Glenview Senior Center Rugen Community Center
Grundy County Health Dept
Hanover Township
Jones Memorial Community Center
Leyden Family Service
Leyden Township Senior Citizens Program
Lincolnwood Senior Services
Lutheran Social Services of Illinois—Elmhurst
Maine Township Senior Services
Medical Personnel Pool—Oak Lawn
Medical Personnel Pool—Oak Park
Howard Mohr Community Center Senior Citizen Program
Morton Grove Senior Center
Niles Senior Citizens Services
North Shore Senior Center
Northbrook Senior Center
Northeastern Illinois Area Agency on Aging—Kankakee
Northeastern Illinois Area Agency on Aging—West Chicago
Park Place Senior Center
Park Ridge Senior Center
Pavilion Senior Center
PLOWS Council on Aging
Rich Township Senior Center
St Joseph Hospital & Health Care Center—Center for Healthy Aging
Senior Citizens of Schaumburg Township Inc
Senior Outreach & Referral
Senior Services Associates Inc—Beecher Community Building
Senior Services Associates Inc—Elgin
Senior Services Associates Inc—McHenry
Senior Services Center of Will County
Albert J Smith Activities Center
Southwest Suburban Center on Aging

Stickney Public Health District
Stickney Township Office on Aging
Suburban Area Agency on Aging
Thornton Township Senior Services
United Charities of Chicago Senior Services
United Way of Chicago—Crusade of Mercy
Kenneth W Young Center for Senior Citizens—Arlington Heights
Kenneth W Young Center for Senior Citizens—Hoffman Estates

Ombudsman services

Area 1 Agency on Aging
Chicago Dept on Aging
Evanston Commission on Aging
Indiana Dept of Human Services

Protective services

Berwyn/Cicero Council on Aging
Cook County Office of the Public Guardian
Family Counseling Service of Evanston & Skokie Valley—Evanston
Family Counseling Service of Evanston & Skokie Valley—Skokie
Illinois Alliance for Aging
Leyden Family Service
Leyden Township Senior Citizens Program
Lutheran Social Services of Illinois—Des Plaines
Lutheran Social Services of Illinois—Home Helps for Seniors
North Shore Senior Center
Oak Park Township Senior Services
Park Place Senior Center
PLOWS Council on Aging
Proviso Council on Aging
Seniors Assistance Center
South Suburban Senior Services—Catholic Charities
Southwest Suburban Center on Aging
Stickney Public Health District
Suburban Area Agency on Aging
Kenneth W Young Center for Senior Citizens—Arlington Heights
Kenneth W Young Center for Senior Citizens—Hoffman Estates

Publications

American Academy of Ophthalmology
American Academy of Physical Medicine & Rehabilitation
American Association of Retired Persons (AARP)—Chicago Area
American Foundation for the Blind
Warren Barr Pavilion of Illinois Masonic Medical Center
Central DuPage Hospital
Citizens Information Service of Illinois
Eldercare America
Hemlock of Illinois
Lutheran Community Services for the Aged
MacNeal Hospital

Mental Health Association of Greater Chicago
Mercy Center for Health Care Services
Mercy Hospital & Medical Center—Eldercare
National Council on the Aging Inc
National Resource Center on Health Promotion & Aging
Northeastern Illinois Area Agency on Aging—Kankakee
Northeastern Illinois Area Agency on Aging—West Chicago
Osteopathic Hospitals & Medical Centers
Rush-Presbyterian-St Luke's Medical Center—Older Adult Services
St Joseph Hospital & Health Care Center—Center for Healthy Aging
St Joseph Hospital of Elgin
Simon Foundation for Continence
Suburban Area Agency on Aging
United Parkinson Foundation
West Suburban Hospital Medical Center

Recreation

Warren Barr Pavilion of Illinois Masonic Medical Center
Berwyn/Cicero Council on Aging
Catholic Charities—Chicago
Chicago Dept on Aging
Chicago Dept on Aging Central/West Region Senior Center
Chicago Dept on Aging Northeast Region—Levy Senior Center
Chicago Dept on Aging Northwest Region—Copernicus Senior Center
Chicago Dept on Aging Southeast Region—Atlas Senior Center
Chicago Dept on Aging Southwest Region Senior Center
Community & Economic Development Association (CEDA)
DuPage Senior Citizens Council
East Chicago Operation Hope
Erie Family Health Center
Fairview Baptist Home
Gottlieb Memorial Hospital
Grant Hospital of Chicago—Prime Life
Greater Hammond Community Services
Hobart Township Community Services
Hyde Park Neighborhood Association
Illinois Masonic Medical Center
Japanese American Service Committee
Meyer Kaplan JCC Senior Program
Korean American Community Service
Korean American Senior Association of Chicagoland
Korean American Senior Center
LaSalle Senior Center
Lithuanian Human Services
Mercy Hospital & Medical Center—Eldercare
Metro Corps of Gary Inc
North Shore Senior Center
Oak Park Senior Center
Palatine Township Senior Citizens Council

Porter County Council on Aging
Presbyterian Home
River Forest Community Center Senior
　Program
Senior Centers of Metropolitan Chicago
South Lake County Community
　Services
Southwest Suburban Center on Aging
Twin Cities Community Services
Veterans Benefits Administration
YMCA of Metropolitan Chicago

Respite services

Central DuPage Hospital
Chicago Dept on Aging
Council for Jewish Elderly
Fairview Baptist Home
Family Care Service of Metropolitan
　Chicago
Gottlieb Memorial Hospital
Help at Home
Hinsdale Hospital—ConfiCare
HomeCorps
Illinois Association of Homes for the
　Aging
Illinois Masonic Medical Center
Kin Care
Lutheran Community Services for the
　Aged
Medical Personnel Pool—Oak Lawn
Medical Personnel Pool—Oak Park
North Shore Senior Center
Nursefinders
Palatine Township Senior Citizens
　Council
Presbyterian Home
Respitecare
St Catherine Hospital
St Joseph Hospital of Elgin
Salvation Army—Family Services
South Suburban Senior
　Services—Catholic Charities
United Charities of Chicago Senior
　Services
Victory Memorial Hospital & Health
　Services
Visiting Nurse Association of Chicago
Wellspring Gerontological Service

Retirement benefits

First National Bank of Geneva
Harris Bank
Retirement Security Inc—An MRM
　Group

Senior center

The Abbey Leisure Center
Antioch Senior Center
Aurora Township Senior Center
Autumn Country Club
Barrington Area Senior Citizens Center
　Inc
Beecher Community Center
Berwyn/Cicero Council on Aging
Bloomingdale Township Senior Center
Bolingbrook Senior Center
Bradley Bourbannais Senior Citizens
Cary Grove Senior Center

Catholic Charities—Chicago
Channahon Park District
Chicago Dept on Aging
Chicago Dept on Aging Central/West
　Region Senior Center
Chicago Dept on Aging Northeast
　Region—Levy Senior Center
Chicago Dept on Aging Northwest
　Region—Copernicus Senior Center
Chicago Dept on Aging Southeast
　Region—Atlas Senior Center
Chicago Dept on Aging Southwest
　Region Senior Center
Coal City Senior Citizens
Community House of Hinsdale Senior
　Center
Community Senior Center
Council for Jewish Elderly
Deatherage-Drdak Senior Center
Deerfield Senior Center
Des Plaines Community Senior Center
Downers Grove Park District Senior
　Center
Dundee Township Park District
East Chicago Operation Hope
Eastern Will County Senior Services
Ela Township Senior Center—Harry
　Knigge Senior Civic Center
Elk Grove Senior Center
Ford Heights Community Service
　Senior Center
Fox Lake Senior Center
Fox River Grove Senior Center
Fox Valley Park District
Geneva Park District
Glen Ellyn Drop-In Center
Glen Ellyn Park District Senior Adult
　Program
Glen Ellyn Senior Service Center
Golden Diners Senior Center
Greater Elgin Senior Center
Greater Hammond Community Services
Hartman Center
Harvard Senior Center
Hebron Senior Center
Highland Park Senior Center
Hobart Township Community Services
Hull House Association
Hyde Park Neighborhood Association
Marie Irwin Community Center
Japanese American Service Committee
Jewish Family & Community Service
　Central & South Chicago
Jewish Family & Community Service
　North Chicago
Kankakee County Senior Citizens
　Center
Korean American Community Service
Lake Forest—Lake Bluff Gorton Senior
　Center
LaSalle Senior Center
Levy Center
Lisle Park District
Lithuanian Human Services
Little Brothers—Friends of the Elderly
Lockport Congregational Church
Lombard Community Senior Center

Lutheran Social Services of
　Illinois—Des Plaines
Mayslake Village Senior Center
Metro Corps of Gary Inc
Morris Senior Center
Mt Prospect Senior Citizens Center
Mundelein Senior Center
Naperville Park District
New Horizon Community Center
North Chicago Senior Center
North Shore Senior Center
Oak Lawn Senior Center
Oak Park Senior Center
Oak Park Township Senior Services
Older Adult Rehabilitation Service
　(OARS)
Palatine Township Senior Citizens
　Council
Park Place Senior Center
Parkside Senior Services—Lutheran
　General Health Care
Pavilion Senior Center
Pembroke Senior Citizens Center
Porter County Council on Aging
Prospect Heights Senior Center
Proviso Council on Aging
Robbins Senior Center
Rolling Meadows Senior Center
Round Lake Area Senior Center
Salvation Army Golden Diners
Salvation Army—Second Horizon
　Senior Center
Salvation Army Senior Services &
　Center
Schaumburg Health & Human Services
Schaumburg Senior Center
Senior Adult Center—Leaning Tower
　YMCA
Senior Centers of Metropolitan Chicago
Senior Citizens Center Golden Age
　Chateau
Senior Service Association of McHenry
　County
Senior Services Center of Will County
　Albert J Smith Activities Center
South Lake County Community
　Services
South Suburban Senior
　Services—Catholic Charities
Southeastern Grundy Senior Citizens
Southwest Suburban Center on Aging
Troy Township Senior Citizens Center
Valley View Community Center
Vernon Hills Senior Citizens
Warren Township Senior Center
Waukegan Park District Older Adult
　Program—Lilac Cottage Senior
　Center
Waukegan Senior Center
Wayne Township Seniors
Westmont Park District Senior Citizens
　Center
Wheaton Park District Senior Center
Willowbrook/Burr Ridge/Pleasant Dale
　Senior Center
YMCA of Metropolitan Chicago
York Township Senior Center

✔ In order to support future editions of this publication would you please mention *Elder Services* each time you contact
any advertiser, facility, or service.

Kenneth W Young Center for Senior
    Citizens—Arlington Heights
Zion Senior Center—Zion Park District

Social services

American Red Cross
Warren Barr Pavilion of Illinois
    Masonic Medical Center
Central DuPage Hospital
Chicago Dept on Aging
Gottlieb Memorial Hospital
Hinsdale Hospital—ConfiCare
HomeCorps
Howard Area Community Center
Lincoln West Hospital—Golden Years
    Program
Living-at-Home Program
MacNeal Hospital
Mercy Center for Health Care Services
Palatine Township Senior Citizens
    Council
Pathways Consultants for Senior Living
    Inc
St Anthony Medical Center
St Joseph Hospital of Elgin
St Mary of Nazareth Hospital Center
University of Chicago
    Hospital—Windemere Senior Health
    Center
Victory Memorial Hospital & Health
    Services
West Suburban Hospital Medical
    Center
Wheeling Township Services

Support groups

Alcoholics Anonymous
Alliance for the Mentally Ill
Arthritis Foundation—Illinois Chapter
Association House of Chicago
Catholic Charities—Chicago
Central DuPage Hospital
Council for Jewish Elderly
Council for Jewish Elderly Adult Day
    Care Center
Epilepsy Foundation of Greater
    Chicago
Erie Family Health Center
Fairview Baptist Home
Family Services Association of Greater
    Elgin Area
Gottlieb Memorial Hospital
Hinsdale Hospital—ConfiCare
Howard Area Community Center
Hull House Association
Illinois Association of Homes for the
    Aging
Illinois Masonic Medical Center
Japanese American Service Committee
Jewish Family & Community Service
    Central & South Chicago
Jewish Family & Community Service
    North Chicago
Korean American Community Service
Lifelink Corporation
Lincoln West Hospital—Golden Years
    Program
Living-at-Home Program

Lutheran Community Services for the
    Aged
MacNeal Hospital
Mercy Center for Health Care Services
Mercy Hospital & Medical
    Center—Eldercare
Mile Square Health Center Inc
North Shore Senior Center
Palatine Township Senior Citizens
    Council
Park Place Senior Center
Parkside Senior Services—Lutheran
    General Health Care
Presbyterian Home
Respitecare
Rush-Presbyterian-St Lukes Medical
    Center—Bowman Center
Rush-Presbyterian-St Luke's Medical
    Center—Older Adult Services
St Joseph Hospital of Elgin
Salvation Army—Family Services
Self-Help Center
Senior Centers of Metropolitan Chicago
Simon Foundation for Continence
Southwest Suburban Center on Aging
Anita Stone Jewish Community Center
United Charities North Center
United Charities of Chicago Senior
    Services
Veterans Benefits Administration
Victory Memorial Hospital & Health
    Services
Weinstein Brothers Memorial Chapels
Wellspring Gerontological Service
West Suburban Hospital Medical
    Center
Kenneth W Young Center for Senior
    Citizens—Arlington Heights
Kenneth W Young Center for Senior
    Citizens—Hoffman Estates

Transportation

Berwyn/Cicero Council on Aging
Bloom Township Senior Citizens
    Services
Chicago Dept on Aging
Community & Economic Development
    Association (CEDA)
East Chicago Operation Hope
Greater Hammond Community Services
Hobart Township Community Services
HomeCorps
Hyde Park Neighborhood Association
Illinois Masonic Medical Center
LaSalle Senior Center
Leyden Family Service
Lincoln West Hospital—Golden Years
    Program
Lithuanian Human Services
Little Brothers—Friends of the Elderly
Lutheran Social Services of
    Illinois—Home Helps for Seniors
Metro Corps of Gary Inc
Mile Square Health Center Inc
North Shore Senior Center
Older Adult Rehabilitation Service
    (OARS)
Orland Township Senior Services

PACE
Palos Area Transportation Services for
    the Elderly
PLOWS Council on Aging
Porter County Council on Aging
PRC Paratransit Services Inc
Presbyterian Home
Proviso Council on Aging
Rich Township Senior Center
Senior Citizens of Schaumburg
    Township Inc
Seniors Assistance Center
South Lake County Community
    Services
South Suburban Senior
    Services—Catholic Charities
Southwest Suburban Center on Aging
Thornton Township Senior Services
Wheeling Township Services
Kenneth W Young Center for Senior
    Citizens—Arlington Heights
Kenneth W Young Center for Senior
    Citizens—Hoffman Estates

Volunteer opportunities

Warren Barr Pavilion of Illinois
    Masonic Medical Center
Berwyn/Cicero Council on Aging
Calumet City Youth & Family Services
Central DuPage Hospital
Chicago Dept on Aging
DuPage County Dept of Human
    Resources
DuPage Senior Citizens Council
Hinsdale Hospital—ConfiCare
Howard Area Community Center
Illinois Alliance for Aging
Lutheran Community Services for the
    Aged
Lutheran Social Services of
    Illinois—Des Plaines
Mercy Center for Health Care Services
North Shore Senior Center
Northeastern Illinois University Student
    Volunteer Corps
Osteopathic Hospitals & Medical
    Centers
Palatine Township Senior Citizens
    Council
Park Place Senior Center
Parkside Senior Services—Lutheran
    General Health Care
Proviso Council on Aging
St Anthony Medical Center
St Joseph Hospital of Elgin
St Mary of Nazareth Hospital Center
Suburban Area Agency on Aging
United Way of Will County Volunteer
    Services
Victory Memorial Hospital & Health
    Services
Volunteer Network
Kenneth W Young Center for Senior
    Citizens—Arlington Heights
Kenneth W Young Center for Senior
    Citizens—Hoffman Estates

Will services
The Center of Concern
Des Plaines Municipal Offices
Evanston Commission on Aging
Niles Senior Citizens Services

Park Ridge Senior Center
PLOWS Council on Aging
Senior Citizens of Schaumburg
  Township Inc
Seniors Assistance Center

Kenneth W Young Center for Senior
  Citizens—Arlington Heights
Kenneth W Young Center for Senior
  Citizens—Hoffman Estates

✔ In order to support future editions of this publication would you please mention *Elder Services* each time you contact any advertiser, facility, or service.

MERCYELDERCARE
Comprehensive Services for Older Adults and Caregivers

In-Patient Care:

- Older Adult Unit
- Rehabilitation Unit
- Older Adult Psychiatry Program
- Skilled Nursing Unit
- Alcohol and Drug Dependency Program
- Diabetes Treatment Center

Out-Patient Care:

- Mercy Home Health Care/Private Duty Services
- Eye Center
- Audiology Services
- Physical Medicine and Rehabilitation Services
- Support and Self-help Groups
- Caregiver Classes
- Health Promotion Lectures and Classes

Long-Term Care:

- Mercy Health Care and Rehabilitation Center in Homewood
- Respite Care

In addition to these services, MercyEldercare also provides:

- Lifepass membership program for people 55 and Up
- Information and referrals about programs and services in the Chicago metropolitan area

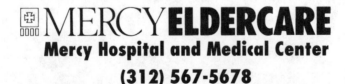

MERCYELDERCARE
Mercy Hospital and Medical Center
(312) 567-5678

Should Your Relative Live Alone?

This checklist may serve as a guide to evaluate if your older relative should continue to live alone.

SAFETY NEEDS

Yes No

- ☐ ☐ Has your relative had accidents because of weakness, dizziness, or inability to get around?
- ☐ ☐ Has use of the stove, oven, or appliances become a safety problem because of forgetfulness?
- ☐ ☐ Are there hazardous conditions in your relative's home, such as the bathroom and bedroom being on separate floors?
- ☐ ☐ Does your relative refuse to use a wheelchair, walker, or other assisting devices necessary for safety?
- ☐ ☐ Does your relative express a desire to die, or seem to be depressed, apathetic, or without an interest in living?

NUTRITIONAL NEEDS

Yes No

- ☐ ☐ Is your relative unable or unwilling to use the kitchen for food preparation?
- ☐ ☐ Is there a demonstrated nutritional problem (weight loss, illness, anemia, etc.)?
- ☐ ☐ Does your relative eat only inappropriate foods that will not supply nutritional needs?
- ☐ ☐ Does your relative "forget" to eat?

PERSONAL HYGIENE

Yes No

- ☐ ☐ Is your relative unwilling or unable to get to the toilet when necessary?
- ☐ ☐ Is your relative unable to change clothing or bed linens as necessary to remain clean and dry?

MEDICAL NEEDS

Yes No

- ☐ ☐ Does your relative forget to take necessary medications?
- ☐ ☐ Is it likely that your relative would take an inappropriate dose of medicine, purposely or accidentally?
- ☐ ☐ Is your relative physically unable to handle medications (spills or drops them) or to give injections?
- ☐ ☐ Is your relative unable to obtain help in case of need?
- ☐ ☐ If hearing is severely impaired, does your relative refuse to use an aid or shut it off?

SOCIAL NEEDS

Yes No

- ☐ ☐ Is your relative unable to handle money?
- ☐ ☐ Does your relative get lost in familiar situations?
- ☐ ☐ Has your relative left home without a destination?
- ☐ ☐ Has your relative behaved inappropriately in public (exposed self, threatened others, etc.)?

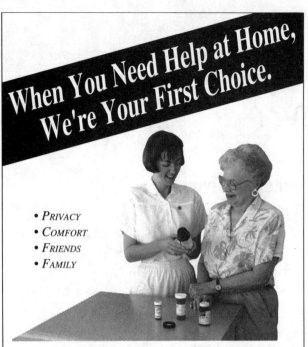
☐ ☐ Does your relative have mental or emotional problems that might be a threat to self or others?

These questions are phrased in such a way that "Yes" answers suggest a problem. If you answered "Yes" to some of them, you should be thinking of, and planning for, the probability that your relative will need additional care and support in the future. If many of your responses were a definite "Yes," a change may be needed very soon. Depending on your relative's needs, the change may mean caring for the person in your own home, in an adult family home, in a congregate-care facility, or choosing a retirement or nursing home.

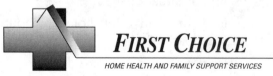

Home Care Needs Checklist

Use as a guide to assess your home care needs. Check those areas where you feel assistance is needed.

Personal and Domestic Needs

☐ Bathing/grooming
☐ Dressing
☐ Shopping
☐ Cooking
☐ Feeding
☐ Getting into and out of bed
☐ Getting to the bathroom
☐ Walking
☐ Transportation
☐ House cleaning
☐ Laundry
☐ Pet care
☐ Other _____

Medical Needs

☐ Taking medication
☐ Using eye drops
☐ Changing dressing
☐ Catheter care
☐ Exercises
☐ Other _____

Questions to Ask about Care for Your Relative within Your Own Home

This checklist may serve as a guide to help you decide if your older relative should be cared for in your home.

HEALTH AND SAFETY

Yes No

☐ ☐ Would your home require major modifications to provide an adequate environment for your relative (heating, plumbing, laundry facilities, accessible bathrooms, etc.)?

☐ ☐ Would it be necessary to modify your home to increase safety (add railings, etc.) or allow mobility?

☐ ☐ Does your relative require nursing services that are too physically difficult or demanding for you (turning, transfer to toilet, etc.)?

☐ ☐ Is your relative likely to regularly disturb the sleep of others by calling out, needing care, or wandering?

☐ ☐ Is your relative likely to wander away from you or the house if left unsupervised?

☐ ☐ Is your relative likely to create safety hazards for other family members because of forgetfulness or carelessness (falling asleep while smoking, misuse of appliances, etc.)?

TIME AND ENERGY

Yes No

☐ ☐ Does your relative require someone available at all times to provide personal care?

☐ ☐ Must clothing and bed linens be changed and laundered so frequently that this becomes an excessive physical demand?

☐ ☐ Do you have other family responsibilities that could result in split loyalties and/or emotional overload?

EMOTIONAL CONSIDERATIONS

Yes No

☐ ☐ Has your relative become emotionally explosive or verbally abusive?

☐ ☐ Has your relative accused you or others of trying to kill him/her (poisoning food, etc.) or stealing money?

☐ ☐ Have you become cut off from friends and other family members because of the demands of caring for your relative?

☐ ☐ Have you given up activities and interests that are important to you because of the demands of caring for your relative?

PERSONAL CONSIDERATIONS

Yes No

☐ ☐ Does your relative interfere with the running of your household?

☐ ☐ Has loss of privacy become a problem for the adult members of the household (a strain on marriage)?

☐ ☐ Is there conflict with younger adults and adolescent family members because of the presence of your relative?

SITUATIONAL CONSIDERATIONS

Yes No

☐ ☐ Is it necessary for the family to change homes or move to another community, making continued care unrealistic?

☐ ☐ Has financial demand made continued employment or longer work hours necessary?

☐ ☐ Has a helping, supportive family member moved out of the household, increasing the burden for remaining caregivers?

☐ ☐ Has an additional family emergency created conflict or competition for time and energy?

These questions are phrased in such a way that "Yes" answers suggest a problem. If you answered "Yes" to very many of these questions, you will probably want to reconsider caring for your relative in your own home and begin to explore a change in living arrangements for your relative. Depending on your relative's needs, the change may mean finding a congregate-care facility, bringing in community services, or choosing an adult foster home or a nursing home. To assist in this, prescreening services are offered by state and other agencies to help you determine what your relative's needs are. Case management programs coordinate services to assist in this effort to obtain the best and most appropriate care.

It is important also to have a current, thorough medical evaluation of some of the apparent medical and social problems of your relative. For example, can appropriate medication assist in alleviating some of the problems? Are drugs prescribed in the proper dosage, that is, too much or too little? Are the combination of drugs being taken harmful in their joint effect?

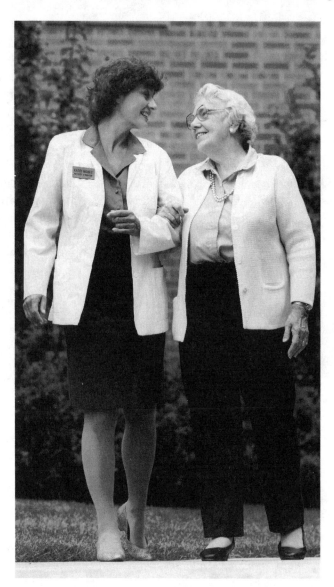

Questions to Ask When Selecting a Nursing Home

This checklist may serve as a guide when looking for a nursing home or evaluating one already being used.

GENERAL

Yes No

☐ ☐ Does the home have a license from the state Board of Health?

☐ ☐ Is the administrator licensed by the state Board of Health?

☐ ☐ Is there a written statement of the resident's rights clearly posted?

☐ ☐ Are visiting hours convenient for residents and visitors?

LOCATION

Yes No

☐ ☐ Is the home near family and friends?

☐ ☐ Is the home reasonably close to a hospital offering emergency services?

☐ ☐ Does the location enable family, friends and the resident's physician to visit?

GENERAL PHYSICAL CHARACTERISTICS

Yes No

☐ ☐ Is the nursing home clean, orderly, and relatively odor-free?

☐ ☐ Is the home well lighted?

☐ ☐ Are the rooms kept at a comfortable temperature and well ventilated?

☐ ☐ Are toilet and bathing facilities accessible to handicapped residents?

☐ ☐ Is the furniture attractive, comfortable, safe, and easy for elderly people to get in and out of?

ATTITUDES AND ATMOSPHERE

Yes No

☐ ☐ Is the general atmosphere of the nursing home warm, pleasant, and cheerful?

☐ ☐ Is the administrator courteous and helpful?

☐ ☐ Are staff members cheerful, courteous, and enthusiastic or do they appear angry and intimidating?

☐ ☐ Do staff members take time to visit with residents?

☐ ☐ Do staff members show residents genuine interest and affection?

☐ ☐ Are residents treated with dignity and respect by staff?

☐ ☐ Do residents look well cared for and generally content?

☐ ☐ Can residents bring any of their own furniture with them?

☐ ☐ Are residents allowed to wear their own clothes, decorate their rooms, and keep a few prized possessions in their rooms?

☐ ☐ Do staff knock on the door before entering a resident's room?

Used with permission from *Nursing Home Life: A Guide for Residents and Families* published by the American Association of Retired Persons.

✔ In order to support future editions of this publication would you please mention **Elder Services** each time you contact any advertiser, facility, or service.

☐ ☐ Do staff speak to residents about their activities and where the residents are being taken?

☐ ☐ Do you see groups of nursing assistants watching television in anyone's room or in the day room or do they seem attentive to residents' needs?

☐ ☐ Do residents, other visitors, and volunteers speak favorably about the home?

☐ ☐ Is there a sense of fellowship among the residents?

SAFETY

Yes No

☐ ☐ Is the nursing home free of obvious risks, such as obstacles to residents, hazards underfoot, unsteady chairs?

☐ ☐ Are there grab bars in the toilet and bathing facilities and handrails on both sides of the hallways?

☐ ☐ Are hallways wide enough to permit wheelchairs to pass each other easily?

☐ ☐ Do bathtubs and showers have nonslip surfaces?

☐ ☐ Are residents prohibited from smoking in their rooms?

☐ ☐ Are smoke detectors, the automatic sprinkler system, and automatic emergency lighting in good operating order?

☐ ☐ Are there portable fire extinguishers?

☐ ☐ Are exits clearly marked and exit signs illuminated?

☐ ☐ Are exit doors unobstructed and unlocked from inside?

☐ ☐ Is an emergency evacuation plan posted in prominent locations?

☐ ☐ Are there fire drills involving staff and residents?

☐ ☐ Are doors to stairways kept closed?

MEDICAL, DENTAL, AND OTHER SERVICES

Yes No

☐ ☐ Is the prospective resident's physician willing to visit the home?

☐ ☐ In the case of medical emergencies, is a physician available at all times, either on staff or on call?

☐ ☐ Does the home have arrangements with a nearby hospital for quick transfer of nursing home residents in an emergency?

☐ ☐ Does the home allow the resident to be treated by a physician of his/her own choice?

☐ ☐ Is the resident involved in developing the care plan?

☐ ☐ Is confidentiality of medical records assured?

☐ ☐ Does the home have an arrangement with an outside dental service to provide residents with dental care when necessary?

☐ ☐ Is at least one registered nurse (RN) or licensed practical nurse (LPN) on duty day and night?

☐ ☐ Is an RN on duty during the day, seven days a week?

☐ ☐ Does an RN serve as director of nursing services?

☐ ☐ If the person to be placed requires special services, such as therapy or a special diet, does the home provide them?

PHARMACEUTICAL SERVICES

Yes No

☐ ☐ Are pharmaceutical services supervised by a qualified pharmacist?

☐ ☐ Is a room set aside for storing and preparing drugs and other pharmaceutical items?

☐ ☐ Does a qualified pharmacist maintain and monitor a record of each resident's drug therapy?

☐ ☐   Are residents allowed to choose their own pharmacist?

FOOD SERVICES

Yes No

☐ ☐   Is the kitchen clean and reasonably tidy? Is perishable food properly refrigerated? Is waste properly disposed of? Do kitchen staff follow good standards of food handling?

☐ ☐   Ask to see the meal schedule. Are at least three meals served each day? Are meals served at normal hours, with plenty of time for leisurely eating?

☐ ☐   Are nutritious between-meal and bedtime snacks available?

☐ ☐   Are residents given enough food? Does the food look appetizing?

☐ ☐   Sample a meal. Is the food tasty and served at the proper temperature?

☐ ☐   Does the meal being served match the posted menu?

☐ ☐   Are special meals prepared for patients on therapeutic diets?

☐ ☐   Are meals planned by a trained dietitian?

☐ ☐   Is the dining room attractive and comfortable?

☐ ☐   Are small tables used rather than mess-hall type tables?

☐ ☐   Can residents have visitors join them at meal time? Is there a charge?

☐ ☐   Do residents who need it get help in eating, whether in the dining room or in their own rooms?

RESIDENTS' ROOMS AND COMMUNAL AREAS

Yes No

☐ ☐   Does each room open onto a hallway?

☐ ☐   Does each room have a window to the outside?

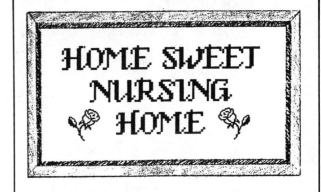
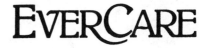
✔ In order to support future editions of this publication would you please mention **Elder Services** each time you contact any advertiser, facility, or service.

☐ ☐ Does each resident have a reading light, a comfortable chair, and a closet and drawers for personal belongings?

☐ ☐ Is fresh drinking water within reach?

☐ ☐ Is there a curtain or screen available to provide privacy for each bed whenever necessary?

☐ ☐ Do bathing and toilet facilities have adequate privacy?

☐ ☐ Does the resident have any input into the assignment of roommates?

☐ ☐ Are nurse and emergency call buttons located at each resident's bed, toilet, and bathing facility?

☐ ☐ Is there a lounge where residents can chat, read, play games, watch television, or just relax away from their rooms?

☐ ☐ Is a public telephone available for residents' use?

☐ ☐ Does the nursing home have an outdoor area where residents can get fresh air and sunshine?

SOCIAL SERVICES AND RESIDENT ACTIVITIES

Yes No

☐ ☐ Are social services available to aid residents and their families?

☐ ☐ Are residents encouraged, but not forced, to participate in activities?

☐ ☐ Do residents have an opportunity to attend religious services and talk with clergy both in and outside the home?

☐ ☐ Do staff assist the residents in getting from their rooms to activities?

☐ ☐ Are residents encouraged to participate in community activities outside the nursing home (health permitting)?

☐ ☐ Does the nursing home have a varied program of recreational, cultural, and intellectual activities for residents?

☐ ☐ Are there group and individual activities?

☐ ☐ Is there an activities coordinator on the staff?

☐ ☐ Is suitable space available for resident activities? Are tools and supplies provided?

☐ ☐ Are activities offered for residents who are relatively inactive or confined to their rooms?

☐ ☐ Look at the activities schedule. Are activities provided each day? Are some activities scheduled in the evenings and weekends? Are those posted activities actually taking place?

TRANSPORTATION

Yes No

☐ ☐ Does the nursing home provide transportation for residents?

☐ ☐ Is the home on a bus route for convenience of residents and visitors?

FINANCIAL CONSIDERATIONS

Yes No

☐ ☐ Is the home certified to participate in the Medicare and/or Medicaid programs?

☐ ☐ Are many of the services needed included in the basic charge?

☐ ☐ Do the estimated monthly costs (including extra charges) compare favorably with the costs of other homes?

☐ ☐ Is a refund made for unused days paid for in advance?

☐ ☐ Is a list of fees for specific services not covered in the basic rate readily available?

✔ In order to support future editions of this publication would you please mention **Elder Services** each time you contact any advertiser, facility, or service.

☐ ☐ Does the contract between the resident and the home clearly state:
    costs?
    date of admission?
    services to be provided?
    discharge and transfer conditions?

☐ ☐ Do the resident's assets remain in his/her control or that of his/her family?

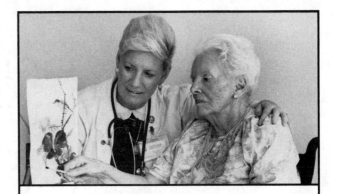

✔ In order to support future editions of this publication would you please mention **Elder Services** each time you contact any advertiser, facility, or service.

Questions to Ask When Inquiring about a Day Care Center

This checklist may serve as a guide when inquiring about a day care center or program for your older relative.

What are the entrance requirements? Is there a waiting list?

What days and hours is the day care center open?

What professional credentials make up the staff of the center: executive director, administrator, social worker, nurse, activities director, aides?

What is the cost of day care? Does it differ depending on the number of days per week the person is there? Are there subsidies available?

What type of transportation serves the center? What does it cost?

Are meals and snacks provided?

What are the components of the program: health monitoring, care plans, etc.?

Are the groups divided by the needs and characteristics of the clients?

What are the safety procedures if a client leaves the building? Are the building and grounds secure?

What is the policy for handling and responding to medical emergencies?

What activities are offered? Are outings away from the center offered?

Are personal care needs available (such as bathing, hair care)?

Are caregiver support groups available? Are other support and referral services available?

WHY BE BOTHERED?

Wrong numbers. Unsolicited solicitations. Pranksters. Nosy neighbors. How do you separate these little annoyances from the phone calls you really care about? Like calls from your favorite friends and family?

The solution is Caller ID, new from Illinois Bell. Caller ID clearly shows the caller's number on a display screen that's attached to your phone. It's incredibly easy to use. And affordable, too.

When the phone rings and you're not sure how to answer, the answer is Caller ID.

CALLER ID.
For information and availability, call
1-800-428-2111
Dept. 89.

During its introduction, Caller ID will give you numbers of calls placed within your local Illinois Bell calling area. Both you and the caller must be in specially-equipped calling areas for numbers to appear on your display screen. Display equipment is purchased separately. If you want to block the appearance of your number when you place a call, dial *67 on your touchtone phone, or 1167 on rotary dials. The activation of your blocking is confirmed with a stutter, followed by a dial tone.

© 1992, Illinois Bell

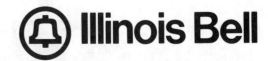

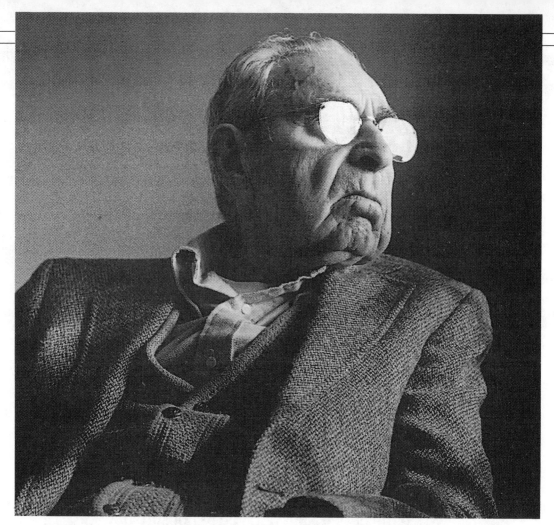

"This is my father, Abe. 77 years old and still too proud to ask for help."

If your father is like most, he'll never admit to needing help. Which is why you should know about Lifeline. A very special service that calls for help when you can't be there. Activated by the press of a button, it puts your father in touch with well-trained professionals who know everything about him: his age, his address, his medical conditions. Plus the phone numbers of neighbors and relatives who can assist when an ambulance isn't necessary. More than a medical alert service, Lifeline is someone you can trust to watch over your loved one every hour of every day. Someone you can call a friend.

For more information about a service your father will one day thank you for, contact:

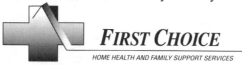

FIRST CHOICE

HOME HEALTH AND FAMILY SUPPORT SERVICES

708/ 383-2500

LIFELINE®

You've got a friend™

Helpline Numbers

AIDS Hotline . . . . available 24 hours a day (800) 342-7514

Alcoholics Anonymous . . . . available 24 hours a day (312) 346-1475

Alzheimers Association . . . . (708) 933-1000
available 24 hours a day (800) 621-0379

American Council of the Blind . . . . (800) 424-8666

American Heart Association . . . . (800) 242-1793

American Red Cross . . . . (312) 440-2000

Arthritis Consulting Services . . . . (800) 327-2027

Arthritis Foundation . . . . (800) 572-2397

Better Hearing Institute . . . . (800) EAR-WELL

Cancer Information . . . . (800) 422-6237

Communicating for Seniors (Health) . . . . (800) 432-3276

Community Caring Helpline (Nationwide) . . . . (800) 252-8966

Community Crisis Center (Elgin) . . . . 24-hour hotline (708) 697-2380

Crisisline . . . . available 24 hours a day (312) 941-0707

Drug Abuse Hotline . . . . (312) 878-3838

Elder Abuse Hotline (Nationwide) . . . . (800) 252-8966
(708) 596-6690 South Suburban Chicago

ELDERLINK Nationwide . . . . (800) 252-8966

Emergency & Referral Services . . . . (800) 782-7860

Healthcare Hotline . . . . (800) 325-9564

Home-Line/Illinois Housing . . . . (800) 942-8439

Hospice Link . . . . (800) 331-1620

Medicare Hotline . . . . (800) 647-8089

National Council on the Aging . . . . (800) 424-9046

National Eye Care Project . . . . (800) 222-EYES

National Parkinsons Disease Foundation . . . . (800) 327-4545

Nursing Home Info . . . . (800) 252-4343

Senior Action Center . . . . (800) 252-6565

Social Security . . . . (800) 772-1213

Suicide Prevention Hotline . . . . (312) 769-6200

Tele-Help (North Suburban Chicago) . . . . (708) 291-0085

Veteran's Benefits Hotline . . . . (800) 827-0466

Helpful Materials for Caregivers

PUBLICATIONS

Helping the Aging Family by Victoria E. Bumagin and Kathryn F. Hirn. Published by Scott, Foresman and Company, 1990. A guide of interactive intervention, counseling, and coping strategies.

How to Care for Your Parents by Nora Jean Levin. Published by Storm King Press, 1990. Compact, inexpensive handbook for adult children.

How to Choose a Retirement Community by Martha S. Schumann. Published by RRP Ltd., 213 Institute Place, Suite 305, Chicago, IL 60610, (312) 664-6672. A guide to choosing a retirement center. Includes all the questions you need to ask.

It's Your Move by Dona Hollifield, 900 N. Lake Shore Drive, Chicago, IL 60611, (312) 335-0504. Detailed how to's of moving from one residence to another.

Taking Care by Mary Roman, M.S.W. Published by the Metropolitan Chicago Coalition on Aging, 1989. A handbook for family caregivers for older adults.

36-Hour Day by Nancy Mace and Peter Rabins, M.D. Published by Johns Hopkins University Press, 1981. A guide to caring for persons with dementing illnesses and memory loss later in life.

When Love Gets Tough by Doug Manning. Published by In-Sight Books, 1985. A guide to making the nursing home decision. Also several booklets available.

ORGANIZATIONS

AARP Publications, Program Resources Dept. BV, 1909 K. Street N.W., Washington, DC 20049. Write and request a listing of publications. AARP has a wide range of topics available.

The Center for Applied Gerontology, 3003 W. Touhy Avenue, Chicago, IL 60645, (312) 508-1073. Programs, seminars, workshops, and educational materials.

Centering Corporation, Box 3367, Omaha, NE 68103. Newsletter and publications on many topics of interest to older people, caregivers, and other professionals. Catalog available.

Elder Press, 731 Treat Avenue, San Francisco, CA 94110. Activity resources for older adults. Memory makers, books, audio and video tapes. Catalogs available.

Rush Alzheimer's Disease Center, 1725 W. Harrison Street, Chicago, IL 60612, (312) 942-6799. Various publications and videos available for free, rent, and purchase.

Terra Nova Films, Inc., 9848 S. Winchester Avenue, Chicago, IL 60643, (312) 881-8491. Over 70 film topics related to aging available for rent and/or purchase.

Abbreviations Used in the Directory

ORGANIZATION OR PROGRAM ABBREVIATIONS

AAA Area Agency on Aging

AAHA American Academy of Health Administration; American Association of Homes for the Aging

ACDD Accreditation Council on Services for People with Developmental Disabilities

ACSM American College of Sports Medicine

ACSW Academy of Certified Social Workers

ADRDA Alzheimer's Disease and Related Disorders Association, also known as The Alzheimer's Association

AFCSP Alzheimer's Family and Caregiver Support Program

AHA American Health Association

AHCA American Health Care Association

AMA American Medical Association

AOA American Osteopathic Association

APA American Psychology Association

APHA American Partial Hospitalization Association

APTA American Physical Therapy Association

ASHA American Speech Language Hearing Association

ATC Athletic Trainer Certified

CAP College of American Pathologists

CARF Commission on Accreditation of Rehabilitative Facilities

CBRF Community Based Residential Facility

CCAC Continuing Care Accreditation Commission

CCP Community Care Program

CHAMPUS Civilian Health and Medical Program of the Uniformed Services

CJE Council for Jewish Elderly

CMHP Community Mental Health Provider

COA Council on Accreditation

CORF Certified Outpatient Rehab Facility

CSALA Community Supervised Apartment Living Arrangements

CSWE Council on Social Work Education

DHS Department of Health Services or Department of Human Services

DPW Department of Public Welfare

HCA Health Care Administration

HCFA Health Care Financing Administration

HFC Health Facilities Council

IAHA Illinois Association of Homes for the Aging; Indiana Hospital Association

IAPRS International Association of Psychosocial Rehabilitation Services

IBH Industries for the Blind and Handicapped
IDOA Illinois Department on Aging
IDPH Illinois Department of Public Health
IHA Indiana Hospital Association
IHCA Illinois Health Care Association
JCAHO Joint Commission on Accreditation of Healthcare Organizations
NAATP National Association of Addiction Treatment Providers
NAC National Accreditation Council
NAPPH National Association of Private Psychiatric Hospitals
NAPRF National Association of Private Residential Facilities
NAPRR National Association of Private Residential Resources
NARF National Association of Rehabilitative Facilities
NASUA National Association of State Units on Aging
NISH National Industries for the Severely Handicapped
SS Social Security
SSI Supplemental Security Income
VA Veterans Administration

CONDITIONS AND FACILITIES ABBREVIATIONS

ADC Adult day care
ADHC Adult day health care
CMI Chronic mental illness
DD Developmental disability
ICF Intensive care facility
ICF/MR Intermediate care facility for mentally retarded
IQ Intelligence quotient
MH Mental health or mental hygiene
MI Mental illness
MPSC Multipurpose senior center

MR Mental retardation
RCF Residential care facility
SNF Skilled nursing facility

OTHER TEXT ABBREVIATIONS

Admin Administration or administrator
Admis Admissions
Amer American
Apt Apartment
Assn Association
Asst Assistant
BSW Bachelor of Social Work
CEO Chief Executive Officer
Cert Certification
Chair Chairperson
CNA Certified Nurse's Aide
Comm Community
Coord Coordinator
CPE Certificate for Physical Education (British)
CSW Certified Social Worker
Dept Department
Dir Director
Div Division
DME Durable Medical Equipment
DON Director of Nursing
EEG Electroencephalogram
Exec Executive
Ft Full-time
Gen General
Hosp Hospital
I & R Information and Referral
LPN Licensed Practical Nurse
LPT Licensed Physical Therapist
LSW Licensed Social Worker
LTC Long-term care insurance
LVN Licensed Visiting Nurse; Licensed Vocational Nurse
Mgr Manager
MSW Master of Social Work
Natl National

✔ In order to support future editions of this publication would you please mention **Elder Services** each time you contact any advertiser, facility, or service.

OT	Occupational Therapist; Occupational Therapy		**Rehab**	Rehabilitation or rehabilitative
OTR	Occupational Therapist, Registered		**Rep**	Representative
Pres	President		**Res**	Residential
Prog	Program		**RN**	Registered Nurse
Proj	Project		**Soc**	Social
Psych	Psychiatric		**Sr**	Senior
Pt	Part-time		**ST**	Speech Therapist; Speech Therapy
PT	Physical Therapist; Physical Therapy		**Supt**	Superintendent
Reg	Regional		**Svc(s)**	Service(s)
			Tech	Technician; Technical

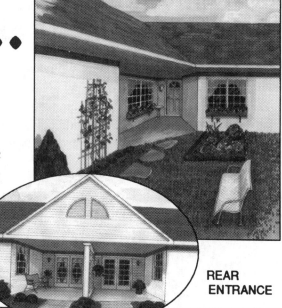
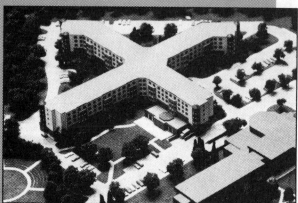

DIRECTORY OF
FACILITIES

You might not be able to give your parents good health, but you can give them good health care.

As your parents grow older, their healthcare requirements will also change. And that is the benefit of having a system of healthcare services working for you. Whether you have concerns about where your parents will reside in the future, or whether you have already identified a need for more comprehensive medical care, Central DuPage Health System has a continuum of services to respond to their needs:

A Life-care Retirement Community   Wyndemere provides a gracious living environment and comprehensive services to its residents. We will be opening our retirement community in 1993. Please call for additional information.

Alzheimer's Assessment Program   Central DuPage Hospital, in conjunction with Community Convalescent Center of Naperville and the Alzheimer's Disease Center of Rush-Presbyterian-St. Luke's Hospital, offers professional and personal resources for the evaluation and management of this disease.

Home Healthcare Services and Home IV Therapy
Community Nursing Service of DuPage brings a full range of healthcare services into the home, including skilled nursing care; therapies; social service; home health aide, homemaker, and Hospice services.

Intermediate/Skilled Care Facility   Community Convalescent Center of Naperville is committed to meeting the distinct needs of older adults, including short-term care for convalescence or rehabilitation, long-term care and Alzheimer's care.

For more information on how Central DuPage Health System can make health care work for you and your parents, please call our Information and Referral Service at **708-260-2685**.

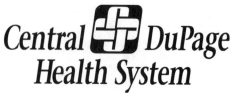

Central DuPage Health System

1151 E. Warrenville Road
Naperville, Illinois 60563

M a k i n g   H e a l t h   C a r e   W o r k   F o r   Y o u .

Adult Day Care Centers

ILLINOIS

Arlington Heights

Northwest Community Hospital Adult Day Care Center at Park Place Senior Center
306 W Park St, Arlington Heights, IL 60005
(708) 392-1015, 577-3677
CONTACT: Becky Vasilakis
CLIENTS SERVED PER MONTH: 50
HOURS OF OPERATION: Mon-Fri, 7:30 am - 5:30 pm
MEALS: Lunch; Snack
SERVICES OFFERED: Rehabilitative and supportive care; Nutritional guidance; Exercise and socialization; Transportation to and from program; Health maintenance and assessment; Financial counseling; Legal counseling; Mental health counseling.

Parkside Adult Day Health Center
811 E Central Rd, Arlington Heights, IL 60005
(708) 439-5900, 439-5912 FAX
CONTACT: Intake specialist
CLIENTS SERVED PER MONTH: 35 per day
HOURS OF OPERATION: Mon-Fri, 7:00 am - 5:30 pm
MEALS: Lunch; Snack
SERVICES OFFERED: Rehabilitative and supportive care; Exercise and socialization; Transportation to and from program; Health maintenance and assessment; Support groups; Periodic educational programs.
See ads pages 140, 202, 301

Aurora

New Encounters Adult Day Care Centre
49 E Downer Pl, Aurora, IL 60505
(708) 896-7474
CONTACT: Rachel Lye
CLIENTS SERVED PER MONTH: 12
HOURS OF OPERATION: Mon-Fri, 7:30 am - 5:30 pm
MEALS: Lunch; Snack
SERVICES OFFERED: Rehabilitative and supportive care; Nutritional guidance; Exercise and socialization; Transportation to and from program; Health maintenance and assessment; Mental health counseling; Physical & mental assessment with continuing observation & care.

Bellwood

Proviso Council on Aging Adult Day Health Center
439 Bohland Ave, Bellwood, IL 60104
(708) 547-5600
CONTACT: Cindy Troutner
CLIENTS SERVED PER MONTH: 40
HOURS OF OPERATION: Mon-Fri, 8:30 am - 4:30 pm
MEALS: Lunch; Snack; Fees: $1.25
SERVICES OFFERED: Rehabilitative and supportive care; Nutritional guidance; Exercise and socialization; Transportation to and from program; Health maintenance and assessment; Legal counseling; Mental health counseling; Podiatry; Support groups; Case management.

Chicago

Adult Day Center Hyde Park Neighborhood Club
5480 S Kenwood Ave, Chicago, IL 60615
(312) 643-4062
CONTACT: Polly Boyajian LSW
CLIENTS SERVED PER MONTH: 40
HOURS OF OPERATION: Mon-Fri, 8:30 am - 5:00 pm
MEALS: Lunch; Snack
SERVICES OFFERED: Nutritional guidance; Exercise and socialization; Transportation to and from program; Health maintenance and assessment; Mental health counseling; Information & referral.

Alzheimer's Family Care Center
5522 N Milwaukee Ave, Chicago, IL 60630
(312) 763-1698
CONTACT: Jane Stansell
CLIENTS SERVED PER MONTH: 30 per day
HOURS OF OPERATION: Mon-Fri, 7:00 am - 4:30 pm
MEALS: Lunch
SERVICES OFFERED: Nutritional guidance; Exercise and socialization; Transportation to and from program; Health maintenance and assessment; Dementia specific programming for clients in the mid to late stages of dementia.

✔ In order to support future editions of this publication would you please mention *Elder Services* each time you contact any advertiser, facility, or service.

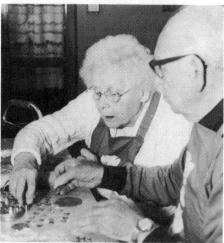

Warren Barr Pavilion of Illinois Masonic Medical Center
66 W Oak St, Chicago, IL 60610
(312) 337-5400 ext 289
CONTACT: Barbara Castro
CLIENTS SERVED PER MONTH: 50
HOURS OF OPERATION: Mon-Fri, 7:00 am - 4:30 pm
MEALS: Lunch; Snack
SERVICES OFFERED: Rehabilitative and supportive care; Nutritional guidance; Exercise and socialization; Transportation to and from program; Health maintenance and assessment; Financial counseling; Legal counseling; Mental health counseling; Beauty/Barber shop; Dentists; Podiatry; Gift shop; Ice cream parlor.

Bethel New Life
4501 W Augusta Blvd, Chicago, IL 60651
(312) 342-6550
CONTACT: Mary Nelson

Casa Central
1401 N California Ave, Chicago, IL 60622
(312) 276-1902
CONTACT: Ann Alvarez
CLIENTS SERVED PER MONTH: 29
HOURS OF OPERATION: Mon-Fri
MEALS: Lunch; Snack
SERVICES OFFERED: Exercise and socialization; Transportation to and from program; Health maintenance and assessment.

Chicago Commons Assn—Mary McDowell East Adult Day Care Center
1258 W 51st St, Chicago, IL 60609
(312) 373-2900
CONTACT: Dorothy Gibbs
CLIENTS SERVED PER MONTH: 60
HOURS OF OPERATION: Mon-Fri, 8:00 am - 5:00 pm
MEALS: Lunch; Snack
SERVICES OFFERED: Rehabilitative and supportive care; Nutritional guidance; Exercise and socialization; Transportation to and from program.

Chicago Osteopathic Hospital & Medical Center
5200 S Ellis Ave, Chicago, IL 60615
(312) 947-3000
See ad page xvii

Dependable Nightingale's Agency
5419 N Sheridan Rd, Chicago, IL 60640
(312) 728-9479

Greek-American Community Services—Northwest Chicago Senior Care
3940 N Pulaski, Chicago, IL 60641
(312) 545-0303
CONTACT: Ethel Kotsovos
CLIENTS SERVED PER MONTH: 12
HOURS OF OPERATION: Mon, Wed, Fri, 8:00 am - 5:00 pm
MEALS: Lunch; Snack

SERVICES OFFERED: Rehabilitative and supportive care; Nutritional guidance; Exercise and socialization; Transportation to and from program; Health maintenance and assessment; Counseling.

Help & Care Providers
3805 N Drake Ave, Chicago, IL 60618
(312) 539-4848

Japanese American Service Committee of Chicago
4427 N Clark St, Chicago, IL 60640
(312) 275-7212
CONTACT: Masaru Nambu
HOURS OF OPERATION: Mon-Fri, 8:00 am - 5:00 pm
MEALS: Lunch; Snack
SERVICES OFFERED: Exercise and socialization; Alzheimer's patients accepted.

Maria Kaupas Adult Day Care Center
2701 W 68th St, Chicago, IL 60629
(312) 471-8032
CONTACT: Rosemary Maria
CLIENTS SERVED PER MONTH: 30-40
HOURS OF OPERATION: Mon-Fri, 7:00 am - 5:30 pm
MEALS: Lunch; Snack
SERVICES OFFERED: Rehabilitative and supportive care; Exercise and socialization.

Ada S Niles Adult Day Care Center
6414 S Halsted St, Chicago, IL 60621
(312) 488-5400
CONTACT: BJ Jones
CLIENTS SERVED PER MONTH: 27
HOURS OF OPERATION: 8:30 am - 4:00 pm
MEALS: Breakfast
SERVICES OFFERED: Exercise and socialization; Transportation to and from program.

Umoja Care Inc
4501 W Augusta, Chicago, IL 60651
(312) 342-6550
CONTACT: Hassan Muhammad

YMCA of Metro Chicago
825 W Chicago, Chicago, IL 60622
(312) 850-6000
CONTACT: Dannette Smith

YWCA—Harriet M Harris Adult Day Care Center
6200 S Drexel Ave, Chicago, IL 60637
(312) 363-3839
CONTACT: Theresa Mims
CLIENTS SERVED PER MONTH: 35
HOURS OF OPERATION: Mon-Fri, 7:30 am - 4:30 pm
MEALS: Lunch; Snack
SERVICES OFFERED: Exercise and socialization; Transportation to and from program; Health maintenance and assessment; Counseling.

Cicero

Older Adult Rehabilitation Services (OARS) Adult Day Care
5817 W Cermak Rd, Cicero, IL 60650
(708) 656-3722
CONTACT: Charles Warner
CLIENTS SERVED PER MONTH: 40
HOURS OF OPERATION: Mon-Fri, 8:00 am - 4:30 pm
MEALS: Lunch; Snack
SERVICES OFFERED: Exercise and socialization; Transportation to and from program; Health maintenance and assessment.

Countryside

Older Adult Rehabilitation Service (OARS) Adult Day Care
6251 S Brainard Ave, Countryside, IL 60525-3949
(708) 352-0417
CONTACT: Charles Warner
CLIENTS SERVED PER MONTH: 25
HOURS OF OPERATION: Mon-Fri, 8:00 am - 4:00 pm
MEALS: Lunch; Snack
SERVICES OFFERED: Exercise and socialization; Transportation to and from program; Health maintenance and assessment.

Des Plaines

Parkside Adult Day Health Center
9375 Church St, Des Plaines, IL 60016
(708) 696-7770, 824-8038 FAX
CONTACT: Intake specialist
CLIENTS SERVED PER MONTH: 60 per day
HOURS OF OPERATION: Mon-Fri, 7:00 am - 5:30 pm
MEALS: Lunch; Snack
SERVICES OFFERED: Rehabilitative and supportive care; Nutritional guidance; Exercise and socialization; Transportation to and from program; Health maintenance and assessment; Counseling; Support groups; Periodic educational programs; Alzheimer's program.
See ads pages 140, 202, 301

Downers Grove

Community Adult Day Care
1005 Grant St, Downers Grove, IL 60515
(708) 968-1060
CONTACT: Pat Rensch
HOURS OF OPERATION: Mon-Fri, 7:30 am - 6:00 pm
MEALS: Lunch; Snack
SERVICES OFFERED: Exercise and socialization.

✔ In order to support future editions of this publication would you please mention *Elder Services* each time you contact any advertiser, facility, or service.

Elgin

Oak Crest Residence Sharing Today
204 S State St, Elgin, IL 60123
(708) 742-2255
CONTACT: Marlene Pokorny
HOURS OF OPERATION: 7 days, 6:30 am - 10:00 pm
MEALS: Breakfast; Lunch; Snack
SERVICES OFFERED: Rehabilitative and supportive care;
    Nutritional guidance; Exercise and socialization;
    First phase Alzheimer's care.

Sunnyside Adult Day Center—Senior Services Associates Inc
101 S Grove St, Elgin, IL 60120
(800) 942-1724; (708) 741-0404
CONTACT: Jean White
CLIENTS SERVED PER MONTH: 20
HOURS OF OPERATION: Mon-Wed, 8:00 am - 4:00 pm
MEALS: Lunch; Snack; Fees: $1.75 per day
SERVICES OFFERED: Nutritional guidance; Exercise and
    socialization; Transportation to and from program;
    Legal counseling; Public aid; Insurance counsel-
    ing; Tax counseling.

Elmhurst

Adult Christian Day Care
314 W Vallette, Elmhurst, IL 60126
(708) 832-1788
CONTACT: Bonnie M Factor
CLIENTS SERVED PER MONTH: 45
HOURS OF OPERATION: Mon-Fri, 8:00 am - 5:00 pm
MEALS: Lunch; Snack; Fees: $2.50
SERVICES OFFERED: Rehabilitative and supportive care;
    Nutritional guidance; Exercise and socialization;
    Transportation to and from program; Counseling.

Adult Christian Day Care—Alzheimer's Center
920 Swain, Elmhurst, IL 60126
(708) 832-0015
CONTACT: Bonnie Factor
CLIENTS SERVED PER MONTH: 23
HOURS OF OPERATION: Mon-Fri, 8:00 am - 5:00 pm
MEALS: Lunch; Fees: $2.50
SERVICES OFFERED: Exercise and socialization; Transpor-
    tation to and from program; Health maintenance
    and assessment; Counseling.

Evanston

Council for Jewish Elderly Adult Day Care Center
1015 W Howard, Evanston, IL 60202
(708) 492-1400
CONTACT: Hedy Ciocci
CLIENTS SERVED PER MONTH: 50 per day
HOURS OF OPERATION: Mon-Fri, 8:30 am - 5:00 pm

MEALS: Lunch; Snack
SERVICES OFFERED: Nutritional guidance; Exercise and
    socialization; Transportation to and from program;
    Health maintenance and assessment; Mental health
    counseling.

Evergreen Park

Little Company of Mary Hospital Adult Day Care
2800 W 95th St, Evergreen Park, IL 60642
(708) 425-3100
CONTACT: Jeanne Kyrouac
HOURS OF OPERATION: Mon-Fri, 7:30 am - 5:30 pm
MEALS: Lunch; Snack

Wellspring Gerontological Services
179 W Washington St, Evergreen Park, IL 60602-2308
(800) 339-9355; (708) 499-0505
CONTACT: Steve C Fox

Frankfort

Autumn Country Club Adult Day Care
627 N LaGrange Rd, Frankfort, IL 60423
(815) 469-0060
CONTACT: Kathy Waterman

Franklin Park

Leyden Adult Day Center
9857 Schiller, Franklin Park, IL 60131
(708) 455-1331
CONTACT: Jo Ann Sawyer
HOURS OF OPERATION: Mon-Fri, 7:30 am - 5:00 pm
MEALS: Lunch; Snack

Glen Ellyn

ESSE Adult Day Care—Ecumenical Support Services for the Elderly
41 N Park Blvd, Glen Ellyn, IL 60137
(708) 858-1005
CONTACT: Bonnie Kuchaes
CLIENTS SERVED PER MONTH: 25
HOURS OF OPERATION: Mon-Fri, 7:30 am - 5:00 pm
MEALS: Lunch; Snack; Fees: $2.50
SERVICES OFFERED: Nutritional guidance; Exercise and
    socialization; Health maintenance and assessment;
    Counseling; Referrals to other agencies.

Hazel Crest

Lutheran Social Services—Home Helps for Seniors
3000 W 170th Pl, Hazel Crest, IL 60429
(708) 335-3800
CONTACT: Dolores Morrow
CLIENTS SERVED PER MONTH: 40
HOURS OF OPERATION: Mon-Fri, 8:00 am - 4:00 pm
MEALS: Breakfast; Lunch
SERVICES OFFERED: Rehabilitative and supportive care; Nutritional guidance; Exercise and socialization; Transportation to and from program; Health maintenance and assessment.

Highland Park

Highland Park Hospital Alternative Adult Day Services
1936 Green Bay Rd, Highland Park, IL 60035
(708) 432-8000
CONTACT: Mark Newton
CLIENTS SERVED PER MONTH: 25
HOURS OF OPERATION: Mon-Fri, 8:00 am - 5:00 pm
MEALS: Breakfast; Lunch; Snack
SERVICES OFFERED: Rehabilitative and supportive care; Nutritional guidance; Exercise and socialization; Transportation to and from program; Health maintenance and assessment; Counseling.

Hoffman Estates

Alden—Poplar Creek Rehabilitation & Health Care Center
1545 Barrington Rd, Hoffman Estates, IL 60194
(708) 884-0011
CONTACT: Phyllis Passarelli
CLIENTS SERVED PER MONTH: 12
HOURS OF OPERATION: 7:00 am - 6:00 pm
MEALS: Lunch; Snack
SERVICES OFFERED: Rehabilitative and supportive care; Nutritional guidance; Exercise and socialization; Health maintenance and assessment; Alzheimer's care; Beauty/barber shop; Outings.

Joliet

Community Adult Day Care Systems Inc
1617 Manhattan Rd, Joliet, IL 60433
(815) 727-0003
CONTACT: Janet Rogers
HOURS OF OPERATION: Mon-Fri, 8:00 am - 5:00 pm
MEALS: Lunch; Snack
SERVICES OFFERED: Exercise and socialization; Transportation to and from program $2.50 each way.

Lake Forest

Lake Forest Hospital Adult Day Care
660 N Westmoreland Rd, Lake Forest, IL 60045
(708) 295-3000 ext 5950
CONTACT: William G Ries
HOURS OF OPERATION: Mon-Fri, 8:00 am - 5:00 pm

Libertyville

Condell Day Center Intergenerational Care
900 Garfield, Libertyville, IL 60048
(708) 816-4585
CONTACT: Brigitte Johnson
CLIENTS SERVED PER MONTH: 30
HOURS OF OPERATION: 7:00 am - 5:00 pm
MEALS: Lunch; Snack
SERVICES OFFERED: Rehabilitative and supportive care; Nutritional guidance; Exercise and socialization; Transportation to and from program.

Lindenhurst

Victory Lakes Adult Day Care Center
1055 E Grand Ave, Lindenhurst, IL 60046
(708) 356-5900
CONTACT: Sandy Smith
CLIENTS SERVED PER MONTH: 12
HOURS OF OPERATION: Mon-Fri, 7:00 am - 4:00 pm
MEALS: Lunch; Snack
SERVICES OFFERED: Rehabilitative and supportive care; Nutritional guidance; Exercise and socialization; Health maintenance and assessment; Medication administration.
See ad page 230

Matteson

Applewood Living Center
21020 S Kostner Ave, Matteson, IL 60443
(708) 747-1300
CONTACT: Roseanne Jansen
CLIENTS SERVED PER MONTH: 3-4
HOURS OF OPERATION: Mon-Fri, 7:00 am - 7:00 pm
MEALS: Breakfast; Lunch; Snack
SERVICES OFFERED: Rehabilitative and supportive care; Exercise and socialization; Transportation to and from program; Health maintenance and assessment.

✔ In order to support future editions of this publication would you please mention *Elder Services* each time you contact any advertiser, facility, or service.

Naperville

Alden Nursing Center—Naperville Rehabilitation & Health Care Center
1525 S Oxford Ln, Naperville, IL 60565
(708) 983-0300
CONTACT: Phyllis Passarelli
CLIENTS SERVED PER MONTH: 12
HOURS OF OPERATION: 7:00 am - 6:00 pm
MEALS: Breakfast; Lunch; Snack; Fees: $3.75 for breakfast
SERVICES OFFERED: Rehabilitative and supportive care; Nutritional guidance; Exercise and socialization; Health maintenance and assessment; Alzheimer's care; Beauty/barber shop; Outings.

Ecumenical Adult Care of Naperville
305 W Jackson, Naperville, IL 60540-5204
(708) 357-8166

CONTACT: Laura Milligan
CLIENTS SERVED PER MONTH: 30
HOURS OF OPERATION: Mon-Fri, 8:00 am - 5:00 pm
MEALS: Lunch; Snack
SERVICES OFFERED: Exercise and socialization; Support & referral service for families; Intergenerational activities; Outings; Crafts; Community education in eldercare.
See ad page 144

North Chicago

Veterans Affairs Medical Center—North Chicago-Adult Day Health Care
3001 Green Bay Rd, North Chicago, IL 60089
(708) 578-3743
CONTACT: Daniel Swiehkow
CLIENTS SERVED PER MONTH: 750
HOURS OF OPERATION: Mon-Fri, 8:00 am - 4:30 pm
MEALS: Lunch
SERVICES OFFERED: Rehabilitative and supportive care; Nutritional guidance; Exercise and socialization; Transportation to and from program; Health maintenance and assessment; Financial counseling; Legal counseling; Mental health counseling; Physician & nurse care management.

Northbrook

House of Welcome
1776 Walters Ave, Northbrook, IL 60062
(708) 441-7775
CONTACT: Julie Lamberti
CLIENTS SERVED PER MONTH: 30
HOURS OF OPERATION: Mon-Wed, 9:00 am - 3:00 pm
MEALS: Lunch; Snack
SERVICES OFFERED: Exercise and socialization; Support groups; Case management; Educational workshops; Information & referral; Intergenerational programs.
See ad page 144

Northfield

Parkside Adult Day Health Center
315 Waukegan Rd, Northfield, IL 60093
(708) 696-7770, 824-8038 FAX
CONTACT: Intake specialist
CLIENTS SERVED PER MONTH: 35 per day
HOURS OF OPERATION: Mon-Fri, 7:00 am - 5:30 pm
MEALS: Lunch; Snack
SERVICES OFFERED: Rehabilitative and supportive care; Nutritional guidance; Exercise and socialization; Transportation to and from program; Health maintenance and assessment; Counseling; Support groups; Periodic educational programs.
See ads pages 140, 202, 301

Oak Park

Suburban Adult Day Care Center
149 W Harrison St, Oak Park, IL 60304
(708) 524-1312, 524-2588 FAX
CONTACT: Julia Casten
CLIENTS SERVED PER MONTH: 25
HOURS OF OPERATION: Mon-Fri, 9:00 am - 4:00 pm
MEALS: Breakfast; Lunch; Snack
SERVICES OFFERED: Rehabilitative and supportive care;
    Nutritional guidance; Exercise and socialization;
    Transportation to and from program; Health main-
    tenance and assessment; Mental health counseling.

Palatine

Little Sisters of the Poor
80 W Northwest Hwy, Palatine, IL 60067
(708) 358-5700
CONTACT: Sr Mary Thomas
HOURS OF OPERATION: Mon-Fri, 8:00 am - 5:00 pm
MEALS: Lunch; Snack

Palos Park

The Club Adult Day Care Centers Inc
8800 W 119th St, Palos Park, IL 60464
(708) 361-2740
CONTACT: Sharon Young
CLIENTS SERVED PER MONTH: 40
HOURS OF OPERATION: Mon-Fri, 7:45 am - 5:00 pm
MEALS: Breakfast; Lunch
SERVICES OFFERED: Rehabilitative and supportive care;
    Exercise and socialization; Health maintenance
    and assessment; Counseling.

Park Forest

The Club Adult Day Care Centers Inc
215 Nashua St, Park Forest, IL 60466
(708) 747-7030
CONTACT: Janet Goodwin
CLIENTS SERVED PER MONTH: 60
HOURS OF OPERATION: 7 days, 24 hours per day
MEALS: Breakfast; Lunch; Snack
SERVICES OFFERED: Rehabilitative and supportive care;
    Nutritional guidance; Exercise and socialization;
    Transportation to and from program; Health main-
    tenance and assessment; Counseling.

Roselle

Parkside—Trinity Adult Day Health Center
405 S Rush St, Roselle, IL 60172
(708) 696-7770, 824-8038 FAX
CONTACT: Intake specialist
CLIENTS SERVED PER MONTH: 10 per day
HOURS OF OPERATION: Mon-Fri, 7:00 am - 5:30 pm
MEALS: Lunch; Snack; Fees: $2.50
SERVICES OFFERED: Rehabilitative and supportive care;
    Nutritional guidance; Exercise and socialization;
    Health maintenance and assessment; Counseling;
    Support groups; Periodic educational programs.
See ads pages 140, 202, 301

Skokie

Great Opportunities Adult Day Care
4555 Church St, Skokie, IL 60076
(708) 679-5610
CONTACT: Joanne Benge
CLIENTS SERVED PER MONTH: 35 per day
HOURS OF OPERATION: Mon-Fri, 7:30 am - 4:30 pm
MEALS: Breakfast; Lunch; Snack
SERVICES OFFERED: Rehabilitative and supportive care;
    Nutritional guidance; Exercise and socialization;
    Transportation to and from program; Health main-
    tenance and assessment; Mental health counseling.

South Holland

Rest Haven South
16300 Wausau, South Holland, IL 60473
(708) 596-5500, 596-6502 FAX
CONTACT: Sally Rock
CLIENTS SERVED PER MONTH: 20-25
HOURS OF OPERATION: Mon-Fri, 7:30 am - 5 pm
MEALS: Lunch
SERVICES OFFERED: Rehabilitative and supportive care;
    Nutritional guidance; Exercise and socialization;
    Counseling.
See ad on page i

Stickney

**Stickney Township Office on Aging—North
Stickney Medical Center**
6721 W 40th St, Stickney, IL 60402
(708) 788-9100

Waukegan

Victory Memorial Hospital—Waukegan Adult Day Care Center
2000 Western Ave, Waukegan, IL 60087
(708) 360-9860
CONTACT: Sandra Cech
CLIENTS SERVED PER MONTH: 15 per day
HOURS OF OPERATION: Mon-Fri, 8:00 am - 5:00 pm
MEALS: Lunch; Snack
SERVICES OFFERED: Rehabilitative and supportive care; Nutritional guidance; Exercise and socialization; Health maintenance and assessment.

Willowbrook

Paulson Center Adult Care
619 Plainfield Rd, Willowbrook, IL 60521
(708) 323-5656, 323-5656 FAX
CONTACT: Pam Shank
HOURS OF OPERATION: Mon-Fri, 7:00 am - 4:30 pm
MEALS: Lunch; Snack
SERVICES OFFERED: Rehabilitative and supportive care; Exercise and socialization; Transportation to and from program.
See ad page 73

Wilmette

House of Welcome
1010 Central Ave, Wilmette, IL 60091
(708) 441-7775
CONTACT: Julie Lamberti
CLIENTS SERVED PER MONTH: 30
HOURS OF OPERATION: Tues & Thurs, 9:00 am - 3:00 pm
MEALS: Lunch; Snack
SERVICES OFFERED: Exercise and socialization; Support group; Case management; Educational workshops; Information & referrals; Intergenerational programs.
See ad page 144

Winnetka

House of Welcome
979 Vine St, Winnetka, IL 60093
(708) 441-7775
CONTACT: Julie Lamberti
CLIENTS SERVED PER MONTH: 30
HOURS OF OPERATION: Mon-Fri, 9:00 am - 3:00 pm
MEALS: Lunch; Snack
SERVICES OFFERED: Exercise and socialization; Support groups; Care management; Educational workshops; Information & referral; Intergenerational programs.
See ad page 144

Woodstock

Family Alliance Inc
670 S Eastwood Dr, Woodstock, IL 60098-4633
(815) 338-3590, 337-4406 FAX
CONTACT: Carol Louise
HOURS OF OPERATION: Mon-Fri, 9:00 am - 3:00 pm
MEALS: Lunch; Snack
SERVICES OFFERED: Outreach counseling; Care management.

INDIANA

Crown Point

Caritas Center Adult Day Care
928 S Court St, Crown Point, IN 46307
(219) 662-7131
CONTACT: Shirley Jean Short
CLIENTS SERVED PER MONTH: 25
HOURS OF OPERATION: Mon-Fri, 7:00 am - 6:00 pm
MEALS: Lunch; Snack
SERVICES OFFERED: Rehabilitative and supportive care; Nutritional guidance; Exercise and socialization; Music therapy; Weekly religious services; Caregiver support group.

Gary

Corinthian Christian Center
667 Van Buren, Gary, IN 46402
(219) 885-5819
CONTACT: Cheryl Rivera

Hammond

Ollie's Adult Day Care
635 165th St, Hammond, IN 46324
(219) 931-3752
CONTACT: JoAnna Lyons

YWCA of the Calumet Area—Adult Day Care
250 Ogden St, Hammond, IN 46320
(219) 931-2922
CONTACT: Joan Rowe
CLIENTS SERVED PER MONTH: 35
HOURS OF OPERATION: Mon-Fri, 8:30 am - 3:30 pm (Extended hrs available)
MEALS: Breakfast; Lunch; Snack
SERVICES OFFERED: Nutritional guidance; Exercise and socialization; Transportation to and from program; Health maintenance and assessment; Field trips; Podiatry services.

Highland

Golden Agers Adult Day Care Inc
2450 Lincoln St, Highland, IN 46322
(219) 923-4747
CONTACT: Beverly Calligan RNC
CLIENTS SERVED PER MONTH: 160
HOURS OF OPERATION: Mon-Fri, 7:00 am - 5:00 pm
MEALS: Breakfast; Lunch; Snack; Fees: $1.00 donation
SERVICES OFFERED: Rehabilitative and supportive care; Nutritional guidance; Exercise and socialization; Transportation to and from program; Health maintenance and assessment; Legal counseling; Mental health counseling.

Hobart

Millers Merry Manor
2901 W 37th Ave, Hobart, IN 46342
(219) 942-2170
CONTACT: Nancy Barnes

I Don't Know Where To Begin

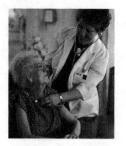

That's how I felt when my mother needed nursing and personal care. Then I found out about home health care from Kimberly Quality Care. By making just one phone call to KQC℠, I arranged for all the services my mom needed. And she's where she most wants to be—at home.

Consulting with her doctors and hospital personnel, KQC's licensed professionals coordinated and managed all aspects of my mom's home care plan. They made sure we knew exactly what to expect, every step of the way. And they worked with us to find the best way to handle costs. My mom and I made the right choice when we selected home health care services from Kimberly Quality Care.

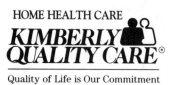

HOME HEALTH CARE

KIMBERLY QUALITY CARE®

Quality of Life is Our Commitment

Belleville/Marion 618-234-6995	**Kankakee/Paxton** 815-935-0046	**Olympia Fields** 708-481-1462
Bloomington 309-829-0008	**Merrillville** 219-769-0215	**Peoria** 309-692-0210
Chicago 312-280-2333	**North Riverside/** **Hickory Hills** 708-447-6220	**Rockford** 815-964-4100
Downers Grove/ **West Chicago** 708-971-1811	**Oak Park** 708-848-0962	**Skokie** 708-965-8150
Joliet/LaSalle/Peru 815-729-4828		**Waukegan** 708-249-5530

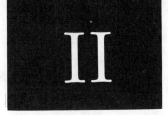

Home Health Care Services

ILLINOIS

Alsip

Abbey Home Healthcare
11600 S Pulaski Rd, Alsip, IL 60658
(708) 597-5454, 597-5255 FAX
CONTACT: John Kovelan
FINANCIAL PLANS ACCEPTED: Medicaid/Medicare certified; Private insurance.
EQUIPMENT & SUPPLIES: Ambulatory assistance equipment; Respiratory equipment; Incontinence and ostomy products; Physical therapy supplies; Nutritional and feeding supplies; Medical equipment; Aerosol therapy; Life support systems.
EQUIPMENT/SUPPLY AVAILABILITY: For rent; For sale; Home delivery & pickup; 24-hour service.

See ad page 153

Dyna Care Home Health Inc
4800 W 129th, Alsip, IL 60658
(708) 389-2700, 389-8160 FAX
CONTACT: Abi Boxwalla
CLIENTS SERVED PER MONTH: 200
FINANCIAL PLANS ACCEPTED: Medicaid/Medicare certified; Private insurance.
SERVICES OFFERED: Skilled nursing; Rehabilitative and supportive care; Help with activities of daily living; Homemaker service; Nutritional guidance; Telephone reassurance/Emergency alert; IV therapy; 24-hour availability; Pharmacy consultation.
EQUIPMENT & SUPPLIES: IV therapy equipment and supplies; Ambulatory assistance equipment; Wheelchairs; Respiratory equipment; Incontinence and ostomy products; Physical therapy supplies; Nutritional and feeding supplies; Ambulatory pumps; Special order equipment.
EQUIPMENT/SUPPLY AVAILABILITY: For rent; For sale; Home delivery & pickup; 24-hour service.

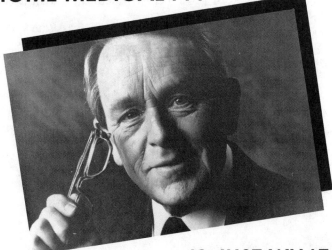
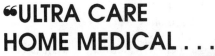
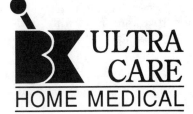

Home Care Service South & West Inc
4839 W 128th Pl Rm 210, Alsip, IL 60658
(708) 371-6170
CONTACT: Mary Ann Slama RN

Argo

Des Plaines Valley Health Center
6138 S Archer Rd, Argo, IL 60501
(708) 458-0831
CONTACT: Dee N Nissen

Arlington Heights

Alpha Home Health Care
1450 S New Wilke Rd, Arlington Heights, IL 60005
(708) 392-2909
FINANCIAL PLANS ACCEPTED: Medicaid/Medicare certified;
Private insurance.
SERVICES OFFERED: Skilled nursing; Rehabilitative and
supportive care; Help with activities of daily living;
Private duty/extended care; Physical therapy;
Speech therapy; Occupational therapy; MSW.

Children's Memorial Home Health Inc
3233 N Arlington Heights Rd, Arlington Heights, IL
60004
(708) 253-2420
CONTACT: Judith Hicks
FINANCIAL PLANS ACCEPTED: Medicaid/Medicare certified;
Private insurance.
SERVICES OFFERED: Skilled nursing; Rehabilitative and
supportive care; Help with activities of daily living;
Telephone reassurance/Emergency alert.

Lifestyle Options Inc
811 E Central, Arlington Heights, IL 60005
(708) 202-0140
CONTACT: Molly Miceli

**Northwest Community Health Services of
Northwest Community Hospital**
800 W Central Rd, Arlington Heights, IL 60005
(708) 577-4048
CONTACT: Catherine J Swick
CLIENTS SERVED PER MONTH: 250
FINANCIAL PLANS ACCEPTED: Medicaid/Medicare certified;
Private insurance.
SERVICES OFFERED: Skilled nursing; Rehabilitative and
supportive care; Help with activities of daily living;
Homemaker service; IV therapy; 24-hour availability.

Nursefinders of Arlington Heights
1101 S Arlington Heights Rd, Arlington Heights, IL
60005
(708) 956-6040
CONTACT: Nancy Saylor
FINANCIAL PLANS ACCEPTED: Private insurance.
SERVICES OFFERED: Skilled nursing; Rehabilitative and
supportive care; Help with activities of daily living;
Homemaker service; Telephone reassurance/Emer-
gency alert; IV therapy; 24-hour availability; Physical therapy; Occupational therapy; Speech therapy; Intermittent visits to round-the-clock care;
Free home care evaluation.
See ad page 167

Orsini Nursing Agency Inc
3403 N Kennicott Ave, Arlington Heights, IL 60004
(708) 259-7985, 259-8591 FAX
CONTACT: Tony Orsini
CLIENTS SERVED PER MONTH: 170
FINANCIAL PLANS ACCEPTED: Private insurance.
SERVICES OFFERED: Skilled nursing; Rehabilitative and
supportive care; Help with activities of daily living;
Homemaker service; Nutritional guidance; Tele-
phone reassurance/Emergency alert; IV therapy;
24-hour availability.
EQUIPMENT & SUPPLIES: IV therapy equipment and sup-
plies; Ambulatory assistance equipment;
Wheelchairs; Respiratory equipment; Incontinence
and ostomy products; Physical therapy supplies;
Nutritional and feeding supplies.
EQUIPMENT/SUPPLY AVAILABILITY: For rent; For sale; Home
delivery & pickup; 24-hour service.

Quality Home Health Care Inc
204 Campus Dr, Arlington Heights, IL 60004
(708) 818-8383, 818-9257 FAX
CONTACT: Barbara Bishov
CLIENTS SERVED PER MONTH: 300
FINANCIAL PLANS ACCEPTED: Medicaid/Medicare certified;
Private insurance.
EQUIPMENT & SUPPLIES: Ambulatory assistance equip-
ment; Wheelchairs; Respiratory equipment; Phys-
ical therapy supplies; Patient room equipment.
EQUIPMENT/SUPPLY AVAILABILITY: For rent; For sale; Home
delivery & pickup; 24-hour service.

Village of Arlington Heights Health Services
33 S Arlington Heights Rd, Arlington Heights, IL
60005
(708) 577-5626, 577-5684 TDD, 577-5634 FAX
CONTACT: Helen Jensen
CLIENTS SERVED PER MONTH: 100-150
SERVICES OFFERED: Skilled nursing; Telephone
reassurance/Emergency alert.

Aurora

Alpha Home Health Care
75 S Stolp, Aurora, IL 60507
(708) 892-2252
CLIENTS SERVED PER MONTH: 45
FINANCIAL PLANS ACCEPTED: Medicaid/Medicare certified;
  Private insurance.
SERVICES OFFERED: Skilled nursing; Rehabilitative and
  supportive care; Help with activities of daily living;
  Private duty/extended care; Physical therapy; So-
  cial work; Speech therapy; Occupational therapy.

Hospitals Home Health Care Services Inc
4255 Westbrook Dr, Aurora, IL 60504
(708) 898-0122
CONTACT: Nancy Baer
FINANCIAL PLANS ACCEPTED: Medicaid/Medicare certified;
  Private insurance.
SERVICES OFFERED: Skilled nursing; Rehabilitative and
  supportive care; Help with activities of daily living;
  Homemaker service; Nutritional guidance; IV ther-
  apy; 24-hour availability; Home medical equip-
  ment.
EQUIPMENT & SUPPLIES: IV therapy equipment and sup-
  plies; Ambulatory assistance equipment;
  Wheelchairs; Respiratory equipment; Incontinence
  and ostomy products; Physical therapy supplies;
  Nutritional and feeding supplies.
EQUIPMENT/SUPPLY AVAILABILITY: For rent; For sale; Home
  delivery & pickup; 24-hour service.

Medical Personnel Pool
912-B N Lake St, Aurora, IL 60507
(708) 896-1212
CONTACT: Susan Faust
FINANCIAL PLANS ACCEPTED: Medicaid/Medicare certified;
  Private insurance.
SERVICES OFFERED: Skilled nursing; Rehabilitative and
  supportive care; Help with activities of daily living;
  Homemaker service; Nutritional guidance; Telephone reassurance/Emergency alert; IV therapy;
  24-hour availability; High-tech home care; Ventilator program; Physical therapy; Speech therapy; Occupational therapy.

Nursefinders of Aurora
1730 N Farnsworth Ave Ste 2, Aurora, IL 60505-1512
(708) 820-9100
FINANCIAL PLANS ACCEPTED: Private insurance.
SERVICES OFFERED: Skilled nursing; Rehabilitative and
  supportive care; Help with activities of daily living;
  Homemaker service; Telephone reassurance/Emer-
  gency alert; IV therapy; 24-hour availability; Physical therapy; Occupational therapy; Speech therapy; Intermittent visits to round-the-clock care;
  Free home care evaluation.

See ad page 167

Visiting Nurse Association of Fox Valley
57 E Downer Pl, Aurora, IL 60505
(708) 892-0646, 892-5290 FAX

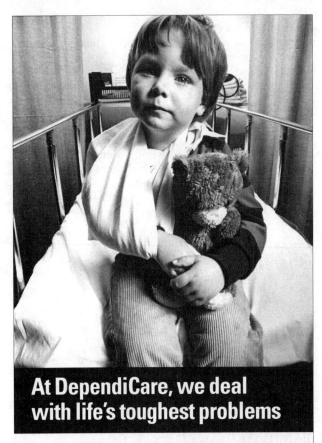
✓ In order to support future editions of this publication would you please mention *Elder Services* each time you contact any advertiser, facility, or service.

CONTACT: Janet S Craft
FINANCIAL PLANS ACCEPTED: Medicaid/Medicare certified; Private insurance.
SERVICES OFFERED: Skilled nursing; Rehabilitative and supportive care; Help with activities of daily living; Nutritional guidance; IV therapy; 24-hour availability; Community health clinics.
EQUIPMENT & SUPPLIES: IV therapy equipment and supplies; Ambulatory assistance equipment; Wheelchairs; Respiratory equipment; Incontinence and ostomy products; Physical therapy supplies; Nutritional and feeding supplies.
EQUIPMENT/SUPPLY AVAILABILITY: For rent; Home delivery & pickup.

Barrington

Caregivers Home Health
33 W Higgins Ste 3000, Barrington, IL 60010
(708) 551-9444, 551-9482 FAX
CONTACT: Anne Melligan
FINANCIAL PLANS ACCEPTED: Medicaid/Medicare certified; Private insurance.
SERVICES OFFERED: Skilled nursing; Rehabilitative and supportive care; Help with activities of daily living; Homemaker service; Nutritional guidance; IV therapy; 24-hour availability.

Farah Medical Group
450 W Hwy 22, Barrington, IL 60010
(708) 382-5350

Batavia

Fox Valley Hospice
113 E Wilson St, Batavia, IL 60510
(708) 879-6064
CONTACT: Vivian J Nimmo
CLIENTS SERVED PER MONTH: 40-50
FINANCIAL PLANS ACCEPTED: Private insurance.
SERVICES OFFERED: 24-hour availability; Psychological & emotional services.
EQUIPMENT & SUPPLIES: Wheelchairs; Incontinence and ostomy products; Nutritional and feeding supplies.
EQUIPMENT/SUPPLY AVAILABILITY: Home delivery & pickup.

Bellwood

Proviso Council on Aging
439 Bohland Ave, Bellwood, IL 60104
(708) 547-5600
CONTACT: Glenn R Green

Berwyn

Abbey Home Healthcare
6833 Roosevelt Rd, Berwyn, IL 60402
(708) 749-7000, 749-0229 FAX
CONTACT: John Kolar
FINANCIAL PLANS ACCEPTED: Medicaid/Medicare certified; Private insurance.
EQUIPMENT & SUPPLIES: Ambulatory assistance equipment; Respiratory equipment; Incontinence and ostomy products; Physical therapy supplies; Nutritional and feeding supplies; Medical equipment; Aerosol therapy; Life support systems.
EQUIPMENT/SUPPLY AVAILABILITY: For rent; For sale; Home delivery & pickup; 24-hour service.
See ad page 153

West Towns Visiting Nurse Service
1441 S Harlem Ave, Berwyn, IL 60402
(708) 749-7171
CONTACT: Sandra Kubik RN

Blue Island

Reach Out in Blue Island
13123 S Western, Blue Island, IL 60406
(708) 389-4029
CONTACT: Connie Motyll

St Francis Home Care Inc
12951 S Western Ave, Blue Island, IL 60406
(708) 371-7777
CONTACT: Beverly Peck
CLIENTS SERVED PER MONTH: 200
FINANCIAL PLANS ACCEPTED: Medicaid/Medicare certified; Private insurance.
SERVICES OFFERED: Skilled nursing; Rehabilitative and supportive care; Help with activities of daily living; Nutritional guidance; IV therapy.

Bridgeview

FirstChoice Home Health & Family Support Services
8080 S Harlem, Bridgeview, IL 60455
(708) 383-2500
CONTACT: Dorothy Butkovich
FINANCIAL PLANS ACCEPTED: Medicaid/Medicare certified; Private insurance.
SERVICES OFFERED: Skilled nursing; Rehabilitative and supportive care; Help with activities of daily living; Homemaker service; Nutritional guidance; Telephone reassurance/Emergency alert; IV therapy; 24-hour availability; Senior family counseling.

ome Medical Equipment

OXYGEN/RESPIRATORY • INCONTINENCE • ENTERAL NUTRITION • AEROSOL THERAPY
SALES • RENTALS • SERVICE • MEDICARE/MEDICAID BILLING

As all medical professionals know, it pays to see a specialist. And that's exactly what you'll find at Abbey Home Healthcare, specialists in homecare and respiratory equipment for the home, along with the largest selection of products and services.

The friendly and knowledgeable people at Abbey Home Healthcare will recommend the proper equipment for all your patients' individual needs, deliver promptly to the

home, set up and throughly demonstrate their equipment, and handle the paperwork for Medicare, Medicaid or other types of healthcare insurance. And we have complete repair capabilities to keep the equipment performing like new.

Abbey Home Healthcare offers you and your patients a one-stop source for homecare and respiratory equipment. We'd like to be a valuable part of your patients' health care team!

Alsip	**Berwyn**	**Crest Hill (Joliet)**	**Lombard**
(708) 597-5454	(708) 749-7000	(815) 439-0066	(708) 629-9850

Merrillville, IN	**Morton Grove**	**Rockford**
(219) 736-6222	(708) 470-2440	(815) 633-7778

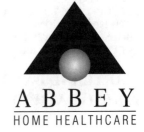

ABBEY
HOME HEALTHCARE

EQUIPMENT & SUPPLIES: IV therapy equipment and supplies; Ambulatory assistance equipment; Wheelchairs; Respiratory equipment; Incontinence and ostomy products; Physical therapy supplies; Nutritional and feeding supplies; Life-line.
EQUIPMENT/SUPPLY AVAILABILITY: For rent; For sale; Home delivery & pickup; 24-hour service.
See ads pages 118, 130, 178

HealthSource Inc
10055 S 76th Ave, Bridgeview, IL 60455
(708) 430-4040
CONTACT: John McGinnis
CLIENTS SERVED PER MONTH: 1,600
FINANCIAL PLANS ACCEPTED: Medicaid/Medicare certified; Private insurance.
SERVICES OFFERED: Skilled nursing; IV therapy; 24-hour availability.
EQUIPMENT & SUPPLIES: IV therapy equipment and supplies; Ambulatory assistance equipment; Wheelchairs; Respiratory equipment; Incontinence and ostomy products; Physical therapy supplies; Nutritional and feeding supplies.
EQUIPMENT/SUPPLY AVAILABILITY: For rent; For sale; Home delivery & pickup; 24-hour service.

Broadview

DependiCare
1815 Gardner Rd, Broadview, IL 60153
(708) 345-7400, 456-1638 FAX
CONTACT: Roger Miller
FINANCIAL PLANS ACCEPTED: Medicaid/Medicare certified; Private insurance.
EQUIPMENT & SUPPLIES: Ambulatory assistance equipment; Wheelchairs; Respiratory equipment; Physical therapy supplies; Aerosol treatments; Bedroom equipment & accessories; Ventilator management.
EQUIPMENT/SUPPLY AVAILABILITY: For rent; For sale; Home delivery & pickup; 24-hour service.
See ads pages 7, 151

Proviso Township Referral Office
2129 Roosevelt Rd, Broadview, IL 60153
(708) 344-7430
CONTACT: Otto D'Angelo, Dir
CLIENTS SERVED PER MONTH: 1,000
SERVICES OFFERED: Telephone reassurance/Emergency alert; Home blood pressure testing; Home delivered meals; Transportation to doctors' offices; Emergency food shopping.
EQUIPMENT & SUPPLIES: Ambulatory assistance equipment; Wheelchairs.
EQUIPMENT/SUPPLY AVAILABILITY: For loan.

✔ In order to support future editions of this publication would you please mention *Elder Services* each time you contact any advertiser, facility, or service.

Burbank

Stickney Township Office on Aging
5635 State Rd, Burbank, IL 60459
(708) 424-9200
CONTACT: Linda Dimengo

Calumet City

Hospice of the Calumet Area Inc
684 State Line, Calumet City, IL 60409
(708) 868-2478
FINANCIAL PLANS ACCEPTED: Medicaid/Medicare certified; Private insurance.
SERVICES OFFERED: Skilled nursing; Homemaker service; Nutritional guidance; Telephone reassurance/ Emergency alert; IV therapy; 24-hour availability; Hospice services.

Carol Stream

Community Nursing Service of DuPage
690 E North Ave, Carol Stream, IL 60188
(708) 665-7000
CONTACT: Debra Murphy

CLIENTS SERVED PER MONTH: Approx 500
FINANCIAL PLANS ACCEPTED: Medicaid/Medicare certified; Private insurance.
SERVICES OFFERED: Skilled nursing; Rehabilitative and supportive care; Help with activities of daily living; Nutritional guidance; Telephone reassurance/ Emergency alert; IV therapy; Chemotherapy; Blood transfusions; Hospice; Social service; Psychiatric program.
See ad page 138

Carpentersville

Family Service—Dundee Township
Huntley Sq, 211 W Main St Ste 218, Carpentersville, IL 60110
(708) 695-3680
CONTACT: Mark Nelson

Cary

Dial-A-Hand
668 Norwood, Cary, IL 60013
(815) 459-6818
CONTACT: Jackie Sherman

Chicago

ABC Home Health of Illinois
5757 N Lincoln Ave, Chicago, IL 60659
(312) 764-2800
CONTACT: Naomi Rubinstein

ABC Home Health Service South
1424 E 53rd St Ste 303, Chicago, IL 60615
(312) 363-4400
CONTACT: Grady Walker

Aetna Nurses Registry
4770 N Lincoln Ave, Chicago, IL 60625
(312) 275-5890
CONTACT: John Flaherty

All Better Care Inc
3530 W Peterson, Chicago, IL 60659
(312) 267-3900
CONTACT: Norma Sanfield

All-Ways Caring Services
2650 W Albion St, Chicago, IL 60645
(312) 764-1313
CONTACT: Jane Sullivan
CLIENTS SERVED PER MONTH: 350
FINANCIAL PLANS ACCEPTED: Private insurance.

SERVICES OFFERED: Skilled nursing; Rehabilitative and supportive care; Help with activities of daily living; Nutritional guidance.

Alverna Home Nursing Center
3215 W 84th St, Chicago, IL 60652
(312) 925-5077
CONTACT: Sr Mary Angela OSF
CLIENTS SERVED PER MONTH: 60-65
FINANCIAL PLANS ACCEPTED: Private insurance.
SERVICES OFFERED: Skilled nursing; Nutritional guidance; Spiritual care.

American Home Care Inc
505 N Lake Shore Dr, Chicago, IL 60611
(312) 644-7300, 644-7423 FAX
CONTACT: Jeremiah Igra, Dir
FINANCIAL PLANS ACCEPTED: Private insurance.
SERVICES OFFERED: Skilled nursing; Rehabilitative and supportive care; Help with activities of daily living; Homemaker service; Nutritional guidance; Telephone reassurance/Emergency alert; 24-hour availability; Private duty nursing; Live-ins.
EQUIPMENT & SUPPLIES: Wheelchairs.
EQUIPMENT/SUPPLY AVAILABILITY: For rent.

ASI Inc
2435 N Western, Chicago, IL 60647
(312) 278-5130, 278-1380 FAX
CONTACT: Awilda Gonzalez
CLIENTS SERVED PER MONTH: 1,000
SERVICES OFFERED: Homemaker service.

Autumn Home Health & Case Management
1625 W Edgewater N-71, Chicago, IL 60660
(312) 769-9030
CONTACT: Andrea Ginsburg
CLIENTS SERVED PER MONTH: 15-20
FINANCIAL PLANS ACCEPTED: Private insurance.
SERVICES OFFERED: Rehabilitative and supportive care; Nutritional guidance; Telephone reassurance/Emergency alert; 24-hour availability; Physician referrals; Family support services; Social workers; Relaxation therapy; Individual case management; Respite care.
EQUIPMENT & SUPPLIES: Ambulatory assistance equipment; Incontinence and ostomy products.
EQUIPMENT/SUPPLY AVAILABILITY: For rent; For sale; Home delivery & pickup; 24-hour service.

Bethel New Life
4501 W Augusta Blvd, Chicago, IL 60651
(312) 342-6550
CONTACT: Mary Nelson

Bruce & Ken's Pharmacy
7150 Addison St, Chicago, IL 60634
(312) 685-6300
CONTACT: Bruce Callahan Jr
CLIENTS SERVED PER MONTH: 310
FINANCIAL PLANS ACCEPTED: Private insurance; Medicare.
SERVICES OFFERED: Rehabilitative and supportive care; IV therapy; 24-hour availability; Blood transfusions.

EQUIPMENT & SUPPLIES: IV therapy equipment and supplies; Ambulatory assistance equipment; Wheelchairs; Respiratory equipment; Incontinence and ostomy products; Physical therapy supplies; Nutritional and feeding supplies; Custom wheelchairs; Seating systems.
EQUIPMENT/SUPPLY AVAILABILITY: For rent; For sale; Home delivery & pickup; 24-hour service.
See ad page 149

Bruce & Ken's Pharmacy
6001 Irving Park Rd, Chicago, IL 60634
(312) 545-6001
CONTACT: Bruce Callahan Jr
CLIENTS SERVED PER MONTH: 310
FINANCIAL PLANS ACCEPTED: Private insurance; Medicare.
SERVICES OFFERED: Rehabilitative and supportive care; IV therapy; 24-hour availability; Blood transfusions.
EQUIPMENT & SUPPLIES: IV therapy equipment and supplies; Ambulatory assistance equipment; Wheelchairs; Respiratory equipment; Incontinence and ostomy products; Physical therapy supplies; Nutritional and feeding supplies; Custom wheelchairs; Seating systems.
EQUIPMENT/SUPPLY AVAILABILITY: For rent; For sale; Home delivery & pickup; 24-hour service.
See ad page 149

Campbell's Personal Care
3357 W Chicago Ave, Chicago, IL 60651
(312) 638-5200
CONTACT: Mae Campbell

✓ In order to support future editions of this publication would you please mention *Elder Services* each time you contact any advertiser, facility, or service.

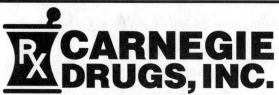

Cardio Care Inc
5915 N Lincoln Ave, Chicago, IL 60659
(312) 989-8117

Carnegie Drugs Inc
100 E Walton, Promenade Area, Chicago, IL 60611
(312) 787-3046
CONTACT: Burton Paley
FINANCIAL PLANS ACCEPTED: Medicaid/Medicare certified;
 Private insurance.
SERVICES OFFERED: Help with activities of daily living;
 Nutritional guidance; Telephone reassurance/
 Emergency alert; Pharmacy services.
EQUIPMENT & SUPPLIES: IV therapy equipment and supplies; Ambulatory assistance equipment;
 Wheelchairs; Respiratory equipment; Incontinence and ostomy products; Physical therapy supplies;
 Nutritional and feeding supplies; Diabetic supplies; Health/Beauty aids; Personal care items.
EQUIPMENT/SUPPLY AVAILABILITY: For rent; For sale; Home
 delivery & pickup; 24-hour service.
See ad page 156

Casa Central
1335 N California Ave, Chicago, IL 60622
(312) 276-1902
CONTACT: Doris Irizarry

Catholic Charities Chicago
126 N Des Plaines, Chicago, IL 60606
(312) 236-5172 ext 216
CONTACT: Laina Lurito
FINANCIAL PLANS ACCEPTED: Medicaid/Medicare certified
 multi home agency not all Medicare/Medicaid.
SERVICES OFFERED: Skilled nursing; Rehabilitative and
 supportive care; Help with activities of daily living.

Catholic Charities Chicago—Senior Case Management Services
5801 N Pulaski Rd, Chicago, IL 60646
(312) 583-9224
CONTACT: Sarah Cohen

Chicago Home Health Services Inc
1229 North Branch St, Chicago, IL 60622-2411
(312) 645-3800, 645-3811 FAX
CONTACT: Susan Breakwell, DON
CLIENTS SERVED PER MONTH: 300
FINANCIAL PLANS ACCEPTED: Medicaid/Medicare;
 Private insurance.
SERVICES OFFERED: Skilled nursing; Nutritional guidance;
 IV therapy; Physical therapy; Occupational therapy;
 Speech therapy; Social worker; Home health aides;
 24-hour availability.
EQUIPMENT & SUPPLIES: Ambulatory assistance equipment; Incontinence and ostomy products; Physical
 therapy supplies; Nutritional and feeding supplies;
 Routine medical supplies.
See ad page 155

Chinese American Services League
310 W 24th Pl, Chicago, IL 60616
(312) 791-0418
CONTACT: Bernarda Wong

Community Care Services Inc
228 S Wabash Ave, Chicago, IL 60604
(312) 786-1481

Comprehensive Home Respiratory Service
4212 N Milwaukee, Chicago, IL 60630
(312) 533-4956
CONTACT: Oscar Muriel

Council for Jewish Elderly
3003 W Touhy, Chicago, IL 60645
(312) 508-1000, 508-1028 FAX
CLIENTS SERVED PER MONTH: 8,000 annually
FINANCIAL PLANS ACCEPTED: Medicaid/Medicare certified.
SERVICES OFFERED: Help with activities of daily living;
 Homemaker service; Nutritional guidance.

Dana Home Care
70 W Erie, Chicago, IL 60610
(312) 266-8291
CONTACT: William Brauer
SERVICES OFFERED: Homemaker service; Alzheimer's programs; In-home care for people with confusional
 disorders; Traditional care for frail elderly.
See ad page 157

Dependable Nightingale's Agency
5419 N Sheridan Rd, Chicago, IL 60640
(312) 728-9479
CONTACT: Dollis C Bowman

DependiCare—North Branch
6320 N Clark St, Chicago, IL 60660
(312) 769-5913, 262-7498 FAX
CONTACT: Roger Miller
FINANCIAL PLANS ACCEPTED: Medicaid/Medicare certified;
    Private insurance.
EQUIPMENT & SUPPLIES: Ambulatory assistance equip-
    ment; Wheelchairs; Respiratory equipment; Phys-
    ical therapy supplies; Aerosol treatments; Bedroom
    equipment & accessories; Ventilator management.
EQUIPMENT/SUPPLY AVAILABILITY: For rent; For sale; Home
    delivery & pickup; 24-hour service.
See ads pages 7, 151

Doubek Pharmacy & Medical Supply
3846 W 63rd St, Chicago, IL 60629
(312) 581-1122, 581-1631 FAX
CONTACT: Dorothy Doubek
CLIENTS SERVED PER MONTH: 1,000
FINANCIAL PLANS ACCEPTED: Medicaid/Medicare certified;
    Private insurance.
EQUIPMENT & SUPPLIES: IV therapy equipment and sup-
    plies; Ambulatory assistance equipment;
    Wheelchairs; Incontinence and ostomy products;
    Nutritional and feeding supplies; Prescriptions.
EQUIPMENT/SUPPLY AVAILABILITY: For rent; For sale; Home
    delivery & pickup; 24-hour service.
See ad page 157

El Dorado Home Health Care
2405 W North Ave, Chicago, IL 60647
(312) 227-2520
CONTACT: Michael Steinhauer

Extended Home Care Services
10555 S Ewing Ave, Chicago, IL 60617
(312) 375-1228
CONTACT: Linda Longoria
CLIENTS SERVED PER MONTH: 30
SERVICES OFFERED: Help with activities of daily living;
    Homemaker service; 24-hour availability.

Family Care Services
234 S Wabash Ave, Chicago, IL 60604
(312) 427-8790
CONTACT: Judy Datz
SERVICES OFFERED: Help with activities of daily living;
    Homemaker service; Nutritional guidance; 24-hour
    availability; Elderly care; Emergency in-home care.

Family Home Health Service Inc
8747 S State St, Chicago, IL 60619
(312) 723-6300
CONTACT: Marland Flemming

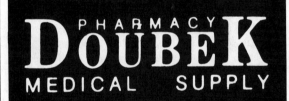

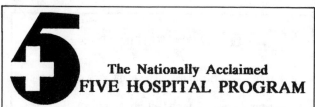
FirstChoice Home Health & Family Support Services
7301 N Sheridan Rd, Chicago, IL 60626
(312) 743-1971
CONTACT: Diane Drews
FINANCIAL PLANS ACCEPTED: Medicaid/Medicare certified;
Private insurance.
SERVICES OFFERED: Skilled nursing; Rehabilitative and
supportive care; Help with activities of daily living;
Homemaker service; Nutritional guidance; Tele-
phone reassurance/Emergency alert; IV therapy;
24-hour availability; Senior family counseling.
EQUIPMENT & SUPPLIES: IV therapy equipment and sup-
plies; Ambulatory assistance equipment;
Wheelchairs; Respiratory equipment; Incontinence
and ostomy products; Physical therapy supplies;
Nutritional and feeding supplies; Life-line.
EQUIPMENT/SUPPLY AVAILABILITY: For rent; For sale; Home
delivery & pickup; 24-hour service.
See ad page 118, 130, 178

Five Hospital Homebound Elderly Program
600 W Diversey Pkwy Ste 200, Chicago, IL 60614
(800) 640-0598; (312) 549-5822
CONTACT: Thomas B Kirkpatrick, Jr
CLIENTS SERVED PER MONTH: 425
FINANCIAL PLANS ACCEPTED: Medicaid/Medicare certified;
Private insurance.
SERVICES OFFERED: Skilled nursing; Rehabilitative and
supportive care; Help with activities of daily living;
Homemaker service; Nutritional guidance; Tele-
phone reassurance/Emergency alert; Infusion ther-
apy; Long-term managed care; Psychiatric RN; Nu-
tritionist; Social work.
See ad page 158

Flash General Help Ltd
5723 W Belmont, Chicago, IL 60634
(312) 637-3031, 637-2904 FAX
CONTACT: Ms Mariola; Ms Helena
CLIENTS SERVED PER MONTH: 15
FINANCIAL PLANS ACCEPTED: Private insurance.
SERVICES OFFERED: Homemaker service; 24-hour avail-
ability; Nurses aides; Housekeepers.

Franciscan Home Health of St Anthony Hospital
2875 W 19th St, Chicago, IL 60623
(312) 762-0771
CONTACT: Cynthia Kyle
CLIENTS SERVED PER MONTH: 90
FINANCIAL PLANS ACCEPTED: Medicaid/Medicare certified;
Private insurance.
SERVICES OFFERED: Skilled nursing; Rehabilitative and
supportive care; Help with activities of daily living;
24-hour availability.

General Health Care Services
3030 W Fullerton Ave, Chicago, IL 60647
(312) 252-4280, 227-1192 FAX
CONTACT: Fredrick E Jacobson, Gen Mgr
EQUIPMENT & SUPPLIES: Incontinence and ostomy products; Linen rental services.
EQUIPMENT/SUPPLY AVAILABILITY: For rent; Home delivery
& pickup.

Habilitative Systems
415 S Kilpatrick St, Chicago, IL 60644
(312) 521-2600
CONTACT: Fran Colman

Hamilton Agency Inc
202 S State, Chicago, IL 60604
(312) 939-1808, 939-1809

Health Connections
500 S Racine Ave, Chicago, IL 60607
(312) 666-0397
CONTACT: Olivea Palmer

Hellenic Family and Community Services, an Agency of the Hellenic Foundation
4940 N Lincoln Ave, Chicago, IL 60625
(312) 769-3838
CONTACT: Angelike Mountanis
SERVICES OFFERED: Help with activities of daily living;
Rehabilitative and supportive care; Telephone
reassurance/Emergency alert; Advocacy; Counseling.

Help & Care Providers
3805 N Drake Ave, Chicago, IL 60618
(312) 539-4848

Help at Home
7429 N Western Ave, Chicago, IL 60649
(312) 508-0000

Holy Cross Hospital
2701 W 68th St, Chicago, IL 60629
(312) 471-8000
CONTACT: Sr Teresa Mary

Home Health & Hospice of Illinois Masonic Medical Center
836 W Wellington, Chicago, IL 60657
(312) 883-7048
CONTACT: Kathleen Woods, Dir
CLIENTS SERVED PER MONTH: 200
FINANCIAL PLANS ACCEPTED: Medicaid/Medicare certified; Private insurance.
SERVICES OFFERED: Skilled nursing; Rehabilitative and supportive care; Help with activities of daily living; Hospice care.

Home Health Care Inc
4324 W Marquette Rd, Chicago, IL 60629
(312) 284-0111, 284-8270 FAX
CONTACT: Mary S Jonker
CLIENTS SERVED PER MONTH: 150
FINANCIAL PLANS ACCEPTED: Medicaid/Medicare certified; Private insurance.
SERVICES OFFERED: Skilled nursing; Rehabilitative and supportive care; Help with activities of daily living; Homemaker service; Nutritional guidance; Telephone reassurance/Emergency alert; 24-hour availability; Physical therapy; Speech therapy; Occupational therapy; Social work; Home health aides.

Home Health Plus
6160 N Cicero, Chicago, IL 60646
(312) 545-6696, 545-3283 FAX
CONTACT: Peter Kapolis
CLIENTS SERVED PER MONTH: 600
FINANCIAL PLANS ACCEPTED: Medicaid/Medicare certified; Private insurance.
SERVICES OFFERED: Skilled nursing; Rehabilitative and supportive care; Help with activities of daily living; Homemaker service; Nutritional guidance; IV therapy; 24-hour availability; Private duty; Intermittent visits.
EQUIPMENT & SUPPLIES: IV therapy equipment and supplies; Nutritional and feeding supplies.

HomeCorps Inc
550 W Jackson Ste 430, Chicago, IL 60661-5716
(800) 745-HOME; (312) 559-9355, 559-0392 FAX
CONTACT: Tommie Lester
FINANCIAL PLANS ACCEPTED: Private insurance.
SERVICES OFFERED: Skilled nursing; Rehabilitative and supportive care; Help with activities of daily living; Homemaker service; Telephone reassurance/Emergency alert; IV therapy; 24-hour availability; Home repair & maintenance; Medication management; Medical claims assistance; Transportation.
EQUIPMENT & SUPPLIES: IV therapy equipment and supplies; Ambulatory assistance equipment;

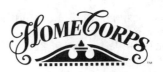
Wheelchairs; Respiratory equipment; Incontinence and ostomy products; Physical therapy supplies; Nutritional and feeding supplies.
EQUIPMENT/SUPPLY AVAILABILITY: For rent; For sale; Home delivery & pickup; 24-hour service.
See ad page 27, 159

Howard Area Community Center
7648 Paulina St, Chicago, IL 60626
(312) 262-6622
CONTACT: Karen Andes

Hull House Association Senior Centers of Metro Chicago
501 W Surf, Chicago, IL 60657
(312) 525-3480
CONTACT: Madeline Armbrust

Illinois Foundation Dentistry for Handicapped
211 E Chicago Ave Ste 820, Chicago, IL 60611
(312) 440-8976
CONTACT: Boris Trukman
FINANCIAL PLANS ACCEPTED: Private insurance.
SERVICES OFFERED: Homebound dental services.
EQUIPMENT & SUPPLIES: Dental equipment for house calls.

Illinois Home Health Care Inc
10325 S Western Ave, Chicago, IL 60643
(312) 233-1900
CONTACT: Barbara McGee

In Home Health Care Service—West Inc
5700 N Sheridan Rd Ste 1001, Chicago, IL 60660
(312) 561-0122; (708) 531-0400
FINANCIAL PLANS ACCEPTED: Medicaid/Medicare certified;
Private insurance.
SERVICES OFFERED: Skilled nursing; Rehabilitative and
supportive care; Help with activities of daily living;
Homemaker service; Nutritional guidance; IV ther-
apy; 24-hour availability; Medical social work.
EQUIPMENT & SUPPLIES: IV therapy equipment and sup-
plies; Ambulatory assistance equipment;
Wheelchairs; Respiratory equipment; Incontinence
and ostomy products; Physical therapy supplies;
Nutritional and feeding supplies; Medical supplies.

Independence Plus Inc
1620 N Normandy Ave, Chicago, IL 60635
(312) 622-8488, (708) 788-4676 TDD, (312) 622-0286
FAX
CONTACT: Ann Adams
CLIENTS SERVED PER MONTH: 30
FINANCIAL PLANS ACCEPTED: Medicaid/Medicare certified;
Private insurance.
SERVICES OFFERED: Skilled nursing; Rehabilitative and
supportive care; Help with activities of daily living;
Homemaker service; Nutritional guidance; IV ther-
apy; 24-hour availability; Physical therapy; Occupa-
tional therapy; Speech therapy; Social work ser-
vices; Home health aides.

**Japanese American Service Committee of
Chicago**
4427 N Clark St, Chicago, IL 60640
(312) 275-7212, 275-0958 FAX
CONTACT: Masaru Nambu
CLIENTS SERVED PER MONTH: 150-250
SERVICES OFFERED: Chore services.

JMK Nursing Resource
2100 S Indiana Ave, Chicago, IL 60616
(312) 326-1750
CONTACT: Mary Harris

Kimberly Quality Care—Chicago
343 W Erie St Ste 420, Chicago, IL 60610
(312) 280-2333, 280-9379 FAX
CONTACT: Penny Duszynski
FINANCIAL PLANS ACCEPTED: Medicaid/Medicare certified;
Private insurance.
SERVICES OFFERED: Skilled nursing; Rehabilitative and
supportive care; Help with activities of daily living;
Homemaker service; IV therapy; 24-hour availability; Physical therapy; Occupational therapy; Speech
therapy.
EQUIPMENT & SUPPLIES: IV therapy equipment and supplies; Incontinence and ostomy products; Nutritional and feeding supplies; Disposable medical
supplies.
EQUIPMENT/SUPPLY AVAILABILITY: For sale; Home delivery
& pickup.
See ad page 148

Kin Care Inc
3318 N Lincoln Ave, Chicago, IL 60657
(312) 975-7777
CLIENTS SERVED PER MONTH: 25
FINANCIAL PLANS ACCEPTED: Private insurance.
SERVICES OFFERED: Rehabilitative and supportive care;
Help with activities of daily living; 24-hour avail-
ability; Care provided in private homes of trained
caregivers; Temporary respite; Convalescent care;
Case management.

Little Brothers—Friends of the Elderly
1658 W Belmont Ave, Chicago, IL 60657
(312) 477-7702
CONTACT: Lawrence Valentine
CLIENTS SERVED PER MONTH: 600 (includes all branch
sites)
SERVICES OFFERED: Help with activities of daily living;
Rehabilitative and supportive care; Nutritional
guidance Emergency food pantries; Telephone
reassurance/Emergency alert; Visitation; Social activities; Free summer vacations; Friendship to
homebound seniors; Holiday parties/visits.

M & R Prescription Center Inc
1959 E 71st, Chicago, IL 60649
(312) 643-4200
CONTACT: Leola Jones

Medical Personnel Pool
30 N Michigan Ave Ste 1206, Chicago, IL 60602
(312) 726-0072
CONTACT: Susan Faust
FINANCIAL PLANS ACCEPTED: Medicaid/Medicare certified;
Private insurance.
SERVICES OFFERED: Skilled nursing; Rehabilitative and
supportive care; Help with activities of daily living;
Homemaker service; Nutritional guidance; Telephone reassurance/Emergency alert; IV therapy;
24-hour availability; High-tech home care; Ventilator program; Physical therapy; Speech therapy; Occupational therapy.

Medical Professionals Home Health Care
162 N State 14th Fl, Chicago, IL 60601
(312) 427-5191
CONTACT: Karen Carr

Mercy Home Health Care—Chatham
8541 S State, Chicago, IL 60619
(312) 874-3500, 874-9461 FAX
CONTACT: Yvonne Keller
CLIENTS SERVED PER MONTH: 350
FINANCIAL PLANS ACCEPTED: Medicaid/Medicare certified;
Private insurance.
SERVICES OFFERED: Skilled nursing; Rehabilitative and
supportive care; Help with activities of daily living;
Homemaker service; Nutritional guidance; Tele-
phone reassurance/Emergency alert; IV therapy;
24-hour availability.
EQUIPMENT & SUPPLIES: Arranged as needed.
See ads pages 116, 161, 351

Metro Portable X-Ray Service
4955 N Milwaukee Ave, Chicago, IL 60630
(312) 736-1401
CONTACT: Dr M Emmanuel

Mt Sinai Hospital Medical Center/Home Health Agency
2720 W 15th St, Chicago, IL 60608
(312) 650-6519, 650-6265 FAX
CONTACT: Joyce Kaires
CLIENTS SERVED PER MONTH: 350-420
FINANCIAL PLANS ACCEPTED: Medicaid/Medicare certified; Private insurance.
SERVICES OFFERED: Skilled nursing; Rehabilitative and supportive care; Help with activities of daily living; Nutritional guidance; Telephone reassurance/ Emergency alert; IV therapy; 24-hour availability; Home health aide; Medical social worker.
EQUIPMENT & SUPPLIES: Arranged as needed.

Northwestern Memorial Home Health Care Services Inc
680 N Lake Shore Dr Ste 815, Chicago, IL 60611
(312) 908-4663, 908-1937 FAX
CONTACT: Adrienne Casanova, Exec Dir
CLIENTS SERVED PER MONTH: 600
FINANCIAL PLANS ACCEPTED: Medicaid/Medicare certified; Private insurance.
SERVICES OFFERED: Skilled nursing; Rehabilitative and supportive care; Help with activities of daily living; Homemaker service; Nutritional guidance; IV therapy; 24-hour availability; In-home psychiatric program; Medical social work.
EQUIPMENT & SUPPLIES: IV therapy equipment and supplies.
See ad page 70

Nursefinders of Central Chicago
8 S Michigan Ave Ste 1500, Chicago, IL 60603-3314
(312) 263-1477, 269-0494 FAX
CONTACT: Jeffrey Siegel
CLIENTS SERVED PER MONTH: 10-20
FINANCIAL PLANS ACCEPTED: Private insurance.
SERVICES OFFERED: Skilled nursing; Rehabilitative and supportive care; Help with activities of daily living; Homemaker service; Nutritional guidance; Telephone reassurance/Emergency alert; IV therapy; 24-hour availability.
See ad page 167

Nursefinders of Hyde Park
1525 E 53rd St Ste 1002, Chicago, IL 60615-4587
(312) 324-4700
CONTACT: Richard Myers
FINANCIAL PLANS ACCEPTED: Medicaid/Medicare certified.
SERVICES OFFERED: Skilled nursing; Rehabilitative and supportive care; Help with activities of daily living; Homemaker service; Telephone reassurance/Emergency alert; IV therapy; 24-hour availability; Physical therapy; Occupational therapy; Speech therapy; Intermittent visits to round-the-clock care; Free home care evaluation.
See ad page 167

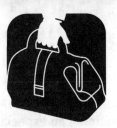
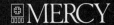
✓ In order to support future editions of this publication would you please mention *Elder Services* each time you contact any advertiser, facility, or service.

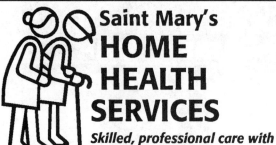
Nursefinders of Lincoln Square
4011 N Damen Ave, Chicago, IL 60618
(312) 404-2056
CONTACT: Jeffery Siegel
FINANCIAL PLANS ACCEPTED: Medicaid/Medicare certified; Private insurance.
SERVICES OFFERED: Skilled nursing; Rehabilitative and supportive care; Help with activities of daily living; Homemaker service; Telephone reassurance/Emergency alert; IV therapy; 24-hour availability; Physical therapy; Occupational therapy; Speech therapy; Intermittent visits to round-the-clock care; Free home care evaluation.
See ad page 167

Nurses on Wheels
3909 W Fullerton Ave, Chicago, IL 60647
(312) 772-1008, 772-7759 FAX
CONTACT: Norma Hepkin
FINANCIAL PLANS ACCEPTED: Medicaid/Medicare certified; Private insurance.
SERVICES OFFERED: Skilled nursing; Homemaker service; Home health aides; Physical therapy; Speech therapy; Medical social workers.

Operation Brotherhood
3745 W Ogden Ave, Chicago, IL 60623
(312) 522-0433
CONTACT: Ray Belin

Osteopathic Home Health Service
5200 S Ellis Ave, Chicago, IL 60615
(312) 947-7463
CONTACT: Diane Shefts
See ad page xvii

Polonia Home Health Care
3301 N Milwaukee, Chicago, IL 60641
(312) 777-1121

Primary Health Care Services
155 N Harbor Dr, Concourse 5, Chicago, IL 60601
(312) 819-1395
CONTACT: Catherine Brown

Professional Nurses Bureau
8420 Bryn Mawr Ste 330, Chicago, IL 60631
(708) 394-0400
CONTACT: Marie Bonzwisk

Ravenswood Home Care
14600 N Ravenswood, Chicago, IL 60640
CONTACT: Madelene R Grimm
CLIENTS SERVED PER MONTH: 200-225
FINANCIAL PLANS ACCEPTED: Medicaid/Medicare certified; Private insurance.
SERVICES OFFERED: Skilled nursing; Rehabilitative and supportive care; Help with activities of daily living; Homemaker service; High-tech nursing; Private-pay aides; Therapy services.

Resurrection Home Health Care Services
7447 W Talcott, Chicago, IL 60631
(312) 792-5020, 594-7991 FAX
CONTACT: Janet M Sullivan
CLIENTS SERVED PER MONTH: 280
FINANCIAL PLANS ACCEPTED: Medicaid/Medicare certified; Private insurance.
SERVICES OFFERED: Skilled nursing; Nutritional guidance; Telephone reassurance/Emergency alert; IV therapy; 24-hour availability; Physical therapy; Occupational therapy; Speech therapy.
EQUIPMENT & SUPPLIES: IV therapy equipment and supplies; Ambulatory assistance equipment; Wheelchairs; Respiratory equipment; Incontinence and ostomy products; Physical therapy supplies; Nutritional and feeding supplies.
EQUIPMENT/SUPPLY AVAILABILITY: For rent; For sale; Home delivery & pickup; 24-hour service.
See ads pages 163, 308

Rush Home Health Service
1700 W Van Buren Ste 325, Chicago, IL 60612
(312) 942-6216
CONTACT: Clara Summerville
CLIENTS SERVED PER MONTH: 700
FINANCIAL PLANS ACCEPTED: Medicaid/Medicare certified; Private insurance.
SERVICES OFFERED: Skilled nursing; Rehabilitative and supportive care; Help with activities of daily living; Homemaker service; Nutritional guidance; Telephone reassurance/Emergency alert; Psychiatric nursing.

St Gregory Socialcare
1634 W Gregory, Chicago, IL 60640
(312) 561-3546
CONTACT: Sr Barbara Quinn

St James Place Ltd
111 N Wabash Ave Ste 703, Chicago, IL 60602
(312) 346-0260
CONTACT: Maryann Zaborsky
FINANCIAL PLANS ACCEPTED: Private insurance.
SERVICES OFFERED: Skilled nursing; Help with activities
of daily living; Homemaker service; Nutritional
guidance; IV therapy; 24-hour availability.
EQUIPMENT & SUPPLIES: IV therapy equipment and supplies.

St Mary's Home Health Services
5306 W Belmont Ave, Chicago, IL 60641
(312) 794-5022, 794-5027 FAX
CONTACT: Terry Mikovich
CLIENTS SERVED PER MONTH: 100
FINANCIAL PLANS ACCEPTED: Medicaid/Medicare certified;
Private insurance.
SERVICES OFFERED: Skilled nursing; Rehabilitative and
supportive care; Homemaker service; Nutritional
guidance; Telephone reassurance/Emergency alert;
Home health aides.
See ad page 162

The Salvation Army—Family Service Division
4800 N Marine Dr, Chicago, IL 60640
(312) 275-6233
CONTACT: Ikuo Yamaguchi
FINANCIAL PLANS ACCEPTED: Private insurance.
SERVICES OFFERED: Rehabilitative and supportive care
(on a limited basis); Counseling for the elderly
and their families.

The Salvation Army
5040 N Pulaski Rd, Chicago, IL 60630
(312) 725-1100
CONTACT: Lt Col Gary L Herndon

Sargent—Water Tower Pharmacy
845 N Michigan Ave 9th Fl, Chicago, IL 60611
(312) 280-1220
CONTACT: Burton Paley
FINANCIAL PLANS ACCEPTED: Medicaid/Medicare certified;
Private insurance.
SERVICES OFFERED: Help with activities of daily living;
Nutritional guidance; Telephone reassurance/
Emergency alert; Pharmacy services.
EQUIPMENT & SUPPLIES: IV therapy equipment and sup-
plies; Ambulatory assistance equipment;
Wheelchairs; Respiratory equipment; Incontinence
and ostomy products; Physical therapy supplies;
Nutritional and feeding supplies; Health/Beauty
aids; Personal care items; Diabetic supplies; Spe-
cialty clothing.
EQUIPMENT/SUPPLY AVAILABILITY: For rent; For sale; Home
delivery & pickup; 24-hour service.
See ad page 164

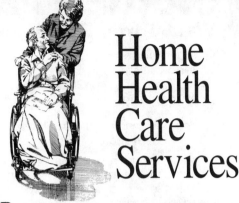
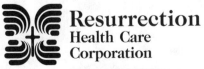
✓ In order to support future editions of this publication would you please mention *Elder Services* each time you contact
any advertiser, facility, or service.

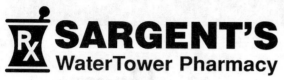
Sauganash Edgebrook Home Nursing Inc
4801 W Peterson Ste 616, Chicago, IL 60646
(312) 777-2590
CONTACT: Martine Munoz

SCH Home-Med North
2760 W Foster Ave, Chicago, IL 60625
(312) 275-9700, 878-6152 FAX
CONTACT: Patricia Sefton
FINANCIAL PLANS ACCEPTED: Medicaid/Medicare certified.
SERVICES OFFERED: Skilled nursing; Rehabilitative and supportive care; Help with activities of daily living; Nutritional guidance; IV therapy; 24-hour availability.
EQUIPMENT & SUPPLIES: IV therapy equipment and supplies; Ambulatory assistance equipment; Wheelchairs; Incontinence and ostomy products; Physical therapy supplies.

Senior Care Inc
4830 W Addison, Chicago, IL 60641
(312) 202-1011
CONTACT: Kay Lavelle

Seniors Home Health Care Ltd
10555 S Ewing Ave Ste 2, Chicago, IL 60617
(312) 768-8100
CONTACT: L Brown
CLIENTS SERVED PER MONTH: 100

FINANCIAL PLANS ACCEPTED: Medicaid/Medicare certified; Private insurance.
SERVICES OFFERED: Skilled nursing; Rehabilitative and supportive care; Help with activities of daily living; Telephone reassurance/Emergency alert.

Society of St Vincent De Paul of Chicago
645 W Randolph St, Chicago, IL 60606
(312) 876-2278
CONTACT: Peggy Gilligan
SERVICES OFFERED: Homemaker service.

Staff Builders Health Services
322 S Green, Chicago, IL 60607
(312) 633-0908, 633-0995 FAX
CONTACT: Mark Richter
CLIENTS SERVED PER MONTH: 60
FINANCIAL PLANS ACCEPTED: Medicaid/Medicare certified; Private insurance.
SERVICES OFFERED: Skilled nursing; Rehabilitative and supportive care; Help with activities of daily living; Homemaker service; Nutritional guidance; Telephone reassurance/Emergency alert; IV therapy; 24-hour availability.

Staff Builders Services
28 E Jackson, Chicago, IL 60604-2215
(312) 986-8358
CONTACT: Jean Bradshaw
SERVICES OFFERED: Homemaker service; Chore service.

Summit Home Health Inc
5331 N Sheridan Rd, Chicago, IL 60640
(312) 275-1500, 275-8245 FAX
CONTACT: Kathleen Lipscomb
CLIENTS SERVED PER MONTH: 350
FINANCIAL PLANS ACCEPTED: Medicaid/Medicare certified; Private insurance.
SERVICES OFFERED: Skilled nursing; Rehabilitative and supportive care; Help with activities of daily living; IV therapy; 24-hour availability.

Third Age Program
825 W Chicago, Chicago, IL 60622
(312) 850-6000

Total Home Health Care of Chicago Inc
1050 N State St, Chicago, IL 60610
(312) 943-0777, 943-7549 FAX
CONTACT: John Aleman, RN
CLIENTS SERVED PER MONTH: 120
FINANCIAL PLANS ACCEPTED: Medicaid/Medicare certified; Private insurance.
SERVICES OFFERED: Skilled nursing; Rehabilitative and supportive care; Help with activities of daily living; Nutritional guidance; IV therapy; 24-hour availability.
EQUIPMENT & SUPPLIES: IV therapy equipment and supplies; Ambulatory assistance equipment; Wheelchairs; Respiratory equipment; Incontinence and ostomy products; Physical therapy supplies; Nutritional and feeding supplies.
EQUIPMENT/SUPPLY AVAILABILITY: For rent; For sale; Home delivery & pickup; 24-hour service.

Ultra Care Home Medical
7065 W Belmont, Chicago, IL 60634
(312) 794-3333
CONTACT: Bruce Callahan Jr
CLIENTS SERVED PER MONTH: 310
FINANCIAL PLANS ACCEPTED: Private insurance; Medicare.
SERVICES OFFERED: Rehabilitative and supportive care; IV therapy; 24-hour availability; Blood transfusions.
EQUIPMENT & SUPPLIES: IV therapy equipment and supplies; Ambulatory assistance equipment; Wheelchairs; Respiratory equipment; Incontinence and ostomy products; Physical therapy supplies; Nutritional and feeding supplies; Custom wheelchairs; Seating systems.
EQUIPMENT/SUPPLY AVAILABILITY: For rent; For sale; Home delivery & pickup; 24-hour service.
See ad page 149

Umoja Care Inc
4501 W Augusta Blvd, Chicago, IL 60651
(312) 342-6550
CONTACT: Hassan Muhammad
CLIENTS SERVED PER MONTH: 200
FINANCIAL PLANS ACCEPTED: Medicaid/Medicare certified.
SERVICES OFFERED: Skilled nursing; Rehabilitative and supportive care; Help with activities of daily living; Homemaker service; Nutritional guidance; Telephone reassurance/Emergency alert; Meals; Transportation; Primary medical care.
EQUIPMENT & SUPPLIES: Ambulatory assistance equipment; Wheelchairs; Incontinence and ostomy products; Physical therapy supplies.

Unlimited Home Care
2939 N Pulaski Rd, Chicago, IL 60641
(312) 725-7881; (708) 998-0045 (Suburban office)

Upjohn HealthCare Services
310 S Peoria Ste 512, Chicago, IL 60607
(312) 829-0600
CONTACT: Gwendolyn Dailey

Visiting Nurse Association of Chicago
322 S Green St, Chicago, IL 60607-3599
(312) 738-8622
CONTACT: Philip M Moore
CLIENTS SERVED PER MONTH: 500-600
FINANCIAL PLANS ACCEPTED: Medicaid/Medicare certified; Private insurance.
SERVICES OFFERED: Skilled nursing; Rehabilitative and supportive care; Help with activities of daily living; Nutritional guidance.

Vital Measurements Inc
4817 W Montrose, Chicago, IL 60641
(312) 282-6232
CONTACT: Rose Vuco

Wishing Well Health Services
5757 N Lincoln Ave, Chicago, IL 60659
(312) 275-4000
CONTACT: Ann Comiskey

Chicago Heights

Alpha Home Health Care
Chicago Heights, IL
(708) 756-2700
FINANCIAL PLANS ACCEPTED: Medicaid/Medicare certified; Private insurance.
SERVICES OFFERED: Skilled nursing; Rehabilitative and supportive care; Help with activities of daily living; Private duty/extended care; Physical therapy; Speech therapy; Occupational therapy; MSW.

Cicero

Berwyn/Cicero Council on Aging
5817 W Cermak Rd, Cicero, IL 60650
(708) 863-3552
CONTACT: Barbara Liscar

Countryside

La Grange Memorial Home Care Services
6406 Joliet Rd, Countryside, IL 60525
(708) 352-6696, 352-9459 FAX
CONTACT: Rita Kopjo, Exec Dir

✔ In order to support future editions of this publication would you please mention *Elder Services* each time you contact any advertiser, facility, or service.

CLIENTS SERVED PER MONTH: 300-320 daily
FINANCIAL PLANS ACCEPTED: Medicaid/Medicare certified;
 Private insurance.
SERVICES OFFERED: Skilled nursing; Rehabilitative and
 supportive care; Help with activities of daily living;
 Homemaker service; Nutritional guidance; IV ther-
 apy; 24-hour availability; Hospice care.

Crest Hill

Abbey Home Healthcare—Crest Hill/Joliet
2416 Plainfield Rd, Crest Hill, IL 60435
(815) 439-0066, 439-0064 FAX
CONTACT: Debbie Wolf
FINANCIAL PLANS ACCEPTED: Medicaid/Medicare certified;
 Private insurance.
EQUIPMENT & SUPPLIES: Ambulatory assistance equip-
 ment; Respiratory equipment; Incontinence and
 ostomy products; Physical therapy supplies; Nutri-
 tional and feeding supplies; Medical equipment;
 Aerosol therapy; Life support systems.
EQUIPMENT/SUPPLY AVAILABILITY: For rent; For sale; Home
 delivery & pickup; 24-hour service.
See ad page 153

Alpha Home Health Care
1520 Rock Run Dr Ste 26, Crest Hill, IL 60435
(815) 741-3502
CONTACT: Laura Dean
FINANCIAL PLANS ACCEPTED: Medicaid/Medicare certified;
 Private insurance.
SERVICES OFFERED: Skilled nursing; Rehabilitative and
 supportive care; Help with activities of daily living;
 Private duty/extended care; Physical therapy;
 Speech therapy; Occupational therapy; MSW.

De Kalb

Alpha Home Health Care
205 N 2nd St, De Kalb, IL 60115
(815) 758-1224
FINANCIAL PLANS ACCEPTED: Medicaid/Medicare certified;
 Private insurance.
SERVICES OFFERED: Skilled nursing; Rehabilitative and
 supportive care; Help with activities of daily living;
 Private duty/extended care; Physical therapy;
 Speech therapy; Occupational therapy; MSW.

Des Plaines

Allcare Health Services Inc
2200 E Devon Ste 157, Des Plaines, IL 60018
(708) 297-0102
CONTACT: Lory Travis

Allcare Home Care
2200 E Devon Ste 154, Des Plaines, IL 60018
(708) 699-8500, 699-7379 FAX
CONTACT: Willa E Hammond
CLIENTS SERVED PER MONTH: 225
FINANCIAL PLANS ACCEPTED: Medicaid/Medicare certified;
 Private insurance.
SERVICES OFFERED: Skilled nursing; Rehabilitative and
 supportive care; Help with activities of daily living;
 Nutritional guidance; Telephone reassurance/
 Emergency alert; IV therapy; 24-hour availability.
EQUIPMENT & SUPPLIES: IV therapy equipment and sup-
 plies; Incontinence and ostomy products.

Concerned Care Inc
1345 Golf Rd, Des Plaines, IL 60016
(708) 635-5666, 296-4335 FAX
FINANCIAL PLANS ACCEPTED: Medicaid/Medicare certified;
 Private insurance.
SERVICES OFFERED: Skilled nursing; Rehabilitative and
 supportive care; Help with activities of daily living;
 Homemaker service; Nutritional guidance; Telephone reassurance/Emergency alert; IV therapy;
 24-hour availability; Live-ins; CNAs; Physical therapy; Occupational therapy; Speech therapy.
See ad page 167

Holy Family Hospital Home Care
100 N River Rd, Des Plaines, IL 60016
(708) 297-1800 ext 2720
CLIENTS SERVED PER MONTH: 600
FINANCIAL PLANS ACCEPTED: Medicaid/Medicare certified;
 Private insurance.
SERVICES OFFERED: Skilled nursing; Rehabilitative and
 supportive care; Help with activities of daily living;
 Nutritional guidance; Telephone reassurance/
 Emergency alert; IV therapy; 24-hour availability.
EQUIPMENT & SUPPLIES: IV therapy equipment and sup-
 plies; Ambulatory assistance equipment;
 Wheelchairs; Respiratory equipment; Incontinence
 and ostomy products; Physical therapy supplies;
 Nutritional and feeding supplies.
EQUIPMENT/SUPPLY AVAILABILITY: For rent; For sale; Home
 delivery & pickup; 24-hour service.

Downers Grove

Health and Human Resources—Downers Grove
842 Curtiss St, Downers Grove, IL 60515
(708) 719-4595
CONTACT: Barbara A Rickerman

Kimberly Quality Care—Downers Grove

1430 Branding Ln Ste 110, Downers Grove, IL 60515
(708) 971-1811, 971-0714 FAX
CONTACT: Jan Fulfs
FINANCIAL PLANS ACCEPTED: Medicaid/Medicare certified;
  Private insurance.
SERVICES OFFERED: Skilled nursing; Rehabilitative and
  supportive care; Help with activities of daily living;
  Homemaker service; IV therapy; 24-hour availabil-
  ity; Specialty rehab & infusion therapy.
EQUIPMENT & SUPPLIES: IV therapy equipment and sup-
  plies; Incontinence and ostomy products; Nutri-
  tional and feeding supplies.
See ad page 148

Nursefinders of Downers Grove

21 W 251 Maple Ave, Downers Grove, IL 60515-4246
(708) 852-4455, 852-9425 FAX
CONTACT: Mark Buck
FINANCIAL PLANS ACCEPTED: Private insurance.
SERVICES OFFERED: Skilled nursing; Rehabilitative and
  supportive care; Help with activities of daily living;
  Homemaker service; Telephone reassurance/Emer-
  gency alert; IV therapy; 24-hour availability; Phys-
  ical therapy; Occupational therapy; Speech ther-
  apy; Intermittent visits to round-the-clock care;
  Free home care evaluation.
See ad page 167

Elgin

Alpha Home Health Care

20 Woodland Ave, Elgin, IL 60123
(708) 931-0930
FINANCIAL PLANS ACCEPTED: Medicaid/Medicare certified;
  Private insurance.
SERVICES OFFERED: Skilled nursing; Rehabilitative and
  supportive care; Help with activities of daily living;
  Private duty/extended care; Physical therapy;
  Speech therapy; Occupational therapy; MSW.

Franciscan Home Health

77 N Airlite St, Elgin, IL 60174
(708) 931-5553
CONTACT: Mary Jo O'Malley
CLIENTS SERVED PER MONTH: 110
FINANCIAL PLANS ACCEPTED: Medicaid/Medicare certified;
  Private insurance.
SERVICES OFFERED: Skilled nursing; Rehabilitative and
  supportive care; Help with activities of daily living;
  Nutritional guidance; IV therapy; 24-hour availabil-
  ity.
See ads pages 18, 168

Sherman Home Care Partners

934 Center St, Elgin, IL 60120
(708) 888-8790, 888-8792 FAX
CONTACT: Katherine Lund
CLIENTS SERVED PER MONTH: 90-100
FINANCIAL PLANS ACCEPTED: Medicaid/Medicare certified;
  Private insurance.

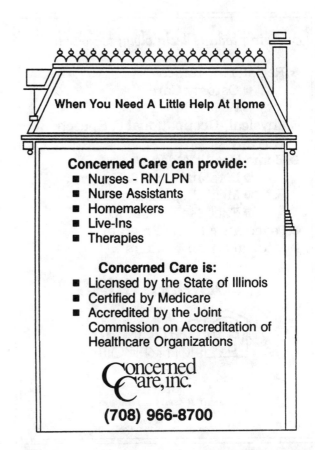

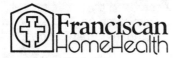

SERVICES OFFERED: Skilled nursing; Rehabilitative and supportive care; Help with activities of daily living; Homemaker service; Nutritional guidance; Telephone reassurance/Emergency alert; IV therapy; 24-hour availability.
EQUIPMENT & SUPPLIES: IV therapy equipment and supplies; Ambulatory assistance equipment; Wheelchairs; Respiratory equipment; Nutritional and feeding supplies; Hospital beds.
EQUIPMENT/SUPPLY AVAILABILITY: For rent; For sale; Home delivery & pickup; 24-hour service.

Visiting Nurse Association of Fox Valley
35 Fountain, Elgin, IL 60120
(708) 888-0505
CONTACT: Mary Tebeau RN
FINANCIAL PLANS ACCEPTED: Medicaid/Medicare certified; Private insurance.
SERVICES OFFERED: Skilled nursing; Rehabilitative and supportive care; Help with activities of daily living; Nutritional guidance; IV therapy; 24-hour availability; Physical therapy; Occupational therapy; Speech therapy; Medical therapy; Social services.
EQUIPMENT & SUPPLIES: IV therapy equipment and supplies; Incontinence and ostomy products; Nutritional and feeding supplies; Supplies needed to provide home care to clients.

Elk Grove Village

Critical Care America
985 Busse Rd, Elk Grove Village, IL 60007
(800) 458-6055
CONTACT: Barbara McMullin
CLIENTS SERVED PER MONTH: 150
FINANCIAL PLANS ACCEPTED: Medicaid/Medicare certified; Private insurance.
SERVICES OFFERED: Nutritional guidance; Telephone reassurance/Emergency alert; IV therapy; 24-hour availability.
EQUIPMENT & SUPPLIES: IV therapy equipment and supplies; Nutritional and feeding supplies.
EQUIPMENT/SUPPLY AVAILABILITY: For rent; For sale; Home delivery & pickup; 24-hour service.

Elmhurst

Care Tech Inc
747 Church Rd Ste A6, Elmhurst, IL 60126
(815) 344-9099

Home Nutritional Support
342 Carol Ln, Elmhurst, IL 60126
(708) 350-2299
CONTACT: Tom Bro

Medical Personnel Pool
453 N York Rd, Elmhurst, IL 60126
(708) 941-1771
CONTACT: Carol Auge
FINANCIAL PLANS ACCEPTED: Medicaid/Medicare certified; Private insurance.
SERVICES OFFERED: Skilled nursing; Rehabilitative and supportive care; Help with activities of daily living; Homemaker service; Nutritional guidance; Telephone reassurance/Emergency alert; IV therapy; 24-hour availability; High-tech home care; Ventilator program; Physical therapy; Speech therapy; Occupational therapy.

Elmwood Park

Alpha Home Health Care
1930 N Harlem Ave, Mont Clare Professional Center, Elmwood Park, IL 60635
(708) 453-9556
FINANCIAL PLANS ACCEPTED: Medicaid/Medicare certified; Private insurance.
SERVICES OFFERED: Skilled nursing; Rehabilitative and supportive care; Help with activities of daily living; Private duty/extended care; Physical therapy; Speech therapy; Occupational therapy; MSW.

Nursefinders of Elmwood Park
7310 W North Ave, Elmwood Park, IL 60635-4234
(708) 452-8800, 452-8724 FAX
CONTACT: Carol Howard
CLIENTS SERVED PER MONTH: 150-200
FINANCIAL PLANS ACCEPTED: Private insurance.
SERVICES OFFERED: Skilled nursing; Rehabilitative and supportive care; Help with activities of daily living; Homemaker service; Telephone reassurance/Emergency alert; IV therapy; 24-hour availability; Physical therapy; Occupational therapy; Speech therapy; Intermittent visits to round-the-clock care; Free home evaluation.
EQUIPMENT & SUPPLIES: Arranged as needed.
See ad page 167

Evanston

Caring Home Aid Program—Seniors Action Service Inc
1610 Maple, Evanston, IL 60201
(708) 864-7274
CONTACT: Phyllis Weiner
SERVICES OFFERED: Help with activities of daily living; Homemaker service.

Home Vision Care
1925 Central, Evanston, IL 60201
(708) 864-0300
CONTACT: Joan Sable

Kimberly Quality Care—Evanston
1609 Sherman Ave Ste 209, Evanston, IL 60201
(708) 328-1625
CONTACT: Elayne Weathersby
FINANCIAL PLANS ACCEPTED: Private insurance.
SERVICES OFFERED: Skilled nursing; Rehabilitative and supportive care; Help with activities of daily living; Homemaker service; IV therapy; 24-hour availability.
EQUIPMENT & SUPPLIES: IV therapy equipment and supplies; Ambulatory assistance equipment; Wheelchairs; Respiratory equipment; Incontinence and ostomy products; Physical therapy supplies; Nutritional and feeding supplies.
See ad page 148

Medical Personnel Pool
990 Grove St 2nd Fl, Evanston, IL 60201
(708) 869-7601
CONTACT: Nancy A Williams RN
FINANCIAL PLANS ACCEPTED: Medicaid/Medicare certified; Private insurance.
SERVICES OFFERED: Skilled nursing; Rehabilitative and supportive care; Help with activities of daily living; Homemaker service; Nutritional guidance; Telephone reassurance/Emergency alert; IV therapy; 24-hour availability; High-tech home care; Ventilator program; Physical therapy; Speech therapy; Occupational therapy.

Mobile Medical Care of St Francis Hospital
355 Ridge Ave, Evanston, IL 60202
(708) 492-6196, 492-7103 FAX
CONTACT: Joyce Johnson
FINANCIAL PLANS ACCEPTED: Medicaid/Medicare certified; Private insurance.
SERVICES OFFERED: Telephone reassurance/Emergency alert; Medical care in the home with lab, x-ray, EKGS.

Alice Toch Nurses Registry
1825 Madison, Evanston, IL 60202
(708) 491-6491
CONTACT: Paula Blue

Visiting Nurse Association North
2008 Dempster St, Evanston, IL 60202
(708) 328-1900, 328-9253 FAX
CONTACT: Phyllis R Anderson
CLIENTS SERVED PER MONTH: 600
FINANCIAL PLANS ACCEPTED: Medicaid/Medicare certified; Private insurance.
SERVICES OFFERED: Skilled nursing; Rehabilitative and supportive care; Help with activities of daily living; Homemaker service; Nutritional guidance; IV therapy; 24-hour availability; Hospice; Respite care.
EQUIPMENT & SUPPLIES: IV therapy equipment and supplies; Ambulatory assistance equipment; Incontinence and ostomy products; Physical therapy supplies; Nutritional and feeding supplies.

Evergreen Park

The Caring Touch
2400 W 95th St Ste 403, Evergreen Park, IL 60642
(312) 738-0299
CONTACT: Frances Free

Health Force
3336 W 95th St, Evergreen Park, IL 60642
(708) 422-7700
CONTACT: Marilynn Lopez
SERVICES OFFERED: Rehabilitative and supportive care; Help with activities of daily living; Homemaker service; Hospital staffing.

Harriet Holmes Health Care Services Inc
9730 S Western Ave Ste 426, Evergreen Park, IL 60642
(708) 422-8575
CONTACT: Dorothy Sims

Little Company of Mary Hospital & Health Care Centers
2800 W 95th St, Evergreen Park, IL 60642
(708) 422-6200
CONTACT: Sister Kathleen McIntyre
CLIENTS SERVED PER MONTH: 180
FINANCIAL PLANS ACCEPTED: Medicaid/Medicare certified; Private insurance.

✔ In order to support future editions of this publication would you please mention *Elder Services* each time you contact any advertiser, facility, or service.

SERVICES OFFERED: Skilled nursing; Rehabilitative and supportive care; Help with activities of daily living; Nutritional guidance; Telephone reassurance/ Emergency alert; Hospice home care; Adult day care; Alzheimer's home care; Care management.

Peace Memorial Home Health Service
10124 S Kedzie Ave, Evergreen Park, IL 60642
(708) 636-0544, 636-7375 FAX
CONTACT: Pat Witte
CLIENTS SERVED PER MONTH: 50
FINANCIAL PLANS ACCEPTED: Private insurance.
SERVICES OFFERED: Skilled nursing; Help with activities of daily living; Homemaker service; Nutritional guidance; Telephone reassurance/Emergency alert; 24-hour availability.

Flossmoor

Home Health Plus
19730 Governors Hwy Ste 2-5, Flossmoor, IL 60422-2040
(708) 799-8896, 799-4327 FAX
CONTACT: Carol Daniels
CLIENTS SERVED PER MONTH: 600
FINANCIAL PLANS ACCEPTED: Medicaid/Medicare certified; Private insurance.
SERVICES OFFERED: Skilled nursing; Rehabilitative and supportive care; Help with activities of daily living; Homemaker service; Nutritional guidance; IV therapy; 24-hour availability; Private duty; Intermittent visits.
EQUIPMENT & SUPPLIES: IV therapy equipment and supplies; Nutritional and feeding supplies.

Franklin Park

Leyden Family Service (Mental Health Center) Senior Citizen Program
10001 W Grand Ave, Franklin Park, IL 60131
(708) 451-0330
CONTACT: Dennis P Vaccaro

Geneva

Carlton Health Care
Box 172, 202 Campbell, Geneva, IL 60134
(708) 232-6908, 232-8477 FAX
CONTACT: Donna Greul
CLIENTS SERVED PER MONTH: 30
FINANCIAL PLANS ACCEPTED: Private insurance.
SERVICES OFFERED: Skilled nursing; Help with activities of daily living; Homemaker service; 24-hour availability.

Community Contacts Inc
1035 E State St, Geneva, IL 60134
(708) 232-9100
CONTACT: Susan Schumpp
SERVICES OFFERED: Homemaker service.

Glen Ellyn

Alpha Home Health Care
489 Taft (2 West), Glen Ellyn, IL 60137
(708) 790-4424
CLIENTS SERVED PER MONTH: 50
FINANCIAL PLANS ACCEPTED: Medicaid/Medicare certified; Private insurance.
SERVICES OFFERED: Skilled nursing; Rehabilitative and supportive care; Help with activities of daily living; Private duty/extended care; Physical therapy; Speech therapy; Occupational therapy; MSW.

Glencoe

Chicagoland Therapy Associates
111 Hogarth Ln, Glencoe, IL 60022-0417
(708) 835-0660

Harvey

South Suburban Senior Services of Catholic Charities
15300 S Lexington Ave, Harvey, IL 60426
(708) 596-2222, 596-9567 FAX
CONTACT: Margaret Latham
CLIENTS SERVED PER MONTH: 1,550
SERVICES OFFERED: Help with activities of daily living; Homemaker service; Telephone reassurance/Emergency alert; Case management; Home-delivered meals; Nutrition site; Counseling; Activity center.

Hazel Crest

Home Health Services of South Suburban Hospital
17800 S Kedzie, Hazel Crest, IL 60429
(708) 799-8000 ext 3267
CONTACT: Sandra Baniewicz
CLIENTS SERVED PER MONTH: 100
FINANCIAL PLANS ACCEPTED: Medicaid/Medicare certified; Private insurance.
SERVICES OFFERED: Skilled nursing; Rehabilitative and supportive care; Help with activities of daily living; IV therapy.

Nursefinders of Hazel Crest
17504 S Carriage Way Ste B, Hazel Crest, IL 60429-
     2006
(708) 799-7999
CONTACT: Pat Graff
FINANCIAL PLANS ACCEPTED: Private insurance.
SERVICES OFFERED: Skilled nursing; Rehabilitative and
     supportive care; Help with activities of daily living;
     Homemaker service; Telephone reassurance/Emer-
     gency alert; IV therapy; 24-hour availability; Phys-
     ical therapy; Occupational therapy; Speech ther-
     apy; Intermittent visits to round-the-clock care;
     Free home care evaluation.
See ad page 167

Hickory Hills

Kimberly Quality Care—Hickory Hills
7667 W 95th St Ste 300, Hickory Hills, IL 60457
(708) 598-1411, 598-2074 FAX
CONTACT: Sandi Vandenbroek
FINANCIAL PLANS ACCEPTED: Medicaid/Medicare certified;
     Private insurance.
SERVICES OFFERED: Skilled nursing; Rehabilitative and
     supportive care; Help with activities of daily living;
     Homemaker service; IV therapy; 24-hour availabil-
     ity.
EQUIPMENT & SUPPLIES: IV therapy equipment and sup-
     plies; Ambulatory assistance equipment;
     Wheelchairs; Respiratory equipment; Incontinence
     and ostomy products; Physical therapy supplies;
     Nutritional and feeding supplies.
See ad page 148

Highland Park

Highland Park Hospital Home Health Services
1936 Greenbay Rd, Highland Park, IL 60035
(708) 480-3749
CONTACT: J Findley
CLIENTS SERVED PER MONTH: 190
FINANCIAL PLANS ACCEPTED: Medicaid/Medicare certified;
     Private insurance.
SERVICES OFFERED: Skilled nursing; Rehabilitative and
     supportive care; Help with activities of daily living;
     Nutritional guidance; Telephone reassurance/
     Emergency alert; IV therapy; 24-hour availability.
EQUIPMENT & SUPPLIES: Incontinence and ostomy pro-
     ducts; Other equipment arranged as needed.

Highwood

Traycee Home Care
448 Sheridan Rd, Highwood, IL 60040
(708) 432-5190
CONTACT: Bonnie Ramis
CLIENTS SERVED PER MONTH: 100

FINANCIAL PLANS ACCEPTED: Private insurance.
SERVICES OFFERED: Rehabilitative and supportive care;
     Help with activities of daily living; Homemaker
     service; Nutritional guidance; Telephone
     reassurance/Emergency alert; 24-hour availability;
     CNA.
EQUIPMENT & SUPPLIES: Ambulatory assistance equip-
     ment; Wheelchairs.
EQUIPMENT/SUPPLY AVAILABILITY: For sale; Home delivery
     & pickup.
See ad page 165

Hinsdale

Health Care at Home
7 Salt Creek Ln Ste 101, Hinsdale, IL 60521
(708) 920-8300, 850-3969 FAX
CONTACT: Bruce Harlow
CLIENTS SERVED PER MONTH: 150-200
FINANCIAL PLANS ACCEPTED: Medicaid/Medicare certified;
     Private insurance.
SERVICES OFFERED: Skilled nursing; Rehabilitative and
     supportive care; Help with activities of daily living;
     Telephone reassurance/Emergency alert; IV ther-
     apy; 24-hour availability.
See ad page 73

Hoffman Estates

Kenneth W Young Center for Senior Services
2500 W Higgins Rd Ste 655, Hoffman Estates, IL
     60195
(708) 885-1631
CONTACT: Barbara Meyer
FINANCIAL PLANS ACCEPTED: Private insurance.
SERVICES OFFERED: Professional counseling; Home deliv-
     ered meals; Case management/Service coordina-
     tion; Chore/Housekeeping; Training and educa-
     tion.

Homewood

Caremark Inc
1125 W 175th, Homewood, IL 60430
(708) 957-9572, 957-8531 FAX
CONTACT: Carol Aronson
CLIENTS SERVED PER MONTH: 900
FINANCIAL PLANS ACCEPTED: Private insurance.
SERVICES OFFERED: Skilled nursing; Nutritional guidance;
     IV therapy; 24-hour availability; Social services.
EQUIPMENT & SUPPLIES: IV therapy equipment and sup-
     plies; Nutritional and feeding supplies.
EQUIPMENT/SUPPLY AVAILABILITY: For rent; Home delivery
     & pickup; 24-hour service.

✔ In order to support future editions of this publication would you please mention *Elder Services* each time you contact any advertiser, facility, or service.

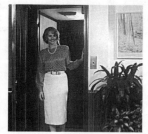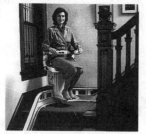
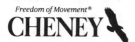
Concerned Care Inc

17924 S Halsted, Homewood, IL 60430
(708) 798-8966, 798-9274 FAX
FINANCIAL PLANS ACCEPTED: Medicaid/Medicare certified; Private insurance.
SERVICES OFFERED: Skilled nursing; Rehabilitative and supportive care; Help with activities of daily living; Homemaker service; Nutritional guidance; Telephone reassurance/Emergency alert; IV therapy; 24-hour availability; Physical therapy; Occupational therapy; Speech therapy; Live-ins; CNAs.
See ad page 167

Ingalls Home Care

2640 W 183rd St, Homewood, IL 60430
(708) 206-1496
CONTACT: Jean LaRoche

Joliet

Care Company Health Care Inc

257 Springfield Ave, Joliet, IL 60435
(815) 725-2902
CONTACT: Peter M Jursinic

Community Care System Inc

407 W Jefferson St, Joliet, IL 60435
(815) 727-0026

Franciscan Home Health of St Joseph Medical Center

333 Madison St, Joliet, IL 60435-9934
(815) 741-7371
CONTACT: Donna Talbot

In Home Health Care Service—West Inc-Joliet Div

310 N Hammes Ave, Joliet, IL 60435
(815) 725-8400
CONTACT: George Deming; Margaret Kolenc RN
CLIENTS SERVED PER MONTH: 165
FINANCIAL PLANS ACCEPTED: Medicaid/Medicare certified; Private insurance.
SERVICES OFFERED: Skilled nursing; Rehabilitative and supportive care; Help with activities of daily living; Nutritional guidance; Telephone reassurance/Emergency alert; IV therapy; 24-hour availability; Physical therapy; Occupational therapy; Speech therapy; Social work services; High-tech services.
EQUIPMENT & SUPPLIES: IV therapy equipment and supplies; Incontinence and ostomy products; Nutritional and feeding supplies; Wound care supplies & dressings.

Kimberly Quality Care—Joliet

3033 W Jefferson Ste 204, Joliet, IL 60435-5252
(815) 729-4828
CONTACT: Helen Smunt
FINANCIAL PLANS ACCEPTED: Medicaid/Medicare certified; Private insurance.
SERVICES OFFERED: Skilled nursing; Rehabilitative and supportive care; Help with activities of daily living; Homemaker service; IV therapy; 24-hour availability; Physical therapy; Occupational therapy; Speech therapy.
EQUIPMENT & SUPPLIES: IV therapy equipment and supplies; Ambulatory assistance equipment; Wheelchairs; Respiratory equipment; Incontinence and ostomy products; Physical therapy supplies; Nutritional and feeding supplies.
See ad page 148

Medical Personnel Pool

2112 W Jefferson Ste 232, Joliet, IL 60435
(815) 725-9091
CONTACT: Cheri Gericke
FINANCIAL PLANS ACCEPTED: Medicaid/Medicare certified; Private insurance.
SERVICES OFFERED: Skilled nursing; Rehabilitative and supportive care; Help with activities of daily living; Homemaker service; Nutritional guidance; Telephone reassurance/Emergency alert; IV therapy; 24-hour availability; High-tech home care; Ventilator program; Physical therapy; Speech therapy; Occupational therapy.

Nursefinders of Joliet

121 Springfield Ave, Joliet, IL 60435
(815) 725-4466, 725-4475 FAX
CONTACT: Susan Welch
FINANCIAL PLANS ACCEPTED: Private insurance.

SERVICES OFFERED: Skilled nursing; Rehabilitative and supportive care; Help with activities of daily living; Homemaker service; Nutritional guidance; IV therapy; 24-hour availability; Intermittent visits to round-the-clock care.
See ad page 167

Upjohn HealthCare Services
2112 W Jefferson Ste 300, Joliet, IL 60435-6622
(815) 741-1440
CONTACT: Cindy Weber
CLIENTS SERVED PER MONTH: 150
FINANCIAL PLANS ACCEPTED: Medicaid/Medicare certified; Private insurance.
SERVICES OFFERED: Skilled nursing; Rehabilitative and supportive care; Help with activities of daily living; Nutritional guidance.

Justice

Mercy Home Health Care
81st & Kean Ave, Justice, IL 60458
(800) 339-0666, 496-8205 FAX
CONTACT: Yvonne Keller
CLIENTS SERVED PER MONTH: 350
FINANCIAL PLANS ACCEPTED: Medicaid/Medicare certified; Private insurance.
SERVICES OFFERED: Skilled nursing; Rehabilitative and supportive care; Help with activities of daily living; Homemaker service; Nutritional guidance; Telephone reassurance/Emergency alert; IV therapy; 24-hour availability.
EQUIPMENT & SUPPLIES: Arranged as needed.
See ads pages 116, 161, 351

La Grange

La Grange Community Nurse & Service Association
27 Calendar Ct, La Grange, IL 60525
(708) 352-0081
CONTACT: Patty Donahue
FINANCIAL PLANS ACCEPTED: Medicaid/Medicare certified; Private insurance.
SERVICES OFFERED: Skilled nursing; Rehabilitative and supportive care; Help with activities of daily living; Telephone reassurance/Emergency alert.

Lake Forest

Lake Forest Hospital Home Health
660 N Westmoreland Rd, Lake Forest, IL 60045
(708) 234-5600
CONTACT: William G Ries

Lake In The Hills

Around the Clock Nursing Registry Inc
1111 Algonquin Rd, Lake In The Hills, IL 60102
(708) 658-8855

Lake Villa

Family Care Services of Lake and McHenry Counties
PO Box 168, Rte 83, Lake Villa, IL 60046
(708) 356-6000
CONTACT: Phil Racette

Lake County Health Dept
121 E Grand Ave, Lake Villa, IL 60046
(708) 360-6711

Lemont

Home Health Care Inc—Lemont
106 Stephens St, Lemont, IL 60439
(708) 257-1111, 257-1115 FAX
FINANCIAL PLANS ACCEPTED: Medicaid/Medicare certified; Private insurance.
SERVICES OFFERED: Skilled nursing; Rehabilitative and supportive care; Help with activities of daily living; Homemaker service; Nutritional guidance; Telephone reassurance/Emergency alert; 24-hour availability.

Libertyville

Caregivers Home Health
800 S Milwaukee Ave, Libertyville, IL 60048
(708) 367-3838
SERVICES OFFERED: Skilled nursing; Rehabilitative and supportive care; Help with activities of daily living; Homemaker service; Nutritional guidance; IV therapy; 24-hour availability.

Medical Personnel Pool
1117 S Milwaukee Ave, Libertyville, IL 60048
(708) 362-7017
CONTACT: Nancy Williams
FINANCIAL PLANS ACCEPTED: Medicaid/Medicare certified; Private insurance.
SERVICES OFFERED: Skilled nursing; Rehabilitative and supportive care; Help with activities of daily living; Homemaker service; Nutritional guidance; Telephone reassurance/Emergency alert; IV therapy; 24-hour availability; High-tech home care; Ventilator program; Physical therapy; Speech therapy; Occupational therapy.

✓ In order to support future editions of this publication would you please mention *Elder Services* each time you contact any advertiser, facility, or service.

Nursefinders of Libertyville
1757 N Milwaukee Ave, Libertyville, IL 60048-1316
(708) 816-8720
CONTACT: Sandy Hackler
FINANCIAL PLANS ACCEPTED: Private insurance.
SERVICES OFFERED: Skilled nursing; Rehabilitative and supportive care; Help with activities of daily living; Homemaker service; Telephone reassurance/Emergency alert; IV therapy; 24-hour availability; Physical therapy; Occupational therapy; Speech therapy; Intermittent visits to round-the-clock care; Free home care evaluation.
See ad page 167

Lombard

Abbey Home Healthcare
219 S Eisenhower Ln, Lombard, IL 60148
(708) 629-9850, 629-8948 FAX
CONTACT: John Kovelan
FINANCIAL PLANS ACCEPTED: Medicaid/Medicare certified; Private insurance.
EQUIPMENT & SUPPLIES: Ambulatory assistance equipment; Respiratory equipment; Incontinence and ostomy products; Physical therapy supplies; Nutritional and feeding supplies; Medical equipment; Aerosol therapy; Life support systems.
EQUIPMENT/SUPPLY AVAILABILITY: For rent; For sale; Home delivery & pickup; 24-hour service.
See ad page 153

Olsten Healthcare
450 E 22nd St Ste 121, Lombard, IL 60148-6170
(800) 244-4075; (312) 565-1706
CONTACT: Linda Dobosz

Lyons

MacNeal Home Health Services
7310 39th St Ste 101, Lyons, IL 60534-1247
(708) 447-3555, 447-3974 FAX
CONTACT: Prudence Ogden
CLIENTS SERVED PER MONTH: 1,400
FINANCIAL PLANS ACCEPTED: Medicaid/Medicare certified; Private insurance.
SERVICES OFFERED: Skilled nursing; Rehabilitative and supportive care; Help with activities of daily living; Homemaker service; Nutritional guidance; IV therapy; 24-hour availability; Occupational therapy; Physical therapy; Speech therapy.
EQUIPMENT & SUPPLIES: IV therapy equipment and supplies; Ambulatory assistance equipment.
EQUIPMENT/SUPPLY AVAILABILITY: For sale; Home delivery & pickup.
See ad page 174

Maywood

NovaCare Inc
1701 S 1st Ave Ste 509, Maywood, IL 60153
(708) 338-1030

McHenry

Northern Illinois Medical Center—Home Health Care
4201 Medical Center Dr, McHenry, IL 60050
(815) 344-6602
CONTACT: Anne Mattson
CLIENTS SERVED PER MONTH: 130
FINANCIAL PLANS ACCEPTED: Medicaid/Medicare certified; Private insurance.
SERVICES OFFERED: Skilled nursing; Rehabilitative and supportive care; Help with activities of daily living; Nutritional guidance; Telephone reassurance/ Emergency alert.

Melrose Park

Gottlieb Memorial Hospital
701 W North Ave, Melrose Park, IL 60160
(708) 450-4956, 681-5412 FAX
CONTACT: Char Olsen

CLIENTS SERVED PER MONTH: 300
FINANCIAL PLANS ACCEPTED: Medicaid/Medicare certified; Private insurance.
SERVICES OFFERED: Skilled nursing; Rehabilitative and supportive care; Help with activities of daily living; Nutritional guidance; Telephone reassurance/ Emergency alert; Medical social services.
See ad page 127

Westlake Community Hospital
1225 Superior St, Melrose Park, IL 60160
(708) 681-3000
CONTACT: Theresa Rogers

Morton Grove

Abbey Home Healthcare
8224 Lehigh Ave, Morton Grove, IL 60053
(708) 470-2440, 470-4713 FAX
CONTACT: Mike Kotlan
FINANCIAL PLANS ACCEPTED: Medicaid/Medicare certified; Private insurance.
EQUIPMENT & SUPPLIES: Ambulatory assistance equipment; Respiratory equipment; Incontinence and ostomy products; Physical therapy supplies; Nutritional and feeding supplies; Medical equipment; Aerosol therapy; Life support systems.
EQUIPMENT/SUPPLY AVAILABILITY: For rent; For sale; Home delivery & pickup; 24-hour service.
See ad page 153

In Home Health Care—Suburban Chicago North
8700 Waukegan Rd, Morton Grove, IL 60053
(708) 965-8250, 965-5161 FAX
FINANCIAL PLANS ACCEPTED: Medicaid/Medicare certified; Private insurance.
SERVICES OFFERED: Skilled nursing; Nutritional guidance; IV therapy; 24-hour availability; Physical therapy; Occupational therapy; Speech therapy; Social worker; Home health aides.

NMC Home Care
8120 Lehigh Ave, Morton Grove, IL 60053
(312) 792-1821
CONTACT: Charlette Johnson

Mount Prospect

Caremark Home Care Inc
1200 Business Center Dr, Mount Prospect, IL 60056
(708) 803-9600
CONTACT: Louise Pickens

Village of Mt Prospect Human Services Division
50 S Emerson St, Mount Prospect, IL 60056
(708) 870-5680
CONTACT: Nancy Morgan
CLIENTS SERVED PER MONTH: 15

SERVICES OFFERED: Skilled nursing (for Mount Prospect residents); Nutritional guidance; Caregivers support group; Nurses lending closet; Coordinate home companion program (fee for companions); Weekly blood pressure and diabetic screening.

Naperville

Health Force
650 S Route 59, Naperville, IL 60540
(708) 357-7400
CONTACT: Marilynn Lopez
SERVICES OFFERED: Help with activities of daily living; Homemaker service.

Niles

The Caring Touch
5940 W Touhy, Niles, IL 60648
(312) 738-0299

Regency Home Health Care
6625 N Milwaukee Ave, Niles, IL 60648
(708) 647-1511, 647-7746 FAX
CONTACT: Carole Wilstein
CLIENTS SERVED PER MONTH: 150-160
FINANCIAL PLANS ACCEPTED: Medicaid/Medicare certified; Private insurance.
SERVICES OFFERED: Skilled nursing; Rehabilitative and supportive care; Help with activities of daily living; Homemaker service; Nutritional guidance; 24-hour availability; Case management; Intermittent skilled to 24-hour live-in care.

Roche Professional Services
6207 W Howard Ave, Niles, IL 60648
(708) 647-0770
CONTACT: Byron Ishima

North Riverside

Kimberly Quality Care—North Riverside
7222 W Cermak Rd Ste 605, North Riverside, IL 60546
(708) 447-6220, 442-0702 FAX
CONTACT: Lois Dick
FINANCIAL PLANS ACCEPTED: Medicaid/Medicare certified; Private insurance.
SERVICES OFFERED: Skilled nursing; Rehabilitative and supportive care; Help with activities of daily living; Homemaker service; IV therapy; 24-hour availability.
EQUIPMENT & SUPPLIES: IV therapy equipment and supplies; Ambulatory assistance equipment; Wheelchairs; Respiratory equipment; Incontinence and ostomy products; Physical therapy supplies; Nutritional and feeding supplies.
See ad page 148

Northbrook

Caring Companions of the North Shore Inc
1856 Walters Ave, Northbrook, IL 60062
(708) 480-0034
CONTACT: Sarah Hill

Northfield

North Shore Senior Center
7 Happ Rd, Northfield, IL 60093
(708) 446-8750
CONTACT: Sandi Johnson
See ad page 144

Northlake

The Caring Center—Casa San Carlo
444 N Wolf Rd, Northlake, IL 60164
(708) 562-0040
CONTACT: Lydia Nunez RN
SERVICES OFFERED: Skilled nursing; Rehabilitative and supportive care; Help with activities of daily living; Nutritional guidance; Telephone reassurance/ Emergency alert.
See ad page 177

Oak Brook

EHS Home Health Care Service Inc
2025 Windsor Dr, Oak Brook, IL 60521
(708) 572-1232, 572-9797 FAX
CONTACT: John McGinnis
CLIENTS SERVED PER MONTH: 1,200
FINANCIAL PLANS ACCEPTED: Medicaid/Medicare certified; Private insurance.
SERVICES OFFERED: Skilled nursing; Rehabilitative and supportive care; Nutritional guidance; IV therapy; 24-hour availability.

Norrell Health Care
1900 Spring Rd Ste 514, Oak Brook, IL 60521
(708) 954-1535
CONTACT: Barbara Bostelmann

Oak Lawn

Medical Personnel Pool
10735 S Cicero Ave Ste 200, Oak Lawn, IL 60453-5400
(708) 422-2934
CONTACT: Susan Faust
FINANCIAL PLANS ACCEPTED: Medicaid/Medicare certified; Private insurance.
SERVICES OFFERED: Skilled nursing; Rehabilitative and supportive care; Help with activities of daily living; Homemaker service; Nutritional guidance; Telephone reassurance/Emergency alert; IV therapy; 24-hour availability; High-tech home care; Ventilator program; Physical therapy; Speech therapy; Occupational therapy.

Nursefinders of Oak Lawn
4239 W 95th St, Oak Lawn, IL 60453-2623
(708) 857-2400
CONTACT: Karl Ellensohn
FINANCIAL PLANS ACCEPTED: Medicaid/Medicare certified; Private insurance.
SERVICES OFFERED: Skilled nursing; Rehabilitative and supportive care; Help with activities of daily living; Homemaker service; Telephone reassurance/Emergency alert; IV therapy; 24-hour availability; Physical therapy; Occupational therapy; Speech therapy; Intermittent visits to round-the-clock care; Free home care evaluation.
See ad page 167

Plows Council on Aging
4700 W 95th St Ste 106, Oak Lawn, IL 60453
(708) 422-6722
CONTACT: Donald Chapman

Oak Park

Ancilla Home Health
1000 W Lake St, Oak Park, IL 60301
(708) 386-1195
CONTACT: Susan Levitt
FINANCIAL PLANS ACCEPTED: Medicaid/Medicare certified; Private insurance.
SERVICES OFFERED: Skilled nursing; Rehabilitative and supportive care; Telephone reassurance/Emergency alert; IV therapy; Home health aides.
EQUIPMENT & SUPPLIES: IV therapy equipment and supplies; Incontinence and ostomy products; Nutritional and feeding supplies.

At Home Health Inc
715 W Lake St Ste 400, Oak Park, IL 60301
(708) 383-2444, 383-9514 FAX
CONTACT: Rosemary Shmet RN
FINANCIAL PLANS ACCEPTED: Medicaid/Medicare certified; Private insurance.
SERVICES OFFERED: Skilled nursing; Rehabilitative and supportive care; Help with activities of daily living; Homemaker service; Nutritional guidance; Tele-

phone reassurance/Emergency alert; IV therapy; 24-hour availability; Ancillary & related therapy; Intermittent or extended basis nursing.

Bruce & Ken's Pharmacy
111 N Oak Park Ave, Oak Park, IL 60301
(708) 386-8002
CONTACT: Bruce Callahan Jr
CLIENTS SERVED PER MONTH: 225
FINANCIAL PLANS ACCEPTED: Private insurance; Medicare.
SERVICES OFFERED: Rehabilitative and supportive care; IV therapy; 24-hour availability; Blood transfusions.
EQUIPMENT & SUPPLIES: IV therapy equipment and supplies; Ambulatory assistance equipment; Wheelchairs; Respiratory equipment; Incontinence and ostomy products; Physical therapy supplies; Nutritional and feeding supplies; Custom wheelchairs; Seating systems.
EQUIPMENT/SUPPLY AVAILABILITY: For rent; For sale; Home delivery & pickup; 24-hour service.
See ad page 149

The Caring Center—Mills Tower
1025 Pleasant Pl, Oak Park, IL 60302
(708) 386-7536
CONTACT: Laurel Ahlenius RN
SERVICES OFFERED: Skilled nursing; Rehabilitative and supportive care; Help with activities of daily living; Nutritional guidance; Telephone reassurance/ Emergency alert.
See ad page 177

The Caring Center—The Oaks
12 S Humphrey, Oak Park, IL 60302
(708) 383-0999
CONTACT: Laurel Ahlenius RN
SERVICES OFFERED: Skilled nursing; Rehabilitative and supportive care; Help with activities of daily living; Nutritional guidance; Telephone reassurance/ Emergency alert.
See ad page 177

Community Nursing Service West
1041 Madison St, Oak Park, IL 60302
(708) 386-4443
CONTACT: Saundra Spilotro
CLIENTS SERVED PER MONTH: 250
FINANCIAL PLANS ACCEPTED: Medicaid/Medicare certified; Private insurance.
SERVICES OFFERED: Skilled nursing; Rehabilitative and supportive care; Help with activities of daily living; Homemaker service; IV therapy; 24-hour availability; Hospice.

FirstChoice Home Health & Family Support Services
414 S Oak Park Ave Ste 28, Oak Park, IL 60302
(708) 383-2500
CONTACT: Dorothy Butkovich
FINANCIAL PLANS ACCEPTED: Medicaid/Medicare certified; Private insurance.

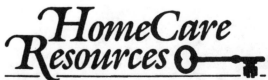
✓ In order to support future editions of this publication would you please mention *Elder Services* each time you contact any advertiser, facility, or service.

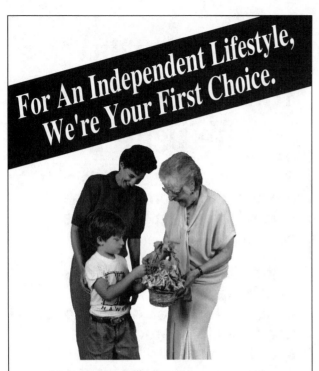

For An Independent Lifestyle, We're Your First Choice.

Maintaining one's independence means a great deal to everyone. The freedom to live in the home that you love. The confidence to continue doing the things you like to do. The security of knowing that assistance is available if you need it.

FirstChoice Health Care offers assisted living options with the flexibility to maintain an independent lifestyle.

- **Home Nursing Care**
- **Assisted Living at Home:**
  - Independent Living
  - Medication Assistance & Supervision
  - Respite Care
  - Live-In Companion
  - Lifeline® Response System
- **Home Delivered Personal Care Products**
- **Home Medical Equipment**
- **Family Retirement Counseling**

To find out more about these and other services, just call and request a complimentary copy of the FirstChoice *Assisted Living Resource Guide*.

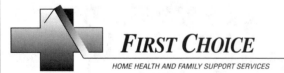

FIRST CHOICE
HOME HEALTH AND FAMILY SUPPORT SERVICES

708/ 383-2500

SERVICES OFFERED: Skilled nursing; Rehabilitative and supportive care; Help with activities of daily living; Homemaker service; Nutritional guidance; Telephone reassurance/Emergency alert; IV therapy; 24-hour availability; Senior family counseling.
EQUIPMENT & SUPPLIES: IV therapy equipment and supplies; Ambulatory assistance equipment; Wheelchairs; Respiratory equipment; Incontinence and ostomy products; Physical therapy supplies; Nutritional and feeding supplies; Life-line.
EQUIPMENT/SUPPLY AVAILABILITY: For rent; For sale; Home delivery & pickup; 24-hour service.
See ads pages 118, 130, 178

Home Companion Service
38 N Austin Blvd, Oak Park, IL 60302
(708) 386-1324
CLIENTS SERVED PER MONTH: 40-50
SERVICES OFFERED: Help with activities of daily living; Homemaker service; 24-hour availability; Caregiver respite.

Home Medical Care Foundation
1100 Lake St Ste 20, Oak Park, IL 60302
(708) 383-0100
CONTACT: Marilyn Oftedahl
FINANCIAL PLANS ACCEPTED: Medicaid/Medicare certified; Private insurance.
SERVICES OFFERED: Skilled nursing; Rehabilitative and supportive care; Help with activities of daily living; Homemaker service; Nutritional guidance; Telephone reassurance/Emergency alert; IV therapy; 24-hour availability; Senior family counseling.
EQUIPMENT & SUPPLIES: IV therapy equipment and supplies; Ambulatory assistance equipment; Wheelchairs; Respiratory equipment; Incontinence and ostomy products; Physical therapy supplies; Nutritional and feeding supplies; Life-line.
EQUIPMENT/SUPPLY AVAILABILITY: For rent; For sale; Home delivery & pickup; 24-hour service.
See ad page 118, 130, 178

HomeCare Resources—An Affiliate of West Suburban Hospital Medical Center
12 W Lake St, Oak Park, IL 60302
(708) 383-4663
CONTACT: Kay Lawrence
CLIENTS SERVED PER MONTH: 300
SERVICES OFFERED: Skilled nursing; Rehabilitative and supportive care; Help with activities of daily living; Homemaker service; Nutritional guidance; Telephone reassurance/Emergency alert; IV therapy; Home health aides; Companion service.
See ad page 177

Kimberly Quality Care—Oak Park
1146 Westgate Ste L104, Oak Park, IL 60301
(708) 848-0962, 848-7530 FAX
CONTACT: Elayne Weathersby
FINANCIAL PLANS ACCEPTED: Private insurance.
SERVICES OFFERED: Skilled nursing; Rehabilitative and supportive care; Help with activities of daily living; Homemaker service; IV therapy; 24-hour availability.

EQUIPMENT & SUPPLIES: IV therapy equipment and supplies; Ambulatory assistance equipment; Wheelchairs; Respiratory equipment; Incontinence and ostomy products; Physical therapy supplies; Nutritional and feeding supplies.

See ad page 148

Medical Personnel Pool

1515 N Harlem Ave Ste 101, Oak Park, IL 60302
(708) 383-7320
CONTACT: Marlene Silenzi
FINANCIAL PLANS ACCEPTED: Medicaid/Medicare certified; Private insurance.
SERVICES OFFERED: Skilled nursing; Rehabilitative and supportive care; Help with activities of daily living; Homemaker service; Nutritional guidance; Telephone reassurance/Emergency alert; IV therapy; 24-hour availability; High-tech home care; Ventilator program; Physical therapy; Speech therapy; Occupational therapy.

Oak Park Township Office

105 S Oak Park Ave, Oak Park, IL 60302
(708) 383-8005
CONTACT: Laslo E Tako

Olympia Fields

Kimberly Quality Care—Olympia Fields

2555 W Lincoln Hwy Ste 213, Olympia Fields, IL 60461
(708) 481-1462, 481-9074 FAX
CONTACT: Betty Gemmato
FINANCIAL PLANS ACCEPTED: Medicaid/Medicare certified; Private insurance.
SERVICES OFFERED: Skilled nursing; Rehabilitative and supportive care; Help with activities of daily living; Homemaker service; IV therapy; 24-hour availability.
EQUIPMENT & SUPPLIES: IV therapy equipment and supplies; Ambulatory assistance equipment; Wheelchairs; Respiratory equipment; Incontinence and ostomy products; Physical therapy supplies; Nutritional and feeding supplies.
EQUIPMENT/SUPPLY AVAILABILITY: For rent; For sale; Home delivery & pickup; 24-hour service.

See ad page 148

Palos Hills

Shay Health Care Services Inc

12600 S Harlem Ave Ste 202, Palos Hills, IL 60463-1448
(708) 361-7990, 361-8074 FAX
CONTACT: Mariann Whitemiller RN
CLIENTS SERVED PER MONTH: 100
FINANCIAL PLANS ACCEPTED: Medicaid/Medicare certified; Private insurance.

SERVICES OFFERED: Skilled nursing; Rehabilitative and supportive care; Help with activities of daily living; Nutritional guidance; IV therapy; 24-hour availability.

Park Forest

Park Forest Health Dept

9 Centre, Park Forest, IL 60466
(708) 748-1118, 748-1630 FAX
CONTACT: Lois Coxworth
CLIENTS SERVED PER MONTH: 500
FINANCIAL PLANS ACCEPTED: Medicaid/Medicare certified; Private insurance.
SERVICES OFFERED: Skilled nursing; Rehabilitative and supportive care; IV therapy.
EQUIPMENT & SUPPLIES: Ambulatory assistance equipment; Wheelchairs.
EQUIPMENT/SUPPLY AVAILABILITY: Through a loan closet.

Park Ridge

A-Abiding Care Inc

PO Box 150, 233 N Northwest Hwy, Park Ridge, IL 60068
(708) 698-2273
CONTACT: Joyce Kernan
FINANCIAL PLANS ACCEPTED: Private insurance.
SERVICES OFFERED: Skilled nursing; Rehabilitative and supportive care; Help with activities of daily living; Homemaker service; Nutritional guidance; Telephone reassurance/Emergency alert; IV therapy; 24-hour availability; Live-in care.

The Center of Concern

1580 N Northwest Hwy Ste 223, Park Ridge, IL 60068
(708) 823-0453
CONTACT: Dorothea Heinrich
CLIENTS SERVED PER MONTH: 20
SERVICES OFFERED: Rehabilitative and supportive care; Help with activities of daily living; Homemaker service.

Omni Home Care

1550 Northwest Hwy, Park Ridge, IL 60068
(708) 297-3720
CONTACT: Patricia Sefton
FINANCIAL PLANS ACCEPTED: Private insurance.
SERVICES OFFERED: Skilled nursing; Rehabilitative and supportive care; Help with activities of daily living; Nutritional guidance; IV therapy; 24-hour availability.
EQUIPMENT & SUPPLIES: IV therapy equipment and supplies; Ambulatory assistance equipment; Wheelchairs; Incontinence and ostomy products; Physical therapy supplies.

✔ In order to support future editions of this publication would you please mention *Elder Services* each time you contact any advertiser, facility, or service.

Richton Park

Rich Township Senior Services
22013 Governor Hwy, Richton Park, IL 60471
(708) 748-5454
CONTACT: George Falaney

River Forest

Home Infusion Therapy
7350 Garden Ct, River Forest, IL 60305
(708) 366-2727
CONTACT: David Krupa

Robbins

Senior Citizens Services
3518 W 139th St, Robbins, IL 60472
(708) 371-7095
CONTACT: Shannon Hunt
SERVICES OFFERED: Help with activities of daily living; Nutritional guidance; Telephone reassurance/Emergency alert; Senior nutrition/recreation activities.

Rolling Meadows

Home Health Plus
1921 Rohlwing Rd, Rolling Meadows, IL 60008
(708) 632-1101, 632-0025 FAX
CONTACT: Julie Thompson
CLIENTS SERVED PER MONTH: 600
FINANCIAL PLANS ACCEPTED: Medicaid/Medicare certified; Private insurance.
SERVICES OFFERED: Skilled nursing; Rehabilitative and supportive care; Help with activities of daily living; Homemaker service; Nutritional guidance; IV therapy; 24-hour availability; Private duty; Intermittent visits.
EQUIPMENT & SUPPLIES: IV therapy equipment and supplies; Nutritional and feeding supplies.

Roselle

Nurses to You Ltd
701 E Irving Park Rd Ste 204, Roselle, IL 60172
(708) 894-1555
CONTACT: Geri Houdek

Saint Charles

Concerned Care Inc
525 Dunham Rd, Saint Charles, IL 60174
(708) 377-2667, 377-8145 FAX
FINANCIAL PLANS ACCEPTED: Medicaid/Medicare certified; Private insurance.
SERVICES OFFERED: Skilled nursing; Rehabilitative and supportive care; Help with activities of daily living; Homemaker service; Nutritional guidance; Telephone reassurance/Emergency alert; IV therapy; 24-hour availability; CNAs; Live-ins; Physical therapy; Occupational therapy; Speech therapy.
See ad page 167

Country Care Inc
1020 Cedar Ave, Saint Charles, IL 60174
(708) 584-7677

Schaumburg

Alexian Home Health
25 E Schaumburg Rd Ste 106, Schaumburg, IL 60193
(708) 386-1195
CONTACT: Jackie Anderson

In Home Health Care Service—West Inc
1699 E Woodfield Rd Ste A-7, Schaumburg, IL 60173
(708) 605-1660
FINANCIAL PLANS ACCEPTED: Medicaid/Medicare certified; Private insurance.
SERVICES OFFERED: Skilled nursing; Rehabilitative and supportive care; Help with activities of daily living; Nutritional guidance; Telephone reassurance/Emergency alert; IV therapy; 24-hour availability; Physical therapy; Occupational therapy; Speech therapy; Social work services; High-tech services.
EQUIPMENT & SUPPLIES: IV therapy equipment and supplies; Incontinence and ostomy products; Nutritional and feeding supplies; Wound care supplies & dressings.

Medical Personnel Pool
1450 E American Ln, Schaumburg, IL 60194
(708) 330-4426
CONTACT: Pat Johnson
FINANCIAL PLANS ACCEPTED: Medicaid/Medicare certified; Private insurance.
SERVICES OFFERED: Skilled nursing; Rehabilitative and supportive care; Help with activities of daily living; Homemaker service; Nutritional guidance; Telephone reassurance/Emergency alert; IV therapy; 24-hour availability; High-tech home care; Ventilator program; Physical therapy; Speech therapy; Occupational therapy.

Skokie

Concerned Care Inc

8950 Gross Point Rd Ste E, Skokie, IL 60077
(708) 966-8700, 966-8586 FAX
FINANCIAL PLANS ACCEPTED: Medicaid/Medicare certified;
    Private insurance.
SERVICES OFFERED: Skilled nursing; Rehabilitative and
    supportive care; Help with activities of daily living;
    Homemaker service; Nutritional guidance; Tele-
    phone reassurance/Emergency alert; IV therapy;
    24-hour availability; Live-ins; Nurse aides; Physical
    therapy; Occupational therapy; Speech therapy.
See ad page 167

Extended Health Services Inc

7434 N Skokie Blvd, Skokie, IL 60077
(708) 679-6565
CONTACT: Greg Schoonover
FINANCIAL PLANS ACCEPTED: Medicaid/Medicare certified;
    Private insurance.
SERVICES OFFERED: Skilled nursing; Rehabilitative and
    supportive care.

Health Connections

7434 N Skokie Blvd, Skokie, IL 60077
(708) 674-4663
CONTACT: Greg Schoonover; Linda Ingram
CLIENTS SERVED PER MONTH: 350-400
FINANCIAL PLANS ACCEPTED: Medicaid/Medicare certified;
    Private insurance.
SERVICES OFFERED: Skilled nursing; Rehabilitative and
    supportive care; Help with activities of daily living;
    Nutritional guidance; Physical therapy; Occupa-
    tional therapy; Speech therapy; Medical social
    worker.

Kelly Assisted Living

8707 Skokie Blvd Ste 109, Skokie, IL 60077
(708) 677-0364
CONTACT: Letitia Jackson
FINANCIAL PLANS ACCEPTED: Private insurance.
SERVICES OFFERED: Help with activities of daily living;
    Homemaker service; 24-hour availability; Compan-
    ionship.

Kimberly Quality Care—Skokie

5225 Old Orchard Rd Ste 4, Skokie, IL 60077
(708) 965-8150, 965-8771 FAX
CONTACT: Shirley Grey
FINANCIAL PLANS ACCEPTED: Medicaid/Medicare certified;
    Private insurance.
SERVICES OFFERED: Skilled nursing; Rehabilitative and
    supportive care; Help with activities of daily living;
    Homemaker service; IV therapy; 24-hour availabil-
    ity.
EQUIPMENT & SUPPLIES: IV therapy equipment and sup-
    plies; Ambulatory assistance equipment;
    Wheelchairs; Respiratory equipment; Incontinence
    and ostomy products; Physical therapy supplies;
    Nutritional and feeding supplies.
See ad page 148

Nursefinders of Skokie

5010 W Dempster St, Skokie, IL 60077
(708) 676-1515, 675-5780 FAX
CONTACT: Terri Pusateria
FINANCIAL PLANS ACCEPTED: Private insurance.
SERVICES OFFERED: Skilled nursing; Rehabilitative and
    supportive care; Help with activities of daily living;
    Homemaker service; Telephone reassurance/Emer-
    gency alert; IV therapy; 24-hour availability; Phys-
    ical therapy; Occupational therapy; Speech ther-
    apy; Intermittent visits to round-the-clock care;
    Free home evaluation.
See ad page 167

Skokie Health Dept

5127 Oakton St, Skokie, IL 60077
(708) 673-0500
CONTACT: Lowell Huckleberry

South Holland

Lutheran Social Services of Illinois—Home Helps for Seniors

640 E 168th Pl, South Holland, IL 60473
(708) 596-6690, 596-8233 FAX
CONTACT: Georgia Veyette
SERVICES OFFERED: Help with activities of daily living;
    Homemaker service; Nutritional guidance.
EQUIPMENT & SUPPLIES: Ambulatory assistance equip-
    ment; Wheelchairs.
EQUIPMENT/SUPPLY AVAILABILITY: For rent; For loan.

Streamwood

Family Service—Hanover Township

519 S Bartlett Rd, Streamwood, IL 60103
(708) 837-8553

Summit

Americanurse Ltd

5712 S Harlem Ave, Summit, IL 60501
(708) 496-0070, (312) 585-6877 TDD, (708) 496-0178
    FAX
CONTACT: Karon Gibson; Marianne Kokalj
FINANCIAL PLANS ACCEPTED: Private insurance.
SERVICES OFFERED: Skilled nursing; Rehabilitative and
    supportive care; Help with activities of daily living;
    Telephone reassurance/Emergency alert; IV ther-
    apy; 24-hour availability; Physical therapy; Case
    management.
EQUIPMENT & SUPPLIES: IV therapy equipment and sup-
    plies; Ambulatory assistance equipment.
EQUIPMENT/SUPPLY AVAILABILITY: Home delivery &
    pickup.

✔   In order to support future editions of this publication would you please mention *Elder Services* each time you contact any advertiser, facility, or service.

Vernon Hills

The Helping Hand Private Duty—DME
6 Phillip Rd Ste 1103, Vernon Hills, IL 60061
(708) 367-9481
CONTACT: Beverly Kelly, Asst Coord
CLIENTS SERVED PER MONTH: 60
SERVICES OFFERED: Skilled nursing; Help with activities of daily living; Homemaker service.
EQUIPMENT & SUPPLIES: Ambulatory assistance equipment; Wheelchairs; Respiratory equipment; Physical therapy supplies.
EQUIPMENT/SUPPLY AVAILABILITY: For rent; For sale; Home delivery & pickup; 24-hour service for respiratory patients only.

Villa Park

Elmhurst Memorial Home Health Care Services
721 E Madison Ste 101, Villa Park, IL 60181
(708) 941-7045, 530-8253 FAX
CONTACT: Laura Ferris
CLIENTS SERVED PER MONTH: 350
FINANCIAL PLANS ACCEPTED: Medicaid/Medicare certified; Private insurance.
SERVICES OFFERED: Skilled nursing; Rehabilitative and supportive care; Help with activities of daily living; Homemaker service; IV therapy; 24-hour availability.
EQUIPMENT & SUPPLIES: IV therapy equipment and supplies; Ambulatory assistance equipment; Wheelchairs; Respiratory equipment; Incontinence and ostomy products; Physical therapy supplies; Nutritional and feeding supplies.
EQUIPMENT/SUPPLY AVAILABILITY: For rent; For sale; Home delivery & pickup; 24-hour service.

Waukegan

Franciscan Home Health
2615 Washington, Waukegan, IL 60085
(708) 360-2480, 249-5897 FAX
CONTACT: Sandra Llewellyn
FINANCIAL PLANS ACCEPTED: Medicaid/Medicare certified; Private insurance.
SERVICES OFFERED: Skilled nursing; Rehabilitative and supportive care; Help with activities of daily living; Nutritional guidance; Telephone reassurance/ Emergency alert; IV therapy; 24-hour availability; MSW.

Helping Care Inc
2424 Washington, Waukegan, IL 60085
(708) 249-8700
CONTACT: Cheryl Perez

Home Health Services of Lake County Health Dept
3010 Grand Ave, Waukegan, IL 60085
(708) 360-6717, 360-3656 FAX
CONTACT: Susan Erickson
CLIENTS SERVED PER MONTH: Approx 150
FINANCIAL PLANS ACCEPTED: Medicaid/Medicare certified; Private insurance.
SERVICES OFFERED: Skilled nursing; Rehabilitative and supportive care; Help with activities of daily living; Nutritional guidance; IV therapy; 24-hour availability.
EQUIPMENT & SUPPLIES: Incontinence and ostomy products.

Kimberly Quality Care—Waukegan
300 Grand Ave Ste 4, Waukegan, IL 60085
(708) 249-5530, 249-4639 FAX
CONTACT: Linda Cisek
FINANCIAL PLANS ACCEPTED: Medicaid/Medicare certified; Private insurance.
SERVICES OFFERED: Skilled nursing; Rehabilitative and supportive care; Help with activities of daily living; Homemaker service; IV therapy; 24-hour availability.
EQUIPMENT & SUPPLIES: IV therapy equipment and supplies; Incontinence and ostomy products; Nutritional and feeding supplies.
See ad page 148

Victory Memorial Hospital Home Health Care
99 Greenwood Ave, Waukegan, IL 60085
(708) 360-4320, 360-4330 FAX
CONTACT: Wendy Koski-Hansen
CLIENTS SERVED PER MONTH: 130
FINANCIAL PLANS ACCEPTED: Medicaid/Medicare certified; Private insurance.
SERVICES OFFERED: Skilled nursing; Rehabilitative and supportive care; Help with activities of daily living; Homemaker service; Nutritional guidance; Telephone reassurance/Emergency alert; IV therapy; 24-hour availability.

West Chicago

Kimberly Quality Care—West Chicago
245 W Roosevelt Rd Ste 125, West Chicago, IL 60185
(708) 293-5611, 293-5695 FAX
FINANCIAL PLANS ACCEPTED: Medicaid/Medicare certified; Private insurance.
SERVICES OFFERED: Skilled nursing; Rehabilitative and supportive care; Help with activities of daily living; Homemaker service; IV therapy; 24-hour availability.
EQUIPMENT & SUPPLIES: IV therapy equipment and supplies; Ambulatory assistance equipment; Wheelchairs; Respiratory equipment; Incontinence and ostomy products; Physical therapy supplies; Nutritional and feeding supplies.
See ad page 148

Westchester

Home Health Plus
2215 Enterprise Dr Ste 1512, Westchester, IL 60154
(708) 531-9339, 531-9680 FAX
CONTACT: Peg Maxon
CLIENTS SERVED PER MONTH: 600
FINANCIAL PLANS ACCEPTED: Medicaid/Medicare certified; Private insurance.
SERVICES OFFERED: Skilled nursing; Rehabilitative and supportive care; Help with activities of daily living; Homemaker service; Nutritional guidance; IV therapy; 24-hour availability; Private duty; Intermittent visits.
EQUIPMENT & SUPPLIES: IV therapy equipment and supplies; Nutritional and feeding supplies.

In Home Health Care Service—West Inc
10526 W 22nd St Ste 301, Westchester, IL 60154-5243
(708) 531-0400, 531-0456 FAX
CONTACT: Eugenia Collias
CLIENTS SERVED PER MONTH: 200
FINANCIAL PLANS ACCEPTED: Medicaid/Medicare certified; Private insurance.
SERVICES OFFERED: Skilled nursing; Rehabilitative and supportive care; Help with activities of daily living; Nutritional guidance; IV therapy; 24-hour availability; Medical social work.
EQUIPMENT & SUPPLIES: IV therapy equipment and supplies; Ambulatory assistance equipment; Wheelchairs; Respiratory equipment; Incontinence and ostomy products; Physical therapy supplies; Nutritional and feeding supplies; Medical supplies.

Westmont

Home Health Care Providers Inc
98 E Naperville Rd, Westmont, IL 60559
(708) 810-1515
SERVICES OFFERED: Skilled nursing; Rehabilitative and supportive care; Help with activities of daily living; Homemaker service; Nutritional guidance; IV therapy; 24-hour availability.
EQUIPMENT & SUPPLIES: IV therapy equipment and supplies; Ambulatory assistance equipment; Wheelchairs; Respiratory equipment; Incontinence and ostomy products; Nutritional and feeding supplies.

Wheaton

Denson Optioncare Pharmacy
200 E Willow, Wheaton, IL 60187
(708) 668-1180, 668-1396 FAX
CONTACT: Tom Denson
FINANCIAL PLANS ACCEPTED: Medicaid/Medicare certified; Private insurance.
SERVICES OFFERED: IV therapy; 24-hour availability.

EQUIPMENT & SUPPLIES: IV therapy equipment and supplies; Incontinence and ostomy products; Nutritional and feeding supplies.
EQUIPMENT/SUPPLY AVAILABILITY: For rent; For sale; Home delivery & pickup.

Denson Shops Inc
509 S Carlton, Wheaton, IL 60189
(708) 665-1488, 668-1396 FAX
CONTACT: Sue Denson; Bob Denson; Pamela Rose
FINANCIAL PLANS ACCEPTED: Medicaid/Medicare certified; Private insurance.
EQUIPMENT & SUPPLIES: Ambulatory assistance equipment; Wheelchairs; Respiratory equipment; Incontinence and ostomy products; Physical therapy supplies; Nutritional and feeding supplies.
EQUIPMENT/SUPPLY AVAILABILITY: For rent; For sale; Home delivery & pickup; 24-hour service.

Wilmette

Altru Nurses Registry
1213 Wilmette Ave, Wilmette, IL 60091
(708) 256-4005
CONTACT: Lorna Mikita

North Shore Visiting Nurse Association
1000 Skokie Blvd Ste 550, Wilmette, IL 60091-1120
(708) 256-7200
CONTACT: Antoinette L Lahart
CLIENTS SERVED PER MONTH: 250-300
FINANCIAL PLANS ACCEPTED: Medicaid/Medicare certified; Private insurance.
SERVICES OFFERED: Skilled nursing; Rehabilitative and supportive care; Help with activities of daily living; Nutritional guidance.

Woodstock

Caregivers Home Health
1065 Lake Ave, Woodstock, IL 60098
(815) 338-8940
CONTACT: Anne Melligan
FINANCIAL PLANS ACCEPTED: Medicaid/Medicare certified; Private insurance.
SERVICES OFFERED: Skilled nursing; Rehabilitative and supportive care; Help with activities of daily living; Homemaker service; Nutritional guidance; IV therapy; 24-hour availability.

Easter Seal Adult & Child Rehabilitation Center
PO Box 326, 708 Washington St, Woodstock, IL 60098
(815) 338-1707, 338-1786 FAX
CONTACT: Susan Martino
CLIENTS SERVED PER MONTH: 2,000 annually
FINANCIAL PLANS ACCEPTED: Medicaid/Medicare certified; Private insurance.

✔ In order to support future editions of this publication would you please mention *Elder Services* each time you contact any advertiser, facility, or service.

SERVICES OFFERED: Skilled nursing; Rehabilitative and supportive care; Help with activities of daily living; Physical therapy; Occupational therapy; Speech therapy.
EQUIPMENT & SUPPLIES: Ambulatory assistance equipment; Wheelchairs; Physical therapy supplies.
EQUIPMENT/SUPPLY AVAILABILITY: For rent.

Healthtrends Ltd
PO Box 157, 1780 E Wood Dr, Woodstock, IL 60098
(815) 338-5050, 338-8707 FAX
CONTACT: Jenny Ramon
CLIENTS SERVED PER MONTH: 80
FINANCIAL PLANS ACCEPTED: Medicaid/Medicare certified; Private insurance.
SERVICES OFFERED: Skilled nursing; Rehabilitative and supportive care; Help with activities of daily living; Homemaker service; Nutritional guidance; Telephone reassurance/Emergency alert; IV therapy; 24-hour availability; High-tech nursing; Physical therapy; Occupational therapy; Speech therapy.
EQUIPMENT & SUPPLIES: Arranged as needed.
See ad page 184

McHenry County Dept of Health
2200 N Seminary Rte 47N, Woodstock, IL 60098
(815) 338-2514
CONTACT: Christine Scanlon

INDIANA

Crown Point

The Caring Co Inc
121 Henderlong Pkwy, Crown Point, IN 46307
(219) 662-7377
CONTACT: Laura J Kruit
CLIENTS SERVED PER MONTH: 20-50

SERVICES OFFERED: Help with activities of daily living; Homemaker service; 24-hour availability; Shopping; Meal-preparation.

ElderCare Services Inc
321 S East, Crown Point, IN 46307
(219) 662-7700
CONTACT: Betty Traves

Meals on Wheels—Northwest Indiana
250 N Main, Crown Point, IN 46307
(219) 769-5858
CONTACT: Margot Clark
CLIENTS SERVED PER MONTH: 395
FINANCIAL PLANS ACCEPTED: Medicaid/Medicare certified; Private insurance.
SERVICES OFFERED: Nutritional guidance; Meals on wheels.
EQUIPMENT & SUPPLIES: Nutritional and feeding supplies.
EQUIPMENT/SUPPLY AVAILABILITY: Home delivery & pickup.

Staff Builders Health Care Services
190 S West St, Crown Point, IN 46307
(219) 662-1870
CONTACT: Sally Wilson

Dyer

Amicare Home Health Services
24 Joliet, Dyer, IN 46311
(219) 322-1323
CONTACT: Maggie Carter

East Chicago

Ancilla Home Health
4320 W 1st Ste 311, East Chicago, IN 46312
(219) 397-1040
CONTACT: Marie Schafbuch

Gary

Gary Neighborhood Services Inc
300 W 21st Ave, Gary, IN 46407
(219) 883-0431
CONTACT: Tom Osborn

Professional Nursing Service—Division of L A Flowers Inc
4485 W 5th Ave, Gary, IN 46406
(219) 944-8633
CONTACT: Dr Lloyd Flower
CLIENTS SERVED PER MONTH: 100
FINANCIAL PLANS ACCEPTED: Private insurance.

SERVICES OFFERED: Skilled nursing; Rehabilitative and supportive care; Help with activities of daily living; Homemaker service; 24-hour availability.

Hammond

Respite Care Service for Handicapped Inc
6525 Columbia Ste B, Hammond, IN 46320
(219) 931-8172

St Margaret Hospital & Health Centers Home Care & Care Connection
5454 Hohman Ave, Hammond, IN 46320
(219) 933-6663, 933-2136 FAX
CONTACT: Karen Wade
CLIENTS SERVED PER MONTH: 285-300
FINANCIAL PLANS ACCEPTED: Medicaid/Medicare certified; Private insurance.
SERVICES OFFERED: Skilled nursing; Rehabilitative and supportive care; Help with activities of daily living; Homemaker service; Nutritional guidance; Telephone reassurance/Emergency alert; IV therapy; 24-hour availability.
EQUIPMENT & SUPPLIES: Arranged as needed.

Visiting Nurse Association of Northwest Indiana Inc
6513 Kennedy Ave, Hammond, IN 46323
(219) 844-1410, 989-4440 FAX
CONTACT: Arlene Jawor
FINANCIAL PLANS ACCEPTED: Medicaid/Medicare certified; Private insurance.
SERVICES OFFERED: Skilled nursing; Rehabilitative and supportive care; Help with activities of daily living; Homemaker service; Nutritional guidance; IV therapy; 24-hour availability; Hospice program.
EQUIPMENT & SUPPLIES: IV therapy equipment and supplies; Ambulatory assistance equipment; Wheelchairs; Nutritional and feeding supplies.
EQUIPMENT/SUPPLY AVAILABILITY: For sale; Home delivery & pickup; 24-hour service.

Highland

Pro Tem Inc
3037 45th St, Highland, IN 46322
(219) 924-9018
CONTACT: Margaret Burger

La Porte

Visiting Nurse Association Home Care Services Inc
1719 State St, La Porte, IN 46350-3172
(219) 362-5914, 325-8616 FAX
CONTACT: Mary Craymer

CLIENTS SERVED PER MONTH: 250
FINANCIAL PLANS ACCEPTED: Medicaid/Medicare certified; Private insurance.
SERVICES OFFERED: Skilled nursing; Rehabilitative and supportive care; Help with activities of daily living; Homemaker service; Nutritional guidance; IV therapy; 24-hour availability; Medicare-certified hospice.

Lake Station

Hi-Tech Home Care of Indiana Inc
3728 Central Ave, Lake Station, IN 46405
(219) 962-4235
CONTACT: Scott Coker

Merrillville

Abbey Home Healthcare
1581 E 90th Pl, Merrillville, IN 46410
(219) 736-6222, 736-0346 FAX
CONTACT: Dave DalCorrobbo
FINANCIAL PLANS ACCEPTED: Medicaid/Medicare certified; Private insurance.
EQUIPMENT & SUPPLIES: Ambulatory assistance equipment; Respiratory equipment; Incontinence and ostomy products; Physical therapy supplies; Nutritional and feeding supplies; Medical equipment; Aerosol therapy; Life support systems.
EQUIPMENT/SUPPLY AVAILABILITY: For rent; For sale; Home delivery & pickup; 24-hour service.
See ad page 153

BHM Health Associates Inc
5490 Broadway, Merrillville, IN 46410-1663
(219) 756-2300
CONTACT: Nancy Rush

HealthInfusion
107 W 79th Ave, Merrillville, IN 46410
(219) 736-7341
CONTACT: Dave Holmes

Home Support Services
5401 Broadway, Merrillville, IN 46410
(219) 980-7180
CONTACT: Pam Jones

Kimberly Quality Care—Merrillville
1000 E 80th Pl Ste 417 S, Merrillville, IN 46410
(219) 769-0215, 736-8414 FAX
CONTACT: Carole Bezat
FINANCIAL PLANS ACCEPTED: Medicaid/Medicare certified; Private insurance.
SERVICES OFFERED: Skilled nursing; Rehabilitative and supportive care; Help with activities of daily living; Homemaker service; IV therapy; 24-hour availability; High-tech services; Ventilator care.

✔ In order to support future editions of this publication would you please mention *Elder Services* each time you contact any advertiser, facility, or service.

EQUIPMENT & SUPPLIES: IV therapy equipment and supplies; Ambulatory assistance equipment; Wheelchairs; Respiratory equipment; Incontinence and ostomy products; Physical therapy supplies; Nutritional and feeding supplies.
See ad page 148

Medical Personnel Pool
7725 Broadway Ste G, Merrillville, IN 46410
(219) 736-1135
CONTACT: Linda Chavez
FINANCIAL PLANS ACCEPTED: Medicaid/Medicare certified; Private insurance.
SERVICES OFFERED: Skilled nursing; Rehabilitative and supportive care; Help with activities of daily living; Homemaker service; Nutritional guidance; Telephone reassurance/Emergency alert; IV therapy; 24-hour availability; High-tech home care; Ventilator program; Physical therapy; Speech therapy; Occupational therapy.

Nursefinders of Merrillville
27 W. 80th Pl, Merrillville, IN 46410-5445
(219) 736-8836
CONTACT: Rhonda Kapler
FINANCIAL PLANS ACCEPTED: Private insurance.
SERVICES OFFERED: Skilled nursing; Rehabilitative and supportive care; Help with activities of daily living; Homemaker service; Telephone reassurance/Emergency alert; IV therapy; 24-hour availability; Physical therapy; Occupational therapy; Speech therapy; Intermittent visits to round-the-clock care; Free home care evaluation.
See ad page 167

Option Care
9111 Broadway Ste AA, Merrillville, IN 46410
(219) 736-1928, 736-0214 FAX
FINANCIAL PLANS ACCEPTED: Medicaid/Medicare certified; Private insurance.
SERVICES OFFERED: IV therapy; 24-hour availability.
EQUIPMENT & SUPPLIES: IV therapy equipment and supplies.

Promed Home Care of Northern Indiana Inc
6111 Harrison Ste 132, Merrillville, IN 46410
(219) 980-0073
CONTACT: Pat Jewitt

Michigan City

Family Association of La Porte County
105 W 5th St, Michigan City, IN 46360
(219) 879-8539
CONTACT: Bert Clemons
CLIENTS SERVED PER MONTH: 140

FINANCIAL PLANS ACCEPTED: Medicaid/Medicare certified; Private insurance.
SERVICES OFFERED: Homemaker service.

St Anthony Hospital Home Health Care
301 W Homer, Michigan City, IN 46360
(219) 874-0605
CONTACT: Kathy Krachinski

Munster

Companion Care
619 Ridge Rd, Munster, IN 46321
(219) 836-2783

Hospice of the Calumet Area Inc
600 Superior Ave, Munster, IN 46321
(219) 922-2732, 922-1947 FAX
CONTACT: Dianna Pandak
FINANCIAL PLANS ACCEPTED: Medicaid/Medicare certified; Private insurance.
SERVICES OFFERED: Skilled nursing; Homemaker service; Nutritional guidance; Telephone reassurance/Emergency alert; IV therapy; 24-hour availability; Hospice services.
EQUIPMENT & SUPPLIES: Arranged as needed.

Valparaiso

Visiting Nurse Association Hospice Home Care
501 Marquette St, Valparaiso, IN 46383-2508
(219) 462-5195, 462-6020 FAX
CONTACT: Jill Jacobson
CLIENTS SERVED PER MONTH: 14
FINANCIAL PLANS ACCEPTED: Medicaid/Medicare certified; Private insurance.
SERVICES OFFERED: Skilled nursing; Help with activities of daily living; Homemaker service; Nutritional guidance; Telephone reassurance/Emergency alert; IV therapy; 24-hour availability; Chaplain; Volunteers.
EQUIPMENT & SUPPLIES: Incontinence and ostomy products; Physical therapy supplies.

Visiting Nurse Association of Porter County Indiana Inc
501 Marquette St, Valparaiso, IN 46383-2508
(219) 462-5195, 462-6020 FAX
CONTACT: Adrianne Jagger
CLIENTS SERVED PER MONTH: 600
FINANCIAL PLANS ACCEPTED: Medicaid/Medicare certified; Private insurance.

SERVICES OFFERED: Skilled nursing; Rehabilitative and supportive care; Help with activities of daily living; Homemaker service; Nutritional guidance; Telephone reassurance/Emergency alert; IV therapy; 24-hour availability; Meals on wheels; Respite care.

EQUIPMENT & SUPPLIES: Incontinence and ostomy products; Physical therapy supplies.

✔ In order to support future editions of this publication would you please mention *Elder Services* each time you contact any advertiser, facility, or service.

Home Health Care Services

Facilities arranged by city.

Home Health Care	Skilled Nursing	Rehabilitative & Supportive Care	Help with Activities of Daily Living	Homemaker Service	Nutritional Guidance	Telephone Reassurance/Emergency Alert	IV Therapy	24-hour Availability
Dyna Care Home Health Inc Alsip, IL	•	•	•	•	•	•	•	•
Alpha Home Health Care Arlington Heights, IL	•	•	•					
Children's Memorial Home Health Inc Arlington Heights, IL	•	•	•			•		
Northwest Community Health Services of Northwest Community Hospital Arlington Heights, IL	•	•	•	•			•	•
Nursefinders of Arlington Heights Arlington Heights, IL	•	•	•	•		•	•	•
Orsini Nursing Agency Inc Arlington Heights, IL	•	•	•	•	•	•	•	•
Village of Arlington Heights Health Services Arlington Heights, IL	•					•		
Alpha Home Health Care Aurora, IL	•	•	•					
Hospitals Home Health Care Services Inc Aurora, IL	•	•	•	•	•		•	•
Medical Personnel Pool Aurora, IL	•	•	•	•	•	•	•	•
Nursefinders of Aurora Aurora, IL	•	•	•	•		•	•	•

Home Health Care	Skilled Nursing	Rehabilitative & Supportive Care	Help with Activities of Daily Living	Homemaker Service	Nutritional Guidance	Telephone Reassurance/Emergency Alert	IV Therapy	24-hour Availability
Visiting Nurse Association of Fox Valley Aurora, IL	•	•	•		•		•	•
Caregivers Home Health Barrington, IL	•	•	•	•			•	•
Fox Valley Hospice Batavia, IL								•
St Francis Home Care Inc Blue Island, IL	•	•	•		•		•	
FirstChoice Home Health & Family Support Services Bridgeview, IL	•	•	•	•	•	•	•	•
HealthSource Inc Bridgeview, IL	•						•	•
Proviso Township Referral Office Broadview, IL						•		
Hospice of the Calumet Area Inc Calumet City, IL	•			•	•	•	•	•
Community Nursing Service of DuPage Carol Stream, IL	•	•	•		•	•	•	
All-Ways Caring Services Chicago, IL	•	•	•		•			
Alverna Home Nursing Center Chicago, IL	•				•			
American Home Care Inc Chicago, IL	•	•	•	•	•	•		•
ASI Inc Chicago, IL				•				
Autumn Home Health & Case Management Chicago, IL		•			•	•		•
Bruce & Ken's Pharmacy Chicago, IL		•					•	•
Carnegie Drugs Inc Chicago, IL			•		•	•		
Catholic Charities Chicago Chicago, IL	•	•	•					

✔ In order to support future editions of this publication would you please mention *Elder Services* each time you contact any advertiser, facility, or service.

Home Health Care

	Skilled Nursing	Rehabilitative & Supportive Care	Help with Activities of Daily Living	Homemaker Service	Nutritional Guidance	Telephone Reassurance/Emergency Alert	IV Therapy	24-hour Availability
Chicago Home Health Services Inc Chicago, IL	•				•		•	•
Council for Jewish Elderly Chicago, IL			•	•	•			
Dana Home Care Chicago, IL				•				
Extended Home Care Services Chicago, IL			•	•				•
Family Care Services Chicago, IL			•	•	•			•
FirstChoice Home Health & Family Support Services Chicago, IL	•	•	•	•	•	•	•	•
Five Hospital Homebound Elderly Program Chicago, IL	•	•	•	•	•	•		
Flash General Help Ltd Chicago, IL				•				•
Franciscan Home Health of St Anthony Hospital Chicago, IL	•	•	•					•
Hellenic Family and Community Services, an Agency of the Hellenic Foundation Chicago, IL		•	•			•		
Home Health & Hospice of Illinois Masonic Medical Center Chicago, IL	•	•	•					
Home Health Care Inc Chicago, IL	•	•	•	•	•	•		•
Home Health Plus Chicago, IL	•	•	•	•	•		•	•
HomeCorps Inc Chicago, IL	•	•	•	•		•	•	•
In Home Health Care Service—West Inc Chicago, IL	•	•	•	•	•		•	•
Independence Plus Inc Chicago, IL	•	•	•	•	•		•	•

Home Health Care	Skilled Nursing	Rehabilitative & Supportive Care	Help with Activities of Daily Living	Homemaker Service	Nutritional Guidance	Telephone Reassurance/Emergency Alert	IV Therapy	24-hour Availability
Kimberly Quality Care—Chicago Chicago, IL	•	•	•	•			•	•
Kin Care Inc Chicago, IL		•	•					•
Little Brothers—Friends of the Elderly Chicago, IL		•	•		•			
Medical Personnel Pool Chicago, IL	•	•	•	•	•	•	•	•
Mercy Home Health Care—Chatham Chicago, IL	•	•	•	•	•	•	•	•
Mt Sinai Hospital Medical Center/ Home Health Agency Chicago, IL	•	•	•		•	•	•	•
Northwestern Memorial Home Health Care Services Inc Chicago, IL	•	•	•	•	•		•	•
Nursefinders of Central Chicago Chicago, IL	•	•	•	•	•	•	•	•
Nursefinders of Hyde Park Chicago, IL	•	•	•	•		•	•	•
Nursefinders of Lincoln Square Chicago, IL	•	•	•	•		•	•	•
Nurses on Wheels Chicago, IL	•			•				
Ravenswood Home Care Chicago, IL	•	•	•	•				
Resurrection Home Health Care Services Chicago, IL	•				•	•	•	•
Rush Home Health Service Chicago, IL	•	•	•	•	•	•		
St James Place Ltd Chicago, IL	•		•	•	•		•	•
St Mary's Home Health Services Chicago, IL	•	•		•	•	•		
The Salvation Army—Family Service Division Chicago, IL		•						

✔ In order to support future editions of this publication would you please mention *Elder Services* each time you contact any advertiser, facility, or service.

Home Health Care	Skilled Nursing	Rehabilitative & Supportive Care	Help with Activities of Daily Living	Homemaker Service	Nutritional Guidance	Telephone Reassurance/Emergency Alert	IV Therapy	24-hour Availability
Sargent—Water Tower Pharmacy Chicago, IL			•		•	•		
SCH Home-Med North Chicago, IL	•	•	•		•		•	•
Seniors Home Health Care Ltd Chicago, IL	•	•	•			•		
Society of St Vincent De Paul of Chicago Chicago, IL				•				
Staff Builders Health Services Chicago, IL	•	•	•	•	•	•	•	•
Staff Builders Services Chicago, IL				•				
Summit Home Health Inc Chicago, IL	•	•	•				•	•
Total Home Health Care of Chicago Inc Chicago, IL	•	•	•		•		•	•
Ultra Care Home Medical Chicago, IL		•					•	•
Umoja Care Inc Chicago, IL	•	•	•	•	•	•		
Visiting Nurse Association of Chicago Chicago, IL	•	•	•		•			
Alpha Home Health Care Chicago Heights, IL	•	•	•					
La Grange Memorial Home Care Services Countryside, IL	•	•	•	•	•		•	•
Alpha Home Health Care Crest Hill, IL	•	•	•					
Alpha Home Health Care De Kalb, IL	•	•	•					
Allcare Home Care Des Plaines, IL	•	•	•		•	•	•	•
Concerned Care Inc Des Plaines, IL	•	•	•	•	•	•	•	•

Home Health Care	Skilled Nursing	Rehabilitative & Supportive Care	Help with Activities of Daily Living	Homemaker Service	Nutritional Guidance	Telephone Reassurance/Emergency Alert	IV Therapy	24-hour Availability
Holy Family Hospital Home Care Des Plaines, IL	•	•	•		•	•	•	•
Kimberly Quality Care—Downers Grove Downers Grove, IL	•	•	•	•			•	•
Nursefinders of Downers Grove Downers Grove, IL	•	•	•	•		•	•	
Alpha Home Health Care Elgin, IL	•	•	•					
Franciscan Home Health Elgin, IL	•	•	•		•		•	
Sherman Home Care Partners Elgin, IL	•	•	•	•	•	•	•	•
Visiting Nurse Association of Fox Valley Elgin, IL	•	•	•		•		•	•
Critical Care America Elk Grove Village, IL					•	•	•	•
Medical Personnel Pool Elmhurst, IL	•	•	•	•	•	•	•	•
Alpha Home Health Care Elmwood Park, IL	•	•	•					
Nursefinders of Elmwood Park Elmwood Park, IL	•	•	•	•		•	•	•
Caring Home Aid Program—Seniors Action Service Inc Evanston, IL			•	•				
Kimberly Quality Care—Evanston Evanston, IL	•	•	•	•			•	•
Medical Personnel Pool Evanston, IL	•	•	•	•	•	•	•	•
Mobile Medical Care of St Francis Hospital Evanston, IL						•		
Visiting Nurse Association North Evanston, IL	•	•	•	•			•	•
Health Force Evergreen Park, IL		•	•	•				

✔ In order to support future editions of this publication would you please mention *Elder Services* each time you contact any advertiser, facility, or service.

Home Health Care	Skilled Nursing	Rehabilitative & Supportive Care	Help with Activities of Daily Living	Homemaker Service	Nutritional Guidance	Telephone Reassurance/Emergency Alert	IV Therapy	24-hour Availability
Little Company of Mary Hospital & Health Care Centers Evergreen Park, IL	●	●	●		●	●		
Peace Memorial Home Health Service Evergreen Park, IL	●		●	●	●	●		●
Home Health Plus Flossmoor, IL	●	●		●	●		●	●
Carlton Health Care Geneva, IL	●		●	●				●
Community Contacts Inc Geneva, IL				●				
Alpha Home Health Care Glen Ellyn, IL	●	●	●					
South Suburban Senior Services of Catholic Charities Harvey, IL			●	●		●		
Home Health Services of South Suburban Hospital Hazel Crest, IL	●	●	●				●	
Nursefinders of Hazel Crest Hazel Crest, IL	●	●	●	●		●	●	●
Kimberly Quality Care—Hickory Hills Hickory Hills, IL	●	●	●	●			●	●
Highland Park Hospital Home Health Services Highland Park, IL	●	●	●		●	●	●	●
Traycee Home Care Highwood, IL		●	●	●	●	●		●
Health Care at Home Hinsdale, IL	●	●	●			●	●	●
Caremark Inc Homewood, IL	●				●		●	●
Concerned Care Inc Homewood, IL	●	●	●	●	●	●	●	●
In Home Health Care Service—West Inc-Joliet Div Joliet, IL	●	●	●		●	●	●	●
Kimberly Quality Care—Joliet Joliet, IL	●	●	●	●			●	●

Home Health Care	Skilled Nursing	Rehabilitative & Supportive Care	Help with Activities of Daily Living	Homemaker Service	Nutritional Guidance	Telephone Reassurance/Emergency Alert	IV Therapy	24-hour Availability
Medical Personnel Pool Joliet, IL	•	•	•	•	•	•	•	•
Nursefinders of Joliet Joliet, IL	•	•	•	•	•		•	•
Upjohn HealthCare Services Joliet, IL	•	•			•			
Mercy Home Health Care Justice, IL	•	•	•	•	•	•	•	•
La Grange Community Nurse & Service Association La Grange, IL	•	•	•			•		
Home Health Care Inc—Lemont Lemont, IL	•	•	•	•	•	•		•
Caregivers Home Health Libertyville, IL	•	•	•	•	•		•	
Medical Personnel Pool Libertyville, IL	•	•	•	•	•	•	•	•
Nursefinders of Libertyville Libertyville, IL	•	•	•	•		•	•	•
MacNeal Home Health Services Lyons, IL	•	•	•	•	•		•	•
Northern Illinois Medical Center—Home Health Care McHenry, IL	•	•	•		•	•		
Gottlieb Memorial Hospital Melrose Park, IL	•	•	•		•	•		
In Home Health Care—Suburban Chicago North Morton Grove, IL	•				•		•	•
Village of Mt Prospect Human Services Division Mount Prospect, IL	•				•			
Health Force Naperville, IL			•	•				
Regency Home Health Care Niles, IL	•	•	•	•	•			•
Kimberly Quality Care—North Riverside North Riverside, IL	•	•	•	•			•	•

✓ In order to support future editions of this publication would you please mention *Elder Services* each time you contact any advertiser, facility, or service.

196 / ILLINOIS / Northlake   II   HOME HEALTH CARE SERVICES

Home Health Care	Skilled Nursing	Rehabilitative & Supportive Care	Help with Activities of Daily Living	Homemaker Service	Nutritional Guidance	Telephone Reassurance/Emergency Alert	IV Therapy	24-hour Availability
The Caring Center—Casa San Carlo Northlake, IL	•	•	•		•	•		
EHS Home Health Care Service Inc Oak Brook, IL	•	•			•		•	•
Medical Personnel Pool Oak Lawn, IL	•	•	•	•	•	•	•	•
Nursefinders of Oak Lawn Oak Lawn, IL	•	•	•	•		•	•	•
Ancilla Home Health Oak Park, IL	•	•				•	•	
At Home Health Inc Oak Park, IL	•	•	•	•	•	•	•	•
Bruce & Ken's Pharmacy Oak Park, IL		•					•	•
The Caring Center—Mills Tower Oak Park, IL	•	•	•		•	•		
The Caring Center—The Oaks Oak Park, IL	•	•	•		•	•		
Community Nursing Service West Oak Park, IL	•	•	•	•			•	•
FirstChoice Home Health & Family Support Services Oak Park, IL	•	•	•	•	•	•	•	•
Home Companion Service Oak Park, IL			•	•				•
Home Medical Care Foundation Oak Park, IL	•	•	•	•	•	•	•	•
HomeCare Resources—An Affiliate of West Suburban Hospital Medical Center Oak Park, IL	•	•	•	•	•	•	•	
Kimberly Quality Care—Oak Park Oak Park, IL	•	•	•	•			•	•
Medical Personnel Pool Oak Park, IL	•	•	•	•	•	•	•	•
Kimberly Quality Care—Olympia Fields Olympia Fields, IL	•	•	•	•			•	•

Home Health Care

	Skilled Nursing	Rehabilitative & Supportive Care	Help with Activities of Daily Living	Homemaker Service	Nutritional Guidance	Telephone Reassurance/Emergency Alert	IV Therapy	24-hour Availability
Shay Health Care Services Inc Palos Hills, IL	●	●	●		●		●	●
Park Forest Health Dept Park Forest, IL	●	●					●	
A-Abiding Care Inc Park Ridge, IL	●	●	●	●	●	●	●	●
The Center of Concern Park Ridge, IL		●	●	●				
Omni Home Care Park Ridge, IL	●	●			●		●	●
Senior Citizens Services Robbins, IL			●		●	●		
Home Health Plus Rolling Meadows, IL	●	●	●	●	●		●	●
Concerned Care Inc Saint Charles, IL	●	●	●	●	●		●	●
In Home Health Care Service—West Inc Schaumburg, IL	●	●	●		●	●	●	●
Medical Personnel Pool Schaumburg, IL	●	●	●	●	●	●	●	●
Concerned Care Inc Skokie, IL	●	●	●	●	●	●	●	●
Extended Health Services Inc Skokie, IL	●	●						
Health Connections Skokie, IL	●	●	●		●			
Kelly Assisted Living Skokie, IL			●	●				●
Kimberly Quality Care—Skokie Skokie, IL	●	●	●	●			●	●
Nursefinders of Skokie Skokie, IL	●	●				●	●	●
Lutheran Social Services of Illinois—Home Helps for Seniors South Holland, IL			●	●	●			
Americanurse Ltd Summit, IL	●	●				●	●	●

✔ In order to support future editions of this publication would you please mention *Elder Services* each time you contact any advertiser, facility, or service.

Home Health Care

	Skilled Nursing	Rehabilitative & Supportive Care	Help with Activities of Daily Living	Homemaker Service	Nutritional Guidance	Telephone Reassurance/Emergency Alert	IV Therapy	24-hour Availability
The Helping Hand Private Duty—DME Vernon Hills, IL	•		•	•				
Elmhurst Memorial Home Health Care Services Villa Park, IL	•	•	•	•			•	•
Franciscan Home Health Waukegan, IL	•	•	•		•	•	•	•
Home Health Services of Lake County Health Dept Waukegan, IL	•	•	•		•		•	•
Kimberly Quality Care—Waukegan Waukegan, IL	•	•	•	•			•	•
Victory Memorial Hospital Home Health Care Waukegan, IL	•	•	•	•	•	•	•	•
Kimberly Quality Care—West Chicago West Chicago, IL	•	•	•	•			•	•
Home Health Plus Westchester, IL	•	•	•	•	•		•	•
In Home Health Care Service—West Inc Westchester, IL	•	•	•		•		•	•
Home Health Care Providers Inc Westmont, IL	•	•	•	•	•		•	•
Denson Optioncare Pharmacy Wheaton, IL							•	•
North Shore Visiting Nurse Association Wilmette, IL	•	•	•		•			
Caregivers Home Health Woodstock, IL	•	•	•	•	•		•	•
Easter Seal Adult & Child Rehabilitation Center Woodstock, IL	•	•	•					
Healthtrends Ltd Woodstock, IL	•	•	•	•	•	•	•	•
The Caring Co Inc Crown Point, IN			•	•				•

Home Health Care	Skilled Nursing	Rehabilitative & Supportive Care	Help with Activities of Daily Living	Homemaker Service	Nutritional Guidance	Telephone Reassurance/Emergency Alert	IV Therapy	24-hour Availability
Meals on Wheels—Northwest Indiana Crown Point, IN					•			
Professional Nursing Service—Division of L A Flowers Inc Gary, IN	•	•	•	•				•
St Margaret Hospital & Health Centers Home Care & Care Connection Hammond, IN	•	•	•	•	•	•	•	•
Visiting Nurse Association of Northwest Indiana Inc Hammond, IN	•	•	•	•	•		•	•
Visiting Nurse Association Home Care Services Inc La Porte, IN	•	•	•	•	•		•	•
Kimberly Quality Care—Merrillville Merrillville, IN	•	•	•	•			•	•
Medical Personnel Pool Merrillville, IN	•	•	•	•	•	•	•	•
Nursefinders of Merrillville Merrillville, IN	•	•	•	•		•	•	•
Option Care Merrillville, IN							•	•
Family Association of La Porte County Michigan City, IN				•				
Hospice of the Calumet Area Inc Munster, IN	•			•	•	•	•	•
Visiting Nurse Association Hospice Home Care Valparaiso, IN	•		•	•		•	•	•
Visiting Nurse Association of Porter County Indiana Inc Valparaiso, IN	•	•	•	•	•	•	•	•

✔ In order to support future editions of this publication would you please mention *Elder Services* each time you contact any advertiser, facility, or service.

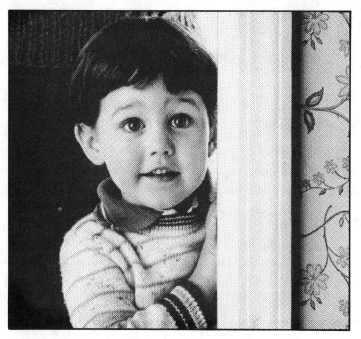

A nursing center so nice he still calls it Grandma's house

Living in a nursing center should be just as nice as living in your own home. And that's why Americana and Monticello Healthcare Centers are dedicated to giving people the same quality of life they've always enjoyed.

But it's not just the warm, relaxed surroundings that make Americana and Monticello so special. It's the attitude which flourishes in such a pleasant environment. Our residents develop a more positive outlook. And this, paired with the best nursing care available, can shorten recovery time.

Visit an Americana or Monticello Healthcare Center soon. It's a place so special even a child can see the difference.

AMERICANA
HEALTHCARE CENTER
A member of the *Manor Healthcare*℠ Community. ©1988 Manor HealthCare Corp.

+ **Americana Healthcare Center of Arlington Heights**
715 W. Central Road
Arlington Heights, IL 60005
(708) 392-2020

* **Americana Healthcare Center of Elgin**
180 S. State Street
Elgin, IL 60123
(708) 742-3310

* **Americana Healthcare Center of Elk Grove**
1920 W. Nerge Rd.
Elk Grove Village, IL 60007
(708) 307-0550

* **Americana-Monticello Healthcare Center of Hinsdale**
600 W. Ogden Avenue
Hinsdale, IL 60521
(708) 325-9630

• **Americana Healthcare Center of Libertyville**
1500 S. Milwaukee Avenue
Libertyville, IL 60048
(708) 816-3200

* **Americana Healthcare Center of Naperville**
200 Martin Avenue
Naperville, IL 60540
(708) 355-4111

+ **Americana Healthcare Center of Oaklawn**
9401 S. Kostner Avenue
Oaklawn, IL 60453
(708) 423-7882

* **Americana-Monticello Healthcare Center of Oaklawn**
6300 W. 95th Street
Oaklawn, IL 60453
(708) 599-8800

* **Americana Healthcare Center**
• **of Palos Heights**
7850 W. College Drive
Palos Heights, IL 60463
(708) 361-6990

* **Americana Healthcare Center of Rolling Meadows**
4225 W. Kirchoff Road
Rolling Meadows, IL 60008
(708) 397-2400

* **Americana Healthcare Center of South Holland**
2145 E. 170th Street
South Holland, IL 60473
(708) 895-3255

* **Americana Healthcare Center of Westmont**
512 E. Ogden Avenue
Westmont, IL 60559
(708) 323-4400

* Specialized Alzheimers Unit   + REACH Subacute Rehabilitation   • Assisted Living

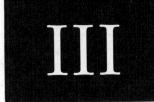

Nursing Homes

ILLINOIS

Arlington Heights

Americana Healthcare Center of Arlington Heights
715 W Central Rd, Arlington Heights, IL 60005
(708) 392-2020, 392-3250 FAX
LICENSURE: Skilled care; Sub-acute rehab.
BEDS: SNF 129.
CERTIFIED: Medicare.
ADMISSIONS REQUIREMENTS: Medical examination; Physician's request.
See ad page 200

Lutheran Home & Services for the Aged
800 W Oakton St, Arlington Heights, IL 60004-4699
(708) 253-3710, 253-1427 FAX
LICENSURE: Skilled care; Intermediate care; Alzheimer's care; Sheltered care.
BEDS: SNF 252 (including 84 Alzheimer's); ICF 60; Sheltered care 167.
CERTIFIED: Medicaid.
ADMISSIONS REQUIREMENTS: Minimum age 60; Medical examination.
STAFF: Physicians 1 (ft), 5 (pt); RNs 19 (ft), 25 (pt); LPNs 15 (ft), 7 (pt); Nurses' aides 76 (ft), 41 (pt); Physical therapists 7 (ft), 2 (pt); Reality therapists 1 (ft); Occupational therapists 1 (pt); Activities coordinators 14 (ft), 1 (pt); Dietitians 1 (ft); Ophthalmologists 1 (pt); Podiatrists 1 (pt); Audiologists 1 (pt); Social workers 3 (ft).
LANGUAGES: Spanish, German
See ads pages 69, 202

Marriott Church Creek Health Care Center
1200 W Central Rd, Arlington Heights, IL 60005
(708) 506-3216, 506-2598 FAX
LICENSURE: Skilled care.
BEDS: SNF 110; ICF 10.
CERTIFIED: Medicare.
ADMISSIONS REQUIREMENTS: Minimum age 18; Medical examination; Physician's request.
STAFF: Physicians; RNs 10 (ft); LPNs 7 (ft); Nurses' aides 30 (ft); Physical therapists 3 (ft); Occupational therapists 1 (ft), 1 (pt); Speech therapists 1 (pt); Activities coordinators 1 (ft), 11 (pt); Dietitians 1 (pt); Ophthalmologists 1 (pt); Podiatrists 1 (pt); Audiologists 1 (pt).

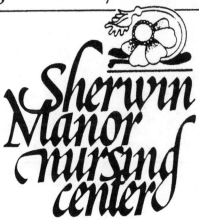

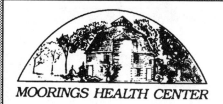

The Moorings Health Center
811 E Central Rd, Arlington Heights, IL 60005
(708) 364-2435
LICENSURE: Intermediate care; Sheltered care.
BEDS: ICF 32; Sheltered care 89.
ADMISSIONS REQUIREMENTS: Minimum age 62; Medical examination; Evaluation.
STAFF: Physicians; RNs; LPNs; Nurses' aides; Physical therapists; Activities coordinators; Dietitians; Food service staff.
See ads pages 140, 202, 301

Northwest Community Continuing Care Center
901 W Kirchoff Rd, Arlington Heights, IL 60005
(708) 259-5850, 577-4064 FAX
LICENSURE: Skilled care; Intermediate care.
BEDS: SNF 150; ICF 50.
CERTIFIED: Medicare.
ADMISSIONS REQUIREMENTS: Minimum age 18; Medical examination.
STAFF: Physicians 1 (ft); RNs 6 (ft), 50 (pt); LPNs 2 (ft), 12 (pt); Nurses' aides 47 (ft), 75 (pt); Physical therapists 3 (ft); Occupational therapists 2 (ft), 1 (pt); Speech therapists 1 (ft); Activities coordinators 4 (ft), 3 (pt); Dietitians 2 (ft); Ophthalmologists; Podiatrists; Audiologists; Physical therapy aides; Rehabilitation aides; Physical therapy techs; Dentists.
LANGUAGES: Polish, Spanish, Tagalog
See ads pages 203, 341

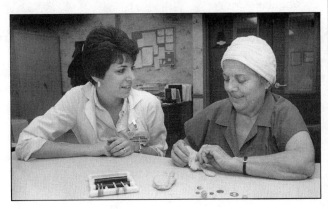

Aurora

Aurora Manor
1601 N Farnsworth, Aurora, IL 60505
(708) 898-1180
LICENSURE: Skilled care; Intermediate care.
BEDS: SNF 54; ICF 151.
CERTIFIED: Medicaid; Medicare.

Countryside Healthcare Centre
2330 W Galena Blvd, Aurora, IL 60506
(708) 896-4686, 896-7868 FAX
LICENSURE: Skilled care; Intermediate care.
BEDS: SNF 107; ICF 102.
CERTIFIED: Medicaid; Medicare.
ADMISSIONS REQUIREMENTS: Minimum age 62; Medical examination; Physician's request.
STAFF: RNs 8 (ft), 2 (pt); LPNs 4 (ft), 4 (pt); Nurses' aides 37 (ft), 37 (pt); Physical therapists 1 (pt) (consultant); Recreational therapists 1 (pt) (consultant); Occupational therapists 1 (pt) (consultant); Speech therapists 1 (pt) (consultant); Activities coordinators 1 (ft); Dietitians 1 (pt) (consultant); Podiatrists 1 (pt) (consultant); Audiologists 1 (pt) (consultant); Dentists (consultant).
See ad on inside back cover

Elmwood Nursing Home
1017 W Galena Blvd, Aurora, IL 60506
(708) 897-3100, 897-1404 FAX
LICENSURE: Skilled care.
BEDS: SNF 64.
CERTIFIED: Medicare.
ADMISSIONS REQUIREMENTS: Minimum age 18; Medical examination.
STAFF: RNs 4 (ft); LPNs 5 (ft); Nurses' aides 20 (ft); Activities coordinators 1 (ft); Dietitians 1 (ft).
LANGUAGES: Greek, Spanish

Jennings Terrace
275 S LaSalle, Aurora, IL 60505
(708) 897-6946
LICENSURE: Skilled care; Intermediate care; Sheltered care.
BEDS: SNF 8; ICF 52; Sheltered care 103.

McAuley Manor
400 W Sullivan Rd, Aurora, IL 60506-1452
(708) 859-3700
LICENSURE: Skilled care; Intermediate care.
BEDS: SNF 32; ICF 56.
ADMISSIONS REQUIREMENTS: Minimum age 52; Medical examination; Physician's request.
STAFF: RNs 6 (ft), 10 (pt); LPNs 2 (ft), 1 (pt); Nurses' aides 28 (ft), 35 (pt); Physical therapists

(contracted); Occupational therapists (contracted); Speech therapists (contracted); Activities coordinators 1 (ft); Dietitians 1 (pt); Ophthalmologists (contracted); Podiatrists (contracted); Audiologists (contracted).

New York Manor Inc
400 E New York, Aurora, IL 60505
(708) 897-8714
LICENSURE: Intermediate care.
BEDS: ICF 121.
ADMISSIONS REQUIREMENTS: Minimum age 22.
STAFF: Physicians 2 (pt); RNs 3 (ft), 2 (pt); LPNs 2 (ft), 3 (pt); Nurses' aides 17 (ft), 8 (pt); Physical therapists 1 (pt); Occupational therapists 1 (pt); Speech therapists 1 (pt); Activities coordinators 1 (pt); Dietitians 1 (pt); Ophthalmologists 1 (pt); Podiatrists 1 (pt); Dentists 1 (pt).

Barrington

Governor's Park Nursing & Rehabilitation Center
1420 S Barrington Rd, Barrington, IL 60010
(708) 382-6664, 382-6693 FAX
LICENSURE: Skilled care; Intermediate care; Alzheimer's care.
BEDS: SNF 75; ICF 75.
CERTIFIED: Medicaid; Medicare.
ADMISSIONS REQUIREMENTS: Minimum age 18; Medical examination; Physician's request.
STAFF: RNs 15 (ft), 6 (pt); LPNs 4 (ft), 3 (pt); Nurses' aides 29 (ft), 6 (pt); Physical therapists 3 (ft), 1 (pt); Occupational therapists 2 (ft), 1 (pt); Speech therapists 1 (pt); Activities coordinators 1 (ft), 3 (pt); Podiatrists (consultant).

Batavia

Firwood Health Care Center
520 Fabyan Pkwy, Batavia, IL 60510
(708) 879-5266, 879-5214 FAX
LICENSURE: Intermediate care.
BEDS: ICF 63.
CERTIFIED: Medicaid.
ADMISSIONS REQUIREMENTS: Medical examination; Physician's request.
STAFF: RNs 1 (ft), 3 (pt); LPNs 2 (ft), 2 (pt); Physical therapists 1 (pt); Recreational therapists 1 (pt); Occupational therapists 1 (pt); Speech therapists 1 (pt); Activities coordinators 1 (ft), 1 (pt); Dietitians 1 (pt); Ophthalmologists 1 (pt); Podiatrists 1 (pt); Audiologists 1 (pt).

Michealsen Health Center
831 N Batavia Ave, Batavia, IL 60510
(708) 879-4300, 879-1153 FAX
LICENSURE: Skilled care; Intermediate care.

BEDS: Total 125.
CERTIFIED: Medicaid; Medicare.
ADMISSIONS REQUIREMENTS: Minimum age 62; Physician's request; Medical evaluation.
STAFF: RNs; LPNs; Physical therapists; Occupational therapists; Activities coordinators; Dietitians Medical director; CNAs; Social workers; Chaplain.
See ads pages iv, 300

Beecher

The Anchorage of Beecher
1201 Dixie Hwy, Beecher, IL 60401
(708) 946-2600, 946-9245 FAX
LICENSURE: Skilled care; Intermediate care.
BEDS: SNF 38; ICF 58.
CERTIFIED: Medicaid; Medicare.
ADMISSIONS REQUIREMENTS: Medical examination.
STAFF: RNs 11 (ft), 3 (pt); LPNs 5 (pt); Nurses' aides 18 (ft), 16 (pt); Physical therapists (contracted); Activities coordinators 1 (ft).

Bensenville

The Anchorage of Bensenville
331 S York Rd, Bensenville, IL 60106
(708) 766-5800, 860-5130 FAX
LICENSURE: Skilled care; Intermediate care.
BEDS: SNF 90; ICF 142.
CERTIFIED: Medicaid; Medicare.
STAFF: Physicians 3 (ft); RNs 6 (ft), 22 (pt); LPNs 7 (ft), 8 (pt); Nurses' aides 44 (ft), 19 (pt); Physical therapists (contracted); Recreational therapists 3 (ft), 1 (pt); Activities coordinators 2 (ft); Dietitians 1 (ft); Podiatrists 1 (ft); Optometrists 1 (pt).

Berwyn

Fairfax Health Care Center
3601 S Harlem Ave, Berwyn, IL 60402
(708) 749-4160, 749-7696 FAX
LICENSURE: Skilled care; Alzheimer's care.
BEDS: SNF 160.
CERTIFIED: Medicaid; Medicare.
ADMISSIONS REQUIREMENTS: Minimum age 65.
STAFF: Physical therapists 1 (ft); Recreational therapists 1 (pt); Occupational therapists 1 (pt); Speech therapists 1 (pt); Activities coordinators 1 (ft); Dietitians 1 (ft); Ophthalmologists 1 (pt); Podiatrists 1 (pt); Audiologists 1 (pt).

Bloomingdale

Alden Nursing Center—Valley Ridge Rehabilitation & Health Care Center
275 Army Trail Rd, Bloomingdale, IL 60108
(708) 893-9616, 924-1059 FAX
LICENSURE: Skilled care; Alzheimer's care.
BEDS: SNF 207; Alzheimer's 69.
CERTIFIED: Medicaid; Medicare.
ADMISSIONS REQUIREMENTS: Minimum age 18.
STAFF: Physicians; RNs; LPNs; Nurses' aides; Physical therapists; Occupational therapists; Speech therapists; Activities coordinators; Dietitians; Ophthalmologists; Podiatrists; Audiologists.

Lexington Health Care Center of Bloomingdale
165 S Bloomingdale Rd, Bloomingdale, IL 60108
(708) 980-8700
LICENSURE: Skilled care.
BEDS: SNF 88.
CERTIFIED: Medicaid; Medicare.

Blue Island

Blue Island Nursing Home Inc
2427 W 127th St, Blue Island, IL 60406
(708) 389-7799
LICENSURE: Intermediate care.
BEDS: ICF 30.
CERTIFIED: Medicaid.

Bridgeview

Bridgeview Convalescent Center
8100 S Harlem Ave, Bridgeview, IL 60455
(708) 594-5440
LICENSURE: Skilled care; Intermediate care.
BEDS: SNF 101; ICF 51.
CERTIFIED: Medicaid; Medicare.
STAFF: Physicians 6 (pt); RNs 8 (ft), 4 (pt); LPNs 6 (ft), 10 (pt); Nurses' aides 77 (ft); Physical therapists 2 (pt); Reality therapists 1 (pt); Recreational therapists 1 (pt); Occupational therapists 1 (pt); Speech therapists 1 (pt); Activities coordinators 1 (ft); Dietitians 1 (pt); Ophthalmologists 1 (pt); Podiatrists 1 (pt); Dentists 1 (pt).

Metropolitan Nursing Center
8540 S Harlem Ave, Bridgeview, IL 60455
(708) 598-2605, 598-5671 FAX
LICENSURE: Skilled care; Intermediate care; Alzheimer's care; Hospice; Respite care.
BEDS: Total 404.
CERTIFIED: Medicaid; VA.
ADMISSIONS REQUIREMENTS: Minimum age per state regulations; "Public Aid Pending" acceptable.

STAFF: Physicians; RNs 11 (ft); LPNs 32 (ft), 8 (pt); Nurses' aides 102 (ft), 3 (pt); Physical therapists 1 (pt); Reality therapists; Recreational therapists; Occupational therapists 1 (pt); Speech therapists 1 (pt); Activities coordinators 11 (ft); Dietitians 1 (pt); Ophthalmologists 1 (pt); Podiatrists 1 (pt); Audiologists 1 (pt); Social services workers; Dentists.
LANGUAGES: Polish

Brookfield

The British Home
31st St & McCormick, Brookfield, IL 60513
(708) 485-0135
LICENSURE: Skilled care; Intermediate care; Sheltered care; Independent living.
BEDS: SNF 46; ICF 26; Sheltered care 64; Independent living 66.
ADMISSIONS REQUIREMENTS: Minimum age 70; Medical examination; Physician's request.
STAFF: Physicians; RNs; LPNs; Nurses' aides; Recreational therapists; Activities coordinators; Dietitians; Podiatrists.

Burbank

Brentwood Nursing & Rehabilitation Center
5400 W 87th St, Burbank, IL 60459
(708) 423-1200
LICENSURE: Skilled care; Alzheimer's care.
BEDS: SNF 165.
CERTIFIED: Medicare.
ADMISSIONS REQUIREMENTS: Medical examination.
STAFF: RNs; LPNs; Nurses' aides; Physical therapists; Recreational therapists; Occupational therapists; Speech therapists; Activities coordinators; Dietitians; Ophthalmologists; Podiatrists.
LANGUAGES: Spanish

Parkside Gardens Nursing Home
5701 W 79th St, Burbank, IL 60459
(708) 636-3850, 636-3897 FAX
LICENSURE: Intermediate care.
BEDS: ICF 78.
ADMISSIONS REQUIREMENTS: Medical examination; Physician's request.
STAFF: LPNs 6 (ft), 3 (pt); Nurses' aides 17 (ft), 7 (pt); Activities coordinators 5 (ft), 1 (pt); Dietitians 5 (ft), 5 (pt).

Burnham

Burnham Terrace Ltd
14500 S Manistee, Burnham, IL 60633
(708) 862-1260
LICENSURE: Skilled care; Intermediate care.
BEDS: SNF 103; ICF 206.
CERTIFIED: Medicaid.

Burr Ridge

King Bruwaert House
6101 S County Line Rd, Burr Ridge, IL 60521
(708) 323-2250
LICENSURE: Skilled care; Sheltered care; Retirement.
BEDS: SNF 35; Sheltered care 83; Retirement home 63.
ADMISSIONS REQUIREMENTS: Minimum age 65; Medical examination.
STAFF: Physicians 1 (pt); RNs 9 (ft), 5 (pt); LPNs 4 (ft); Nurses' aides 20 (ft), 5 (pt); Activities coordinators 4 (ft), 1 (pt); Dietitians 1 (ft); Ophthalmologists 1 (pt); Podiatrists 1 (pt); Audiologists 1 (pt).

Carol Stream

Windsor Park Manor
124 Windsor Park Dr, Carol Stream, IL 60188
(708) 682-4491, 682-4609 FAX
LICENSURE: Skilled care.
BEDS: SNF 60.
CERTIFIED: Medicare.
STAFF: RNs 4 (ft), 9 (pt); LPNs 3 (ft), 3 (pt); Nurses' aides 23 (ft), 8 (pt); Activities coordinators 1 (ft); Dietitians 1 (pt); Ophthalmologists 1 (pt); Podiatrists 1 (pt); Audiologists 1 (pt).

Chicago

The Admiral
909 W Foster Ave, Chicago, IL 60640
(312) 561-2900
LICENSURE: Intermediate care; Sheltered care.
BEDS: ICF 50; Sheltered care 85.

Alden Nursing Center—Lakeland Rehabilitation & Health Care Center
820 W Lawrence Ave, Chicago, IL 60640
(312) 769-2570, 769-0607 FAX
LICENSURE: Skilled care; Intermediate care; Alzheimer's care.
BEDS: Total 300.
CERTIFIED: Medicaid; Medicare; VA.

ADMISSIONS REQUIREMENTS: Minimum age 18; Physician's request.
STAFF: Physicians; RNs; LPNs; Nurses' aides; Physical therapists; Occupational therapists; Speech therapists; Activities coordinators; Dietitians; Ophthalmologists; Podiatrists; Audiologists.

Alden Nursing Center—Morrow Rehabilitation & Health Care Center
5001 S Michigan, Chicago, IL 60615
(312) 924-9292, 924-1308 FAX
LICENSURE: Skilled care.
BEDS: SNF 192.
CERTIFIED: Medicaid; Medicare.
ADMISSIONS REQUIREMENTS: Minimum age 18.
STAFF: Physicians; RNs; LPNs; Nurses' aides; Physical therapists; Reality therapists; Occupational therapists; Speech therapists; Activities coordinators; Dietitians; Ophthalmologists; Podiatrists; Audiologists.

Alden Nursing Center—Princeton Rehabilitation & Health Care Center
255 W 69th St, Chicago, IL 60621
(312) 224-5900, 224-7157 FAX
LICENSURE: Skilled care; Intermediate care; Alzheimer's care.
BEDS: Total 225.
CERTIFIED: Medicaid; Medicare; VA.
ADMISSIONS REQUIREMENTS: Minimum age 18; Medical examination.
STAFF: Physicians; RNs; LPNs; Nurses' aides; Physical therapists; Occupational therapists; Speech therapists; Activities coordinators; Dietitians; Ophthalmologists; Podiatrists; Audiologists.

Alden Nursing Center—Wentworth Rehabilitation & Health Care Center
201 W 69th St, Chicago, IL 60621
(312) 487-1200, 487-4782 FAX
LICENSURE: Skilled care; Intermediate care; Alzheimer's care.
BEDS: SNF 238; ICF 62.
CERTIFIED: Medicaid; Medicare; VA.
ADMISSIONS REQUIREMENTS: Minimum age 18; Physician's request.
STAFF: Physicians; RNs; LPNs; Nurses' aides; Physical therapists; Occupational therapists; Speech therapists; Activities coordinators; Dietitians; Ophthalmologists; Podiatrists; Audiologists.

All American Nursing Home
5448 N Broadway St, Chicago, IL 60640
(312) 334-2224
LICENSURE: Skilled care; Intermediate care.
BEDS: SNF 48; ICF 96.
CERTIFIED: Medicaid.
ADMISSIONS REQUIREMENTS: Minimum age 23.
STAFF: Physicians 4 (pt); RNs 5 (ft); LPNs 12 (ft); Nurses' aides 38 (ft); Physical therapists 1 (pt); Reality therapists 1 (pt); Recreational therapists 1 (pt); Occupational therapists 1 (pt); Speech therapists 1 (pt); Activities coordinators 1 (ft); Dietitians 1 (pt); Podiatrists 1 (pt); Dentists 1 (pt).

Alshore House

2840 W Foster Ave, Chicago, IL 60625
(312) 561-2040
LICENSURE: Intermediate care.
BEDS: ICF 48.
CERTIFIED: Medicaid.
ADMISSIONS REQUIREMENTS: Minimum age 65; Medical examination; Physician's request.
STAFF: Physicians 2 (ft); RNs 3 (ft); LPNs 5 (ft); Nurses' aides 16 (ft); Physical therapists 2 (ft); Reality therapists 2 (ft); Recreational therapists 2 (ft); Occupational therapists 1 (ft); Speech therapists 1 (pt); Activities coordinators 2 (ft); Dietitians 1 (ft); Ophthalmologists 1 (pt); Podiatrists 1 (pt); Audiologists 1 (pt).
LANGUAGES: Romanian, Russian, Yiddish

Ambassador Nursing Center Inc

4900 N Bernard St, Chicago, IL 60625
(312) 583-7130, 583-3929 FAX
LICENSURE: Skilled care.
BEDS: SNF 190.
CERTIFIED: Medicaid; Medicare.
ADMISSIONS REQUIREMENTS: Minimum age 50.
STAFF: Physicians 5 (pt); RNs 13 (ft), 3 (pt); LPNs 3 (ft); Nurses' aides 40 (ft); Physical therapists 1 (pt); Reality therapists 1 (pt); Recreational therapists 5 (ft); Activities coordinators 1 (ft); Dietitians 1 (ft); Ophthalmologists 1 (pt); Podiatrists 1 (pt); Audiologists 1 (pt).
LANGUAGES: Korean, Spanish, Russian, Polish, Yiddish, Hebrew, Lithuanian

Arbour Health Care Center Ltd

1512 W Fargo, Chicago, IL 60626
(312) 465-7751
LICENSURE: Skilled care; Intermediate care.
BEDS: SNF 70; ICF 29.
CERTIFIED: Medicaid.
ADMISSIONS REQUIREMENTS: Minimum age 60; Medical examination; Physician's request.
STAFF: RNs; LPNs; Nurses' aides; Physical therapists; Reality therapists; Recreational therapists; Occupational therapists; Activities coordinators; Dietitians.

Atrium Health Care Center Ltd

1425 W Estes Ave, Chicago, IL 60626
(312) 973-4780, 973-1895 FAX
LICENSURE: Skilled care.
BEDS: SNF 160.
CERTIFIED: Medicaid; Medicare; VA.
ADMISSIONS REQUIREMENTS: Minimum age 22.
STAFF: Physicians 18 (pt); RNs 6 (ft); LPNs 8 (ft); Nurses' aides 30 (ft); Physical therapists 1 (pt); Reality therapists 2 (ft); Recreational therapists 1 (pt); Occupational therapists 1 (pt); Speech therapists 1 (pt); Activities coordinators 5 (ft), 1 (pt); Dietitians 1 (pt); Ophthalmologists 1 (pt); Podiatrists 3 (pt); Audiologists 1 (pt).

Avenue Care Center Inc

4505 S Drexel, Chicago, IL 60653
(312) 285-0550, 285-5618 FAX
LICENSURE: Skilled care.

BEDS: SNF 155.
CERTIFIED: Medicaid.

Balmoral Nursing Centre Inc

2055 W Balmoral Ave, Chicago, IL 60625
(312) 561-8661
LICENSURE: Skilled care.
BEDS: SNF 213.
CERTIFIED: Medicaid.

Warren Barr Pavilion of Illinois Masonic Medical Center

66 W Oak St, Chicago, IL 60610
(312) 337-5400, 337-6438 FAX
LICENSURE: Skilled care; Alzheimer's care.
BEDS: SNF 330.
CERTIFIED: Medicaid; Medicare; VA.
ADMISSIONS REQUIREMENTS: Minimum age 18; Medical examination.
STAFF: Physicians 1 (ft), 3 (pt); RNs 23 (ft), 2 (pt); LPNs 27 (ft); Nurses' aides 115 (ft), 4 (pt); Physical therapists 2 (ft); Recreational therapists 6 (ft), 1 (pt); Occupational therapists 2 (ft); Speech therapists 1 (ft), 1 (pt); Activities coordinators 1 (ft); Dietitians 1 (ft); Ophthalmologists 1 (pt); Podiatrists 1 (pt); Audiologists 1 (pt); Certified occupational therapy aides 1 (ft).
LANGUAGES: Polish, Spanish

Belhaven Inc

11401 S Oakley Ave, Chicago, IL 60643
(312) 233-6311
LICENSURE: Skilled care; Intermediate care.
BEDS: SNF 154; ICF 76.
CERTIFIED: Medicaid; Medicare.

Belmont Nursing Home Inc

1936 W Belmont Ave, Chicago, IL 60657
(312) 525-7176, 525-8929 FAX
LICENSURE: Intermediate care.
BEDS: ICF 61.
CERTIFIED: Medicaid.
ADMISSIONS REQUIREMENTS: Minimum age 18; Medical examination; Mental illness diagnosis.
STAFF: LPNs 4 (ft), 2 (pt); Nurses' aides; Activities coordinators 1 (ft), 2 (pt); Occupational rehabilitation aides 1 (ft), 1 (pt).
LANGUAGES: Spanish, Polish, Swedish, Ethiopian

Bethesda Home & Retirement Center

2833 N Nordica Ave, Chicago, IL 60634
(312) 622-6144, 745-1396 FAX
LICENSURE: Skilled care; Intermediate care; Assisted living.
BEDS: SNF 15; ICF 64; Assisted living 67.
CERTIFIED: Medicaid.
ADMISSIONS REQUIREMENTS: Minimum age 62; Medical examination.
STAFF: Physicians (consultant); RNs 5 (ft), 2 (pt); LPNs 4 (ft), 3 (pt); Nurses' aides 24 (ft), 1 (pt); Occupational therapists (consultant); Speech therapists

(consultant); Activities coordinators 2 (ft); Dietitians (consultant); Ophthalmologists (consultant); Podiatrists (consultant); Audiologists (consultant).

Birchwood Plaza Nursing Home
1426 W Birchwood Ave, Chicago, IL 60626
(312) 274-4405, 274-4763 FAX
LICENSURE: Skilled care; Alzheimer's care.
BEDS: SNF 192.
CERTIFIED: Medicaid; Medicare.
ADMISSIONS REQUIREMENTS: Minimum age 62.
STAFF: RNs 8 (ft), 2 (pt); LPNs 7 (ft), 1 (pt); Nurses' aides 42 (ft), 5 (pt); Activities coordinators 4 (ft), 1 (pt); Dietitians 1 (ft); Physical rehabilitation aides 2 (ft); Social services workers 3 (ft).
LANGUAGES: Russian, Yiddish

Bohemian Home for the Aged
5061 N Pulaski Rd, Chicago, IL 60630
(312) 588-1220
LICENSURE: Skilled care; Intermediate care.
BEDS: SNF 33; ICF 185.
CERTIFIED: Medicaid.
ADMISSIONS REQUIREMENTS: Minimum age 75; Medical examination.
STAFF: Physicians 1 (pt); RNs 14 (ft), 7 (pt); LPNs 11 (ft); Nurses' aides 50 (ft); Activities coordinators 1 (ft); Dietitians 1 (ft).
LANGUAGES: Czech, Polish

Boulevard Care Center Inc
3405 S Michigan Ave, Chicago, IL 60616
(312) 791-0035
LICENSURE: Skilled care.
BEDS: SNF 155.
CERTIFIED: Medicaid.
ADMISSIONS REQUIREMENTS: Medical examination; Physician's request.
STAFF: Physicians 3 (pt); RNs 2 (ft), 2 (pt); LPNs 10 (ft), 4 (pt); Nurses' aides 30 (ft), 5 (pt); Physical therapists 1 (pt); Recreational therapists 2 (ft); Occupational therapists 1 (pt); Speech therapists 1 (pt); Activities coordinators 1 (ft); Dietitians 1 (pt); Ophthalmologists 1 (pt); Podiatrists 1 (pt); Dentists 1 (pt).

Brightview Care Center Inc
4538 N Beacon, Chicago, IL 60640
(312) 275-7200, 275-7543 FAX
LICENSURE: Skilled care.
BEDS: SNF 143.
CERTIFIED: Medicaid.
ADMISSIONS REQUIREMENTS: Medical examination; Physician's request.
STAFF: RNs; LPNs; Nurses' aides; Recreational therapists; Activities coordinators.
LANGUAGES: Spanish

Bryn Mawr Care Inc
5547 N Kenmore, Chicago, IL 60640
(312) 561-7040
LICENSURE: Intermediate care.
BEDS: ICF 174.

Buckingham Pavilion Nursing & Rehabilitation Center
2625 W Touhy Ave, Chicago, IL 60645
(312) 764-6850
LICENSURE: Skilled care; Intermediate care; Alzheimer's care.
BEDS: SNF 34; ICF 88; Alzheimer's 48; Assisted living 80.
CERTIFIED: Medicaid; Medicare.
ADMISSIONS REQUIREMENTS: Minimum age 65.
LANGUAGES: Yiddish, German, Hungarian, Polish, Czech

California Gardens Nursing Center
2829 S California Blvd, Chicago, IL 60608
(312) 847-8061
LICENSURE: Skilled care.
BEDS: SNF 306.
CERTIFIED: Medicaid; Medicare.
ADMISSIONS REQUIREMENTS: Minimum age 21.
STAFF: Physicians 10 (ft); RNs 4 (ft), 8 (pt); LPNs 24 (ft), 4 (pt); Nurses' aides 90 (ft), 5 (pt); Physical therapists 2 (pt); Reality therapists 1 (pt); Recreational therapists 1 (pt); Occupational therapists 2 (pt); Speech therapists 2 (pt); Activities coordinators 1 (ft), 1 (pt); Dietitians 1 (ft), 1 (pt); Ophthalmologists 1 (pt); Podiatrists 2 (pt); Audiologists 1 (pt).
LANGUAGES: Spanish, Lithuanian

Carlton House Nursing Center—CH Nursing Center Inc
725 W Montrose Ave, Chicago, IL 60613
(312) 929-1700
LICENSURE: Skilled care.
BEDS: SNF 244.
CERTIFIED: Medicaid; Medicare.
STAFF: Physicians 16 (ft); RNs; LPNs; Nurses' aides; Physical therapists; Recreational therapists; Occupational therapists; Speech therapists; Activities coordinators; Dietitians; Ophthalmologists; Podiatrists; Audiologists.
LANGUAGES: Spanish, Italian, Tagalog

Carmen Manor Nursing Home
1470 W Carmen, Chicago, IL 60640
(312) 878-7000, 878-8335 FAX
LICENSURE: Intermediate care.
BEDS: ICF 113.
CERTIFIED: Medicaid.
ADMISSIONS REQUIREMENTS: Medical examination; Physician's request.
STAFF: LPNs 9 (ft); Nurses' aides 20 (ft); Activities coordinators 1 (ft); Social workers 1 (ft).

Casa Central Home
1401 N California Ave, Chicago, IL 60622
(312) 276-1902
LICENSURE: Skilled care; Intermediate care.
BEDS: SNF 91; ICF 49.
CERTIFIED: Medicaid.

Central Nursing

2450 N Central Ave, Chicago, IL 60639
(312) 889-1333, 889-1516 FAX
LICENSURE: Skilled care.
BEDS: Total 245.
CERTIFIED: Medicaid; Medicare; VA.

Central Plaza Residential Home

321-327 N Central, Chicago, IL 60644
(312) 626-2300
LICENSURE: Intermediate care.
BEDS: ICF 260.
CERTIFIED: Medicaid.
ADMISSIONS REQUIREMENTS: Minimum age 21; Medical
    examination.
STAFF: Physicians 6 (pt); RNs 2 (ft); LPNs 12 (ft), 1
    (pt); Nurses' aides 45 (ft); Physical therapists 1
    (pt); Recreational therapists 1 (pt); Occupational
    therapists 2 (ft); Speech therapists 1 (pt); Activities
    coordinators 1 (ft); Dietitians 1 (ft), 1 (pt); Oph-
    thalmologists 1 (pt); Podiatrists 1 (pt);
    Audiologists 1 (pt).

Chevy Chase Nursing Center

3400 S Indiana Ave, Chicago, IL 60616
(312) 842-5000, 842-3790 FAX
LICENSURE: Skilled care.
BEDS: SNF 322.
CERTIFIED: Medicaid; Medicare.
ADMISSIONS REQUIREMENTS: Medical examination.
STAFF: Physicians 7 (pt); RNs 4 (ft), 2 (pt); LPNs 28
    (ft), 3 (pt); Nurses' aides 95 (ft), 10 (pt); Physical
    therapists 2 (pt); Recreational therapists 1 (pt);
    Occupational therapists 2 (pt); Speech therapists 2
    (pt); Activities coordinators 1 (ft); Dietitians 1
    (pt); Ophthalmologists 1 (pt); Podiatrists 1 (pt);
    Audiologists 1 (pt).

Clark Manor Convalescent Center

7433 N Clark St, Chicago, IL 60626
(312) 338-8778
LICENSURE: Skilled care.
BEDS: SNF 273.
CERTIFIED: Medicaid; Medicare.
ADMISSIONS REQUIREMENTS: Minimum age 55.
STAFF: Physicians 14 (pt); RNs 20 (ft); LPNs 3 (pt);
    Nurses' aides 50 (ft); Physical therapists 1 (pt);
    Recreational therapists 1 (ft); Occupational thera-
    pists 1 (pt); Speech therapists 1 (pt); Activities
    coordinators 1 (ft); Dietitians 1 (pt); Ophthalmol-
    ogists 1 (pt); Podiatrists 1 (pt); Dentists 1 (pt).

Clayton Residential Home

2026 N Clark St, Chicago, IL 60614
(312) 549-1840
LICENSURE: Intermediate care.
BEDS: ICF 252.
CERTIFIED: Medicaid.
ADMISSIONS REQUIREMENTS: Minimum age 18; Medical
    examination.
STAFF: Physicians 3 (pt); LPNs 9 (ft); Nurses' aides 20
    (ft); Physical therapists 1 (ft), 1 (pt); Reality thera-

pists 2 (ft); Recreational therapists 1 (ft); Occupa-
    tional therapists 1 (ft); Activities coordinators 1
    (ft); Dietitians 1 (ft); Podiatrists 1 (pt).

Cojeunaze Nursing Center

3311 S Michigan Ave, Chicago, IL 60616
(312) 326-5700
LICENSURE: Skilled care; Intermediate care; Retirement.
BEDS: SNF 74; ICF 126.
CERTIFIED: Medicaid.
ADMISSIONS REQUIREMENTS: Minimum age 60; Medical
    examination; Physician's request.
STAFF: Physicians 4 (pt); RNs 2 (ft), 5 (pt); LPNs 9
    (ft), 4 (pt); Nurses' aides 45 (ft), 3 (pt); Physical
    therapists; Reality therapists; Recreational thera-
    pists 1 (pt); Occupational therapists 1 (pt); Activi-
    ties coordinators 1 (ft), 2 (pt); Dietitians 1 (pt);
    Ophthalmologists 1 (pt); Dentists 1 (pt).
LANGUAGES: French

Columbus Manor Residential Care Home

5107-5121 W Jackson Blvd, Chicago, IL 60644
(312) 378-5490
LICENSURE: Intermediate care.
BEDS: ICF 189.
CERTIFIED: Medicaid.
ADMISSIONS REQUIREMENTS: Minimum age 35; Medical
    examination.
STAFF: Physicians; RNs; LPNs; Nurses' aides; Recrea-
    tional therapists; Activities coordinators; Dietitians.
LANGUAGES: Spanish, Polish

Community Care Center Inc

4314 S Wabash Ave, Chicago, IL 60653
(312) 538-8300
LICENSURE: Skilled care; Intermediate care.
BEDS: SNF 145; ICF 59.
CERTIFIED: Medicaid.
ADMISSIONS REQUIREMENTS: Medical examination; Physi-
    cian's request.
STAFF: RNs; LPNs; Nurses' aides; Activities coordinators;
    Dietitians.

Congress Care Center

901 S Austin Ave, Chicago, IL 60644
(312) 287-5959, 287-7909 FAX
LICENSURE: Skilled care; Intermediate care.
BEDS: SNF 70; ICF 70.
CERTIFIED: Medicaid.
ADMISSIONS REQUIREMENTS: Medical examination; Physi-
    cian's request.
STAFF: RNs; LPNs; Nurses' aides; Occupational thera-
    pists; Activities coordinators.

Continental Care Center Inc

5336 N Western Ave, Chicago, IL 60625
(312) 271-5600
LICENSURE: Skilled care.
BEDS: SNF 208.
CERTIFIED: Medicaid; VA.

ADMISSIONS REQUIREMENTS: Minimum age 65.
STAFF: Physicians 38 (pt); RNs 2 (ft), 2 (pt); LPNs 18 (ft), 2 (pt); Nurses' aides 43 (ft); Occupational therapists 3 (ft); Activities coordinators 5 (ft), 1 (pt); Dietitians 1 (ft).

Covenant Home of Chicago
2725 W Foster Ave, Chicago, IL 60625
(312) 878-8200, 334-7516 FAX
LICENSURE: Skilled care; Intermediate care; Alzheimer's care; Sheltered care.
BEDS: SNF 52; Sheltered care 70.
CERTIFIED: Medicaid; Medicare.
ADMISSIONS REQUIREMENTS: Minimum age 62; Physician's request.
STAFF: RNs; LPNs; Physical therapists; Occupational therapists; Activities coordinators; Dietitians; CNAs.
LANGUAGES: Swedish
See ads pages iv, 300

William L Dawson Nursing Home
3500 S Giles Ave, Chicago, IL 60653
(312) 326-2000
LICENSURE: Skilled care.
BEDS: SNF 245.
CERTIFIED: Medicaid.

Deauville Healthcare Center
7445 N Sheridan Rd, Chicago, IL 60626
(312) 338-3300
LICENSURE: Skilled care; Intermediate care.
BEDS: SNF 51; ICF 98.
CERTIFIED: Medicaid; Medicare.
ADMISSIONS REQUIREMENTS: Minimum age 65; Medical examination.
STAFF: Physicians 31 (ft); RNs 6 (ft), 1 (pt); LPNs 7 (ft), 1 (pt); Nurses' aides 52 (ft), 8 (pt); Physical therapists 1 (ft), 1 (pt); Reality therapists 3 (ft); Recreational therapists 5 (ft); Occupational therapists 3 (ft); Speech therapists 1 (ft); Activities coordinators 1 (ft); Dietitians 1 (ft); Ophthalmologists 1 (ft); Podiatrists 1 (ft); Audiologists 1 (ft).
LANGUAGES: Spanish, Yiddish

Edgewater Nursing & Geriatric Center
5838 N Sheridan Rd, Chicago, IL 60660
(312) 769-2230
LICENSURE: Skilled care; Intermediate care; Alzheimer's care; Hospice; Respite care.
BEDS: SNF 127; ICF 61.
CERTIFIED: Medicaid; Medicare; IDPH Exceptional Care.
ADMISSIONS REQUIREMENTS: Minimum age per state regulations; "Public Aid Pending" acceptable.
STAFF: Physicians (contracted); RNs 16 (ft); LPNs 12 (ft); Nurses' aides 38 (ft); Physical therapists (contracted); Reality therapists; Recreational therapists (contracted); Occupational therapists (contracted); Speech therapists (contracted); Activities coordinators 1 (ft); Dietitians (contracted); Ophthalmologists (contracted); Podiatrists (contracted); Audiologists (contracted); Social services workers; Dentists.
LANGUAGES: Spanish, Tagalog

Elston Home Inc
4340 N Keystone, Chicago, IL 60641
(312) 545-8700
LICENSURE: Skilled care; Intermediate care.
BEDS: SNF 84; ICF 33.
CERTIFIED: Medicaid; Medicare.
ADMISSIONS REQUIREMENTS: Minimum age 18; Medical examination; Physician's request.
STAFF: Physicians 10 (ft); RNs 6 (ft), 2 (pt); LPNs 7 (ft), 1 (pt); Nurses' aides 33 (ft), 3 (pt); Physical therapists 1 (ft); Reality therapists 4 (ft); Recreational therapists 3 (ft); Occupational therapists 1 (ft); Activities coordinators 1 (ft); Dietitians 1 (ft); Ophthalmologists 1 (ft); Dentists 1 (ft); Occupational aides 1 (ft).
LANGUAGES: Polish, German, Tagalog

Garden View Home Inc
6450 N Ridge Ave, Chicago, IL 60626
(312) 743-8700, 743-8407 FAX
LICENSURE: Skilled care; Intermediate care.
BEDS: SNF 110; ICF 26.
CERTIFIED: Medicaid.
STAFF: Physicians; RNs; LPNs; Nurses' aides; Physical therapists; Reality therapists; Recreational therapists; Occupational therapists; Speech therapists; Activities coordinators; Dietitians; Ophthalmologists; Podiatrists; Audiologists; Dentists.

Glencrest Nursing Rehabilitation Center Ltd
2451 W Touhy Ave, Chicago, IL 60645
(312) 338-6800
LICENSURE: Skilled care; Intermediate care; Alzheimer's care.
BEDS: SNF 154; ICF 158.
CERTIFIED: Medicaid; Medicare; VA.
ADMISSIONS REQUIREMENTS: Minimum age 50.
STAFF: Physical therapists; Activities coordinators; Dietitians; Speech therapists; Occupational therapists; Respiratory therapists; Social workers; Geriatric therapists.

Grasmere Resident Home Inc
4621 N Sheridan Rd, Chicago, IL 60640
(312) 334-6601
LICENSURE: Intermediate care.
BEDS: ICF 216.
CERTIFIED: Medicaid.
ADMISSIONS REQUIREMENTS: Minimum age 18.
STAFF: Physicians 6 (pt); RNs 1 (ft); LPNs 7 (ft), 3 (pt); Nurses' aides 37 (ft), 1 (pt); Occupational therapists 1 (pt); Activities coordinators 4 (ft), 2 (pt); Dietitians 1 (pt).

Halsted Terrace Nursing Center
10935 S Halsted St, Chicago, IL 60628
(312) 928-2000
LICENSURE: Skilled care.
BEDS: SNF 300.
CERTIFIED: Medicaid.
ADMISSIONS REQUIREMENTS: Physician's request.
STAFF: Physicians 6 (pt); RNs 6 (ft), 2 (pt); LPNs 20 (ft), 5 (pt); Nurses' aides 76 (ft), 3 (pt); Physical

therapists 1 (pt); Occupational therapists 1 (pt); Speech therapists 1 (pt); Activities coordinators; Dietitians 1 (pt).

Heritage Healthcare Centre

5888 N Ridge Ave, Chicago, IL 60660
(312) 769-2626, 769-1799 FAX
LICENSURE: Skilled care; Intermediate care; Alzheimer's care.
BEDS: SNF 44; ICF 84.
CERTIFIED: Medicaid.
ADMISSIONS REQUIREMENTS: Minimum age 60; Medical examination.
STAFF: Physicians 10 (ft); RNs 4 (ft), 2 (pt); LPNs 3 (ft), 4 (pt); Nurses' aides 23 (ft), 6 (pt); Physical therapists 1 (ft), 1 (pt); Recreational therapists 1 (ft); Occupational therapists 1 (ft); Speech therapists 1 (pt); Activities coordinators 4 (ft); Dietitians 1 (ft), 1 (pt); Ophthalmologists 1 (ft); Podiatrists 1 (ft); Audiologists 1 (ft); Social workers 1 (ft).

The Imperial Convalescent & Geriatric Center Inc

1366 W Fullerton Ave, Chicago, IL 60614
(312) 935-7474, 935-0036 FAX
LICENSURE: Skilled care.
BEDS: SNF 248.
CERTIFIED: Medicaid; Medicare; VA.
ADMISSIONS REQUIREMENTS: Minimum age 21; Medical examination.
STAFF: RNs 10 (ft), 4 (pt); LPNs 11 (ft), 4 (pt); Nurses' aides 58 (ft), 12 (pt); Physical therapists 1 (pt); Reality therapists 1 (pt); Occupational therapists 1 (pt); Speech therapists 1 (pt); Activities coordinators 3 (ft), 1 (pt); Dietitians 1 (ft), 1 (pt); Ophthalmologists 1 (pt); Podiatrists 1 (pt); Audiologists 1 (pt).

Jackson Square Nursing Center

5130 W Jackson Blvd, Chicago, IL 60644
(312) 921-8000
LICENSURE: Skilled care.
BEDS: SNF 234.
CERTIFIED: Medicaid; Medicare.

Johnson Rehabilitation Nursing Home

3456 W Franklin Blvd, Chicago, IL 60624
(312) 533-3033
LICENSURE: Skilled care.
BEDS: SNF 76.
CERTIFIED: Medicaid; Medicare.
ADMISSIONS REQUIREMENTS: Minimum age 18; Medical examination; Physician's request.
STAFF: Physicians 4 (pt); RNs 2 (ft); LPNs 8 (ft); Nurses' aides 17 (ft); Physical therapists 1 (pt); Recreational therapists 1 (ft); Dietitians 1 (pt); Podiatrists 1 (pt); Dentists 1 (pt).

Kenwood Healthcare Center Inc

6125 S Kenwood Ave, Chicago, IL 60637
(312) 752-6000
LICENSURE: Skilled care; Intermediate care.

BEDS: SNF 128; ICF 190.
CERTIFIED: Medicaid.

Lake Front Healthcare Center Inc

7618 N Sheridan Rd, Chicago, IL 60626
(312) 743-7711
LICENSURE: Skilled care.
BEDS: SNF 99.
ADMISSIONS REQUIREMENTS: Minimum age 40.
STAFF: Physicians 8 (ft); RNs 7 (ft), 2 (pt); LPNs 8 (ft), 3 (pt); Nurses' aides 40 (ft); Physical therapists 1 (ft); Reality therapists 1 (ft); Recreational therapists 1 (pt); Occupational therapists 1 (ft); Speech therapists 1 (pt); Activities coordinators 1 (ft); Dietitians 1 (ft); Ophthalmologists 2 (ft); Podiatrists 2 (ft); Audiologists 1 (pt).
LANGUAGES: Polish, Italian, Tagalog

Lake Shore Nursing Centre Ltd

7200 N Sheridan Rd, Chicago, IL 60626
(312) 973-7200, 973-7188 FAX
LICENSURE: Skilled care; Intermediate care; Alzheimer's care; Assisted living.
BEDS: Total 328; SNF 31.
CERTIFIED: Medicaid; Medicare; VA.
ADMISSIONS REQUIREMENTS: Minimum age 60; Must need geriatric facility.
STAFF: Physicians; RNs; LPNs; Nurses' aides; Physical therapists; Reality therapists; Recreational therapists; Occupational therapists; Speech therapists; Activities coordinators; Dietitians; Ophthalmologists; Podiatrists; Audiologists; Social workers.
LANGUAGES: Spanish, Yiddish, Russian, French, Polish, Tagalog, Japanese, Chinese
See ad on inside front cover

Lakeview Nursing & Geriatric Center Inc

735 W Diversey Pkwy, Chicago, IL 60614
(312) 348-4055
LICENSURE: Skilled care; Intermediate care; Alzheimer's care.
BEDS: SNF 63; ICF 117.
CERTIFIED: Medicaid; Medicare.
ADMISSIONS REQUIREMENTS: Minimum age 60; Medical examination; Physician's request.
STAFF: Physicians; RNs 12 (ft); LPNs 8 (ft); Nurses' aides 52 (ft); Physical therapists 2 (ft); Reality therapists; Recreational therapists 3 (ft); Occupational therapists; Speech therapists; Activities coordinators 1 (ft); Dietitians; Ophthalmologists; Podiatrists; Audiologists; Dentists.
LANGUAGES: Spanish, Tagalog

Lincoln Park Terrace Inc

2732 N Hampden Ct, Chicago, IL 60614
(312) 248-6000
LICENSURE: Skilled care; Intermediate care.
BEDS: SNF 90; ICF 19.
ADMISSIONS REQUIREMENTS: Minimum age 21.
STAFF: Physicians 6 (pt); RNs 5 (ft), 4 (pt); LPNs 8 (ft), 3 (pt); Nurses' aides 25 (ft), 3 (pt); Physical therapists 1 (pt); Occupational therapists 1 (pt); Speech therapists 1 (pt); Activities coordinators 2

(ft); Dietitians 1 (pt); Ophthalmologists 1 (pt); Podiatrists 1 (pt); Audiologists 1 (pt); Dentists 1 (pt).

Little Sisters of the Poor Center for the Aging
2325 N Lakewood Ave, Chicago, IL 60614
(312) 935-9600
LICENSURE: Skilled care; Intermediate care; Retirement.
BEDS: SNF 25; ICF 77.
CERTIFIED: Medicaid.
ADMISSIONS REQUIREMENTS: Minimum age 60.
STAFF: RNs 7 (ft), 5 (pt); LPNs 3 (ft), 3 (pt); Nurses' aides 18 (ft), 15 (pt); Physical therapists 1 (ft); Occupational therapists 1 (ft); Activities coordinators 1 (ft).

Margaret Manor
1121 N Orleans, Chicago, IL 60610
(312) 943-4300
LICENSURE: Intermediate care.
BEDS: ICF 135.
CERTIFIED: Medicaid.
ADMISSIONS REQUIREMENTS: Medical examination.
STAFF: RNs 1 (ft); LPNs 4 (ft); Nurses' aides 16 (ft); Activities coordinators 1 (ft).
LANGUAGES: Polish, Spanish

Margaret Manor—North Branch
940 W Cullom Ave, Chicago, IL 60613
(312) 525-9000
LICENSURE: Intermediate care.
BEDS: ICF 99.
CERTIFIED: Medicaid.
ADMISSIONS REQUIREMENTS: Minimum age 21; Medical examination; Physician's request.
STAFF: Physicians 4 (pt); RNs 3 (ft), 3 (pt); LPNs 1 (pt); Nurses' aides 11 (ft), 4 (pt); Occupational therapists 1 (pt); Activities coordinators 1 (ft); Dietitians 1 (pt); Ophthalmologists 1 (pt); Laboratory technicians 1 (pt).
LANGUAGES: Spanish, German

Maxwell Manor
4537 S Drexel Blvd, Chicago, IL 60653
(312) 268-8950, 268-9801 FAX
LICENSURE: Intermediate care.
BEDS: ICF 276.
CERTIFIED: Medicaid; Medicare.
ADMISSIONS REQUIREMENTS: Medical examination; Physician's request.
STAFF: Physicians 3 (pt); RNs 1 (ft); LPNs 25 (ft); Nurses' aides 56 (ft), 6 (pt); Physical therapists 1 (ft); Recreational therapists 1 (ft); Occupational therapists 1 (ft); Activities coordinators 6 (ft); Dietitians 15 (ft); Ophthalmologists 1 (pt); Podiatrists 1 (pt); Audiologists 1 (pt).

Mayfield Care Center
5905 W Washington, Chicago, IL 60644
(312) 261-7074
LICENSURE: Skilled care; Intermediate care.
BEDS: SNF 104; ICF 52.

The Methodist Home
1415 W Foster Ave, Chicago, IL 60640
(312) 769-5500 ext 221, 769-6287 FAX
LICENSURE: Skilled care; Intermediate care; Alzheimer's care; Sheltered care.
BEDS: SNF 23; ICF 83; Sheltered care 23.
CERTIFIED: Medicaid; Medicare.
ADMISSIONS REQUIREMENTS: Minimum age 60.
STAFF: Physicians 3 (pt); RNs 2 (ft), 2 (pt); LPNs 4 (ft), 1 (pt); Nurses' aides 30 (ft), 2 (pt); Physical therapists 2 (pt); Recreational therapists 2 (pt); Activities coordinators 1 (ft); Dietitians 1 (ft); Ophthalmologists 1 (pt); Podiatrists 1 (pt); Audiologists 1 (pt).
LANGUAGES: Spanish

Mid-America Convalescent Centers Inc
4920 N Kenmore Ave, Chicago, IL 60640
(312) 769-2700, 769-3226 FAX
LICENSURE: Skilled care.
BEDS: SNF 310.
CERTIFIED: Medicaid; Medicare.
ADMISSIONS REQUIREMENTS: Medical examination; Physician's request.
STAFF: RNs; LPNs; Nurses' aides; Activities coordinators.
LANGUAGES: Spanish, Chinese, Vietnamese

Monroe Pavilion Health Center Inc
1400 W Monroe St, Chicago, IL 60607
(312) 666-4090
LICENSURE: Intermediate care; Alzheimer's care.
BEDS: ICF 136.
CERTIFIED: Medicaid.
ADMISSIONS REQUIREMENTS: Minimum age 18; Medical examination; Physician's request.
STAFF: Physicians 3 (pt); RNs 1 (ft); LPNs 10 (ft), 1 (pt); Nurses' aides 23 (ft); Physical therapists 1 (ft), 2 (pt); Reality therapists 1 (pt); Recreational therapists 1 (pt); Occupational therapists 1 (pt); Speech therapists 1 (pt); Activities coordinators 1 (ft); Dietitians 1 (ft); Ophthalmologists 1 (pt); Podiatrists 1 (pt); Dentists 1 (pt); Psychiatrists 2 (pt).

Montgomery Place
5550 S Shore Dr, Chicago, IL 60637
(312) 753-4100, 752-0056 FAX
LICENSURE: Skilled care; Intermediate care.
BEDS: SNF 47; ICF 46.
ADMISSIONS REQUIREMENTS: Minimum age 60.
STAFF: Physicians; RNs; Physical therapists; Occupational therapists; Activities coordinators; Dietitians; Ophthalmologists; Podiatrists.
LANGUAGES: Greek

Northwest Home for the Aged
6300 N California Ave, Chicago, IL 60659
(312) 973-1900
LICENSURE: Skilled care.
BEDS: SNF 158.
CERTIFIED: Medicaid; Medicare.
ADMISSIONS REQUIREMENTS: Minimum age 65; Medical examination.

STAFF: Physicians 2 (pt); RNs 15 (ft), 10 (pt); LPNs 8 (ft); Nurses' aides 59 (ft), 1 (pt); Physical therapists 1 (pt); Recreational therapists 5 (ft); Occupational therapists 1 (pt); Speech therapists 1 (pt); Activities coordinators 1 (ft); Dietitians 1 (pt); Ophthalmologists 1 (pt); Podiatrists 1 (pt); Dentists 1 (pt).
LANGUAGES: Yiddish, Hebrew

Norwood Park Home
6016 N Nina Ave, Chicago, IL 60631
(312) 631-4856
LICENSURE: Intermediate care; Sheltered care; Adult day care.
BEDS: ICF 131; Sheltered care 200.
CERTIFIED: Medicaid.
ADMISSIONS REQUIREMENTS: Minimum age 65; Medical examination.
STAFF: Physicians 1 (pt); RNs 3 (ft), 6 (pt); LPNs 8 (ft), 2 (pt); Nurses' aides 35 (ft), 6 (pt); Recreational therapists 4 (ft), 2 (pt); Activities coordinators 1 (ft); Dietitians 1 (pt); Podiatrists.

Our Lady of the Resurrection—Extended Care Unit
5645 W Addison Ave, Chicago, IL 60634
(312) 282-7000, 794-7671 FAX
LICENSURE: Skilled care.
BEDS: SNF 46.
CERTIFIED: Medicare.
ADMISSIONS REQUIREMENTS: Medical examination; Physician's request.
STAFF: Physicians 1 (pt); RNs 10 (ft), 4 (pt); LPNs 4 (ft), 3 (pt); Nurses' aides 12 (ft), 4 (pt); Physical therapists 2 (ft); Recreational therapists 1 (pt); Occupational therapists 1 (pt); Speech therapists 1 (pt); Activities coordinators 1 (ft); Dietitians 1 (pt); Podiatrists 1 (pt); Audiologists 1 (pt).
LANGUAGES: Polish
See ads pages 163, 308

Park House Ltd
2320 S Lawndale, Chicago, IL 60623
(312) 522-0400, 522-1692 FAX
LICENSURE: Intermediate care.
BEDS: ICF 106.
CERTIFIED: Medicaid.
ADMISSIONS REQUIREMENTS: Minimum age 18; Medical examination.
STAFF: Physicians; RNs 1 (ft); LPNs 6 (ft); Nurses' aides 24 (ft); Physical therapists; Occupational therapists; Activities coordinators 1 (ft); Dietitians; Ophthalmologists; Podiatrists; Activities aides 2 (ft).

Peterson Park Health Care Center
6141 N Pulaski Rd, Chicago, IL 60646
(312) 478-2000
LICENSURE: Skilled care; Intermediate care.
BEDS: SNF 93; ICF 95.
CERTIFIED: Medicaid; VA.
ADMISSIONS REQUIREMENTS: Minimum age 45.
STAFF: Physicians 30 (pt); RNs 18 (ft); LPNs 9 (ft); Nurses' aides 49 (ft); Physical therapists 2 (ft); Reality therapists 8 (ft); Recreational therapists 5

(ft); Occupational therapists 2 (ft); Speech therapists 1 (pt); Activities coordinators 1 (ft); Dietitians 1 (ft); Ophthalmologists 1 (pt); Podiatrists 1 (pt); Audiologists 1 (pt).
LANGUAGES: Korean, Tagalog, Polish, Spanish, Yiddish, Farsi

Rainbow Beach Nursing Center Inc
7325 S Exchange, Chicago, IL 60649
(312) 731-7300
LICENSURE: Intermediate care.
BEDS: ICF 111.
CERTIFIED: Medicaid.
ADMISSIONS REQUIREMENTS: Minimum age 18.
STAFF: LPNs 9 (ft); Nurses' aides 30 (ft); Activities coordinators 1 (ft).

Sacred Heart Home
1550 S Albany, Chicago, IL 60623
(312) 277-6868
LICENSURE: Intermediate care.
BEDS: ICF 172.
CERTIFIED: Medicaid.

St Agnes Health Care Center
60 E 18th St, Chicago, IL 60616
(312) 922-2777
LICENSURE: Skilled care; Intermediate care.
BEDS: SNF 129; ICF 68.
CERTIFIED: Medicaid; Medicare.

St Joseph Home of Chicago Inc
2650 N Ridgeway Ave, Chicago, IL 60647-1199
(312) 235-8600, 235-2933 FAX
LICENSURE: Skilled care.
BEDS: SNF 173.
CERTIFIED: Medicaid; Medicare.
ADMISSIONS REQUIREMENTS: Minimum age 65; Medical examination.
STAFF: RNs 10 (ft), 7 (pt); LPNs 9 (ft), 4 (pt); Nurses' aides 67 (ft), 10 (pt); Activities coordinators 3 (ft), 2 (pt).
LANGUAGES: Polish

St Joseph Hospital & Health Care Center—Skilled Nursing Unit
2900 N Lake Shore Dr, Chicago, IL 60657
(312) 975-3317
LICENSURE: Skilled care.
BEDS: SNF 65.
CERTIFIED: Medicare.
ADMISSIONS REQUIREMENTS: Physician's order.
STAFF: Physicians 1 (ft); RNs 13 (ft), 21 (pt); LPNs 11 (ft), 16 (pt); Nurses' aides 30 (ft); Recreational therapists 1 (ft); Dietitians 1 (ft); Social workers 1 (ft).
See ad page 11

St Martha Manor
4621 N Racine Ave, Chicago, IL 60640
(312) 784-2300
LICENSURE: Skilled care; Intermediate care.
BEDS: SNF 57; ICF 75.

CERTIFIED: Medicaid.
ADMISSIONS REQUIREMENTS: Minimum age 18.
STAFF: Physicians 5 (pt); RNs 17 (ft); LPNs 4 (ft); Nurses' aides 20 (ft); Physical therapists 3 (pt); Reality therapists 1 (ft); Recreational therapists 1 (ft); Occupational therapists 1 (ft); Speech therapists 1 (ft), 1 (pt); Activities coordinators 5 (ft); Dietitians 1 (pt); Podiatrists 1 (pt); Dentists 1 (pt).

St Paul's House & Health Care Center
3831 N Mozart St, Chicago, IL 60618
(312) 478-4222, 478-4516 FAX
LICENSURE: Skilled care; Intermediate care.
BEDS: SNF 90; ICF 51.
CERTIFIED: Medicaid; Medicare.
ADMISSIONS REQUIREMENTS: Minimum age 18.
STAFF: Physicians; RNs; LPNs; Nurses' aides; Physical therapists; Reality therapists; Recreational therapists; Occupational therapists; Speech therapists; Activities coordinators; Dietitians; Ophthalmologists; Podiatrists; Audiologists.
LANGUAGES: German
See ad page 9

Selfhelp Home for the Aged
908 W Argyle St, Chicago, IL 60640
(312) 271-0300
LICENSURE: Intermediate care.
BEDS: ICF 65.
CERTIFIED: Medicaid.
ADMISSIONS REQUIREMENTS: Minimum age 65; Medical examination; Physician's request.
STAFF: RNs 1 (ft); LPNs 2 (ft), 5 (pt); Nurses' aides 17 (ft), 6 (pt); Physical therapists 1 (pt); Recreational therapists 1 (pt); Occupational therapists 1 (pt).
LANGUAGES: German

Sherwin Manor Nursing Center
7350 N Sheridan Rd, Chicago, IL 60626
(312) 274-1000
LICENSURE: Skilled care.
BEDS: SNF 219.
CERTIFIED: Medicaid; Medicare.
See ad page 201

Washington & Jane Smith Home
2340 W 113th Pl, Chicago, IL 60643
(312) 779-8010, 779-8648 FAX
LICENSURE: Skilled care; Sheltered care.
BEDS: SNF 44.
CERTIFIED: Medicaid.
ADMISSIONS REQUIREMENTS: Minimum age 62; Medical examination.
STAFF: Physicians 2 (pt); RNs 6 (ft), 1 (pt); LPNs 3 (ft), 1 (pt); Nurses' aides 17 (ft), 2 (pt); Physical therapists 1 (ft); Activities coordinators 1 (ft); Dietitians 1 (pt); Podiatrists 1 (pt); Audiologists 1 (pt).

Society for Danish Old People's Home
5656 N Newcastle Ave, Chicago, IL 60631
(312) 775-7383
LICENSURE: Skilled care; Sheltered care; Retirement.

BEDS: SNF 17; Sheltered care 57.
ADMISSIONS REQUIREMENTS: Minimum age 62; Medical examination.
LANGUAGES: Danish

Somerset House
5009 N Sheridan, Chicago, IL 60640
(312) 561-0700, 275-4212 FAX
LICENSURE: Intermediate care; ICF/Developmentally disabled.
BEDS: ICF 375; ICF/DD 75.
CERTIFIED: Medicaid.
ADMISSIONS REQUIREMENTS: Minimum age 18.
STAFF: Physicians 9 (ft); RNs 3 (ft); LPNs 20 (ft), 2 (pt); Nurses' aides 56 (ft); Physical therapists 1 (ft); Recreational therapists 1 (ft); Occupational therapists 1 (ft); Speech therapists 1 (ft); Activities coordinators 1 (ft); Dietitians 1 (ft); Ophthalmologists 1 (ft); Podiatrists 1 (ft); Audiologists 1 (ft).

The Sovereign Home
6159 N Kenmore Ave, Chicago, IL 60660
(312) 761-9050
LICENSURE: Intermediate care.
BEDS: ICF 55.
CERTIFIED: Medicaid.

Warren Park Nursing Pavilion
6700 N Damen Ave, Chicago, IL 60645
(312) 465-5000, 743-5983 FAX
LICENSURE: Skilled care; Intermediate care.
BEDS: SNF 51; ICF 76.
CERTIFIED: Medicaid.
ADMISSIONS REQUIREMENTS: Minimum age 60; Physician's request; Recommendation from Dept on Aging.
STAFF: Physicians 8 (ft); RNs 7 (ft), 4 (pt); LPNs 6 (ft), 3 (pt); Nurses' aides 26 (ft); Physical therapists 2 (ft); Reality therapists 4 (ft); Recreational therapists 4 (ft), 1 (pt); Occupational therapists 2 (ft); Speech therapists 1 (ft); Activities coordinators 1 (ft); Dietitians 1 (ft); Ophthalmologists 2 (ft); Podiatrists 1 (ft); Audiologists 1 (ft).
LANGUAGES: Russian, Spanish

Waterfront Terrace
7750 S Shore Dr, Chicago, IL 60649
(312) 731-4200, 731-9048 FAX
LICENSURE: Intermediate care; Alzheimer's care.
BEDS: ICF 110; Alzheimer's 8.
CERTIFIED: Medicaid; VA.
ADMISSIONS REQUIREMENTS: Minimum age 55; Physician's request.
STAFF: Physicians 4 (ft), 1 (pt); RNs 1 (ft), 1 (pt); LPNs 8 (ft), 5 (pt); Nurses' aides 20 (ft), 10 (pt); Physical therapists 1 (pt); Occupational therapists 1 (pt); Speech therapists 1 (pt); Activities coordinators 1 (ft); Dietitians 1 (pt); Ophthalmologists 3 (pt); Podiatrists 3 (pt); Audiologists 2 (pt).
LANGUAGES: Spanish

Wedgewood Nursing Pavilion Ltd
8001 S Western Ave, Chicago, IL 60620
(312) 436-6600

LICENSURE: Skilled care; Intermediate care.
BEDS: SNF 220; ICF 108.
CERTIFIED: Medicaid.

Wellington Plaza Nursing & Therapy Center
504 W Wellington St, Chicago, IL 60657
(312) 281-6200
LICENSURE: Skilled care; Intermediate care; Alzheimer's care.
BEDS: SNF 34; ICF 62.
CERTIFIED: Medicare.
ADMISSIONS REQUIREMENTS: Minimum age 50; Medical examination; Physician's request.
STAFF: Physicians 4 (pt); RNs 7 (ft), 14 (pt); LPNs 3 (ft), 4 (pt); Nurses' aides 30 (ft), 5 (pt); Physical therapists 1 (ft); Reality therapists 3 (ft); Recreational therapists 1 (ft); Occupational therapists 1 (pt); Speech therapists 1 (pt); Activities coordinators 1 (ft); Dietitians 1 (ft); Ophthalmologists 1 (pt); Podiatrists 1 (pt); Dentists 1 (pt); Social workers 1 (pt).
LANGUAGES: Hebrew, Yiddish, Spanish, Tagalog, Portuguese, German, Estonian

The Westwood Manor Inc
2444 W Touhy Ave, Chicago, IL 60645
(312) 274-7705
LICENSURE: Skilled care; Intermediate care.
BEDS: SNF 26; ICF 89.
CERTIFIED: Medicaid.
ADMISSIONS REQUIREMENTS: Minimum age 18.

The Whitehall Convalescent and Nursing Home
1901 N Lincoln Park W, Chicago, IL 60614
(312) 943-2846, 787-2559 FAX
LICENSURE: Skilled care.
BEDS: SNF 76.
ADMISSIONS REQUIREMENTS: Minimum age 60.
STAFF: Physicians 1 (pt); RNs 6 (ft), 1 (pt); LPNs 7 (ft), 3 (pt); Nurses' aides 32 (ft), 14 (pt); Physical therapists 1 (pt); Occupational therapists 1 (pt); Speech therapists 1 (pt); Activities coordinators 2 (ft); Dietitians 1 (pt); Ophthalmologists 1 (pt); Podiatrists 1 (pt); Social workers 1 (pt) (consultant).
LANGUAGES: German, Spanish

Wilson Care Inc
4544 N Hazel St, Chicago, IL 60640
(312) 561-7241
LICENSURE: Intermediate care.
BEDS: ICF 198.
CERTIFIED: Medicaid.

Wincrest Nursing Center
6326 N Winthrop Ave, Chicago, IL 60660
(312) 338-7800
LICENSURE: Intermediate care; Retirement.
BEDS: ICF 82.
CERTIFIED: Medicaid.
ADMISSIONS REQUIREMENTS: Minimum age 50; Medical examination; Physician's request.
STAFF: RNs 1 (ft); LPNs 5 (ft), 6 (pt); Nurses' aides 11

(ft), 6 (pt); Physical therapists 1 (ft); Recreational therapists 1 (ft); Occupational therapists 1 (ft); Dietitians.

Winston Manor Convalescent & Nursing Home
2155 W Pierce Ave, Chicago, IL 60622
(312) 252-2066
LICENSURE: Intermediate care.
BEDS: ICF 180.

Woodbridge Nursing Pavilion
2242 N Kedzie Ave, Chicago, IL 60647
(312) 486-7700
LICENSURE: Skilled care; Alzheimer's care.
BEDS: SNF 222.
CERTIFIED: Medicaid.
STAFF: Physicians 8 (pt); RNs 9 (ft); LPNs 14 (ft); Nurses' aides 44 (ft); Physical therapists 2 (ft), 1 (pt); Reality therapists 1 (pt); Occupational therapists 1 (ft), 1 (pt); Speech therapists 1 (ft), 1 (pt); Activities coordinators 5 (ft); Dietitians 1 (pt); Ophthalmologists 1 (pt); Podiatrists 2 (pt); Dentists 1 (pt).
LANGUAGES: Spanish

Chicago Heights

Prairie Manor Health Care Center
345 Dixie Hwy, Chicago Heights, IL 60411
(708) 754-7601, 754-8904 FAX
LICENSURE: Skilled care; Intermediate care.
BEDS: SNF 51; ICF 97.
CERTIFIED: Medicare.
ADMISSIONS REQUIREMENTS: Minimum age 18.
STAFF: Physicians; RNs 6 (ft), 2 (pt); LPNs 10 (ft), 4 (pt); Nurses' aides 40 (ft), 16 (pt); Physical therapists 2 (ft); Reality therapists 1 (ft); Recreational therapists 1 (ft); Occupational therapists 1 (ft); Speech therapists 1 (ft); Activities coordinators 1 (ft); Dietitians 1 (pt); Ophthalmologists; Podiatrists 1 (pt); Audiologists.
LANGUAGES: Spanish, Italian

Riviera Manor Inc
490 W 16th Pl, Chicago Heights, IL 60411
(708) 481-4444, 481-4606 FAX
LICENSURE: Skilled care; Intermediate care; Alzheimer's care.
BEDS: SNF 95; ICF 95.
CERTIFIED: Medicaid; Medicare; VA.
ADMISSIONS REQUIREMENTS: Minimum age 21 (prefer over 50); Medical examination; Physician's request.
STAFF: Physicians; RNs; LPNs; Nurses' aides; Physical therapists; Recreational therapists; Occupational therapists; Speech therapists; Activities coordinators; Dietitians; Ophthalmologists; Podiatrists; Psychiatrists.
LANGUAGES: Spanish

Thornton Heights Terrace Ltd
160 W 10th St, Chicago Heights, IL 60411
(708) 754-2220
LICENSURE: Intermediate care.
BEDS: ICF 222.
CERTIFIED: Medicaid.
ADMISSIONS REQUIREMENTS: Minimum age 18.

Chicago Ridge

Chicago Ridge Nursing Center
10602 Southwest Hwy, Chicago Ridge, IL 60415
(708) 448-1540, 448-0118 FAX
LICENSURE: Skilled care; Intermediate care; Alzheimer's care; Hospice; Respite care.
BEDS: Total 231.
CERTIFIED: Medicaid; Medicare; VA.
ADMISSIONS REQUIREMENTS: Minimum age per state regulations; "Public Aid Pending" acceptable.
STAFF: Physicians 5 (pt); RNs 8 (ft); LPNs 21 (ft); Nurses' aides 53 (ft); Physical therapists 1 (pt); Reality therapists; Recreational therapists 1 (pt); Occupational therapists 1 (pt); Speech therapists 1 (pt); Activities coordinators 6 (ft); Dietitians 1 (pt); Ophthalmologists 1 (pt); Podiatrists 1 (pt); Audiologists 1 (pt); Dentists 1 (pt); Social services workers.

Lexington Health Care Center of Chicago Ridge
10300 Southwest Hwy, Chicago Ridge, IL 60415
(708) 425-1100, 425-0779 FAX
LICENSURE: Skilled care; Intermediate care; Alzheimer's care.
BEDS: Total 400.
CERTIFIED: Medicaid; Medicare.

Cicero

Alden Nursing Center—Town Manor Rehabilitation & Health Care Center
6120 W Ogden, Cicero, IL 60650
(708) 863-0500
LICENSURE: Skilled care; Intermediate care; Alzheimer's care.
BEDS: Total 249.
ADMISSIONS REQUIREMENTS: Minimum age 18; Medical examination.

Westshire Retirement & Healthcare Centre
5825 W Cermak Rd, Cicero, IL 60650
(708) 656-9120, 656-9128 FAX
LICENSURE: Skilled care; Intermediate care; Alzheimer's care; Hospice.
BEDS: SNF 76; ICF 409.
CERTIFIED: Medicaid.
ADMISSIONS REQUIREMENTS: Minimum age 18; Medical examination.

STAFF: Physicians 68 (pt); RNs 9 (ft); LPNs 35 (ft); Nurses' aides 78 (ft); Physical therapists 1 (pt); Occupational therapists 1 (pt); Speech therapists 1 (pt); Activities coordinators 9 (ft); Dietitians 1 (ft); Podiatrists 1 (pt); Audiologists 1 (pt).
LANGUAGES: Spanish, Polish, Lithuanian, Czech, Farsi
See ad on inside back cover

Crestwood

Crestwood Heights Nursing Centre
14255 S Cicero Ave, Crestwood, IL 60445
(708) 371-0400, 371-5871 FAX
LICENSURE: Skilled care; Intermediate care; Alzheimer's care.
BEDS: SNF 108; ICF 216.
CERTIFIED: Medicaid; VA; Private pay.
ADMISSIONS REQUIREMENTS: Minimum age 60.
STAFF: RNs 12 (ft), 6 (pt); LPNs 9 (ft), 4 (pt); Nurses' aides 61 (ft), 10 (pt); Physical therapists 2 (ft); Recreational therapists 1 (ft); Occupational therapists 1 (ft); Speech therapists 1 (ft); Activities coordinators 1 (ft); Dietitians 2 (ft) (consultant); Ophthalmologists 2 (ft); Podiatrists 2 (ft); Audiologists 1 (ft); Activity aides 24; Rehabilitation aides 18; Rehabilitation coordinators 2.
LANGUAGES: Spanish, Polish
See ad on inside back cover

Crete

St James Manor
1251 E Richton Rd, Crete, IL 60417
(708) 672-6700, 672-4939 FAX
LICENSURE: Skilled care.
BEDS: SNF 110.
CERTIFIED: Medicaid; Medicare; VA.
ADMISSIONS REQUIREMENTS: Minimum age 21; Medical examination.
STAFF: Physicians (contracted); RNs 4 (ft), 6 (pt); LPNs 6 (ft), 2 (pt); Nurses' aides 25 (ft), 8 (pt); Physical therapists (contracted); Occupational therapists (contracted); Speech therapists (contracted); Activities coordinators 1 (ft), 2 (pt); Dietitians (contracted); Ophthalmologists (contracted); Podiatrists (contracted); Audiologists (contracted).

Crystal Lake

Canterbury Care Center
1000 E Brighton Ln, Crystal Lake, IL 60012
(815) 477-6400
LICENSURE: Skilled care.
BEDS: SNF 99.
CERTIFIED: Medicare.
ADMISSIONS REQUIREMENTS: Minimum age 18; Medical examination; Physician's request.

STAFF: RNs; LPNs; Nurses' aides; Physical therapists; Occupational therapists; Speech therapists; Activities coordinators; Dietitians; Ophthalmologists; Podiatrists; Audiologists.
LANGUAGES: Spanish

Crystal Pines Health Care Center
335 N Illinois Ave, Crystal Lake, IL 60014
(815) 459-7791
LICENSURE: Skilled care.
BEDS: SNF 83.
CERTIFIED: Medicare.
ADMISSIONS REQUIREMENTS: Physician's request.
STAFF: RNs; LPNs; Nurses' aides; Activities coordinators.

Fair Oaks Health Care Center
471 Terra Cotta Ave, Crystal Lake, IL 60014
(815) 455-0550, 455-0608 FAX
LICENSURE: Skilled care; Alzheimer's care.
BEDS: SNF 46.
ADMISSIONS REQUIREMENTS: Minimum age 18; Medical examination; Physician's request.
STAFF: Physicians 1 (pt) (contracted); RNs 4 (ft), 7 (pt); Nurses' aides 13 (ft), 4 (pt); Physical therapists 1 (pt) (contracted); Recreational therapists 1 (pt) (contracted); Speech therapists 1 (pt) (contracted); Activities coordinators 1 (ft); Dietitians 1 (ft); Podiatrists 1 (pt) (contracted).
LANGUAGES: Spanish

De Kalb

De Kalb County Nursing Home
2331 Sycamore Rd, De Kalb, IL 60115
(815) 758-2477, 758-3176 FAX
LICENSURE: Skilled care.
BEDS: SNF 194.
CERTIFIED: Medicaid; Medicare.
ADMISSIONS REQUIREMENTS: Minimum age 18; Medical examination; Physician's request.
STAFF: RNs; LPNs; Nurses' aides; Activities coordinators.

Oak Crest—De Kalb Area Retirement Center
2944 Greenwood Acres Dr, De Kalb, IL 60115
(815) 756-8461
LICENSURE: Intermediate care; Sheltered care; Retirement.
BEDS: ICF 60; Sheltered care 49.
ADMISSIONS REQUIREMENTS: Minimum age 62; Medical examination.
STAFF: RNs 1 (ft), 8 (pt); Nurses' aides 13 (ft), 13 (pt); Recreational therapists 2 (ft); Activities coordinators 1 (ft).

Pine Acres Care Center
1212 S 2nd St, De Kalb, IL 60115
(815) 758-8151, 758-6832 FAX
LICENSURE: Skilled care; Intermediate care; Alzheimer's care.
BEDS: SNF 83; ICF 20; Alzheimer's 16.
CERTIFIED: Medicaid; Medicare.

ADMISSIONS REQUIREMENTS: Medical examination.
STAFF: RNs 2 (ft), 12 (pt); LPNs 8 (ft), 4 (pt); Nurses' aides 20 (ft), 20 (pt); Physical therapists 1 (pt); Activities coordinators 1 (ft).

Deerfield

The Whitehall North
300 Waukegan Rd, Deerfield, IL 60015
(708) 945-4600, 945-6492 FAX
LICENSURE: Skilled care; Alzheimer's care; Sheltered care; Respite care.
BEDS: SNF 180.
CERTIFIED: Medicare.
STAFF: Physicians 2 (pt); RNs 26 (ft); LPNs 3 (ft); Nurses' aides 70 (ft); Physical therapists 1 (ft); Occupational therapists 1 (pt); Speech therapists 1 (pt); Activities coordinators 3 (ft), 1 (pt); Dietitians 1 (pt); Ophthalmologists 1 (pt); Podiatrists 1 (pt); Audiologists 1 (pt).

Des Plaines

Ballard Nursing Center Inc
9300 Ballard Rd, Des Plaines, IL 60016
(708) 294-2300, 229-4012 FAX
LICENSURE: Skilled care; Intermediate care; Alzheimer's care.
BEDS: Total 231.
CERTIFIED: Medicaid; Medicare; VA.
ADMISSIONS REQUIREMENTS: Must be older adult.
STAFF: Physicians; RNs; LPNs; Nurses' aides; Physical therapists; Reality therapists; Recreational therapists; Occupational therapists; Speech therapists; Activities coordinators; Dietitians; Ophthalmologists (consultant); Podiatrists (consultant); Audiologists (consultant).
See ad page 218

Holy Family Health Center
2380 Dempster St, Des Plaines, IL 60016
(708) 296-3335, 296-2027 FAX
LICENSURE: Skilled care; Intermediate care; Alzheimer's care.
BEDS: SNF 106; ICF 232; Alzheimer's 53.
CERTIFIED: Medicaid; Medicare.
STAFF: RNs; LPNs; Nurses' aides; Physical therapists; Recreational therapists; Occupational therapists; Speech therapists; Activities coordinators; Dietitians.

Lee Manor Health Care Residence
1301 Lee St, Des Plaines, IL 60018
(708) 827-9450, 827-5796 FAX
LICENSURE: Skilled care.
BEDS: SNF 282.
CERTIFIED: Medicaid; Medicare.
ADMISSIONS REQUIREMENTS: Minimum age 21; Medical examination.

✔ In order to support future editions of this publication would you please mention *Elder Services* each time you contact any advertiser, facility, or service.

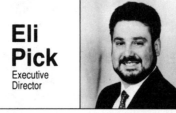
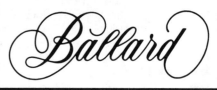
STAFF: RNs 12 (ft); LPNs 10 (ft); Nurses' aides 52 (ft); Recreational therapists 7 (ft); Activities coordinators 1 (ft); Dietitians 1 (ft).
LANGUAGES: Polish, Spanish

Nazarethville
300 N River Rd, Des Plaines, IL 60016
(708) 297-5900
LICENSURE: Intermediate care; Sheltered care.
BEDS: ICF 68; Sheltered care 15.
CERTIFIED: Medicaid.
ADMISSIONS REQUIREMENTS: Minimum age 62; Medical examination; Physician's request.
STAFF: Physicians 2 (pt); RNs 7 (ft); LPNs 5 (pt); Nurses' aides 21 (ft); Physical therapists 1 (ft); Occupational therapists 1 (ft); Speech therapists 1 (pt); Activities coordinators 1 (ft); Dietitians 1 (ft); Ophthalmologists 1 (pt); Podiatrists 1 (pt).
LANGUAGES: Polish

Oakton Pavilion Healthcare Facility Inc
1660 Oakton Pl, Des Plaines, IL 60018
(708) 299-5588, 298-6017 FAX
LICENSURE: Skilled care; Alzheimer's care; Retirement.
BEDS: SNF 294; Retirement 102.
CERTIFIED: Medicaid; Medicare.
ADMISSIONS REQUIREMENTS: Minimum age 18.
STAFF: Physicians 4 (ft), 35 (pt); RNs 37 (ft), 3 (pt); LPNs 6 (ft); Nurses' aides 145 (ft); Physical therapists 1 (pt); Recreational therapists 12 (ft); Occupational therapists 1 (pt); Speech therapists 1

(pt); Activities coordinators 1 (ft); Dietitians 1 (ft); Ophthalmologists 1 (pt); Podiatrists 1 (pt); Audiologists 1 (pt).
LANGUAGES: German, Polish

Dolton

Countryside Healthcare Center
1635 E 154th St, Dolton, IL 60419
(708) 841-9550
LICENSURE: Skilled care; Intermediate care.
BEDS: SNF 100; ICF 97.
CERTIFIED: Medicaid.

Dolton Healthcare Center Inc
14325 S Blackstone, Dolton, IL 60419
(708) 849-5000
LICENSURE: Skilled care; Intermediate care.
BEDS: SNF 25; ICF 42.
CERTIFIED: Medicaid.
ADMISSIONS REQUIREMENTS: Medical examination.
STAFF: Physicians 8 (pt); RNs 3 (ft), 4 (pt); LPNs 2 (ft), 1 (pt); Nurses' aides 12 (ft), 9 (pt); Physical therapists 1 (ft), 1 (pt); Reality therapists 1 (ft), 1 (pt); Recreational therapists 1 (ft), 1 (pt); Occupational therapists 1 (ft), 1 (pt); Activities coordinators 1 (ft), 1 (pt); Dietitians 1 (pt); Ophthalmologists 1 (pt); Dentists 1 (pt).

One of the best alternatives to a nursing home

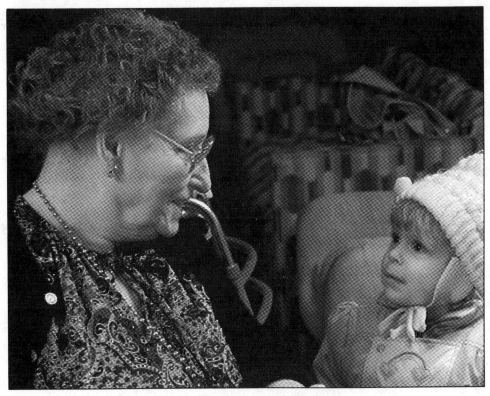

Fairview Baptist Home offers sheltered care, which is a level of care designed for those who need help but are not helpless. Some of our residents had been turned down by retirement centers yet were not ready for a nursing home. In fact many of the elderly who receive assistance with the little things of life never have need of a skilled nursing facility.

If you would like more information about Fairview Baptist Home for yourself or someone you love call:

(708) 852-4350

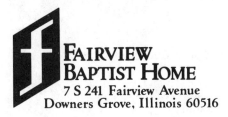

FAIRVIEW BAPTIST HOME
7 S 241 Fairview Avenue
Downers Grove, Illinois 60516

A not for profit corporation

Downers Grove

Fairview Baptist Home
7 S 241 Fairview Ave, Downers Grove, IL 60516
(708) 852-0426, 852-0761 FAX
LICENSURE: Skilled care; Intermediate care.
BEDS: SNF 40; ICF 66.
ADMISSIONS REQUIREMENTS: Minimum age 60; Medical examination; Financial information.
STAFF: Physicians 33 (pt); RNs 10 (ft), 10 (pt); LPNs 4 (ft), 2 (pt); Physical therapists 1 (ft); Recreational therapists 2 (ft), 1 (pt); Occupational therapists 1 (ft); Speech therapists 1 (ft); Activities coordinators 1 (ft); Dietitians 1 (pt); Ophthalmologists 1 (pt); Podiatrists 1 (pt); Audiologists 1 (pt).
See ads pages 136, 219

Rest Haven West Skilled Nursing Center
3450 Saratoga Ave, Downers Grove, IL 60515
(708) 969-2900, 241-0615 FAX
LICENSURE: Skilled care; Intermediate care; Alzheimer's care.
BEDS: SNF 145.
CERTIFIED: Medicaid; Medicare.
STAFF: Physicians 6 (pt); RNs 9 (ft), 2 (pt); LPNs 6 (ft), 6 (pt); Nurses' aides 42 (ft), 26 (pt); Physical therapists 2 (pt); Occupational therapists 1 (pt); Speech therapists 1 (pt); Activities coordinators 3 (ft), 3 (pt); Dietitians 1 (ft); Ophthalmologists 1 (pt); Podiatrists 1 (pt); Audiologists 1 (pt); Dentists 1 (pt).
LANGUAGES: Polish, Spanish, German
See ad on page i

Dwight

Fernwood Health Care Center
300 E Mazon Ave, Dwight, IL 60420
(815) 584-1240
LICENSURE: Skilled care.
BEDS: SNF 92.
CERTIFIED: Medicaid; Medicare.
ADMISSIONS REQUIREMENTS: Medical examination.
STAFF: RNs 2 (ft), 1 (pt); LPNs 6 (ft), 1 (pt); Nurses' aides 15 (ft), 8 (pt); Physical therapists 1 (pt); Occupational therapists 1 (pt); Activities coordinators 1 (ft).

Elgin

Americana Healthcare Center of Elgin
180 S State St, Elgin, IL 60123
(708) 742-3310, 742-8112 FAX
LICENSURE: Skilled care; Alzheimer's care.
BEDS: SNF 51; Alzheimer's 21.
CERTIFIED: Medicare.
ADMISSIONS REQUIREMENTS: Medical examination; Physician's orders.
See ad page 200

Apostolic Christian Resthaven
2750 W Highland Ave, Elgin, IL 60123
(708) 741-4543
LICENSURE: Skilled care; Retirement.
BEDS: SNF 50.
CERTIFIED: Medicaid.
ADMISSIONS REQUIREMENTS: Minimum age 18; Medical examination.
STAFF: RNs 6 (ft), 3 (pt); LPNs 1 (ft); Nurses' aides 18 (ft), 8 (pt); Activities coordinators 1 (ft).
LANGUAGES: Spanish

Ashwood Health Care Center
134 N McLean Blvd, Elgin, IL 60123
(708) 742-8822
LICENSURE: Skilled care; Intermediate care.
BEDS: SNF 50; ICF 56.

Heritage Manor of Elgin
355 Raymond St, Elgin, IL 60120
(708) 697-6636
LICENSURE: Skilled care.
BEDS: SNF 90.
CERTIFIED: Medicaid; Medicare.
ADMISSIONS REQUIREMENTS: Minimum age 21; Medical examination.
STAFF: Physical therapists 1 (pt); Recreational therapists 1 (pt); Occupational therapists 1 (pt); Speech therapists 1 (pt); Activities coordinators 1 (ft), 1 (pt); Dietitians 1 (pt); Ophthalmologists 1 (pt); Podiatrists 1 (pt); Audiologists 1 (pt).
LANGUAGES: Spanish

Metropolitan Nursing Center of Elgin
50 N Jane Dr, Elgin, IL 60123
(708) 697-3750, 697-5385 FAX
LICENSURE: Skilled care; Intermediate care; Alzheimer's care; Hospice; Respite care.
BEDS: Total 203.
CERTIFIED: Medicaid; Medicare; VA.
ADMISSIONS REQUIREMENTS: Minimum age per state regulations; "Public Aid Pending" acceptable.
STAFF: Physicians 2 (pt); RNs 10 (ft), 9 (pt); LPNs 8 (ft), 1 (pt); Nurses' aides 45 (ft), 5 (pt); Physical therapists 1 (pt); Recreational therapists 1 (ft); Occupational therapists 1 (pt); Speech therapists 1 (pt); Activities coordinators 3 (ft), 1 (pt); Dietitians 1 (pt); Ophthalmologists 1 (pt); Podiatrists 1 (pt); Audiologists 1 (pt); Dentists 1 (pt); Social services workers.
LANGUAGES: Spanish

Sherman West Court
1950 Larkin Ave, Elgin, IL 60123
(708) 742-7070, 742-7248 FAX
LICENSURE: Skilled care; Sheltered care.
BEDS: SNF 92; Sheltered care 28.
CERTIFIED: Medicare.
ADMISSIONS REQUIREMENTS: Medical examination; Physician's request.

STAFF: Physicians 23 (pt); RNs 10 (ft), 12 (pt); LPNs 3 (ft), 4 (pt); Nurses' aides 26 (ft), 4 (pt); Physical therapists 4 (ft), 1 (pt); Occupational therapists 2 (ft); Speech therapists 1 (ft); Activities coordinators 2 (ft); Dietitians 1 (ft); Podiatrists 4 (pt).
LANGUAGES: Spanish, Tagalog

Elk Grove Village

Americana Healthcare Center of Elk Grove
1920 Nerge Rd, Elk Grove Village, IL 60007
(708) 307-0550, 307-0735 FAX
LICENSURE: Skilled care; Alzheimer's care.
BEDS: SNF 90; ICF 30.
CERTIFIED: Medicaid; Medicare.
ADMISSIONS REQUIREMENTS: Medical examination; Physician's orders.
See ad page 200

Elmhurst

Elmhurst Extended Care Center Inc
200 E Lake St, Elmhurst, IL 60126
(708) 834-4337
LICENSURE: Skilled care; Alzheimer's care.
BEDS: SNF 112.
CERTIFIED: Medicare.
ADMISSIONS REQUIREMENTS: Minimum age 18.
STAFF: Physicians 4 (pt); RNs 9 (ft), 4 (pt); LPNs 5 (ft), 4 (pt); Nurses' aides 28 (ft), 29 (pt); Physical therapists 1 (pt); Recreational therapists 1 (ft); Occupational therapists 1 (pt); Speech therapists 1 (pt); Activities coordinators 2 (pt); Dietitians 1 (ft); Ophthalmologists 1 (pt); Podiatrists 1 (pt); Dentists 1 (pt).

York Convalescent Center
127 W Diversey, Elmhurst, IL 60126
(708) 530-5225, 530-7775 FAX
LICENSURE: Skilled care; Alzheimer's care.
BEDS: SNF 125; ICF 63.
CERTIFIED: Medicaid; Medicare; VA.
ADMISSIONS REQUIREMENTS: No ventilators.
STAFF: RNs 13 (ft); LPNs 13 (ft); Nurses' aides 56 (ft); Physical therapists 1 (pt); Occupational therapists 1 (pt); Activities coordinators 6 (ft); Dietitians 1 (ft); Ophthalmologists 1 (pt); Podiatrists 1 (pt).
LANGUAGES: Polish, Indian, Tagalog, Spanish

Elmwood Park

Royal Elm Convalescent & Geriatric Center Inc
7733 W Grand Ave, Elmwood Park, IL 60635
(708) 452-9200, 452-7214 FAX
LICENSURE: Skilled care; Intermediate care; Alzheimer's care; Respite care; Hospice.

BEDS: Total 245.
CERTIFIED: Medicaid; Medicare; IDPH Exceptional Care.
ADMISSIONS REQUIREMENTS: Minimum age per state regulations; "Public Aid Pending" acceptable.
STAFF: Physicians 24 (pt); RNs 10 (ft), 6 (pt); LPNs 17 (ft), 10 (pt); Nurses' aides 68 (ft), 2 (pt); Physical therapists 1 (pt); Reality therapists; Recreational therapists 1 (pt); Occupational therapists 1 (pt); Speech therapists 1 (pt); Activities coordinators 5 (ft); Dietitians 1 (pt); Ophthalmologists 1 (pt); Podiatrists 1 (pt); Audiologists 1 (pt); Social services workers; Dentists.
LANGUAGES: Italian, Lithuanian, Polish, Spanish

Evanston

Albany House
901 Maple Ave, Evanston, IL 60202
(708) 475-4000
LICENSURE: Intermediate care.
BEDS: ICF 437.
CERTIFIED: Medicaid.

Dobson Plaza
120 Dodge Ave, Evanston, IL 60202
(708) 869-7744, 869-2931 FAX
LICENSURE: Skilled care; Intermediate care; Alzheimer's care; Sheltered care.
BEDS: Total 93.
CERTIFIED: Medicaid; Medicare.
ADMISSIONS REQUIREMENTS: Minimum age 65.
STAFF: RNs 10 (ft), 8 (pt); LPNs 4 (ft); Nurses' aides 20 (ft), 5 (pt); Physical therapists; Recreational therapists (consultant); Occupational therapists (consultant); Speech therapists (consultant); Activities coordinators 1 (ft); Dietitians 1 (ft) (consultant); Ophthalmologists (consultant); Podiatrists (consultant); Audiologists (consultant).
LANGUAGES: Yiddish

Greenwood Care Center
1406 Chicago Ave, Evanston, IL 60202
(708) 328-6503
LICENSURE: Intermediate care.
BEDS: ICF 145.
CERTIFIED: Medicaid.

Kensington Health Care Center
820 Foster Ave, Evanston, IL 60201
(708) 869-0142
LICENSURE: Skilled care; Intermediate care.
BEDS: SNF 130; ICF 170.

The King Home
1555 Oak Ave, Evanston, IL 60201
(708) 864-5460
LICENSURE: Intermediate care.
BEDS: ICF 20.

ADMISSIONS REQUIREMENTS: Minimum age 60; Males only.

STAFF: Physicians 1 (pt); RNs 5 (ft), 2 (pt); LPNs 3 (ft), 2 (pt); Nurses' aides 6 (ft), 2 (pt); Physical therapists 1 (pt); Recreational therapists 1 (pt); Occupational therapists 1 (pt); Activities coordinators 1 (ft); Dietitians 1 (pt); Ophthalmologists 1 (pt); Podiatrists 1 (pt).

McGaw Health Care Center

3200 Grant St, Evanston, IL 60201
(708) 570-3422
LICENSURE: Skilled care; Intermediate care; Alzheimer's care.
BEDS: Total 210.
CERTIFIED: Medicare.
ADMISSIONS REQUIREMENTS: Minimum age 65.
STAFF: Physicians 1 (ft), 3 (pt) (and consultants); RNs 25 (ft), 39 (pt); LPNs 7 (ft), 2 (pt); Nurses' aides 68 (ft), 10 (pt); Physical therapists 1 (ft); Occupational therapists 1 (ft), 1 (pt); Speech therapists 1 (pt); Activities coordinators 1 (ft); Dietitians 2 (ft); Ophthalmologists 1 (pt); Podiatrists 1 (pt); Audiologists 1 (pt); Physicians 15 (pt) (consultant); Social workers 1 (ft), 3 (pt); Activity therapists 2 (ft), 3 (pt); Physical therapy aides 2 (pt); Physical therapy assistants 2 (ft), 1 (pt).
LANGUAGES: Spanish

Oakwood Terrace Nursing Home

1300 Oak Ave, Evanston, IL 60201
(708) 869-1300, 869-1378 FAX
LICENSURE: Skilled care; Intermediate care.
BEDS: SNF 4; ICF 53.
STAFF: Physicians 2 (ft) (consultant); RNs 2 (ft), 8 (pt); LPNs 1 (ft); Nurses' aides 23 (ft), 8 (pt); Physical therapists 1 (pt) (consultant); Recreational therapists 1 (ft); Occupational therapists 1 (pt) (consultant); Speech therapists 1 (pt) (consultant); Activities coordinators 1 (ft); Dietitians 1 (pt) (consultant); Podiatrists 1 (pt) (consultant); Audiologists 1 (pt) (consultant).

St Francis Extended Care Center

500 Asbury St, Evanston, IL 60202
(708) 492-3320
LICENSURE: Skilled care; Intermediate care.
BEDS: SNF 78; ICF 46.
CERTIFIED: Medicaid; Medicare.
ADMISSIONS REQUIREMENTS: Minimum age 18; Medical examination.
STAFF: Physicians (consultant); RNs 12 (ft), 2 (pt); LPNs 3 (ft), 1 (pt); Nurses' aides 41 (ft); Physical therapists 2 (ft); Reality therapists 1 (ft); Recreational therapists 2 (ft), 1 (pt); Occupational therapists (consultant); Speech therapists (consultant); Activities coordinators 1 (ft); Dietitians 1 (ft); Ophthalmologists (consultant); Podiatrists (consultant); Audiologists (consultant).
LANGUAGES: Spanish

Swedish Retirement Association

2320 Pioneer Pl, Evanston, IL 60202
(708) 328-8700

LICENSURE: Intermediate care; Sheltered care.
BEDS: ICF 50; Sheltered care 99.
ADMISSIONS REQUIREMENTS: Minimum age 60; Medical examination.
STAFF: Physicians; RNs; LPNs; Nurses' aides; Physical therapists; Recreational therapists; Occupational therapists; Activities coordinators; Dietitians; Ophthalmologists; Podiatrists; Dentists.

Evergreen Park

Park Lane Nursing Center Association

9125 S Pulaski, Evergreen Park, IL 60642
(708) 425-3400
LICENSURE: Skilled care.
BEDS: SNF 249.
CERTIFIED: Medicaid.
ADMISSIONS REQUIREMENTS: Minimum age 45.
STAFF: RNs 3 (ft); LPNs 17 (ft); Nurses' aides 80 (ft); Recreational therapists 6 (ft); Activities coordinators 1 (ft).

Peace Memorial Home

10124 S Kedzie Ave, Evergreen Park, IL 60642
(708) 636-9200
LICENSURE: Skilled care; Retirement.
BEDS: SNF 242.
CERTIFIED: Medicaid.
ADMISSIONS REQUIREMENTS: Minimum age 18; Medical examination; Physician's request.
STAFF: Physicians 1 (pt); RNs 15 (ft); LPNs 18 (ft); Nurses' aides 107 (ft); Physical therapists 1 (pt); Reality therapists 1 (pt); Recreational therapists 1 (pt); Occupational therapists 1 (pt); Speech therapists 1 (pt); Activities coordinators 1 (pt); Dietitians 1 (pt); Podiatrists 1 (pt); Dentists 1 (pt).

Forest Park

Altenheim

7824 Madison St, Forest Park, IL 60130
(708) 366-2206, 366-2235 FAX
LICENSURE: Intermediate care; Sheltered care.
BEDS: ICF 99; Sheltered care 52.
CERTIFIED: Medicaid.
ADMISSIONS REQUIREMENTS: Minimum age 62; Medical examination.
STAFF: Physicians; RNs; LPNs; Nurses' aides; Physical therapists; Recreational therapists; Occupational therapists; Speech therapists; Activities coordinators; Dietitians; Ophthalmologists; Podiatrists; Audiologists.
LANGUAGES: German, Spanish

Frankfort

Frankfort Terrace
PO Box 460, 40 N Smith, Frankfort, IL 60423
(815) 469-3156
LICENSURE: Intermediate care.
BEDS: ICF 120.
CERTIFIED: Medicaid.

Franklin Park

Westlake Pavilion
10500 Grand Ave, Franklin Park, IL 60131
(708) 451-1520, 451-1503 FAX
LICENSURE: Skilled care; Intermediate care; Alzheimer's
care.
BEDS: SNF 129; ICF 25.
CERTIFIED: Medicaid; Medicare.
ADMISSIONS REQUIREMENTS: Minimum age 18; Medical
examination.
STAFF: RNs; LPNs; Nurses' aides; Physical therapists;
Recreational therapists; Occupational therapists;
Activities coordinators; Dietitians.

Geneva

Geneva Care Center
1101 E State St, Geneva, IL 60134
(708) 232-7544
LICENSURE: Intermediate care.
BEDS: ICF 107.
ADMISSIONS REQUIREMENTS: Medical examination.
STAFF: Physicians 3 (pt); RNs 5 (ft); LPNs 5 (ft);
Nurses' aides 14 (ft); Physical therapists 1 (pt);
Reality therapists 1 (pt); Recreational therapists 1
(pt); Occupational therapists 1 (pt); Speech therapists 1 (pt); Activities coordinators 3 (ft); Dietitians 1 (pt); Ophthalmologists 1 (pt); Podiatrists 1
(pt); Audiologists 1 (pt).

Glenview

The Abington of Glenview
3901 Glenview Rd, Glenview, IL 60025
(708) 729-0000, 729-1552 FAX
LICENSURE: Skilled care; Intermediate care.
BEDS: SNF 100; ICF 100.
CERTIFIED: Medicare; Private.
ADMISSIONS REQUIREMENTS: Minimum age 18; Medical
examination.
STAFF: Physicians 10 (ft), 20 (pt); RNs 15 (ft), 9 (pt);
LPNs 5 (ft), 3 (pt); Nurses' aides 50 (ft), 8 (pt);
Physical therapists 4 (ft), 1 (pt); Reality therapists;
Recreational therapists 1 (ft); Occupational thera-
pists 2 (ft); Speech therapists 1 (ft); Activities co-

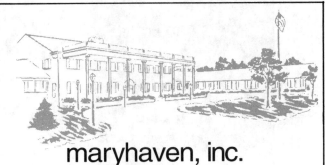
ordinators 54 (ft); Dietitians 1 (ft); Ophthalmol-
ogists 1 (ft); Podiatrists 2 (ft); Audiologists 1 (ft);
Medical directors 1 (pt); Directors of nursing 1
(ft); Asst directors of nursing 2 (ft); Nursing supervisors 3 (ft); Licensed social workers 1 (ft), 1
(pt).
See ad page 225

Glenview Terrace Nursing Center
1511 Greenwood Rd, Glenview, IL 60025
(708) 729-9090, 729-9135 FAX
LICENSURE: Skilled care; Alzheimer's care.
BEDS: SNF 293.
CERTIFIED: Medicaid; Medicare; VA.
ADMISSIONS REQUIREMENTS: Minimum age 18; Physician's
request.
STAFF: Physicians 1 (ft); RNs 28 (ft); LPNs 4 (ft);
Nurses' aides 86 (ft); Physical therapists 2 (ft);
Reality therapists 5 (ft); Recreational therapists 1
(ft); Occupational therapists 1 (ft); Speech thera-
pists 2 (ft); Activities coordinators 8 (ft); Dietitians
1 (ft); Ophthalmologists 1 (ft); Podiatrists 1 (ft);
Audiologists 1 (ft).
LANGUAGES: Polish, Tagalog
See ad page 224

Maryhaven Inc
1700 E Lake Ave, Glenview, IL 60025
(708) 729-1300

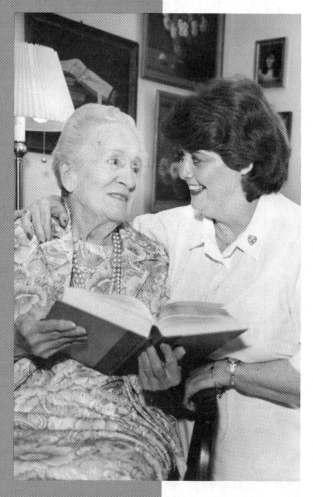
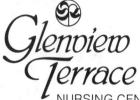

LICENSURE: Skilled care; Intermediate care.
BEDS: SNF 42; ICF 105.
CERTIFIED: Medicaid.
ADMISSIONS REQUIREMENTS: Minimum age 65; Medical
    examination.
STAFF: RNs 7 (ft), 8 (pt); Nurses' aides 27 (ft), 3 (pt);
    Activities coordinators 3 (ft), 5 (pt).
See ad page 223

Glenwood

Glenwood Terrace Nursing Center
19330 S Cottage Grove, Glenwood, IL 60425
(708) 758-6200
LICENSURE: Skilled care; Intermediate care; Alzheimer's
    care.
BEDS: SNF 92; ICF 92.
CERTIFIED: Medicaid; VA.
ADMISSIONS REQUIREMENTS: Medical examination.
STAFF: Physicians 3 (ft); RNs 6 (ft); LPNs 5 (ft);
    Nurses' aides 53 (ft); Physical therapists 4 (ft);
    Reality therapists 4 (ft); Recreational therapists 4
    (ft), 3 (pt); Occupational therapists 4 (ft); Activi-
    ties coordinators 1 (ft); Dietitians 1 (ft); Ophthal-
    mologists 1 (ft); Podiatrists 1 (ft).

Harvey

Alden Nursing Center—Heather Rehabilitation & Health Care Center
15600 S Honore St, Harvey, IL 60426
(708) 333-9550, 333-9554 FAX
LICENSURE: Skilled care; Intermediate care; Alzheimer's
    care.
BEDS: Total 173.
CERTIFIED: Medicaid; Medicare; VA.
ADMISSIONS REQUIREMENTS: Minimum age 18; Medical
    examination.
STAFF: Physicians; RNs; LPNs; Nurses' aides; Physical
    therapists; Recreational therapists; Occupational
    therapists; Speech therapists; Activities coordina-
    tors; Dietitians; Ophthalmologists; Podiatrists;
    Audiologists.

Hazel Crest

Imperial Nursing Center of Hazel Crest
3300 W 175th St, Hazel Crest, IL 60429
(708) 335-2400, 335-0668 FAX
LICENSURE: Skilled care; Intermediate care; Alzheimer's
    care; Hospice; Respite care.
BEDS: Total 204.
CERTIFIED: Medicaid; Medicare; VA.
ADMISSIONS REQUIREMENTS: Minimum age per state regu-
    lations; "Public Aid Pending" acceptable.
STAFF: Physicians 3 (ft); RNs 11 (ft), 4 (pt); LPNs 5
    (ft), 3 (pt); Nurses' aides 45 (ft), 10 (pt); Physical
    therapists 1 (ft); Reality therapists; Recreational
    therapists 1 (ft); Occupational therapists 1 (ft);

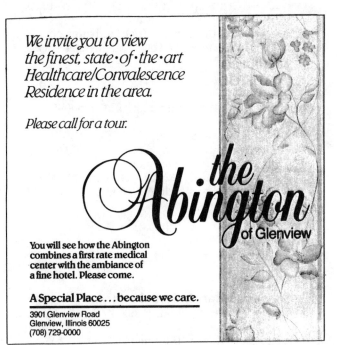
Speech therapists 1 (pt); Activities coordinators 5
    (ft); Dietitians 1 (ft); Ophthalmologists 1 (pt);
    Podiatrists 1 (pt); Audiologists 1 (pt); Dentists;
    Social services workers.

Hickory Hills

Hickory Nursing Pavilion Inc
9246 S Roberts Rd, Hickory Hills, IL 60457
(708) 598-4040, 598-0365 FAX
LICENSURE: Intermediate care.
BEDS: ICF 74.
CERTIFIED: Medicaid.
STAFF: RNs 2 (ft); LPNs 3 (ft), 3 (pt); Nurses' aides 16
    (ft).

Highland Park

Abbott House
405 Central Ave, Highland Park, IL 60035
(708) 432-6080, 432-7286 FAX
LICENSURE: Intermediate care; ICF/MI.
BEDS: ICF 106.
CERTIFIED: Medicaid; VA.
ADMISSIONS REQUIREMENTS: Minimum age 16; Medical
    examination.

✔ In order to support future editions of this publication would you please mention *Elder Services* each time you contact any advertiser, facility, or service.

STAFF: RNs 4 (ft), 6 (pt); LPNs 2 (ft), 2 (pt); Nurses' aides 16 (ft), 2 (pt); Recreational therapists 1 (pt); Occupational therapists 1 (pt); Activities coordinators 1 (ft); Dietitians 1 (pt); Podiatrists 1 (pt).
See ad page 239

Villa St Cyril
1111 Saint Johns Ave, Highland Park, IL 60035
(708) 432-9104
LICENSURE: Intermediate care.
BEDS: ICF 82.
ADMISSIONS REQUIREMENTS: Minimum age 65.
STAFF: Physicians 7 (pt); RNs 7 (ft), 4 (pt); LPNs 1 (ft), 2 (pt); Nurses' aides 12 (ft); Dietitians 1 (ft); Podiatrists 1 (pt).

Highwood

Highland Park Health Care Center Inc
50 Pleasant Ave, Highwood, IL 60040
(708) 432-9142
LICENSURE: Skilled care; Intermediate care.
BEDS: SNF 82; ICF 13.
CERTIFIED: Medicaid.
ADMISSIONS REQUIREMENTS: Minimum age 21; Medical examination.
STAFF: Physicians; RNs 5 (ft), 6 (pt); LPNs 1 (ft); Nurses' aides 20 (ft), 5 (pt); Physical therapists (consultant); Reality therapists; Recreational therapists; Occupational therapists; Activities coordinators 1 (ft); Dietitians (consultant); Ophthalmologists; Podiatrists.

Hillside

Oakridge Convalescent Home Inc
323 Oakridge Ave, Hillside, IL 60162
(708) 547-6595
LICENSURE: Skilled care; Intermediate care.
BEDS: SNF 58; ICF 15.
CERTIFIED: Medicaid.

Hinsdale

Americana-Monticello Healthcare Center of Hinsdale
600 W Ogden Ave, Hinsdale, IL 60521
(708) 325-9630, 325-9648 FAX
LICENSURE: Skilled care; Intermediate care; Alzheimer's care.
BEDS: SNF 148; Alzheimer's 34.
CERTIFIED: Medicare.
ADMISSIONS REQUIREMENTS: Medical examination.

STAFF: Physical therapists 1 (ft); Recreational therapists 1 (ft); Occupational therapists 1 (ft); Speech therapists 1 (pt); Activities coordinators 1 (ft); Dietitians 1 (ft); Podiatrists 1 (pt).
See ad page 200

Hoffman Estates

Alden—Poplar Creek Rehabilitation & Health Care Center
1545 Barrington Rd, Hoffman Estates, IL 60194
(708) 884-0011, 884-0121 FAX
LICENSURE: Skilled care; Intermediate care; Alzheimer's care; Hospice.
BEDS: SNF 154; ICF 63.
CERTIFIED: Medicaid; Medicare; VA.
ADMISSIONS REQUIREMENTS: Minimum age 18; Medical examination.
STAFF: Physicians; RNs; LPNs; Nurses' aides; Physical therapists; Reality therapists; Recreational therapists; Occupational therapists; Speech therapists; Activities coordinators; Dietitians; Ophthalmologists; Podiatrists; Audiologists; Chaplain.

Homewood

Heartland Health Care Center—Homewood
940 Maple Ave, Homewood, IL 60430
(708) 799-0244
LICENSURE: Skilled care.
BEDS: SNF 120.

Mercy Health Care & Rehabilitation Center
19000 Halsted St, Homewood, IL 60430
(708) 957-9200, 799-4787 FAX
LICENSURE: Skilled care; Alzheimer's care.
BEDS: SNF 259.
CERTIFIED: Medicaid; Medicare; VA.
ADMISSIONS REQUIREMENTS: Medical examination.
STAFF: RNs 15 (ft), 2 (pt); LPNs 21 (ft), 7 (pt); Nurses' aides 74 (ft), 4 (pt); Physical therapists 2 (ft); Occupational therapists 1 (ft), 1 (pt); Speech therapists 1 (ft); Activities coordinators 5 (ft), 1 (pt); Dietitians 2 (pt); Ophthalmologists 1 (pt); Podiatrists 1 (pt); Psychiatrists 1 (pt); Dentists 1 (pt); Psychologists 1 (pt).
LANGUAGES: Spanish, Italian, Polish
See ads pages 116, 161, 351

Indian Head Park

Briar Place Ltd
6800 W Joliet Rd, Indian Head Park, IL 60525
(708) 246-8500
LICENSURE: Skilled care; Intermediate care.
BEDS: SNF 88; ICF 157.

CERTIFIED: Medicaid.
ADMISSIONS REQUIREMENTS: Minimum age 21; Medical examination; Physician's request.
STAFF: RNs 5 (ft), 2 (pt); LPNs 10 (ft), 6 (pt); Nurses' aides 48 (ft), 9 (pt); Physical therapists (consultant); Activities coordinators 1 (ft); Dietitians.
LANGUAGES: Spanish

Island Lake

Sheltering Oak
PO Box 367, Island Lake, IL 60042
(708) 526-3636
LICENSURE: Intermediate care.
BEDS: ICF 70.
CERTIFIED: Medicaid.

Itasca

The Arbor
535 S Elm St, Itasca, IL 60143
(708) 773-9416
LICENSURE: Intermediate care.
BEDS: ICF 80.
ADMISSIONS REQUIREMENTS: Minimum age 18; Medical examination.
STAFF: Physicians; RNs; LPNs; Nurses' aides; Recreational therapists; Activities coordinators; Dietitians; Ophthalmologists.

Joliet

Deerbrook Nursing Centre
306 N Larkin Ave, Joliet, IL 60435
(815) 744-5560, 744-6914 FAX
LICENSURE: Skilled care.
BEDS: SNF 224.
CERTIFIED: Medicaid; Medicare; VA.
ADMISSIONS REQUIREMENTS: Minimum age 18; Medical examination.
STAFF: RNs 6 (ft), 1 (pt); LPNs 10 (ft), 4 (pt); Nurses' aides 44 (ft), 10 (pt); Physical therapists 1 (pt) (consultant); Recreational therapists 1 (pt) (consultant); Occupational therapists 1 (pt) (consultant); Speech therapists 1 (pt) (consultant); Activities coordinators 1 (ft); Dietitians 1 (pt) (consultant); Ophthalmologists 2 (pt) (consultant); Podiatrists 2 (pt) (consultant); Audiologists 1 (pt) (consultant).
LANGUAGES: Spanish, German, Polish
See ad on inside back cover

Draper Plaza
777 Draper Ave, Joliet, IL 60432
(815) 727-4794

LICENSURE: Skilled care; Intermediate care; Alzheimer's care.
BEDS: SNF 84; ICF 84.
CERTIFIED: Medicaid; Medicare.
ADMISSIONS REQUIREMENTS: Minimum age 18; Medical examination; Physician's request.
STAFF: Physicians 1 (ft); RNs 5 (ft); LPNs 12 (ft); Nurses' aides 60 (ft), 5 (pt); Physical therapists 1 (pt); Recreational therapists 1 (ft); Occupational therapists 1 (pt); Speech therapists 1 (pt); Activities coordinators 1 (ft); Dietitians 1 (pt); Podiatrists 1 (pt).
LANGUAGES: Spanish

Joliet Terrace
2230 McDonough, Joliet, IL 60436
(815) 729-3801
LICENSURE: Intermediate care.
BEDS: ICF 120.
CERTIFIED: Medicaid.

Metropolitan Nursing Center of Joliet
222 N Hammes, Joliet, IL 60435
(815) 725-0443, 725-1079 FAX
LICENSURE: Skilled care; Intermediate care; Alzheimer's care; Hospice; Respite care.
BEDS: SNF 203.
CERTIFIED: Medicaid; Medicare; VA.
ADMISSIONS REQUIREMENTS: Minimum age per state regulations; "Public Aid Pending" acceptable.
STAFF: Physicians; RNs; LPNs; Nurses' aides; Physical therapists; Reality therapists; Recreational therapists; Occupational therapists; Speech therapists; Activities coordinators; Dietitians; Ophthalmologists; Podiatrists; Audiologists; Dentists; Social services workers.

Our Lady of Angels Retirement Home
1201 Wyoming Ave, Joliet, IL 60435
(815) 725-6631
LICENSURE: Intermediate care; Sheltered care.
BEDS: ICF 50; Sheltered care 50.
CERTIFIED: Medicaid.
ADMISSIONS REQUIREMENTS: Minimum age 65; Medical examination; Ambulatory.
STAFF: RNs 1 (ft), 5 (pt); LPNs 2 (pt); Nurses' aides 21 (ft), 12 (pt); Physical therapists 1 (pt); Activities coordinators 1 (ft); Dietitians 1 (ft).

Rosewood Care Center Inc—Joliet
3401 Hennepin Dr, Joliet, IL 60435
(815) 436-5900
LICENSURE: Skilled care; Intermediate care.
BEDS: SNF 60; ICF 60.

Salem Village
1314 Rowell Ave, Joliet, IL 60433
(815) 727-5451
LICENSURE: Skilled care; Intermediate care; Alzheimer's care; Sheltered care; Retirement.
BEDS: SNF 36; ICF 246.
CERTIFIED: Medicaid.

✔ In order to support future editions of this publication would you please mention *Elder Services* each time you contact any advertiser, facility, or service.

ADMISSIONS REQUIREMENTS: Minimum age 62; Medical examination.

STAFF: Physicians 1 (pt); RNs 6 (ft), 5 (pt); LPNs 20 (ft), 8 (pt); Nurses' aides 55 (ft), 39 (pt); Physical therapists 1 (pt); Reality therapists 1 (pt); Recreational therapists 1 (pt); Occupational therapists 1 (pt); Activities coordinators 1 (ft), 6 (pt); Dietitians 1 (ft).

Sunny Hill Nursing Home
Doris & Neal Sts, Joliet, IL 60433
(815) 727-8710, 727-8637 FAX
LICENSURE: Skilled care; Intermediate care.
BEDS: SNF 50; ICF 250.
CERTIFIED: Medicaid.
ADMISSIONS REQUIREMENTS: Minimum age 18; Medical examination.
STAFF: RNs 8 (ft), 3 (pt); LPNs 25 (ft), 10 (pt); Nurses' aides 91 (ft), 13 (pt); Recreational therapists 6 (ft); Activities coordinators 1 (ft); Dietitians 1 (ft).

Villa Franciscan
210 N Springfield Ave, Joliet, IL 60435
(815) 725-3400
LICENSURE: Skilled care; Alzheimer's care.
BEDS: SNF 176.
CERTIFIED: Medicaid; Medicare.
ADMISSIONS REQUIREMENTS: Medical examination; Physician's request.
STAFF: RNs 6 (ft), 1 (pt); LPNs 12 (ft), 6 (pt); Nurses' aides 34 (ft), 8 (pt); Activities coordinators 2 (ft), 3 (pt).
LANGUAGES: Spanish

Justice

Rosary Hill Home
9000 W 81st St, Justice, IL 60458
(708) 458-3040
LICENSURE: Intermediate care; Sheltered care.
BEDS: ICF 18; Sheltered care 50.
ADMISSIONS REQUIREMENTS: Females only; Medical examination; Must be ambulatory.
STAFF: Physicians 1 (ft); RNs 1 (ft); LPNs 1 (ft); Nurses' aides 6 (ft); Physical therapists 1 (pt); Activities coordinators 1 (ft); Dietitians 1 (pt); Ophthalmologists 1 (pt); Podiatrists 1 (pt).
LANGUAGES: Polish

La Grange

Colonial Manor Healthcare Center
339 S 9th Ave, La Grange, IL 60525
(708) 354-4660
LICENSURE: Skilled care; Intermediate care; Alzheimer's care.
BEDS: SNF 96; ICF 107.
CERTIFIED: Medicaid; Medicare.

ADMISSIONS REQUIREMENTS: Medical examination; Physician's request.
STAFF: Physicians; RNs; LPNs; Nurses' aides; Physical therapists; Reality therapists; Recreational therapists; Occupational therapists; Speech therapists; Activities coordinators; Dietitians.

Fairview Health Care Center
701 N La Grange Rd, La Grange, IL 60525
(708) 354-7300, 354-8928 FAX
LICENSURE: Skilled care; Hospice.
BEDS: SNF 131.
CERTIFIED: Medicare.
ADMISSIONS REQUIREMENTS: Minimum age 19; Medical examination.
STAFF: Physicians (consultant); RNs 7 (ft), 9 (pt); LPNs 11 (ft), 1 (pt); Nurses' aides 45 (ft), 8 (pt); Physical therapists 1 (ft); Reality therapists 1 (ft); Recreational therapists 3 (ft), 2 (pt); Occupational therapists 1 (pt) (contracted); Speech therapists 1 (pt) (contracted); Activities coordinators 1 (ft); Dietitians 1 (pt) (consultant); Ophthalmologists 1 (pt) (consultant); Podiatrists 1 (pt) (consultant); Audiologists 1 (pt) (consultant).

La Grange Park

Plymouth Place
315 N La Grange Rd, La Grange Park, IL 60525
(708) 354-0340
LICENSURE: Intermediate care; Sheltered care.
BEDS: ICF 76; Sheltered care 300.
ADMISSIONS REQUIREMENTS: Minimum age 60; Medical examination.
STAFF: Physicians 8 (pt); RNs 6 (ft), 5 (pt); LPNs 7 (ft), 6 (pt); Nurses' aides 26 (ft), 4 (pt); Physical therapists (contracted); Recreational therapists 2 (ft); Occupational therapists (contracted); Speech therapists (contracted); Activities coordinators 1 (ft); Dietitians 1 (pt); Ophthalmologists; Podiatrists; Audiologists (contracted).

Lake Bluff

Hill Top Sanitorium
502 Waukegan Rd, Lake Bluff, IL 60044
(708) 295-1550 295-1652 FAX
LICENSURE: Skilled care; Intermediate care; Non-medical nursing care.
BEDS: Total 23.
CERTIFIED: Medicare.
ADMISSIONS REQUIREMENTS: Membership in Church of Christian Science.
STAFF: LPNs 13 (ft); Nurses' aides 8 (ft).

Lake Bluff Healthcare Centre
700 Jenkisson Ave, Lake Bluff, IL 60044
(708) 295-3900, (708) 295-3989 FAX

LICENSURE: Skilled care; Intermediate care; Alzheimer's care; Hospice.
BEDS: SNF 160; ICF 71.
CERTIFIED: Medicaid; Medicare; VA.
ADMISSIONS REQUIREMENTS: Medical examination.
STAFF: RNs 20 (ft), 3 (pt); LPNs 9 (ft), 4 (pt); Nurses' aides 50 (ft), 11 (pt); Activities coordinators 5 (ft), 1 (pt); Dietitians 2 (ft), 1 (pt).

Lansing

Tri State Manor Nursing Home
2500 E 175th St, Lansing, IL 60438
(708) 474-7330
LICENSURE: Intermediate care.
BEDS: ICF 56.

Lemont

Holy Family Villa
12375 McCarthy Rd, Lemont, IL 60439
(708) 257-2291, 257-1259 FAX
LICENSURE: Intermediate care.
BEDS: ICF 99.
CERTIFIED: Medicaid.
ADMISSIONS REQUIREMENTS: Minimum age 65; Medical examination.
STAFF: Physicians 1 (ft); RNs 2 (ft), 2 (pt); LPNs 7 (ft), 2 (pt); Nurses' aides 28 (ft), 12 (pt); Physical therapists 1 (ft); Activities coordinators 3 (ft), 1 (pt); Dietitians 1 (ft); Podiatrists 1 (pt).
LANGUAGES: Lithuanian

Mother Theresa Home
1270 Franciscan Dr, Lemont, IL 60439
(708) 257-5801, 257-8615 FAX
LICENSURE: Skilled care; Intermediate care; Sheltered care.
BEDS: SNF 60; ICF 60; Sheltered care 30.
CERTIFIED: Medicaid.
ADMISSIONS REQUIREMENTS: Minimum age 65; Medical examination.
STAFF: Physicians 1 (pt); RNs 6 (ft), 4 (pt); LPNs 7 (ft), 3 (pt); Nurses' aides 65 (ft), 13 (pt); Recreational therapists 1 (ft); Activities coordinators 4 (ft); Dietitians 1 (pt).

Libertyville

Americana Healthcare Center of Libertyville
1500 S Milwaukee Ave, Libertyville, IL 60048
(708) 816-3200, 816-6874 FAX
LICENSURE: Skilled care; Intermediate care; Assisted living.
BEDS: SNF 121; Assisted living facility 28.
CERTIFIED: Medicaid; Medicare.

ADMISSIONS REQUIREMENTS: Medical examination; Physical history.
See ad page 200

Libertyville Manor Extended Care Facility
610 Peterson Rd, Libertyville, IL 60048
(708) 367-6100
LICENSURE: Skilled care.
BEDS: SNF 174.
CERTIFIED: Medicare.
ADMISSIONS REQUIREMENTS: Minimum age 21; Medical examination.
STAFF: Physicians; RNs; LPNs; Nurses' aides; Physical therapists; Reality therapists; Occupational therapists; Speech therapists; Activities coordinators; Dietitians; Ophthalmologists; Podiatrists; Audiologists.

Winchester House
1125 N Milwaukee Ave, Libertyville, IL 60048
(708) 362-4340
LICENSURE: Skilled care.
BEDS: SNF 359.
CERTIFIED: Medicaid; Medicare.
ADMISSIONS REQUIREMENTS: Minimum age 18; Must be a Lake County resident.
STAFF: RNs 30 (ft); LPNs 13 (ft); Nurses' aides 146 (ft); Physical therapists 1 (pt); Recreational therapists 1 (ft); Occupational therapists 1 (ft); Speech therapists 1 (pt); Activities coordinators 1 (ft); Dietitians 2 (ft).

Lincolnwood

Regency Park Manor
7000 N McCormick Blvd, Lincolnwood, IL 60645
(708) 673-7166, 673-7185 FAX
LICENSURE: Skilled care; Sheltered care.
BEDS: SNF 40; Sheltered care 25.
STAFF: Physicians 1 (pt); RNs 6 (ft), 3 (pt); LPNs 3 (ft), 2 (pt); Nurses' aides 4 (ft), 4 (pt); Activities coordinators 1 (ft).
See ad page 291

Lindenhurst

Victory Lakes Continuing Care Center
1055 E Grand Ave, Lindenhurst, IL 60046
(708) 356-5900, 356-4570 FAX
LICENSURE: Skilled care; Alzheimer's care.
BEDS: SNF 100; Alzheimer's 20.
CERTIFIED: Medicare.
ADMISSIONS REQUIREMENTS: Medical examination.
STAFF: RNs 8 (ft); LPNs 7 (ft); Nurses' aides 44 (ft); Physical therapists 1 (pt); Recreational therapists 2 (pt); Occupational therapists 1 (pt); Speech therapists 1 (pt); Activities coordinators 1 (ft); Dietitians 1 (pt); Podiatrists 1 (pt).
See ad page 230

✔ In order to support future editions of this publication would you please mention *Elder Services* each time you contact any advertiser, facility, or service.

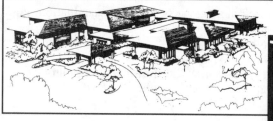

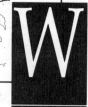

When someone you love requires full-time attention.

Victory Lakes offers a special Alzheimer's unit.
Adults suffering from Alzheimer's disease and related disorders need a nurturing, non-challenging environment where they can be comfortable and secure. In the "Sunshine Wing" at Victory Lakes, we have created a serene atmosphere where patients, guided by familiar faces, can move through their daily routine at their own pace. Meals are served in a private dining room, and outdoor and indoor activities are an integral part of the program.

Come, visit anytime. Meet our professional staff. Get to know firsthand what you can expect from a quality, nursing home environment.

Victory Lakes provides a variety of skilled nursing care programs to suit your needs.
• Long-term Continuing Care
• Adult Day Care program - daily basis
• Respite program - overnight to 30 days
• Rehabilitation/Medicare unit - short term
• Alzheimer's and related disorders unit

At Victory Lakes, our goal is to motivate and assist residents in maintaining their optimal level of mental and physical function.

For a tour or complimentary brochure, call Mary Riggs at **708/ 356-5900.**

VICTORY LAKES
CONTINUING CARE CENTER

1055 E. Grand Avenue • Lindenhurst, IL
7 miles west of Rt. 94 • Affiliated with Victory Memorial Hospital, Waukegan.

Lisle

Snow Valley Living Center
5000 Lincoln, Lisle, IL 60532
(708) 852-5100
LICENSURE: Skilled care.
BEDS: SNF 51.
ADMISSIONS REQUIREMENTS: Minimum age 19.

Lombard

Beacon Hill
2400 S Finley Rd, Lombard, IL 60148
(708) 620-5850, 691-8715 FAX
LICENSURE: Skilled care; Intermediate care.
BEDS: SNF 45; ICF 21.
CERTIFIED: Medicare.
ADMISSIONS REQUIREMENTS: Physician's request.
STAFF: RNs 5 (ft), 6 (pt); LPNs 5 (ft), 6 (pt); Nurses' aides 22 (ft), 4 (pt); Physical therapists 1 (ft), 5 (pt); Recreational therapists 2 (ft), 5 (pt); Occupational therapists 1 (ft), 5 (pt); Speech therapists 1 (ft), 5 (pt); Activities coordinators 1 (ft); Dietitians 1 (ft); Podiatrists 1 (ft).

Bloomingdale Pavilion
1050 Shedron Way, Lombard, IL 60108
(708) 894-7400, 894-8528 FAX
LICENSURE: Skilled care.
BEDS: SNF 259.
CERTIFIED: Medicaid; Medicare.
ADMISSIONS REQUIREMENTS: Medical examination.
STAFF: Physicians; RNs; LPNs; Nurses' aides; Physical therapists; Occupational therapists; Speech therapists; Speech therapists; Activities coordinators; Dietitians; Ophthalmologists; Podiatrists; Audiologists.

Lexington Health Care Center of Lombard
2100 S Finley Rd, Lombard, IL 60148
(708) 495-4000
LICENSURE: Skilled care; Intermediate care.
BEDS: SNF 175; ICF 40.
CERTIFIED: Medicaid; Medicare.

Long Grove

Maple Hill Nursing Home Ltd
RFD Box 2308, 2308 N Old Hicks Rd, Long Grove, IL 60047
(708) 438-8275, 438-3254 FAX
LICENSURE: Skilled care; Intermediate care; Alzheimer's care.
BEDS: Total 200.
CERTIFIED: Medicaid; Medicare; VA.

ADMISSIONS REQUIREMENTS: Medical examination.
STAFF: RNs 12 (ft), 11 (pt); LPNs 4 (ft), 2 (pt); Activities coordinators 8 (ft), 2 (pt).

Marengo

Florence Nursing Home
546 E Grant Hwy, Marengo, IL 60152
(815) 568-8322
LICENSURE: Intermediate care; Alzheimer's care.
BEDS: ICF 49.
ADMISSIONS REQUIREMENTS: Minimum age 22; Medical examination.
STAFF: RNs 1 (ft); LPNs 4 (ft); Nurses' aides 11 (ft); Activities coordinators 1 (ft).

Matteson

Applewood Living Center
21020 S Kostner Ave, Matteson, IL 60443
(708) 747-1300, 747-6282 FAX
LICENSURE: Skilled care; Intermediate care.
BEDS: SNF 105.
CERTIFIED: VA.
ADMISSIONS REQUIREMENTS: Minimum age 18; Medical examination.
STAFF: RNs; LPNs; Nurses' aides; Activities coordinators.

Maywood

Baptist Retirement Home
316 W Randolph, Maywood, IL 60153
(708) 344-1541
LICENSURE: Intermediate care; Retirement.
BEDS: ICF 69.
CERTIFIED: Medicaid.
ADMISSIONS REQUIREMENTS: Medical examination.
STAFF: Physicians 2 (ft); RNs 3 (ft); LPNs 5 (ft); Nurses' aides 24 (ft); Physical therapists 1 (pt); Reality therapists 1 (pt); Recreational therapists 2 (ft); Occupational therapists 1 (pt); Speech therapists 1 (pt); Activities coordinators 2 (ft); Dietitians 1 (ft); Ophthalmologists 1 (pt); Podiatrists 1 (pt); Audiologists 1 (pt); Dentists 1 (pt).

McHenry

Royal Terrace
803 Royal Dr, McHenry, IL 60050
(815) 344-2600, 344-8418 FAX
LICENSURE: Skilled care.
BEDS: SNF 316.
CERTIFIED: Medicaid; Medicare.

✔ In order to support future editions of this publication would you please mention *Elder Services* each time you contact any advertiser, facility, or service.

ADMISSIONS REQUIREMENTS: Minimum age 18; Medical examination; Physician's request.

STAFF: RNs; LPNs; Nurses' aides; Physical therapists; Reality therapists; Recreational therapists; Occupational therapists; Speech therapists; Activities coordinators; Dietitians.

LANGUAGES: Spanish, Polish

Melrose Park

Gottlieb Memorial Hospital Extended Care Unit

701 W North Ave, Melrose Park, IL 60160
(708) 450-4923
LICENSURE: Skilled care.
BEDS: SNF 34.
CERTIFIED: Medicaid; Medicare.
ADMISSIONS REQUIREMENTS: Medical examination; Physician's request; Pre-screening by admissions coordinator.
STAFF: RNs; LPNs; Nurses' aides; Physical therapists; Recreational therapists; Occupational therapists; Speech therapists; Dietitians; Social workers; Physiatrists; Respiratory therapists.
See ad page 127

Midlothian

Bowman Nursing Home

3249 W 147th St, Midlothian, IL 60445
(708) 389-3141
LICENSURE: Intermediate care; Alzheimer's care.
BEDS: ICF 92.
CERTIFIED: Medicaid.
ADMISSIONS REQUIREMENTS: Minimum age 65.
STAFF: Physicians 3 (pt); RNs 4 (ft); LPNs 6 (ft); Nurses' aides 20 (ft); Physical therapists 1 (pt); Reality therapists 2 (pt); Recreational therapists 2 (ft); Occupational therapists 1 (pt); Speech therapists 1 (pt); Activities coordinators 2 (ft); Dietitians 1 (pt); Ophthalmologists 1 (pt); Podiatrists 1 (pt); Audiologists 1 (pt).

Crestwood Terrace

13301 S Central Ave, Midlothian, IL 60445
(708) 597-5251
LICENSURE: Intermediate care.
BEDS: ICF 126.
CERTIFIED: Medicaid.
ADMISSIONS REQUIREMENTS: Medical examination.
STAFF: Physicians 1 (ft), 10 (pt); RNs 2 (ft), 2 (pt); LPNs 3 (ft), 6 (pt); Nurses' aides 14 (ft), 10 (pt); Reality therapists 3 (ft); Recreational therapists 3 (ft); Occupational therapists 1 (pt); Speech therapists 1 (pt); Activities coordinators 1 (ft); Dietitians 1 (pt); Ophthalmologists 1 (pt); Podiatrists 1 (pt); Dentists 2 (pt).
LANGUAGES: Polish, Italian

Morris

Grundy County Home

PO Box 669, Clay & Quarry Sts, Morris, IL 60450
(815) 942-3255
LICENSURE: Intermediate care; Alzheimer's care.
BEDS: ICF 143.
CERTIFIED: Medicaid.
ADMISSIONS REQUIREMENTS: Minimum age 18; Medical examination; Physician's request.

Morris Lincoln Nursing Home

916 Fremont Ave, Morris, IL 60450
(815) 942-1202
LICENSURE: Intermediate care; Sheltered care.
BEDS: ICF 47; Sheltered care 34.
CERTIFIED: Medicaid.
ADMISSIONS REQUIREMENTS: Medical examination.
STAFF: RNs 2 (ft), 2 (pt); LPNs 3 (ft), 1 (pt); Nurses' aides 14 (ft), 4 (pt); Recreational therapists 2 (ft); Physical therapy aides 1 (ft); Dietitian supervisors 1 (ft).

Walnut Grove Village

Twilight Dr, Morris, IL 60450
(815) 942-5108
LICENSURE: Skilled care; Intermediate care; Sheltered care.
BEDS: SNF 50; ICF 17; Sheltered care 30.
CERTIFIED: Medicaid; Medicare.

Morton Grove

Bethany Terrace Nursing Centre

8425 N Waukegan Rd, Morton Grove, IL 60053
(708) 965-8100
LICENSURE: Skilled care; Intermediate care; Alzheimer's care; Sheltered care.
BEDS: SNF 103; ICF 160; Alzheimer's 91; Sheltered care 12.
CERTIFIED: Medicaid; Medicare.
ADMISSIONS REQUIREMENTS: Minimum age 18.
STAFF: Physicians 3 (pt); RNs 13 (ft), 18 (pt); LPNs 10 (ft), 11 (pt); Nurses' aides 86 (ft), 43 (pt); Physical therapists 1 (ft), 1 (pt); Recreational therapists 7 (ft), 5 (pt); Occupational therapists 1 (pt); Speech therapists 1 (ft); Dietitians 1 (ft); Ophthalmologists 1 (pt); Podiatrists 1 (pt); Audiologists 1 (pt).
See ad page 233

Naperville

Alden Nursing Center—Naperville Rehabilitation & Health Care Center

1525 S Oxford Ln, Naperville, IL 60565
(708) 983-0300, 983-9360 FAX

LICENSURE: Skilled care; Intermediate care; Alzheimer's care; Hospice.
BEDS: Total 203.
CERTIFIED: Medicaid; Medicare; VA.
ADMISSIONS REQUIREMENTS: Minimum age 18; Medical examination.
STAFF: Physicians; RNs; LPNs; Nurses' aides; Physical therapists; Reality therapists; Recreational therapists; Occupational therapists; Speech therapists; Activities coordinators; Dietitians; Ophthalmologists; Podiatrists; Audiologists; Chaplain.

Americana Healthcare Center of Naperville

200 W Martin Ave, Naperville, IL 60540
(708) 355-4111, 355-1792 FAX
LICENSURE: Skilled care; Intermediate care; Alzheimer's care.
BEDS: SNF 90; Alzheimer's 24.
CERTIFIED: Medicare.
ADMISSIONS REQUIREMENTS: Medical examination.
STAFF: Physicians 1 (ft); RNs 7 (ft); LPNs 3 (ft), 4 (pt); Nurses' aides 20 (ft), 12 (pt); Physical therapists 1 (ft); Recreational therapists 1 (ft); Occupational therapists 1 (ft); Speech therapists 1 (pt); Activities coordinators 1 (ft); Dietitians 1 (ft); Podiatrists 1 (pt).
See ad page 200

Community Convalescent Center of Naperville

1136 N Mill St, Naperville, IL 60563
(708) 355-3300 355-1417 FAX
LICENSURE: Skilled care; Intermediate care; Alzheimer's care.
BEDS: SNF 125; Alzheimer's 25.
CERTIFIED: Medicaid; Medicare; JCAHO.
ADMISSIONS REQUIREMENTS: Medical examination.
STAFF: RNs 10 (ft), 2 (pt); LPNs 10 (ft), 4 (pt); Nurses' aides 31 (ft), 18 (pt); Physical therapists 1 (pt); Recreational therapists 3 (ft), 5 (pt); Occupational therapists 1 (pt); Speech therapists 1 (pt); Activities coordinators 1 (ft); Dietitians 1 (ft), 1 (pt); Ophthalmologists 1 (pt); Podiatrists 1 (pt); Audiologists 1 (pt); Dentists 1 (pt).
See ad page 138

St Patrick's Residence

1400 Brookdale Rd, Naperville, IL 60563-2126
(708) 416-6565
LICENSURE: Skilled care; Intermediate care; Alzheimer's care; Sheltered care.
BEDS: SNF 42; ICF 107; Sheltered care 61.
CERTIFIED: Medicaid.
ADMISSIONS REQUIREMENTS: Minimum age 65.
STAFF: Physicians 5 (pt); RNs 10 (ft), 3 (pt); LPNs 10 (ft), 4 (pt); Nurses' aides 90 (ft); Occupational therapists; Activities coordinators 4 (ft); Dietitians 1 (ft).

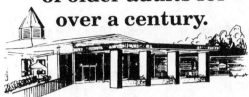
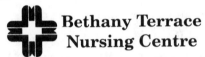
Niles

Forest Villa Nursing Center

6840 W Touhy Ave, Niles, IL 60648
(708) 647-8994, 647-1539 FAX
LICENSURE: Skilled care; Intermediate care.
BEDS: SNF 55; ICF 151.
CERTIFIED: Medicaid; Medicare.
ADMISSIONS REQUIREMENTS: Minimum age 62; Medical examination.
STAFF: Physicians 1 (pt); RNs 15 (ft), 4 (pt); LPNs 5 (ft), 2 (pt); Nurses' aides 45 (ft), 3 (pt); Physical therapists 1 (ft); Recreational therapists 1 (ft); Occupational therapists 1 (ft); Speech therapists 1 (ft); Activities coordinators 1 (ft); Dietitians 1 (ft); Ophthalmologists 1 (pt); Podiatrists 1 (pt); Audiologists 1 (pt).
LANGUAGES: Polish

Glen Bridge Nursing & Rehabilitation Center

8333 W Golf Rd, Niles, IL 60648
(708) 966-9190
LICENSURE: Skilled care; Intermediate care; Alzheimer's care.
BEDS: SNF 151; ICF 151.
CERTIFIED: Medicaid.
STAFF: Physicians 7 (ft); RNs 14 (ft); LPNs 9 (ft); Nurses' aides 72 (ft); Physical therapists 1 (ft); Recreational therapists 6 (ft); Occupational therapists 2 (ft); Speech therapists 1 (ft); Activities co-

✔ In order to support future editions of this publication would you please mention *Elder Services* each time you contact any advertiser, facility, or service.

ordinators 1 (ft); Dietitians 1 (pt); Ophthalmologists 1 (pt); Podiatrists 1 (pt); Audiologists 1 (pt).
LANGUAGES: Polish, Spanish, Yiddish, German

George J Goldman Memorial Home for the Aged
6601 W Touhy Ave, Niles, IL 60648
(708) 647-9875, 647-7969 FAX
LICENSURE: Skilled care; Intermediate care.
BEDS: SNF 101.
CERTIFIED: Medicaid; Medicare.
ADMISSIONS REQUIREMENTS: Must be older adult.
STAFF: Physicians 2 (pt); RNs 5 (ft), 1 (pt); LPNs 2 (ft), 4 (pt); Nurses' aides 30 (ft), 2 (pt); Physical therapists 1 (ft); Activities coordinators 1 (ft); Dietitians 1 (ft).
LANGUAGES: Yiddish, Spanish

Hampton Plaza
8555 Maynard Rd, Niles, IL 60648
(708) 967-7000
LICENSURE: Skilled care; Intermediate care.
BEDS: SNF 150; ICF 150.
CERTIFIED: Medicaid.
ADMISSIONS REQUIREMENTS: Minimum age 21; Medical examination; Physician's request.
STAFF: Physicians 30 (pt); RNs 10 (pt); LPNs 10 (pt); Nurses' aides 80 (pt); Physical therapists 1 (pt); Recreational therapists 1 (pt); Occupational therapists 1 (pt); Speech therapists 1 (pt); Activities coordinators 5 (pt); Dietitians 1 (pt); Ophthalmologists 1 (pt); Podiatrists 2 (pt); Audiologists 1 (pt).
LANGUAGES: Spanish, Polish, Russian

Regency Nursing Centre
6631 Milwaukee Ave, Niles, IL 60648
(708) 647-7444, 647-6403 FAX
LICENSURE: Skilled care; Alzheimer's care.
BEDS: SNF 300.
CERTIFIED: Medicaid; Medicare; VA.
ADMISSIONS REQUIREMENTS: Minimum age 60; Medical examination.

St Andrew Home for the Aged
7000 N Newark, Niles, IL 60648
(708) 647-8332
LICENSURE: Intermediate care; Sheltered care.
BEDS: ICF 33; Sheltered care 57.
CERTIFIED: Medicaid.

St Benedict Home for Aged
6930 W Touhy Ave, Niles, IL 60648
(708) 774-1440
LICENSURE: Skilled care.
BEDS: ICF 99.
ADMISSIONS REQUIREMENTS: Minimum age 70; Medical examination.
STAFF: Physicians; RNs; LPNs 3 (ft), 2 (pt); Nurses' aides 3 (ft), 2 (pt); Reality therapists 1 (pt); Occupational therapists 1 (pt); Dietitians 1 (ft); Ophthalmologists 1 (pt); Dentists 1 (pt).

Norridge

Central Baptist Home for the Aged
4750 N Orange Ave, Norridge, IL 60656
(708) 452-3800, 452-3840 FAX
LICENSURE: Skilled care; Intermediate care; Sheltered care.
BEDS: SNF 29; ICF 93; Sheltered care 29.
CERTIFIED: Medicaid.
ADMISSIONS REQUIREMENTS: Medical examination.

Norridge Nursing Centre Inc
7001 W Cullom, Norridge, IL 60634
(708) 457-0700, 457-8852 FAX
LICENSURE: Skilled care; Intermediate care; Alzheimer's care; Assisted living; Hospice.
BEDS: SNF 210; ICF 105.
CERTIFIED: Medicaid; Medicare; VA; JCAH.
ADMISSIONS REQUIREMENTS: Minimum age 60; Medical examination.
STAFF: Physicians; RNs; LPNs; Nurses' aides; Physical therapists; Reality therapists; Recreational therapists; Occupational therapists; Speech therapists; Dietitians; Ophthalmologists; Podiatrists; Audiologists; Social workers.
LANGUAGES: Spanish, Polish, Italian, Greek
See ad on inside front cover

North Aurora

Maplewood Health Care Center
310 Banbury Rd, North Aurora, IL 60542
(708) 892-7627
LICENSURE: Intermediate care; Alzheimer's care.
BEDS: ICF 129.
CERTIFIED: Medicaid.
ADMISSIONS REQUIREMENTS: Medical examination; Physician's request.
STAFF: Physicians 2 (ft); RNs 4 (ft); LPNs 6 (ft); Nurses' aides 40 (ft); Physical therapists 1 (pt); Reality therapists 6 (ft); Recreational therapists 1 (ft); Occupational therapists 1 (pt); Speech therapists 1 (pt); Activities coordinators 3 (ft); Dietitians 1 (ft); Ophthalmologists 1 (pt); Podiatrists 1 (pt).
LANGUAGES: Spanish, Polish

North Riverside

The Scottish Home
2800 Des Plaines Ave, North Riverside, IL 60546
(708) 447-5092, 447-5269 FAX
LICENSURE: Intermediate care; Sheltered care.
BEDS: ICF 14; Sheltered care 49.
ADMISSIONS REQUIREMENTS: Minimum age 62.

Northbrook

Brandel Care Center

2155 Pfingsten Rd, Northbrook, IL 60062
(708) 480-6350
LICENSURE: Skilled care.
BEDS: SNF 102.
CERTIFIED: Medicaid; Medicare.
ADMISSIONS REQUIREMENTS: Minimum age 18; Medical examination; Physician's request.
STAFF: Physicians; RNs; LPNs; Physical therapists; Occupational therapists; Activities coordinators; Dietitians; Social workers; Chaplain; CNAs; Medical director.
See ads pages iv, 300

GAF/Lake Cook Terrace

222 Dennis Dr, Northbrook, IL 60062
(708) 564-0505
LICENSURE: Skilled care; Intermediate care.
BEDS: SNF 90; ICF 50.
CERTIFIED: Medicaid.
ADMISSIONS REQUIREMENTS: Minimum age 50.
STAFF: Physicians 1 (ft), 3 (pt); RNs 6 (ft), 3 (pt); LPNs 4 (ft), 1 (pt); Nurses' aides 31 (ft), 3 (pt); Reality therapists 1 (pt); Occupational therapists 2 (pt); Activities coordinators 1 (ft); Dietitians 1 (pt).

Glen Oaks Nursing Home Inc

270 Skokie Hwy, Northbrook, IL 60062
(708) 498-9320
LICENSURE: Skilled care; Intermediate care.
BEDS: SNF 164; ICF 130.
CERTIFIED: Medicaid; Medicare.
STAFF: Physicians 7 (pt); RNs 38 (ft); LPNs 14 (ft); Nurses' aides 64 (ft), 3 (pt); Physical therapists 5 (ft), 2 (pt); Reality therapists 2 (ft); Recreational therapists 7 (ft); Occupational therapists 1 (ft); Speech therapists 1 (pt); Activities coordinators 1 (ft); Dietitians 1 (pt); Ophthalmologists 1 (pt); Podiatrists 2 (pt); Dentists 1 (pt); Art therapists 1 (ft).

Northlake

Villa Scalabrini

480 N Wolf Rd, Northlake, IL 60164
(708) 562-0040, 562-3955 FAX
LICENSURE: Skilled care; Intermediate care; Alzheimer's care.
BEDS: SNF 120; ICF 62; Alzheimer's 20; Sheltered care 63.
CERTIFIED: Medicaid; Medicare.
ADMISSIONS REQUIREMENTS: Minimum age 60; Medical examination.
STAFF: Physicians; RNs; LPNs; Nurses' aides; Physical therapists; Recreational therapists; Occupational therapists; Speech therapists; Activities coordina-

tors; Dietitians; Ophthalmologists; Podiatrists; Audiologists.
LANGUAGES: Italian

Oak Brook

Oak Brook Healthcare Centre

2013 Midwest Rd, Oak Brook, IL 60521
(708) 495-0220, 495-9150 FAX
LICENSURE: Skilled care; Intermediate care.
BEDS: SNF 110; ICF 28.
CERTIFIED: Medicaid; Medicare.
ADMISSIONS REQUIREMENTS: Minimum age 65; Medical examination.
STAFF: RNs 4 (ft), 2 (pt); LPNs 6 (ft), 5 (pt); Nurses' aides 40 (ft); Physical therapists 1 (ft), 1 (pt); Recreational therapists 1 (pt); Occupational therapists 2 (ft), 1 (pt); Activities coordinators 3 (ft); Dietitians 1 (pt); Ophthalmologists 1 (pt); Podiatrists 1 (pt).
See ad on inside front cover

Oak Lawn

Americana Healthcare Center of Oak Lawn

9401 S Kostner Ave, Oak Lawn, IL 60453
(708) 423-7882, 423-5779 FAX
LICENSURE: Skilled care; Intermediate care; Sub-acute rehab.
BEDS: SNF 143.
CERTIFIED: Medicare.
ADMISSIONS REQUIREMENTS: Minimum age 18; Medical examination; Physician's request.
See ad page 200

Americana-Monticello Healthcare Center of Oak Lawn

6300 W 95th St, Oak Lawn, IL 60453
(708) 599-8800, 598-7135 FAX
LICENSURE: Skilled care; Intermediate care; Alzheimer's care.
BEDS: SNF 130; Alzheimer's 53.
CERTIFIED: Medicare.
ADMISSIONS REQUIREMENTS: Medical examination.
See ad page 200

Concord Extended Care

9401 S Ridgeland Ave, Oak Lawn, IL 60453
(708) 599-6700
LICENSURE: Skilled care; Alzheimer's care.
BEDS: SNF 134.
CERTIFIED: Medicaid; Medicare.
ADMISSIONS REQUIREMENTS: Minimum age 45; Medical examination.
STAFF: Physicians 1 (pt); RNs 4 (ft), 2 (pt); LPNs 7 (ft), 5 (pt); Nurses' aides 30 (ft), 17 (pt); Physical therapists 1 (pt); Recreational therapists 2 (ft), 2 (pt); Occupational therapists 1 (pt); Speech thera-

pists 1 (pt); Dietitians 1 (pt); Ophthalmologists 1 (pt); Podiatrists 1 (pt).
LANGUAGES: Polish, Spanish

Oak Lawn Convalescent Home
9525 S Mayfield, Oak Lawn, IL 60453
(708) 636-7000
LICENSURE: Skilled care; Intermediate care.
BEDS: SNF 75; ICF 68.
CERTIFIED: Medicaid.
ADMISSIONS REQUIREMENTS: Minimum age 18; Medical examination; Physician's request.
STAFF: Physicians; RNs; LPNs; Nurses' aides; Physical therapists; Reality therapists; Occupational therapists; Activities coordinators; Dietitians; Ophthalmologists; Podiatrists; Audiologists.

Oak Park

Metropolitan Nursing Center of Oak Park
625 N Harlem Ave, Oak Park, IL 60302
(708) 848-5966, 848-1257 FAX
LICENSURE: Skilled care; Intermediate care; Alzheimer's care; Respite care.
BEDS: SNF 176; ICF 28.
ADMISSIONS REQUIREMENTS: Minimum age per state regulations.
STAFF: Physicians 15 (pt); RNs 5 (ft); LPNs 15 (ft); Nurses' aides 35 (ft); Physical therapists 1 (pt); Reality therapists 2 (ft), 1 (pt); Recreational therapists 4 (ft); Occupational therapists 1 (ft), 1 (pt); Speech therapists 1 (pt); Activities coordinators; Dietitians 1 (pt); Ophthalmologists 1 (pt); Podiatrists 1 (pt); Audiologists 1 (pt); Social services workers; Dentists.
LANGUAGES: Spanish, Tagalog, Italian

The Woodbine Convalescent Home
6909 W North Ave, Oak Park, IL 60302
(708) 386-1112
LICENSURE: Skilled care.
BEDS: SNF 66.
ADMISSIONS REQUIREMENTS: Minimum age 65; Medical examination.
STAFF: Physicians 2 (ft); RNs 6 (ft), 2 (pt); LPNs 3 (ft), 2 (pt); Nurses' aides 24 (ft); Physical therapists 1 (ft); Speech therapists (consultant); Activities coordinators 2 (ft); Dietitians 1 (pt); Podiatrists 1 (pt).

Oswego

The Tillers Nursing Home
PO Box 950, 4390 Rte 71, Oswego, IL 60543
(708) 554-1001, 554-9650 FAX
LICENSURE: Skilled care; Intermediate care.
BEDS: Swing beds SNF/ICF 85; Sheltered care 14.

ADMISSIONS REQUIREMENTS: Medical examination.
STAFF: Physicians 13 (pt); RNs 5 (ft), 6 (pt); LPNs 1 (ft); Nurses' aides 24 (ft), 15 (pt); Physical therapists 2 (pt); Recreational therapists 1 (ft); Occupational therapists; Activities coordinators 2 (ft), 3 (pt); Dietitians 1 (ft); Podiatrists 1 (pt).

Palatine

Little Sisters of the Poor
80 W Northwest Hwy, Palatine, IL 60067-3580
(708) 358-5700
LICENSURE: Intermediate care; Long-term care nursing.
BEDS: ICF 107.
CERTIFIED: Medicaid.
ADMISSIONS REQUIREMENTS: Medical examination; Must be older adult.
STAFF: Physicians 3 (pt); RNs 6 (ft), 14 (pt); LPNs 1 (ft), 2 (pt); Nurses' aides 21 (ft), 6 (pt).
LANGUAGES: French

Plum Grove Nursing Home
24 S Plum Grove Rd, Palatine, IL 60067
(708) 358-0311, 358-8875 FAX
LICENSURE: Skilled care; Intermediate care; Alzheimer's care.
BEDS: SNF 35; ICF 34.
CERTIFIED: Medicare.
ADMISSIONS REQUIREMENTS: Minimum age 18; Medical examination.
STAFF: RNs; LPNs; Nurses' aides; Physical therapists; Reality therapists; Recreational therapists; Occupational therapists; Speech therapists; Activities coordinators; Dietitians; Ophthalmologists; Podiatrists; Audiologists.
LANGUAGES: Spanish, Polish

Palos Heights

Americana Healthcare Center of Palos Heights
7850 W College Dr, Palos Heights, IL 60463
(708) 361-6990, 361-9512 FAX
LICENSURE: Skilled care; Intermediate care; Alzheimer's care; Long-term residential.
BEDS: SNF 117; Alzheimer's 30; Assisted living facility 30.
CERTIFIED: Medicare.
ADMISSIONS REQUIREMENTS: Medical examination; Physician's orders.
See ad page 200

Rest Haven Central Nursing Home
13259 S Central Ave, Palos Heights, IL 60463
(708) 597-1000, 389-9990 FAX
LICENSURE: Skilled care; Intermediate care.
BEDS: SNF 96; ICF 97.
CERTIFIED: Medicaid; Medicare.
ADMISSIONS REQUIREMENTS: Medical examination.

STAFF: Physicians 12 (pt); RNs 6 (ft), 16 (pt); LPNs 6 (ft), 7 (pt); Nurses' aides 53 (ft), 97 (pt); Physical therapists 1 (pt); Reality therapists 1 (pt); Recreational therapists 1 (pt); Occupational therapists 1 (pt); Speech therapists 1 (pt); Activities coordinators 1 (ft); Dietitians 1 (ft), 1 (pt); Podiatrists 1 (pt).

See ad on page i

Ridgeland Living Center
12550 S Ridgeland Ave, Palos Heights, IL 60463
(708) 597-9300, 371-4818 FAX
LICENSURE: Skilled care.
BEDS: SNF 92.
ADMISSIONS REQUIREMENTS: Minimum age 19; Medical examination; Physician's request.

Palos Hills

Windsor Manor Nursing & Rehabilitation Center
10426 S Roberts Rd, Palos Hills, IL 60465
(708) 598-3460, 598-2520 FAX
LICENSURE: Skilled care; Intermediate care.
BEDS: SNF 83; ICF 120.
CERTIFIED: Medicaid; Medicare; VA.
ADMISSIONS REQUIREMENTS: Medical examination.
STAFF: Physicians 1 (ft), 6 (pt); RNs 4 (ft), 1 (pt); LPNs 11 (ft), 1 (pt); Nurses' aides 8 (pt); Physical therapists 1 (pt); Reality therapists 1 (pt); Recreational therapists 1 (ft); Occupational therapists 1 (pt); Speech therapists 1 (pt); Activities coordinators 1 (ft); Dietitians 1 (ft); Ophthalmologists 1 (pt); Podiatrists 1 (pt); Audiologists 1 (pt).
LANGUAGES: Polish, Spanish

Park Ridge

Park Ridge Healthcare Center
665 Busse Hwy, Park Ridge, IL 60068
(708) 825-5517
LICENSURE: Intermediate care.
BEDS: ICF 49.
ADMISSIONS REQUIREMENTS: Minimum age 21; Medical examination.
STAFF: Physicians 8 (pt); RNs 1 (ft), 1 (pt); LPNs 3 (ft), 2 (pt); Nurses' aides 10 (ft), 5 (pt); Physical therapists 1 (pt); Recreational therapists 1 (ft); Occupational therapists 1 (pt); Speech therapists 1 (pt); Activities coordinators 1 (ft); Dietitians 1 (pt); Ophthalmologists 1 (pt); Social services workers 1 (pt).

Resurrection Nursing Pavilion
1001 N Greenwood Ave, Park Ridge, IL 60068
(708) 692-5600, 692-2305 FAX
LICENSURE: Skilled care.
BEDS: SNF 298.
CERTIFIED: Medicaid; Medicare.

ADMISSIONS REQUIREMENTS: Minimum age 22; Medical examination; Physician's request.
See ads pages 163, 308

St Matthew Lutheran Home
1601 N Western Ave, Park Ridge, IL 60068
(708) 825-5531, 318-6659 FAX
LICENSURE: Skilled care; Intermediate care; Alzheimer's care.
BEDS: SNF 130; ICF 53.
CERTIFIED: Medicaid.
ADMISSIONS REQUIREMENTS: Minimum age 65; Medical examination.
STAFF: Physicians 1 (pt); RNs 13 (ft), 5 (pt); LPNs 4 (ft), 2 (pt); Nurses' aides 46 (ft), 29 (pt); Activities coordinators 1 (ft); Dietitians 1 (pt).

Plainfield

Lakewood Living Center
1112 N Eastern Ave, Plainfield, IL 60544
(815) 436-3400
LICENSURE: Skilled care.
BEDS: SNF 50.
ADMISSIONS REQUIREMENTS: Minimum age 18; Medical examination; Physician's request.
STAFF: Physicians 1 (pt); RNs 2 (ft), 10 (pt); LPNs 2 (pt); Nurses' aides 5 (ft), 21 (pt); Activities coordinators 1 (ft), 2 (pt); Dietitians 1 (pt).

Richton Park

Richton Crossing Convalescent Center
APO Box B345, Imperial Dr & Cicero Ave, Richton Park, IL 60471
(708) 747-6120
LICENSURE: Skilled care; Intermediate care.
BEDS: SNF 142; ICF 152.
CERTIFIED: Medicaid; Medicare.
ADMISSIONS REQUIREMENTS: Medical examination.
STAFF: Physicians 16 (pt); RNs 9 (ft), 6 (pt); LPNs 14 (ft), 10 (pt); Nurses' aides 54 (ft), 13 (pt); Physical therapists 2 (ft), 1 (pt); Reality therapists 2 (ft); Recreational therapists 2 (ft); Occupational therapists 1 (pt); Speech therapists 1 (ft); Activities coordinators 8 (ft); Dietitians 1 (pt); Ophthalmologists 1 (pt); Podiatrists 1 (pt); Dentists 1 (pt).

Riverwoods

Brentwood North Nursing & Rehabilitation Center
3705 Deerfield Rd, Riverwoods, IL 60015
(708) 459-1200, 459-0113 FAX
LICENSURE: Skilled care; Alzheimer's care.
BEDS: Swing beds SNF/ICF/Alzheimer's care 248.
CERTIFIED: Medicare.

✔ In order to support future editions of this publication would you please mention *Elder Services* each time you contact any advertiser, facility, or service.

ADMISSIONS REQUIREMENTS: Minimum age 21; Medical examination; Physician's request.
STAFF: RNs 38 (ft), 27 (pt); LPNs 3 (ft), 3 (pt); Nurses' aides 44 (ft), 13 (pt); Physical therapists 5 (ft), 2 (pt); Recreational therapists 5 (ft), 2 (pt); Occupational therapists 3 (ft), 1 (pt); Activities coordinators 1 (ft); Dietitians 2 (ft).
LANGUAGES: Spanish, German

Robbins

Lydia Healthcare
13901 S Lydia Ave, Robbins, IL 60472
(708) 385-8700, 385-5642 FAX
LICENSURE: Intermediate care.
BEDS: ICF 262.
CERTIFIED: Medicaid; VA.
ADMISSIONS REQUIREMENTS: Minimum age 18; Medical examination.
LANGUAGES: Spanish

Rolling Meadows

Americana Healthcare Center of Rolling Meadows
4225 Kirchoff Rd, Rolling Meadows, IL 60008
(708) 397-2400, 397-2914 FAX
LICENSURE: Skilled care; Intermediate care; Alzheimer's care.
BEDS: SNF 108; Alzheimer's 38.
CERTIFIED: Medicaid; Medicare.
ADMISSIONS REQUIREMENTS: Medical examination.
See ad page 200

Roselle

Abbington House
31 W Central, Roselle, IL 60172
(708) 894-5058
LICENSURE: Intermediate care.
BEDS: ICF 82.
CERTIFIED: Medicaid.
ADMISSIONS REQUIREMENTS: Minimum age 65; Medical examination.
STAFF: Physicians 5 (pt); RNs 3 (ft); LPNs 3 (pt); Nurses' aides 6 (ft), 5 (pt); Physical therapists 1 (pt); Activities coordinators 1 (ft); Dietitians 1 (pt); Ophthalmologists 1 (pt); Dentists 1 (pt).

Round Lake Beach

Hillcrest Nursing Center
1740 N Circuit Dr, Round Lake Beach, IL 60073
(708) 546-5301, 546-7563 FAX
LICENSURE: Intermediate care; Alzheimer's care.

BEDS: ICF 123.
CERTIFIED: Medicaid; VA.
ADMISSIONS REQUIREMENTS: Minimum age 65; Medical examination.
STAFF: Physicians 1 (ft); RNs 3 (ft), 1 (pt); LPNs 7 (ft), 2 (pt); Nurses' aides 20 (ft), 5 (pt); Activities coordinators 1 (ft), 3 (pt); Dietitians 1 (pt); Ophthalmologists 1 (pt); Podiatrists 1 (pt).
See ad page 239

Saint Charles

Pine View Care Center
611 Allen Ln, Saint Charles, IL 60174
(708) 377-2211
LICENSURE: Skilled care.
BEDS: SNF 120.
CERTIFIED: Medicare.
ADMISSIONS REQUIREMENTS: Minimum age 22; Medical examination.
STAFF: Physicians 3 (pt); RNs 8 (ft); LPNs 12 (ft); Nurses' aides 25 (ft); Physical therapists 4 (pt); Occupational therapists 1 (pt); Speech therapists 1 (pt); Activities coordinators 1 (ft); Dietitians 1 (pt); Ophthalmologists 1 (pt); Podiatrists 1 (pt); Dentists 1 (pt).
LANGUAGES: Spanish

Sandwich

Dogwood Health Care Center
902 E Arnold St, Sandwich, IL 60548
(815) 786-8409
LICENSURE: Intermediate care; Retirement.
BEDS: ICF 63; Retirement apartments 20.
CERTIFIED: Medicaid.
ADMISSIONS REQUIREMENTS: Minimum age 55; Medical examination; Physician's request.
STAFF: RNs; LPNs; Nurses' aides; Activities coordinators.

Willow Crest Nursing Pavilion
515 N Main St, Sandwich, IL 60548
(815) 786-8426
LICENSURE: Skilled care; Intermediate care.
BEDS: SNF 58; ICF 58.
CERTIFIED: Medicaid.

Schaumburg

Friendship Village of Schaumburg
350 W Schaumburg Rd, Schaumburg, IL 60194
(708) 884-5005, 843-4271 FAX
LICENSURE: Skilled care; Alzheimer's care; Retirement.
BEDS: SNF 190; Assisted living 76; Retirement apartments 546.
CERTIFIED: Medicaid; Medicare.

ADMISSIONS REQUIREMENTS: Minimum age 62; Medical examination; Physician's request.
STAFF: Physicians 3 (pt); RNs 16 (ft), 14 (pt); LPNs 4 (ft), 2 (pt); Nurses' aides 40 (ft), 36 (pt); Physical therapists 1 (pt); Occupational therapists 1 (pt); Speech therapists 1 (pt); Activities coordinators 2 (ft), 3 (pt); Dietitians 1 (pt); Ophthalmologists 1 (pt); Podiatrists 1 (pt).
See ad page 317

Lexington Health Care Center of Schaumburg
653 S Roselle Rd, Schaumburg, IL 60193
(708) 351-5500
LICENSURE: Skilled care; Intermediate care.
BEDS: SNF 150; ICF 65.

Shabbona

Shabbona Health Care Center Inc
W Comanche Rd, Shabbona, IL 60550
(815) 824-2194, 824-2196 FAX
LICENSURE: Skilled care.
BEDS: SNF 91.
CERTIFIED: Medicaid; Medicare.
ADMISSIONS REQUIREMENTS: Minimum age 50; Medical examination; Physician's request.
STAFF: Physicians 4 (pt); RNs 8 (ft), 2 (pt); LPNs 1

(ft), 1 (pt); Nurses' aides 25 (ft), 12 (pt); Physical therapists 1 (pt); Activities coordinators 2 (ft); Dietitians 1 (pt); Podiatrists 1 (pt).

Skokie

Lieberman Geriatric Health Centre
9700 Gross Point Rd, Skokie, IL 60076
(708) 674-7210, 674-6366 FAX
LICENSURE: Skilled care; Alzheimer's care.
BEDS: SNF 240.
CERTIFIED: Medicaid.
ADMISSIONS REQUIREMENTS: Medical examination.
STAFF: Physicians 3 (pt); RNs 35 (ft); LPNs 10 (ft); Nurses' aides 118 (ft); Physical therapists 1 (pt); Recreational therapists 2 (ft); Speech therapists 1 (pt); Activities coordinators 6 (ft), 1 (pt); Dietitians 1 (ft), 2 (pt); Ophthalmologists 1 (pt); Podiatrists 1 (pt); Audiologists 1 (pt); Social workers 5 (ft), 2 (pt).
LANGUAGES: Yiddish, Hebrew, Russian

Old Orchard Manor
4660 Old Orchard Rd, Skokie, IL 60076
(708) 676-4800
LICENSURE: Skilled care.
BEDS: SNF 61.
ADMISSIONS REQUIREMENTS: Minimum age 22; Medical examination; Physician's request.

✔ In order to support future editions of this publication would you please mention *Elder Services* each time you contact any advertiser, facility, or service.

STAFF: RNs 8 (ft), 5 (pt); LPNs 1 (ft); Nurses' aides 21 (ft), 1 (pt); Physical therapists 2 (pt); Activities coordinators 1 (ft), 3 (pt); Dietitians 1 (pt); Ophthalmologists 1 (pt); Podiatrists 1 (pt).
LANGUAGES: French, German, Polish, Japanese, Chinese, Russian

Skokie Meadows Nursing Center 1
9615 N Knox Ave, Skokie, IL 60076
(708) 679-4161
LICENSURE: Skilled care.
BEDS: SNF 113.
CERTIFIED: Medicaid; Medicare.
ADMISSIONS REQUIREMENTS: Minimum age 20; Medical examination.
STAFF: RNs; LPNs; Nurses' aides; Physical therapists; Reality therapists; Recreational therapists; Occupational therapists; Speech therapists; Activities coordinators; Dietitians; Ophthalmologists; Podiatrists; Audiologists; Dentists.

Skokie Meadows Nursing Center 2
4600 W Golf Rd, Skokie, IL 60076
(708) 679-1157
LICENSURE: Intermediate care.
BEDS: ICF 111.
CERTIFIED: Medicaid.

Village Nursing Home Inc
9000 Lavergne Ave, Skokie, IL 60077
(708) 679-2322
LICENSURE: Skilled care; Intermediate care.
BEDS: SNF 98; ICF 51.
CERTIFIED: Medicaid.

South Chicago Heights

Woodside Manor
120 W 26th St, South Chicago Heights, IL 60411
(708) 756-5200
LICENSURE: Skilled care; Intermediate care.
BEDS: SNF 64; ICF 48.
CERTIFIED: Medicaid.

South Elgin

Alderwood Health Care Center
746 Spring St, South Elgin, IL 60177
(708) 697-0565
LICENSURE: Skilled care; Intermediate care.
BEDS: SNF 14; ICF 76.
CERTIFIED: Medicaid.

Fox Valley Healthcare Inc
759 Kane St, South Elgin, IL 60177
(708) 697-3310
LICENSURE: Skilled care; Intermediate care.
BEDS: SNF 107; ICF 99.

CERTIFIED: Medicaid; Medicare.
ADMISSIONS REQUIREMENTS: Minimum age 18.
STAFF: RNs 10 (ft); LPNs 2 (ft); Nurses' aides 30 (ft); Physical therapists 1 (ft); Occupational therapists 1 (pt); Speech therapists 1 (pt); Activities coordinators 1 (ft).
LANGUAGES: French, Italian, Polish

South Holland

Americana Healthcare Center of South Holland
2145 E 170th St, South Holland, IL 60473
(708) 895-3255, 895-3867 FAX
LICENSURE: Skilled care; Intermediate care; Alzheimer's care.
BEDS: SNF 150; Alzheimer's 30.
CERTIFIED: Medicare.
ADMISSIONS REQUIREMENTS: Medical examination.
See ad page 200

Rest Haven South
16300 Wausau Ave, South Holland, IL 60473
(708) 596-5500, 596-6527 FAX
LICENSURE: Skilled care; Intermediate care; Alzheimer's care; Day care.
BEDS: SNF 86; ICF 50; Alzheimer's 30.
CERTIFIED: Medicare.
ADMISSIONS REQUIREMENTS: Minimum age 60; Medical examination.
STAFF: Physicians 8 (pt); RNs 8 (ft), 12 (pt); LPNs 3 (ft), 5 (pt); Nurses' aides 26 (ft), 53 (pt); Physical therapists 3 (pt); Occupational therapists 1 (pt); Speech therapists 1 (pt); Activities coordinators 2 (ft), 1 (pt); Dietitians 1 (ft); Ophthalmologists 1 (pt); Podiatrists 1 (pt); Audiologists 1 (pt).
LANGUAGES: Spanish, Dutch
See ad on page i

Windmill Nursing Pavilion Ltd
16000 S Wabash Ave, South Holland, IL 60473
(708) 339-0600
LICENSURE: Skilled care; Intermediate care; Alzheimer's care.
BEDS: SNF 100; ICF 50.
CERTIFIED: Medicaid.
ADMISSIONS REQUIREMENTS: Minimum age 21; Physician's request.
STAFF: Physicians; RNs; LPNs; Nurses' aides; Physical therapists; Occupational therapists; Speech therapists; Activities coordinators; Dietitians; Ophthalmologists; Podiatrists; Dentists.

Stickney

Pershing Convalescent Home Inc
3900 S Oak Park Ave, Stickney, IL 60402
(708) 484-7543, 484-7586 FAX
LICENSURE: Intermediate care.
BEDS: ICF 51.

CERTIFIED: Medicaid.
STAFF: Physicians (consultant); RNs 3 (ft); LPNs 4 (pt); Nurses' aides 8 (ft), 3 (pt); Physical therapists (consultant); Speech therapists (consultant); Dietitians (consultant); Ophthalmologists (consultant); Podiatrists (consultant); Audiologists (consultant).

Tinley Park

The McAllister Nursing Home Inc
18300 S Lavergne Ave, Tinley Park, IL 60477
(708) 798-2272
LICENSURE: Skilled care; Intermediate care.
BEDS: SNF 59; ICF 42.
CERTIFIED: Medicaid; Medicare.
ADMISSIONS REQUIREMENTS: Minimum age 18; Medical examination; Physician's request.
STAFF: Physicians 2 (pt); RNs 6 (ft), 2 (pt); LPNs 5 (ft), 2 (pt); Physical therapists 1 (ft), 1 (pt); Reality therapists 1 (pt); Recreational therapists 2 (ft); Occupational therapists 1 (ft), 1 (pt); Speech therapists 1 (pt); Activities coordinators 1 (pt); Dietitians 1 (ft), 1 (pt); Ophthalmologists 1 (pt); Audiologists 1 (pt); Dentists 1 (pt).

Wauconda

Town Hall Estates—Wauconda Inc
176 Thomas Ct, Wauconda, IL 60084
(708) 526-5551, 526-4231 FAX
LICENSURE: Intermediate care.
BEDS: ICF 98.
CERTIFIED: Medicaid.
ADMISSIONS REQUIREMENTS: Physician's request.
STAFF: Physicians 10 (pt); RNs 3 (ft), 2 (pt); LPNs 2 (ft); Nurses' aides 15 (ft); Physical therapists 1 (pt); Reality therapists 1 (ft); Recreational therapists 1 (pt); Activities coordinators 2 (ft); Dietitians 1 (pt); Podiatrists 1 (pt).

Waukegan

Bayside Terrace
1100 S Lewis Ave, Waukegan, IL 60085
(708) 244-8196, 244-7647 FAX
LICENSURE: Intermediate care; ICF/MI.
BEDS: Total 168.
CERTIFIED: Medicaid; VA.
ADMISSIONS REQUIREMENTS: Minimum age 21; Medical examination; Physician's request.
STAFF: Physicians 3 (pt); RNs 1 (ft); LPNs 11 (ft), 3 (pt); Nurses' aides 30 (ft), 4 (pt); Activities coordinators 5 (ft); Dietitians 1 (pt); Podiatrists 1 (pt).
See ad page 239

Lake Park Center
919 Washington Park, Waukegan, IL 60085
(708) 623-9100
LICENSURE: Intermediate care.
BEDS: ICF 210.
CERTIFIED: Medicaid.
ADMISSIONS REQUIREMENTS: Mental illness.

Northshore Terrace
2222 14th St, Waukegan, IL 60085
(708) 249-2400, 249-8409 FAX
LICENSURE: Skilled care; Intermediate care.
BEDS: SNF 125; ICF 146.
CERTIFIED: Medicaid.
ADMISSIONS REQUIREMENTS: Minimum age 30.
STAFF: Physicians 10 (pt); RNs 16 (ft); LPNs 8 (ft); Nurses' aides 70 (ft), 8 (pt); Physical therapists 1 (pt); Reality therapists 1 (pt); Recreational therapists 1 (pt); Occupational therapists 1 (pt); Speech therapists 1 (pt); Activities coordinators 1 (ft); Dietitians 1 (ft); Ophthalmologists 1 (pt); Podiatrists 1 (pt); Audiologists 1 (pt); Dentists 1 (pt).
LANGUAGES: Polish, Spanish

Pavilion of Waukegan Inc
2217 Washington St, Waukegan, IL 60085
(708) 244-4100
LICENSURE: Skilled care.
BEDS: SNF 99.
CERTIFIED: Medicaid; Medicare.

The Terrace Nursing Home Inc
1615 Sunset Ave, Waukegan, IL 60087
(708) 244-6700
LICENSURE: Skilled care.
BEDS: SNF 112.
CERTIFIED: Medicaid; Medicare; VA.
ADMISSIONS REQUIREMENTS: Minimum age 18; Medical examination.
STAFF: Physicians 17 (pt); RNs 12 (ft), 2 (pt); LPNs 4 (ft), 3 (pt); Nurses' aides 38 (ft), 7 (pt); Physical therapists 1 (pt); Reality therapists 2 (ft); Recreational therapists 1 (ft); Occupational therapists 2 (pt); Speech therapists 1 (pt); Activities coordinators 1 (ft); Dietitians 1 (pt); Ophthalmologists 1 (pt); Podiatrists 1 (pt); Dentists 1 (pt).
LANGUAGES: Spanish

West Chicago

Arbor Terrace Health Care Center
30 W 300 North Ave, West Chicago, IL 60185
(708) 231-4050, 231-1278 FAX
LICENSURE: Skilled care; Intermediate care; Assisted & independent living.
BEDS: SNF 70; ICF 70; Hospice & respite care 44; Retirement 178.
CERTIFIED: Medicaid; Medicare.

ADMISSIONS REQUIREMENTS: Minimum age 18; Medical examination.
STAFF: RNs; LPNs; Nurses' aides; Physical therapists; Recreational therapists; Activities coordinators.

West Chicago Terrace
928 Joliet Rd, West Chicago, IL 60185
(708) 231-9292, 231-6797 FAX
LICENSURE: Intermediate care.
BEDS: ICF 120.
CERTIFIED: Medicaid.
STAFF: Physicians 2 (pt); RNs 2 (ft), 1 (pt); LPNs 4 (ft), 2 (pt); Nurses' aides 27 (ft), 2 (pt); Physical therapists 1 (pt); Recreational therapists 1 (pt); Occupational therapists 1 (pt); Speech therapists 1 (pt); Activities coordinators 3 (ft), 1 (pt); Dietitians 1 (pt); Ophthalmologists 1 (pt); Podiatrists 1 (pt); Audiologists 1 (pt).

Westchester

Westchester Manor
2901 S Wolf Rd, Westchester, IL 60154
(708) 531-1441, 409-1271 FAX
LICENSURE: Skilled care.
BEDS: SNF 120.
CERTIFIED: Medicare.

Westmont

Americana Healthcare Center of Westmont
512 E Ogden Ave, Westmont, IL 60559
(708) 323-4400, 323-2083 FAX
LICENSURE: Skilled care; Intermediate care; Alzheimer's care.
BEDS: SNF 97; Alzheimer's 30.
CERTIFIED: Medicaid; Medicare.
ADMISSIONS REQUIREMENTS: Medical examination; Physician's request.
See ad page 200

Burgess Square Healthcare Centre
5801 S Cass Ave, Westmont, IL 60559
(708) 971-2645
LICENSURE: Skilled care; Intermediate care.
BEDS: SNF 106; ICF 105.
CERTIFIED: Medicaid; Medicare.
ADMISSIONS REQUIREMENTS: Minimum age 50; Medical examination; Physician's request.
STAFF: RNs 3 (ft); LPNs 9 (ft), 4 (pt); Nurses' aides 37 (ft), 9 (pt); Activities coordinators 4 (ft), 2 (pt).
LANGUAGES: Polish, Spanish, German

Westmont Convalescent Center
6501 S Cass Ave, Westmont, IL 60559
(708) 960-2026
LICENSURE: Skilled care; Intermediate care; Alzheimer's care.

BEDS: SNF 108; ICF 107.
CERTIFIED: Medicaid; Medicare.
ADMISSIONS REQUIREMENTS: Minimum age 60.
STAFF: Physicians; RNs; LPNs; Nurses' aides; Physical therapists; Occupational therapists; Speech therapists; Activities coordinators; Dietitians; Ophthalmologists; Podiatrists; Dentists.
LANGUAGES: Polish, Spanish

Wheaton

Du Page Convalescent Center
PO Box 708, 400 N County Farm Rd, Wheaton, IL 60187
(708) 665-6400
LICENSURE: Skilled care.
BEDS: SNF 408.
CERTIFIED: Medicaid.
ADMISSIONS REQUIREMENTS: Minimum age 18.
STAFF: Physicians; RNs; LPNs; Nurses' aides; Physical therapists; Recreational therapists; Occupational therapists; Speech therapists; Activities coordinators; Dietitians; Ophthalmologists; Podiatrists.

Parkway Healthcare Center
219 E Parkway Dr, Wheaton, IL 60187
(708) 668-4635, 690-0260 FAX
LICENSURE: Skilled care; Intermediate care; Alzheimer's care.
BEDS: SNF 14; ICF 35; Medicare 20.
CERTIFIED: Medicaid; Medicare.
ADMISSIONS REQUIREMENTS: Minimum age 60; Medical examination; Physician's request.
STAFF: RNs 5 (ft); LPNs 6 (ft); Nurses' aides 21 (ft); Physical therapists 3 (ft); Occupational therapists 2 (ft); Speech therapists 2 (ft); Activities coordinators 2 (ft); Dietitians 1 (ft); Ophthalmologists 1 (pt); Podiatrists 1 (pt); Audiologists 1 (pt).
LANGUAGES: Spanish

Sandalwood Healthcare Centre
2180 W Manchester Rd, Wheaton, IL 60187
(708) 665-4330
LICENSURE: Skilled care; Intermediate care; Alzheimer's care.
BEDS: SNF 106; ICF 103.
CERTIFIED: Medicaid; Medicare.
ADMISSIONS REQUIREMENTS: Minimum age 55; Medical examination.
STAFF: Physicians 37 (ft); RNs 9 (ft), 3 (pt); LPNs 6 (ft), 3 (pt); Nurses' aides 39 (ft), 6 (pt).

Wheaton Convalescent Center
1325 Manchester Rd, Wheaton, IL 60187
(708) 668-2500
LICENSURE: Skilled care; Intermediate care.
BEDS: SNF 82; ICF 41.
CERTIFIED: Medicaid.

Wheeling

Addolorata Villa
555 McHenry Rd, Wheeling, IL 60090
(708) 537-2900, 215-5805 FAX
LICENSURE: Skilled care; Intermediate care; Alzheimer's care; Sheltered care.
BEDS: SNF 20; ICF 60; Sheltered care 45.
CERTIFIED: Medicaid.
ADMISSIONS REQUIREMENTS: Minimum age 60; Medical examination.
STAFF: Physicians 4 (pt); RNs 5 (ft), 6 (pt); LPNs 2 (ft), 1 (pt); Nurses' aides 12 (ft), 5 (pt); Physical therapists 1 (pt); Occupational therapists 1 (pt); Speech therapists 1 (pt); Activities coordinators 1 (ft); Dietitians 1 (ft); Podiatrists 1 (pt).
LANGUAGES: Polish, Italian, Spanish

Willowbrook

Chateau Village Living Center
7050 Madison St, Willowbrook, IL 60521
(708) 323-6380, 323-6387 FAX
LICENSURE: Skilled care; Intermediate care.
BEDS: SNF 100; ICF 50.
CERTIFIED: Medicare.
ADMISSIONS REQUIREMENTS: Minimum age 18; Medical examination.
STAFF: Physicians 4 (pt); RNs 5 (ft); LPNs 11 (ft); Nurses' aides 31 (ft), 5 (pt); Physical therapists 2 (pt); Reality therapists 1 (ft); Recreational therapists 1 (ft); Occupational therapists 1 (pt); Speech therapists 1 (pt); Activities coordinators 3 (ft); Dietitians 1 (pt); Ophthalmologists 1 (pt); Podiatrists 1 (pt); Audiologists 1 (pt).
LANGUAGES: Spanish, German, Polish, Lithuanian

Wilmette

Normandy House
432 Poplar Dr, Wilmette, IL 60091
(708) 256-5000
LICENSURE: Skilled care; Intermediate care; Alzheimer's care.
BEDS: SNF 28; ICF 26; Alzheimer's 26.
ADMISSIONS REQUIREMENTS: Minimum age 22; Medical examination; Physician's request.
STAFF: Physicians 2 (pt); RNs 10 (ft), 8 (pt); LPNs 2 (ft); Nurses' aides 20 (ft); Physical therapists 1 (pt); Speech therapists 1 (pt); Activities coordinators 1 (ft), 3 (pt); Dietitians 1 (pt); Podiatrists 3 (pt).

Wilmington

Royal Willow Nursing Care Center
555 Kahler Rd, Wilmington, IL 60481
(815) 476-7931
LICENSURE: Skilled care; Intermediate care.
BEDS: SNF 98; ICF 98.
CERTIFIED: Medicaid; Medicare.
ADMISSIONS REQUIREMENTS: Medical examination.
STAFF: Physicians; RNs; LPNs; Nurses' aides; Physical therapists; Occupational therapists; Speech therapists; Activities coordinators; Dietitians; Ophthalmologists; Podiatrists.

Winfield

Liberty Hill Healthcare Center
28 W 141 Liberty Rd, Winfield, IL 60190
(708) 668-2928
LICENSURE: Intermediate care; Alzheimer's care; Retirement.
BEDS: ICF 115.
CERTIFIED: Medicaid.
ADMISSIONS REQUIREMENTS: Minimum age 55.
STAFF: Physicians 4 (ft); RNs 8 (ft); LPNs 9 (ft), 2 (pt); Nurses' aides 16 (ft); Physical therapists 2 (ft); Reality therapists 2 (ft); Recreational therapists 2 (ft); Occupational therapists 1 (ft); Activities coordinators 2 (ft); Dietitians 1 (pt); Ophthalmologists 1 (pt); Podiatrists 1 (pt); Dentists 1 (pt).
LANGUAGES: Spanish, Polish

Woodstock

Sunset Manor
PO Box 520, 920 N Seminary Ave, Woodstock, IL 60098
(815) 338-1749, 338-0062 FAX
LICENSURE: Skilled care; Intermediate care; Alzheimer's care; Sheltered care.
BEDS: SNF 29; ICF 46; Sheltered care 63.
CERTIFIED: Medicaid.
ADMISSIONS REQUIREMENTS: Minimum age 60; Medical examination.
STAFF: RNs 7 (ft), 1 (pt); LPNs 5 (ft), 2 (pt); Nurses' aides 25 (ft), 5 (pt); Activities coordinators 2 (ft), 5 (pt).

Valley Hi Nursing Home
2406 Hartland Rd, Woodstock, IL 60098
(815) 338-0312
LICENSURE: Skilled care; Intermediate care.
BEDS: SNF 97; ICF 20.
CERTIFIED: Medicaid.
ADMISSIONS REQUIREMENTS: Minimum age 18; Medical examination; Physician's request.
STAFF: RNs 9 (ft), 5 (pt); LPNs 3 (ft); Nurses' aides 28 (ft), 4 (pt); Activities coordinators 1 (ft).

✔ In order to support future editions of this publication would you please mention *Elder Services* each time you contact any advertiser, facility, or service.

The Woodstock Residence
309 McHenry Rd, Woodstock, IL 60098
(815) 338-1700
LICENSURE: Skilled care.
BEDS: SNF 114.
CERTIFIED: Medicaid; Medicare.
ADMISSIONS REQUIREMENTS: Minimum age 21; Medical examination; Physician's request.
STAFF: Physicians 1 (ft), 12 (pt); RNs 15 (ft); LPNs 1 (ft); Nurses' aides 44 (ft), 4 (pt); Physical therapists 3 (ft), 1 (pt); Reality therapists 2 (ft), 1 (pt); Recreational therapists 2 (ft), 1 (pt); Occupational therapists 2 (ft); Speech therapists 1 (ft); Activities coordinators 3 (ft); Dietitians 1 (ft); Ophthalmologists 1 (pt); Podiatrists 1 (pt); Dentists 1 (pt).

Yorkville

Hillside Health Care Center
PO Box 459, Rte 34 & Game Farm Rd, Yorkville, IL 60560
(708) 553-5811, 553-6155 FAX
LICENSURE: Skilled care.
BEDS: SNF 79.
CERTIFIED: Medicaid; Medicare.
ADMISSIONS REQUIREMENTS: Minimum age 18; Medical examination.
STAFF: Physicians; RNs; LPNs; Nurses' aides; Physical therapists; Recreational therapists; Occupational therapists; Speech therapists; Activities coordinators; Dietitians; Ophthalmologists; Podiatrists.

Zion

Crown Manor Healthcare Center
1805 27th St, Zion, IL 60099
(708) 746-3736, 746-7218 FAX
LICENSURE: Skilled care; Alzheimer's care.
BEDS: SNF 113.
CERTIFIED: Medicaid; Medicare; VA.
ADMISSIONS REQUIREMENTS: Minimum age 18; Medical examination.
STAFF: Physicians; RNs 2 (ft), 4 (pt); LPNs 7 (ft), 8 (pt); Nurses' aides 54 (ft), 17 (pt); Recreational therapists 1 (ft); Speech therapists 1 (pt); Activities coordinators 3 (ft), 2 (pt); Podiatrists 1 (pt).
LANGUAGES: Spanish

Rolling Hills Manor
3615 16th St, Zion, IL 60099
(708) 746-8382
LICENSURE: Skilled care.
BEDS: SNF 135.
CERTIFIED: Medicaid; Medicare.
ADMISSIONS REQUIREMENTS: Minimum age 63; Medical examination.
STAFF: RNs 3 (ft), 3 (pt); LPNs 8 (ft), 4 (pt); Nurses' aides 33 (ft), 1 (pt); Physical therapists 1 (pt); Reality therapists 1 (pt); Recreational therapists 2

(ft); Occupational therapists 1 (pt); Speech therapists 1 (pt); Activities coordinators 1 (ft); Dietitians 1 (pt); Ophthalmologists 1 (pt); Podiatrists 1 (pt); Dentists 1 (pt).
LANGUAGES: Slovak

Sheridan Health Care Center
2534 Elim Ave, Zion, IL 60099
(708) 746-8435, 746-1744 FAX
LICENSURE: Skilled care; Intermediate care.
BEDS: SNF 95; ICF 193.
CERTIFIED: Medicaid; Medicare.
ADMISSIONS REQUIREMENTS: Minimum age 40; Medical examination.
STAFF: Physicians; RNs; LPNs; Nurses' aides; Physical therapists; Recreational therapists; Occupational therapists; Speech therapists; Activities coordinators; Dietitians; Ophthalmologists.

INDIANA

Chesterton

Chesterton Health Care Facility
PO Box 598, 1620 S Country Rd 100 E, Chesterton, IN 46304
(219) 926-8387
LICENSURE: Skilled care; Intermediate care.
BEDS: SNF 53; ICF 47.

Crown Point

Colonial Nursing Home
119 N Indiana Ave, Crown Point, IN 46307
(219) 663-2532, 663-2533 FAX
LICENSURE: Intermediate care.
BEDS: ICF 40.
CERTIFIED: Medicare.
STAFF: Physicians 1 (pt); RNs 1 (ft); LPNs 2 (ft), 3 (pt); Nurses' aides 14 (ft), 8 (pt); Activities coordinators 1 (ft); Dietitians 1 (ft); Podiatrists 1 (pt).

Lake County Convalescent Home
2900 W 93rd Ave, Crown Point, IN 46307
(219) 663-5118, 769-1708 FAX
LICENSURE: Skilled care; Intermediate care; Alzheimer's care; Residential care.
BEDS: SNF 45; ICF 405; Residential care 34.
CERTIFIED: Medicaid; Medicare.
ADMISSIONS REQUIREMENTS: Minimum age 18; Medical examination.
STAFF: Physicians 1 (ft), 3 (pt); RNs 16 (ft), 7 (pt); LPNs 15 (ft), 1 (pt); Nurses' aides 161 (ft), 15 (pt); Physical therapists; Recreational therapists 6 (ft), 1 (pt); Activities coordinators 1 (ft); Dietitians 1 (pt); Pharmacists 1 (ft), 1 (pt); Pharmacy techni-

cians 2 (ft); Lab technicians 1 (ft).
LANGUAGES: Polish, German, Serbo-Croatian, Lithuanian, Italian, Spanish

Lutheran Home of Northwest Indiana Inc
1200 E Luther Dr, Crown Point, IN 46307-5099
(219) 663-3860, 769-1145 Merrillville, (312) 895-8866
    Chicago, (219) 662-3070 FAX
LICENSURE: Intermediate care; Retirement.
BEDS: ICF 191.
CERTIFIED: Medicaid.
ADMISSIONS REQUIREMENTS: Medical examination.
STAFF: Physicians 2 (pt); RNs 5 (ft), 8 (pt); LPNs 4
    (ft), 2 (pt); Nurses' aides 32 (ft), 24 (pt); Physical
    therapists 1 (pt); Recreational therapists 3 (ft), 2
    (pt); Occupational therapists 1 (pt); Speech thera-
    pists 1 (pt); Activities coordinators 1 (ft); Dieti-
    tians 1 (pt); Podiatrists 1 (pt).

St Anthony Home
Main & Franciscan Rd, Crown Point, IN 46307
(219) 663-8100, 757-6365 FAX
LICENSURE: Skilled care; Intermediate care; Alzheimer's
    care.
BEDS: SNF 31; ICF 160; Alzheimer's 38.
CERTIFIED: Medicaid; Medicare.
STAFF: Physicians 1 (ft); RNs 15 (ft); LPNs 15 (ft);
    Nurses' aides 110 (ft); Recreational therapists 3
    (ft); Dietitians 1 (ft).
See ad page 245

Demotte

Lake Holiday Manor
PO Box 230, 10325 County Line Rd, Demotte, IN
    46372
(219) 345-5211, 345-2465 FAX
LICENSURE: Intermediate care; Alzheimer's care; Resi-
    dential care.
BEDS: Total 115.
CERTIFIED: Medicaid.
ADMISSIONS REQUIREMENTS: Minimum age 18; Medical
    examination; Physician's request.
STAFF: RNs 2 (ft); LPNs 1 (ft), 2 (pt); Nurses' aides 20
    (ft), 20 (pt); Activities coordinators 1 (ft), 1 (pt);
    Dietitians 1 (pt).

Dyer

Meridian Nursing Center—Dyer
601 Sheffield Ave, Dyer, IN 46311
(219) 322-2273
LICENSURE: Skilled care; Intermediate care.
BEDS: SNF 70; ICF 58.
CERTIFIED: Medicaid; Medicare.
ADMISSIONS REQUIREMENTS: Minimum age 21.

Our Lady of Mercy Hospital Transitional Care Center
US Hwy 30, Dyer, IN 46311-1799
(219) 865-2141
LICENSURE: Skilled care.
BEDS: SNF 20.

Regency Place
2300 Great Lakes Dr, Dyer, IN 46311
(219) 322-3555
LICENSURE: Skilled care; Intermediate care; Comprehen-
    sive care.
BEDS: SNF 52; ICF 92; Comprehensive care 6.
STAFF: RNs; LPNs; Nurses' aides.

East Chicago

Lake County Rehabilitation Center Inc
5025 McCook Ave, East Chicago, IN 46312
(219) 397-0380
LICENSURE: Skilled care; Intermediate care.
BEDS: SNF 60; ICF 62.
CERTIFIED: Medicaid; Medicare.
ADMISSIONS REQUIREMENTS: Minimum age 18; Medical
    examination; Physician's request.

✓ In order to support future editions of this publication would you please mention *Elder Services* each time you contact
any advertiser, facility, or service.

STAFF: Physicians 3 (pt); RNs 2 (ft), 3 (pt); LPNs 5 (ft), 6 (pt); Nurses' aides 29 (ft), 3 (pt); Physical therapists; Activities coordinators 2 (ft); Dietitians 1 (pt).
LANGUAGES: Spanish

Gary

Green's Geriatric Health Center
2052 Delaware St, Gary, IN 46407
(219) 886-1511
LICENSURE: Intermediate care; Retirement.
BEDS: ICF 35.
CERTIFIED: Medicaid.
ADMISSIONS REQUIREMENTS: Medical examination; Physician's request.
STAFF: Physicians; RNs; LPNs 8 (ft); Nurses' aides 12 (ft), 8 (pt); Activities coordinators 1 (ft); Dietitians 1 (pt); Podiatrists 1 (pt).

Simmons Loving Care Health Facility
PO Box 1675, 700 E 21st Ave, Gary, IN 46407
(219) 886-9029
LICENSURE: Intermediate care.
BEDS: ICF 46.
CERTIFIED: Medicaid.

West Side Health Care Center
353 Tyler St, Gary, IN 46402
(219) 886-7070, 886-0810 FAX
LICENSURE: Skilled care; Intermediate care.
BEDS: Total 214.
CERTIFIED: Medicaid; VA.
STAFF: RNs 3 (ft), 2 (pt); LPNs 13 (ft), 4 (pt); Nurses' aides 51 (ft), 14 (pt); Recreational therapists 2 (ft); Occupational therapists 1 (pt); Activities coordinators 1 (ft); Dietitians 1 (pt).
LANGUAGES: Spanish

Wildwood Manor—Clark
1964 Clark Rd, Gary, IN 46404
(219) 949-9640
LICENSURE: Skilled care; Intermediate care.
BEDS: SNF 82; ICF 38.
CERTIFIED: Medicaid; Medicare.
ADMISSIONS REQUIREMENTS: Minimum age 21; Medical examination; Physician's request.
STAFF: Physicians 5 (pt); RNs 3 (ft), 1 (pt); LPNs 12 (ft), 2 (pt); Nurses' aides 41 (ft), 10 (pt); Physical therapists 1 (pt); Occupational therapists 2 (pt); Activities coordinators 2 (ft); Dietitians 1 (ft), 2 (pt); Ophthalmologists 1 (pt).

Wildwood Manor—Mount
386 Mount St, Gary, IN 46406
(219) 949-5600
LICENSURE: Intermediate care.
BEDS: ICF 69.
CERTIFIED: Medicaid.
ADMISSIONS REQUIREMENTS: Minimum age 18; Medical examination; Physician's request.

STAFF: Physicians 2 (pt); RNs 1 (ft); LPNs 4 (ft), 3 (pt); Nurses' aides 18 (ft), 5 (pt); Physical therapists 1 (pt); Occupational therapists 1 (pt); Speech therapists 1 (pt); Activities coordinators 1 (ft); Dietitians 1 (pt); Ophthalmologists 1 (pt); Podiatrists 1 (pt); Dentists 1 (pt).
LANGUAGES: Spanish

Hammond

Hammond Nursing Home
1402 E 173rd St, Hammond, IN 46324
(219) 844-4534
LICENSURE: Intermediate care.
BEDS: ICF 40.
CERTIFIED: Medicaid.

Highland

Highland Nursing Home
9630 5th St, Highland, IN 46322
(219) 924-6953, 922-1957
LICENSURE: Intermediate care.
BEDS: ICF 40.
CERTIFIED: Medicaid.
ADMISSIONS REQUIREMENTS: Medical examination; Physician's request.
STAFF: Physicians 1 (pt); RNs 1 (pt); LPNs 6 (ft); Nurses' aides 12 (ft), 6 (pt); Activities coordinators 1 (pt); Dietitians 1 (pt).
LANGUAGES: Spanish

Hobart

Miller's Merry Manor
2901 W 37th Ave, Hobart, IN 46342
(219) 942-2170
LICENSURE: Skilled care; Intermediate care.
BEDS: SNF 31; ICF 129.
CERTIFIED: Medicaid; Medicare.
ADMISSIONS REQUIREMENTS: Minimum age 18; Medical examination; Physician's request.
STAFF: Physicians 1 (pt); RNs 10 (ft), 2 (pt); LPNs 3 (ft), 9 (pt); Nurses' aides 29 (ft), 29 (pt); Physical therapists 1 (pt); Occupational therapists 1 (pt); Speech therapists 1 (pt); Activities coordinators 2 (ft), 1 (pt); Dietitians 1 (pt); Ophthalmologists 1 (pt); Podiatrists 1 (pt); Dentists 1 (pt); Medication aides 8 (ft), 3 (pt).
LANGUAGES: Spanish

Sebo's Heritage Manor
4410 W 49th Ave, Hobart, IN 46342
(219) 947-1507, 942-3279 FAX
LICENSURE: Intermediate care; Alzheimer's care.
BEDS: ICF 54.

CERTIFIED: Medicaid; VA.
ADMISSIONS REQUIREMENTS: Minimum age 21; Medical examination; Physician's request.
STAFF: Physicians 2 (pt); RNs 2 (ft), 2 (pt); LPNs 3 (ft), 3 (pt); Nurses' aides 12 (ft), 6 (pt); Recreational therapists 1 (pt); Activities coordinators 1 (ft); Dietitians 1 (pt); Ophthalmologists 1 (pt); Podiatrists 1 (pt).
LANGUAGES: Spanish, Slavic languages

La Porte

Continuing Care Center of La Porte
1007 Lincolnway, La Porte, IN 46350
(219) 326-1234
LICENSURE: Skilled care; Intermediate care.
BEDS: SNF 36; ICF 9.

Countryside Place
1700 I St, La Porte, IN 46350
(219) 362-6234
LICENSURE: Skilled care; Intermediate care.
BEDS: SNF 39; ICF 60.
CERTIFIED: Medicaid; Medicare.

Fountainview Terrace
1900 Andrew Ave, La Porte, IN 46350
(219) 362-7014
LICENSURE: Skilled care; Intermediate care; Residential care.
BEDS: SNF 64; ICF 114; Residential care 16.
CERTIFIED: Medicaid; Medicare.
ADMISSIONS REQUIREMENTS: Medical examination; Physician's request.
STAFF: RNs 6 (ft), 1 (pt); LPNs 5 (ft), 2 (pt); Nurses' aides 35 (ft), 25 (pt); Physical therapists 1 (pt); Speech therapists 1 (pt); Activities coordinators 1 (ft); Dietitians 1 (pt).
LANGUAGES: Spanish, German, Polish

Lowell

Lowell Health Care Center
255 Burnham St, Lowell, IN 46356
(219) 696-7791
LICENSURE: Intermediate care; Comprehensive care.
BEDS: ICF 100; Comprehensive care 44.
CERTIFIED: Medicaid.
ADMISSIONS REQUIREMENTS: Minimum age 18; Medical examination.
STAFF: Physicians 1 (ft), 2 (pt); RNs 3 (ft), 1 (pt); LPNs 6 (ft); Nurses' aides 20 (ft), 20 (pt); Activities coordinators 1 (ft), 1 (pt); Dietitians 1 (ft); Ophthalmologists 1 (pt); Podiatrists 1 (pt).

Merrillville

Lincolnshire Health Care Center
8380 Virginia St, Merrillville, IN 46410
(219) 769-9009
LICENSURE: Intermediate care.
BEDS: ICF 100.

Merrillville Manor
601 W 61st Ave, Merrillville, IN 46410
(219) 980-5950
LICENSURE: Skilled care; Intermediate care.
BEDS: SNF 120; ICF 60.
CERTIFIED: Medicaid; Medicare.

Southlake Care Center
8800 Virginia Pl, Merrillville, IN 46410
(219) 736-1310
LICENSURE: Intermediate care; Residential care.
BEDS: ICF 223; Residential care 6.

Towne Centre
7250 Arthur Blvd, Merrillville, IN 46410
(219) 736-2900, 736-2209 FAX
LICENSURE: Skilled care; Intermediate care; Assisted living; Retirement care.
BEDS: SNF 28; ICF 36; Assisted living 34; Retirement apts 148.
CERTIFIED: Medicaid; Medicare.
ADMISSIONS REQUIREMENTS: Minimum age 65; Medical examination; Physician's request.
STAFF: Physicians 4 (pt); RNs 3 (ft); LPNs 3 (ft), 3 (pt); Nurses' aides 20 (ft), 20 (pt); Physical therapists 1 (pt); Occupational therapists 1 (pt); Speech therapists 1 (pt); Activities coordinators 1 (ft), 2 (pt); Dietitians 1 (ft), 1 (pt); Ophthalmologists 1 (pt); Podiatrists 1 (pt); Audiologists 1 (pt).

Michigan City

Life Care Center of Michigan City
802 US Hwy 20 E, Michigan City, IN 46360
(219) 872-7251
LICENSURE: Intermediate care.
BEDS: ICF 129.
CERTIFIED: Medicaid.

Michigan City Health Care
1101 E Coolspring Ave, Michigan City, IN 46360
(219) 874-5211
LICENSURE: Skilled care; Intermediate care; Alzheimer's care.
BEDS: SNF 66; ICF 198.
CERTIFIED: Medicaid; Medicare.
ADMISSIONS REQUIREMENTS: Medical examination.
STAFF: Physicians 1 (ft); RNs 7 (ft), 5 (pt); LPNs; Nurses' aides; Physical therapists 1 (ft); Reality therapists; Recreational therapists 1 (ft); Occupa-

tional therapists 1 (ft); Speech therapists 2 (ft); Activities coordinators 1 (ft); Dietitians 2 (ft); Ophthalmologists; Podiatrists 1 (ft).

Red Oaks Healthcare Center

910 S Carroll Ave, Michigan City, IN 46360
(219) 872-0696
LICENSURE: Skilled care; Intermediate care.
BEDS: SNF 58; ICF 58.
CERTIFIED: Medicaid; Medicare.
ADMISSIONS REQUIREMENTS: Minimum age 18; Medical examination; Physician's request.
STAFF: RNs 6 (ft), 3 (pt); LPNs 5 (ft), 2 (pt); Nurses' aides 31 (ft), 6 (pt); Physical therapists (contracted); Occupational therapists (contracted); Speech therapists (contracted); Activities coordinators 1 (ft), 1 (pt); Dietitians (contracted); Ophthalmologists (contracted); Podiatrists (contracted).

Munster

Munster Med-Inn

7935 Calumet Ave, Munster, IN 46321
(219) 836-8300
LICENSURE: Skilled care; Intermediate care; Residential care; Comprehensive care.
BEDS: SNF 208; ICF 48; Residential care 30; Comprehensive care 2.
CERTIFIED: Medicaid; Medicare.
ADMISSIONS REQUIREMENTS: Minimum age 18; Medical examination; Physician's request.
STAFF: RNs 4 (ft), 7 (pt); LPNs 19 (ft), 2 (pt); Nurses' aides 106 (ft), 23 (pt); Physical therapists 1 (ft); Occupational therapists 1 (ft); Speech therapists 1 (ft); Activities coordinators 1 (ft); Dietitians 1 (ft), 1 (pt); Certified occupational therapy aides 2 (ft); Physical therapy aides 5 (ft), 2 (pt); Activities aides 2 (ft), 2 (pt).
LANGUAGES: Spanish, Polish

Portage

Fountainview Place

3175 Lancer St, Portage, IN 46368
(219) 762-9571
LICENSURE: Skilled care; Intermediate care; Residential care.
BEDS: SNF 71; ICF 149; Residential care 6.
CERTIFIED: Medicaid; Medicare.
ADMISSIONS REQUIREMENTS: Minimum age 18.
STAFF: Physicians 1 (pt); RNs 8 (ft), 2 (pt); LPNs 16 (ft), 4 (pt); Nurses' aides 70 (ft), 10 (pt); Physical therapists 1 (ft), 1 (pt); Occupational therapists 1 (pt); Speech therapists 1 (pt); Activities coordinators 2 (ft); Dietitians 1 (pt); Podiatrists 1 (pt).
LANGUAGES: Spanish

Miller's Merry Manor

5909 Lute Rd, Portage, IN 46368
(219) 763-2273, 763-7218 FAX
LICENSURE: Skilled care; Intermediate care.
BEDS: SNF 22; ICF 44.
CERTIFIED: Medicaid; Medicare.
ADMISSIONS REQUIREMENTS: Minimum age 18; Medical examination; Physician's request.
STAFF: RNs 3 (ft), 3 (pt); LPNs 3 (ft), 3 (pt); Nurses' aides 20 (ft), 10 (pt); Physical therapists 2 (pt); Recreational therapists 1 (pt); Occupational therapists 1 (pt); Speech therapists 1 (pt); Activities coordinators 1 (ft); Dietitians 1 (pt).

San Pierre

Little Company of Mary Health Facility Inc

Rte 1 Box 22A, San Pierre, IN 46374-9714
(219) 828-4111
LICENSURE: Intermediate care; Alzheimer's care.
BEDS: ICF 200.
CERTIFIED: Medicaid.
ADMISSIONS REQUIREMENTS: Minimum age 18; Medical examination.
STAFF: RNs 3 (ft), 3 (pt); LPNs 2 (ft), 1 (pt); Nurses' aides 60 (ft), 30 (pt); Activities coordinators 1 (ft).
LANGUAGES: Polish, Czech

Valparaiso

Canterbury Place

251 East Dr, Valparaiso, IN 46383
(219) 462-6158, 465-7680 FAX
LICENSURE: Skilled care; Intermediate care.
BEDS: SNF 51; ICF 51.
CERTIFIED: Medicaid; Medicare; VA.
ADMISSIONS REQUIREMENTS: Minimum age 18.
STAFF: RNs 3 (ft), 2 (pt); LPNs 6 (ft), 4 (pt); Nurses' aides 20 (ft), 15 (pt); Recreational therapists 1 (ft); Activities coordinators 1 (ft).

Life Care Center of Valparaiso

3405 Campbell Rd, Valparaiso, IN 46383
(219) 462-1023
LICENSURE: Skilled care; Intermediate care.
BEDS: SNF 31; ICF 41.

Pavilion Health Care Center

606 Wall St, Valparaiso, IN 46383
(219) 464-4976, 464-3612 FAX
LICENSURE: Skilled care; Intermediate care.
BEDS: SNF 96; ICF 96.
CERTIFIED: Medicaid; Medicare.
ADMISSIONS REQUIREMENTS: Minimum age 18; Medical examination; Physician's request.
STAFF: RNs 9 (ft), 2 (pt); LPNs 11 (ft); Nurses' aides 48 (ft), 12 (pt); Physical therapists 1 (pt); Recreational therapists 1 (pt); Occupational therapists 1 (pt); Speech therapists 1 (pt); Activities coordina-

tors 1 (ft); Dietitians 1 (pt); Ophthalmologists 1
(pt); Podiatrists 1 (pt); Audiologists 1 (pt); Respiratory therapists 8 (ft), 3 (pt).

Whispering Pines Health Care Center
3301 N Calumet Ave, Valparaiso, IN 46383
(219) 462-0508
LICENSURE: Skilled care; Intermediate care.
BEDS: SNF 39; ICF 152.
CERTIFIED: Medicaid; Medicare.
ADMISSIONS REQUIREMENTS: Medical examination; Physician's request.
STAFF: Physicians 1 (ft); RNs 7 (ft), 5 (pt); LPNs 6 (ft),
5 (pt); Nurses' aides 60 (ft), 45 (pt); Physical
therapists 1 (ft); Occupational therapists 1 (ft);
Speech therapists 1 (pt); Activities coordinators 3
(ft), 1 (pt); Dietitians 1 (pt).

The Willow Rehabilitation Center
1000 Elizabeth St, Valparaiso, IN 46383
(219) 464-4858, 477-4746 FAX
LICENSURE: Skilled care; Intermediate care.
BEDS: SNF 50; ICF 50.
CERTIFIED: Medicaid; Medicare.
ADMISSIONS REQUIREMENTS: Physician's request.
STAFF: RNs 9 (ft); LPNs 3 (ft); Nurses' aides 60 (ft);
Physical therapists 2 (pt); Occupational therapists
1 (pt); Speech therapists 1 (pt); Activities coordi-
nators 1 (ft); Dietitians 1 (pt); Ophthalmologists 1
(pt); Podiatrists 1 (pt); Audiologists 1 (pt).

Whiting

Hammond-Whiting Convalescent Center
1000 114th St, Whiting, IN 46394
(219) 659-2770
LICENSURE: Intermediate care.
BEDS: ICF 80.
CERTIFIED: Medicaid.
ADMISSIONS REQUIREMENTS: Minimum age 65; Medical
examination; Physician's request.
STAFF: RNs 2 (ft), 6 (pt); LPNs 1 (ft); Nurses' aides 20
(ft), 12 (pt); Activities coordinators 1 (ft).

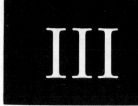

Nursing Homes

Facilities arranged by city.

Activities	Arts & Crafts	Cards	Games	Reading Groups	Religious Activities	Movies	Shopping Trips	Dances/Social/Cultural Gatherings	Intergenerational Programs	Pet Therapy	Outings/Sight-seeing	Group Exercise
Americana Healthcare Center of Arlington Heights Arlington Heights, IL	•	•	•	•	•	•	•	•	•	•	•	•
Lutheran Home & Services for the Aged Arlington Heights, IL	•	•	•	•	•	•	•	•	•	•	•	•
Marriott Church Creek Health Care Center Arlington Heights, IL	•	•	•	•	•	•	•	•	•	•	•	•
The Moorings Health Center Arlington Heights, IL	•	•	•	•	•	•	•	•	•	•	•	•
Northwest Community Continuing Care Center Arlington Heights, IL	•	•	•	•	•	•	•	•	•	•	•	•
Countryside Healthcare Centre Aurora, IL	•	•	•	•	•	•	•	•	•	•	•	•
Elmwood Nursing Home Aurora, IL	•	•	•	•	•	•	•	•	•	•	•	•
McAuley Manor Aurora, IL	•	•	•		•	•	•			•	•	•
New York Manor Inc Aurora, IL	•			•	•		•		•			
Governor's Park Nursing & Rehabilitation Center Barrington, IL	•	•	•	•	•	•	•	•	•	•	•	•
Firwood Health Care Center Batavia, IL	•	•	•		•	•	•	•	•	•	•	•
Michealsen Health Center Batavia, IL	•	•	•	•	•	•	•	•	•	•	•	•
The Anchorage of Beecher Beecher, IL	•	•	•	•		•				•		

Activities	Arts & Crafts	Cards	Games	Reading Groups	Religious Activities	Movies	Shopping Trips	Dances/Social/Cultural Gatherings	Intergenerational Programs	Pet Therapy	Outings/Sight-seeing	Group Exercise
The Anchorage of Bensenville Bensenville, IL	•	•	•		•	•	•	•	•	•		
Fairfax Health Care Center Berwyn, IL	•		•		•	•	•	•		•	•	•
Alden Nursing Center—Valley Ridge Rehabilitation & Health Care Center Bloomingdale, IL	•	•	•	•	•	•	•	•		•		•
Bridgeview Convalescent Center Bridgeview, IL	•	•	•	•	•	•	•	•				
Metropolitan Nursing Center Bridgeview, IL	•	•	•	•	•	•	•	•	•	•		•
The British Home Brookfield, IL	•	•	•	•	•	•	•	•	•	•		
Brentwood Nursing & Rehabilitation Center Burbank, IL	•	•	•		•	•						
Parkside Gardens Nursing Home Burbank, IL	•		•	•	•	•	•			•	•	•
King Bruwaert House Burr Ridge, IL	•	•	•	•	•	•	•	•		•		
Windsor Park Manor Carol Stream, IL	•	•	•	•	•	•		•	•	•	•	•
Alden Nursing Center—Lakeland Rehabilitation & Health Care Center Chicago, IL	•	•	•	•	•	•	•	•	•	•	•	•
Alden Nursing Center—Morrow Rehabilitation & Health Care Center Chicago, IL	•	•	•	•	•	•	•	•		•		
Alden Nursing Center—Princeton Rehabilitation & Health Care Center Chicago, IL	•	•	•	•	•	•		•	•	•	•	•
Alden Nursing Center—Wentworth Rehabilitation & Health Care Center Chicago, IL	•	•	•	•	•	•	•	•				•
All American Nursing Home Chicago, IL	•	•	•	•	•	•	•	•				
Alshore House Chicago, IL	•	•	•	•	•	•	•	•	•	•	•	•
Ambassador Nursing Center Inc Chicago, IL	•	•	•		•	•	•	•	•	•		
Arbour Health Care Center Ltd Chicago, IL	•	•										
Atrium Health Care Center Ltd Chicago, IL	•	•	•	•	•	•	•	•			•	•

✔ In order to support future editions of this publication would you please mention *Elder Services* each time you contact any advertiser, facility, or service.

Activities	Arts & Crafts	Cards	Games	Reading Groups	Religious Activities	Movies	Shopping Trips	Dances/Social/Cultural Gatherings	Intergenerational Programs	Pet Therapy	Outings/Sight-seeing	Group Exercise
Avenue Care Center Inc Chicago, IL	•	•	•	•	•	•	•	•	•			
Warren Barr Pavilion of Illinois Masonic Medical Center Chicago, IL	•	•	•	•	•	•	•	•	•	•	•	•
Belmont Nursing Home Inc Chicago, IL	•	•	•	•	•	•	•	•		•		•
Bethesda Home & Retirement Center Chicago, IL	•	•	•		•	•	•	•			•	•
Birchwood Plaza Nursing Home Chicago, IL	•	•	•	•	•	•	•	•	•		•	•
Bohemian Home for the Aged Chicago, IL	•		•	•	•	•	•					
Boulevard Care Center Inc Chicago, IL	•	•	•	•	•			•				
Brightview Care Center Inc Chicago, IL	•	•	•	•	•	•	•	•	•	•		
Buckingham Pavilion Nursing & Rehabilitation Center Chicago, IL	•	•	•	•	•	•	•	•	•	•	•	•
California Gardens Nursing Center Chicago, IL	•	•	•	•	•	•	•	•	•	•		
Carlton House Nursing Center—CH Nursing Center Inc Chicago, IL	•	•	•	•	•	•	•	•	•		•	•
Carmen Manor Nursing Home Chicago, IL	•	•	•		•	•	•	•			•	•
Central Nursing Chicago, IL	•	•	•	•	•	•	•	•			•	•
Central Plaza Residential Home Chicago, IL	•	•	•	•	•	•	•	•		•		
Chevy Chase Nursing Center Chicago, IL	•	•	•	•	•	•	•	•	•			
Clark Manor Convalescent Center Chicago, IL	•	•	•	•	•	•	•	•				
Clayton Residential Home Chicago, IL	•		•	•		•	•	•				
Cojeunaze Nursing Center Chicago, IL	•	•	•	•	•	•	•	•				
Columbus Manor Residential Care Home Chicago, IL	•	•	•	•	•	•	•	•				
Community Care Center Inc Chicago, IL	•	•	•	•	•	•	•	•	•	•		

Activities	Arts & Crafts	Cards	Games	Reading Groups	Religious Activities	Movies	Shopping Trips	Dances/Social/Cultural Gatherings	Intergenerational Programs	Pet Therapy	Outings/Sight-seeing	Group Exercise
Congress Care Center Chicago, IL	•	•	•	•	•	•	•	•	•	•		
Continental Care Center Inc Chicago, IL	•	•	•		•	•	•	•		•	•	•
Covenant Home of Chicago Chicago, IL	•		•	•	•	•	•	•	•	•	•	•
Deauville Healthcare Center Chicago, IL	•	•	•	•	•	•	•	•	•	•		
Edgewater Nursing & Geriatric Center Chicago, IL	•	•	•	•	•	•	•	•	•	•		•
Elston Home Inc Chicago, IL	•	•	•	•	•	•	•					
Garden View Home Inc Chicago, IL	•	•	•	•	•	•	•	•	•	•		
Glencrest Nursing Rehabilitation Center Ltd Chicago, IL	•	•	•	•	•	•	•	•				
Grasmere Resident Home Inc Chicago, IL	•	•	•			•	•	•				
Halsted Terrace Nursing Center Chicago, IL	•	•	•			•	•	•				
Heritage Healthcare Centre Chicago, IL	•	•	•	•	•	•	•	•		•		
The Imperial Convalescent & Geriatric Center Inc Chicago, IL	•	•	•	•	•	•	•	•	•	•	•	•
Johnson Rehabilitation Nursing Home Chicago, IL	•	•	•	•	•	•	•	•				
Lake Front Healthcare Center Inc Chicago, IL	•	•	•	•	•	•	•	•	•	•		
Lake Shore Nursing Centre Ltd Chicago, IL	•	•	•	•	•	•	•	•	•	•	•	•
Lakeview Nursing & Geriatric Center Inc Chicago, IL	•	•	•	•	•	•	•	•	•	•		
Lincoln Park Terrace Inc Chicago, IL	•	•	•	•		•	•	•				
Little Sisters of the Poor Center for the Aging Chicago, IL	•	•	•	•	•	•	•	•				
Margaret Manor Chicago, IL	•	•	•	•	•	•	•	•				

✔ In order to support future editions of this publication would you please mention *Elder Services* each time you contact any advertiser, facility, or service.

Activities	Arts & Crafts	Cards	Games	Reading Groups	Religious Activities	Movies	Shopping Trips	Dances/Social/Cultural Gatherings	Intergenerational Programs	Pet Therapy	Outings/Sight-seeing	Group Exercise
Margaret Manor—North Branch Chicago, IL	•	•	•	•	•	•	•	•				
Maxwell Manor Chicago, IL	•	•	•	•	•	•	•	•	•		•	•
The Methodist Home Chicago, IL	•	•	•	•	•	•	•	•	•	•	•	•
Mid-America Convalescent Centers Inc Chicago, IL	•	•	•	•	•	•	•	•	•	•		
Monroe Pavilion Health Center Inc Chicago, IL	•	•	•	•	•	•	•	•				
Montgomery Place Chicago, IL	•	•	•	•	•	•	•	•			•	•
Northwest Home for the Aged Chicago, IL	•	•	•	•	•	•		•				
Norwood Park Home Chicago, IL	•	•	•			•	•	•				
Our Lady of the Resurrection—Extended Care Unit Chicago, IL	•	•	•		•							
Park House Ltd Chicago, IL	•	•	•	•	•		•	•				
Peterson Park Health Care Center Chicago, IL	•	•	•	•	•	•	•	•	•	•		
Rainbow Beach Nursing Center Inc Chicago, IL	•	•	•	•	•	•	•	•	•	•		
St Joseph Home of Chicago Inc Chicago, IL	•	•	•	•	•	•	•	•	•	•	•	•
St Joseph Hospital & Health Care Center—Skilled Nursing Unit Chicago, IL	•	•	•	•	•	•	•	•	•	•	•	•
St Martha Manor Chicago, IL	•	•	•	•	•	•		•				
St Paul's House & Health Care Center Chicago, IL	•	•	•	•	•	•	•	•	•	•	•	•
Selfhelp Home for the Aged Chicago, IL	•	•	•	•	•	•		•				
Washington & Jane Smith Home Chicago, IL	•	•	•	•	•	•	•	•	•	•	•	•
Society for Danish Old People's Home Chicago, IL	•	•	•			•	•	•				

Activities	Arts & Crafts	Cards	Games	Reading Groups	Religious Activities	Movies	Shopping Trips	Dances/Social/Cultural Gatherings	Intergenerational Programs	Pet Therapy	Outings/Sight-seeing	Group Exercise
Somerset House Chicago, IL	•	•	•	•	•	•	•	•	•	•		
Warren Park Nursing Pavilion Chicago, IL	•	•	•	•	•	•	•	•	•	•	•	•
Waterfront Terrace Chicago, IL	•	•	•	•	•	•	•	•			•	•
Wellington Plaza Nursing & Therapy Center Chicago, IL	•	•	•	•	•	•	•	•				
The Westwood Manor Inc Chicago, IL	•	•	•		•	•		•				
The Whitehall Convalescent and Nursing Home Chicago, IL	•		•	•	•	•		•		•	•	
Wincrest Nursing Center Chicago, IL	•	•	•		•	•	•	•				
Woodbridge Nursing Pavilion Chicago, IL	•	•	•	•	•	•	•	•				
Prairie Manor Health Care Center Chicago Heights, IL	•	•	•	•	•	•	•	•	•	•	•	•
Riviera Manor Inc Chicago Heights, IL	•	•	•	•	•	•	•	•	•	•	•	•
Thornton Heights Terrace Ltd Chicago Heights, IL	•	•	•	•	•	•	•	•				
Chicago Ridge Nursing Center Chicago Ridge, IL	•	•	•	•	•	•	•	•	•	•		•
Lexington Health Care Center of Chicago Ridge Chicago Ridge, IL	•		•		•			•				•
Alden Nursing Center—Town Manor Rehabilitation & Health Care Center Cicero, IL	•	•	•	•	•	•	•	•		•		•
Westshire Retirement & Healthcare Centre Cicero, IL	•	•	•	•	•	•	•	•	•	•	•	•
Crestwood Heights Nursing Centre Crestwood, IL	•	•	•	•	•	•	•	•	•	•	•	•
St James Manor Crete, IL	•	•	•	•	•	•					•	•
Canterbury Care Center Crystal Lake, IL	•		•	•	•	•		•			•	•
Crystal Pines Health Care Center Crystal Lake, IL	•	•			•	•	•	•				

✔ In order to support future editions of this publication would you please mention *Elder Services* each time you contact any advertiser, facility, or service.

Activities	Arts & Crafts	Cards	Games	Reading Groups	Religious Activities	Movies	Shopping Trips	Dances/Social/Cultural Gatherings	Intergenerational Programs	Pet Therapy	Outings/Sight-seeing	Group Exercise
Fair Oaks Health Care Center Crystal Lake, IL	•	•	•	•	•	•	•	•	•	•	•	•
De Kalb County Nursing Home De Kalb, IL	•	•	•	•	•	•	•	•		•	•	•
Oak Crest—De Kalb Area Retirement Center De Kalb, IL	•	•	•	•	•	•	•	•				
Pine Acres Care Center De Kalb, IL	•	•	•	•	•	•		•	•	•		
The Whitehall North Deerfield, IL	•	•	•	•	•	•		•		•		•
Ballard Nursing Center Inc Des Plaines, IL	•	•	•	•	•	•	•	•	•	•	•	•
Holy Family Health Center Des Plaines, IL	•	•	•	•	•	•	•	•	•	•	•	•
Lee Manor Health Care Residence Des Plaines, IL	•	•	•	•	•	•	•	•	•	•	•	•
Nazarethville Des Plaines, IL	•	•	•							•		
Oakton Pavilion Healthcare Facility Inc Des Plaines, IL	•	•	•	•	•	•	•	•	•			
Dolton Healthcare Center Inc Dolton, IL	•	•	•	•	•	•	•					
Fairview Baptist Home Downers Grove, IL	•	•	•	•	•	•	•	•	•	•	•	•
Rest Haven West Skilled Nursing Center Downers Grove, IL	•	•	•	•	•	•	•	•	•	•	•	
Fernwood Health Care Center Dwight, IL	•	•	•	•	•	•	•	•				
Americana Healthcare Center of Elgin Elgin, IL	•	•	•	•	•	•	•	•		•		•
Apostolic Christian Resthaven Elgin, IL	•		•	•	•	•	•			•	•	
Heritage Manor of Elgin Elgin, IL	•	•	•	•	•			•	•	•		
Metropolitan Nursing Center of Elgin Elgin, IL	•	•	•	•	•	•	•	•	•	•	•	•
Sherman West Court Elgin, IL	•	•	•	•	•	•	•	•	•	•		•

Activities	Arts & Crafts	Cards	Games	Reading Groups	Religious Activities	Movies	Shopping Trips	Dances/Social/Cultural Gatherings	Intergenerational Programs	Pet Therapy	Outings/Sight-seeing	Group Exercise
Americana Healthcare Center of Elk Grove Elk Grove Village, IL	•	•	•	•	•	•	•	•	•	•	•	•
Elmhurst Extended Care Center Inc Elmhurst, IL	•	•	•	•	•	•	•	•				
York Convalescent Center Elmhurst, IL	•	•	•	•	•	•	•	•	•	•	•	•
Royal Elm Convalescent & Geriatric Center Inc Elmwood Park, IL	•	•	•	•	•	•	•	•	•	•	•	•
Albany House Evanston, IL	•	•	•	•	•	•	•					
Dobson Plaza Evanston, IL	•	•	•	•	•	•		•			•	•
The King Home Evanston, IL	•		•			•			•			
McGaw Health Care Center Evanston, IL	•	•	•	•	•	•	•	•	•	•		•
Oakwood Terrace Nursing Home Evanston, IL	•		•	•	•	•	•	•	•	•		
St Francis Extended Care Center Evanston, IL	•	•	•	•	•	•		•	•			
Swedish Retirement Association Evanston, IL	•	•	•	•	•	•	•					
Park Lane Nursing Center Association Evergreen Park, IL	•	•	•	•	•	•	•	•	•			
Peace Memorial Home Evergreen Park, IL	•	•	•	•	•	•		•				
Altenheim Forest Park, IL	•	•	•	•	•	•	•			•		
Westlake Pavilion Franklin Park, IL	•	•		•	•	•		•	•	•	•	•
Geneva Care Center Geneva, IL	•	•	•	•	•	•	•	•	•			•
The Abington of Glenview Glenview, IL	•	•	•	•	•	•	•			•	•	
Glenview Terrace Nursing Center Glenview, IL	•	•	•	•	•	•	•	•	•	•		•
Maryhaven Inc Glenview, IL	•	•	•	•	•	•	•	•	•	•	•	•
Glenwood Terrace Nursing Center Glenwood, IL	•	•	•	•	•	•	•	•	•	•	•	•

✔ In order to support future editions of this publication would you please mention *Elder Services* each time you contact any advertiser, facility, or service.

Activities	Arts & Crafts	Cards	Games	Reading Groups	Religious Activities	Movies	Shopping Trips	Dances/Social/Cultural Gatherings	Intergenerational Programs	Pet Therapy	Outings/Sight-seeing	Group Exercise
Alden Nursing Center—Heather Rehabilitation & Health Care Center Harvey, IL	•	•	•	•	•	•	•	•	•	•	•	•
Imperial Nursing Center of Hazel Crest Hazel Crest, IL	•	•	•	•	•	•	•	•	•	•	•	•
Hickory Nursing Pavilion Inc Hickory Hills, IL	•	•	•	•	•	•	•	•	•			
Abbott House Highland Park, IL	•	•	•		•	•	•	•	•	•	•	•
Villa St Cyril Highland Park, IL	•	•	•	•	•	•	•	•		•	•	
Highland Park Health Care Center Inc Highwood, IL	•	•	•	•	•	•	•	•	•			
Americana-Monticello Healthcare Center of Hinsdale Hinsdale, IL	•	•	•	•	•	•	•	•	•	•		•
Alden—Poplar Creek Rehabilitation & Health Care Center Hoffman Estates, IL	•	•	•	•	•	•	•	•	•	•	•	•
Mercy Health Care & Rehabilitation Center Homewood, IL	•	•	•	•	•	•	•	•	•	•	•	
Briar Place Ltd Indian Head Park, IL	•	•	•	•	•	•	•	•	•	•		
The Arbor Itasca, IL	•	•	•	•	•	•	•		•	•	•	
Deerbrook Nursing Centre Joliet, IL	•	•	•	•	•	•	•	•	•	•	•	•
Draper Plaza Joliet, IL	•	•	•	•	•	•	•	•	•	•		
Metropolitan Nursing Center of Joliet Joliet, IL	•	•		•	•	•	•	•	•		•	•
Our Lady of Angels Retirement Home Joliet, IL	•	•	•	•	•	•	•	•				
Salem Village Joliet, IL	•	•		•	•		•	•	•			
Sunny Hill Nursing Home Joliet, IL	•	•	•	•	•	•	•	•		•		
Villa Franciscan Joliet, IL	•	•	•	•	•	•	•	•	•	•		

Activities	Arts & Crafts	Cards	Games	Reading Groups	Religious Activities	Movies	Shopping Trips	Dances/Social/Cultural Gatherings	Intergenerational Programs	Pet Therapy	Outings/Sight-seeing	Group Exercise
Rosary Hill Home Justice, IL	•	•	•		•	•						•
Colonial Manor Healthcare Center La Grange, IL	•	•	•	•	•	•	•	•				
Fairview Health Care Center La Grange, IL	•	•	•	•	•	•	•	•	•	•		
Plymouth Place La Grange Park, IL	•	•	•	•	•	•	•	•	•	•		
Hill Top Sanitorium Lake Bluff, IL					•	•					•	
Lake Bluff Healthcare Centre Lake Bluff, IL	•	•	•	•	•	•	•	•		•		•
Holy Family Villa Lemont, IL	•		•	•	•	•	•	•	•	•	•	•
Mother Theresa Home Lemont, IL	•	•	•	•	•	•	•	•	•	•	•	•
Americana Healthcare Center of Libertyville Libertyville, IL	•	•	•	•	•	•	•	•	•	•	•	•
Libertyville Manor Extended Care Facility Libertyville, IL	•	•	•	•	•	•	•	•	•	•	•	•
Winchester House Libertyville, IL	•	•	•	•	•	•	•	•				
Regency Park Manor Lincolnwood, IL	•	•	•	•		•	•	•			•	•
Victory Lakes Continuing Care Center Lindenhurst, IL	•	•	•	•	•	•	•	•	•	•	•	•
Snow Valley Living Center Lisle, IL	•	•	•		•	•	•			•		•
Beacon Hill Lombard, IL	•	•	•	•	•	•	•	•		•		•
Bloomingdale Pavilion Lombard, IL	•	•	•	•	•	•	•	•	•	•	•	•
Maple Hill Nursing Home Ltd Long Grove, IL	•	•	•	•	•	•	•	•	•	•	•	•
Florence Nursing Home Marengo, IL	•	•	•	•	•	•			•	•	•	•
Applewood Living Center Matteson, IL	•	•	•	•	•	•	•	•	•	•	•	•
Baptist Retirement Home Maywood, IL	•	•		•	•	•	•	•	•	•		

✔ In order to support future editions of this publication would you please mention *Elder Services* each time you contact any advertiser, facility, or service.

Activities	Arts & Crafts	Cards	Games	Reading Groups	Religious Activities	Movies	Shopping Trips	Dances/Social/Cultural Gatherings	Intergenerational Programs	Pet Therapy	Outings/Sight-seeing	Group Exercise
Royal Terrace McHenry, IL	•	•	•	•	•	•	•	•	•	•		
Bowman Nursing Home Midlothian, IL	•	•	•	•	•	•	•	•	•	•	•	•
Crestwood Terrace Midlothian, IL	•	•	•	•	•	•	•	•		•		
Grundy County Home Morris, IL	•	•	•	•	•	•	•	•	•	•		
Morris Lincoln Nursing Home Morris, IL	•	•	•		•	•	•	•		•		
Bethany Terrace Nursing Centre Morton Grove, IL	•	•	•	•	•	•	•	•	•	•	•	•
Alden Nursing Center—Naperville Rehabilitation & Health Care Center Naperville, IL	•	•	•	•	•	•	•	•	•	•		•
Americana Healthcare Center of Naperville Naperville, IL	•	•	•	•	•	•	•	•	•	•	•	•
Community Convalescent Center of Naperville Naperville, IL	•	•	•	•	•	•	•	•	•	•		
St Patrick's Residence Naperville, IL	•	•	•	•	•	•	•	•				
Forest Villa Nursing Center Niles, IL	•	•	•	•	•	•	•	•	•	•	•	•
Glen Bridge Nursing & Rehabilitation Center Niles, IL	•	•	•	•	•	•	•	•	•	•		
George J Goldman Memorial Home for the Aged Niles, IL	•	•	•		•	•	•	•	•	•	•	•
Hampton Plaza Niles, IL	•	•	•	•	•	•	•	•	•	•		
Regency Nursing Centre Niles, IL	•	•	•	•	•	•	•	•	•	•	•	•
St Benedict Home for Aged Niles, IL	•	•	•	•	•	•	•	•				
Central Baptist Home for the Aged Norridge, IL	•		•	•	•	•	•		•		•	•
Norridge Nursing Centre Inc Norridge, IL	•	•	•	•	•	•	•	•	•	•	•	•
Maplewood Health Care Center North Aurora, IL	•	•	•	•	•	•	•	•	•	•	•	•

Activities	Arts & Crafts	Cards	Games	Reading Groups	Religious Activities	Movies	Shopping Trips	Dances/Social/Cultural Gatherings	Intergenerational Programs	Pet Therapy	Outings/Sight-seeing	Group Exercise
The Scottish Home North Riverside, IL	•	•	•	•	•	•	•			•	•	•
Brandel Care Center Northbrook, IL	•	•	•	•	•	•		•			•	•
GAF/Lake Cook Terrace Northbrook, IL	•	•	•	•	•	•	•	•				
Glen Oaks Nursing Home Inc Northbrook, IL	•	•	•	•	•	•	•	•				
Villa Scalabrini Northlake, IL	•	•	•		•			•			•	•
Oak Brook Healthcare Centre Oak Brook, IL	•	•	•	•	•	•				•	•	
Americana Healthcare Center of Oak Lawn Oak Lawn, IL	•	•	•	•	•	•	•	•		•		
Americana-Monticello Healthcare Center of Oak Lawn Oak Lawn, IL	•	•	•		•	•	•	•	•	•	•	•
Concord Extended Care Oak Lawn, IL	•	•	•	•	•	•	•	•	•	•		
Oak Lawn Convalescent Home Oak Lawn, IL	•	•	•	•	•	•	•		•	•		
Metropolitan Nursing Center of Oak Park Oak Park, IL	•	•	•	•	•	•	•	•	•	•	•	•
The Woodbine Convalescent Home Oak Park, IL	•	•	•	•	•					•		•
The Tillers Nursing Home Oswego, IL	•	•	•		•	•			•	•	•	•
Little Sisters of the Poor Palatine, IL	•	•	•	•	•	•	•	•	•	•	•	•
Plum Grove Nursing Home Palatine, IL	•	•	•	•	•	•	•	•	•	•		
Americana Healthcare Center of Palos Heights Palos Heights, IL	•	•	•	•	•	•	•	•	•	•	•	•
Rest Haven Central Nursing Home Palos Heights, IL	•		•		•	•		•	•	•	•	•
Ridgeland Living Center Palos Heights, IL	•	•	•	•	•	•	•	•	•	•	•	•
Windsor Manor Nursing & Rehabilitation Center Palos Hills, IL	•	•	•	•	•	•	•	•			•	•

✔ In order to support future editions of this publication would you please mention *Elder Services* each time you contact any advertiser, facility, or service.

Activities	Arts & Crafts	Cards	Games	Reading Groups	Religious Activities	Movies	Shopping Trips	Dances/Social/Cultural Gatherings	Intergenerational Programs	Pet Therapy	Outings/Sight-seeing	Group Exercise
Park Ridge Healthcare Center Park Ridge, IL	•	•	•	•	•	•		•				
Resurrection Nursing Pavilion Park Ridge, IL	•	•	•	•	•	•	•	•	•	•	•	•
St Matthew Lutheran Home Park Ridge, IL	•	•	•	•	•	•	•	•	•	•		
Lakewood Living Center Plainfield, IL	•	•	•	•	•	•	•	•				
Richton Crossing Convalescent Center Richton Park, IL	•	•	•	•		•	•	•				
Brentwood North Nursing & Rehabilitation Center Riverwoods, IL	•	•	•	•	•	•	•	•	•	•	•	•
Lydia Healthcare Robbins, IL	•	•	•	•	•	•	•	•	•		•	•
Americana Healthcare Center of Rolling Meadows Rolling Meadows, IL	•	•	•	•	•	•	•	•	•	•		•
Abbington House Roselle, IL	•	•	•	•	•	•	•	•				
Hillcrest Nursing Center Round Lake Beach, IL	•	•	•	•	•	•	•	•	•	•	•	
Pine View Care Center Saint Charles, IL	•	•	•	•	•	•	•	•				
Dogwood Health Care Center Sandwich, IL	•	•	•	•	•	•	•	•				
Willow Crest Nursing Pavilion Sandwich, IL	•	•	•	•	•	•	•	•	•	•	•	•
Friendship Village of Schaumburg Schaumburg, IL	•	•	•	•	•	•	•	•				
Shabbona Health Care Center Inc Shabbona, IL	•	•	•	•		•	•	•				
Lieberman Geriatric Health Centre Skokie, IL	•	•	•	•	•	•	•	•	•	•	•	•
Old Orchard Manor Skokie, IL	•	•	•	•	•	•	•	•	•	•	•	•
Skokie Meadows Nursing Center 1 Skokie, IL	•	•	•	•	•	•	•	•				
Fox Valley Healthcare Inc South Elgin, IL	•	•	•	•	•	•	•	•				
Americana Healthcare Center of South Holland South Holland, IL	•	•		•	•	•	•	•		•	•		•

Activities	Arts & Crafts	Cards	Games	Reading Groups	Religious Activities	Movies	Shopping Trips	Dances/Social/Cultural Gatherings	Intergenerational Programs	Pet Therapy	Outings/Sight-seeing	Group Exercise
Rest Haven South South Holland, IL	•	•	•	•	•	•	•	•	•	•	•	•
Windmill Nursing Pavilion Ltd South Holland, IL	•	•	•	•	•	•	•	•				
Pershing Convalescent Home Inc Stickney, IL	•	•	•	•	•	•	•		•	•		
The McAllister Nursing Home Inc Tinley Park, IL	•	•	•	•	•	•	•	•				
Town Hall Estates—Wauconda Inc Wauconda, IL	•	•	•	•	•	•	•	•	•	•		•
Bayside Terrace Waukegan, IL	•	•	•		•	•	•	•				•
Lake Park Center Waukegan, IL	•	•	•		•	•	•	•			•	
Northshore Terrace Waukegan, IL	•	•	•	•	•	•	•	•		•		
The Terrace Nursing Home Inc Waukegan, IL	•	•	•	•	•	•	•	•				
Arbor Terrace Health Care Center West Chicago, IL	•	•	•	•	•	•	•	•				•
West Chicago Terrace West Chicago, IL	•	•	•	•	•	•	•	•	•	•	•	•
Americana Healthcare Center of Westmont Westmont, IL	•	•	•	•	•	•	•	•	•	•	•	
Burgess Square Healthcare Centre Westmont, IL	•	•	•	•	•	•	•	•				
Westmont Convalescent Center Westmont, IL	•		•	•	•	•	•	•				
Du Page Convalescent Center Wheaton, IL	•	•	•	•	•	•	•	•				
Parkway Healthcare Center Wheaton, IL	•	•	•	•	•	•	•		•	•	•	•
Sandalwood Healthcare Centre Wheaton, IL	•	•	•	•	•	•	•	•				
Addolorata Villa Wheeling, IL	•	•	•	•	•	•	•	•	•	•	•	•
Chateau Village Living Center Willowbrook, IL	•	•	•	•	•	•	•	•	•	•	•	
Normandy House Wilmette, IL	•	•	•	•	•	•		•			•	•
Royal Willow Nursing Care Center Wilmington, IL	•	•	•		•	•	•			•		

✔ In order to support future editions of this publication would you please mention *Elder Services* each time you contact any advertiser, facility, or service.

Activities	Arts & Crafts	Cards	Games	Reading Groups	Religious Activities	Movies	Shopping Trips	Dances/Social/Cultural Gatherings	Intergenerational Programs	Pet Therapy	Outings/Sight-seeing	Group Exercise
Liberty Hill Healthcare Center Winfield, IL	•	•	•	•	•	•	•	•				
Sunset Manor Woodstock, IL	•	•	•	•	•	•	•		•	•	•	•
Valley Hi Nursing Home Woodstock, IL	•	•	•			•	•					
The Woodstock Residence Woodstock, IL	•	•	•		•	•	•	•				
Hillside Health Care Center Yorkville, IL	•	•		•				•	•	•	•	•
Crown Manor Healthcare Center Zion, IL	•	•	•	•	•	•	•	•	•	•		•
Rolling Hills Manor Zion, IL	•	•	•	•	•	•	•	•	•	•		
Sheridan Health Care Center Zion, IL	•	•	•	•	•	•	•	•	•			•
Colonial Nursing Home Crown Point, IN	•	•	•	•	•	•	•	•	•		•	
Lake County Convalescent Home Crown Point, IN	•	•	•	•	•	•	•	•	•	•		
Lutheran Home of Northwest Indiana Inc Crown Point, IN	•	•	•	•	•	•	•	•	•	•	•	•
St Anthony Home Crown Point, IN	•	•	•		•	•	•	•	•	•		•
Lake Holiday Manor Demotte, IN	•	•	•	•		•	•	•		•		
Meridian Nursing Center—Dyer Dyer, IN	•	•	•	•	•	•	•	•	•	•	•	•
Lake County Rehabilitation Center Inc East Chicago, IN	•	•	•	•	•	•	•	•	•	•		
Green's Geriatric Health Center Gary, IN	•	•	•	•		•	•	•		•		
West Side Health Care Center Gary, IN	•	•	•	•	•	•	•	•	•	•	•	•
Wildwood Manor—Clark Gary, IN	•	•	•	•	•	•	•	•				
Wildwood Manor—Mount Gary, IN	•	•	•	•	•	•	•	•				
Highland Nursing Home Highland, IN	•	•	•	•	•	•	•	•			•	•

Activities

	Arts & Crafts	Cards	Games	Reading Groups	Religious Activities	Movies	Shopping Trips	Dances/Social/Cultural Gatherings	Intergenerational Programs	Pet Therapy	Outings/Sight-seeing	Group Exercise
Miller's Merry Manor — Hobart, IN	•	•	•	•	•	•	•	•				
Sebo's Heritage Manor — Hobart, IN	•	•	•	•	•	•	•	•		•	•	•
Fountainview Terrace — La Porte, IN	•	•	•	•	•	•	•	•	•			
Lowell Health Care Center — Lowell, IN	•	•	•	•	•	•	•	•	•	•		
Towne Centre — Merrillville, IN	•	•	•	•	•	•	•	•	•	•	•	•
Michigan City Health Care — Michigan City, IN	•	•			•							
Red Oaks Healthcare Center — Michigan City, IN	•	•	•	•	•		•	•	•	•		
Munster Med-Inn — Munster, IN	•	•	•		•			•	•	•		
Fountainview Place — Portage, IN	•	•	•	•	•	•	•	•	•	•		
Miller's Merry Manor — Portage, IN	•	•	•	•	•	•	•	•		•		
Little Company of Mary Health Facility Inc — San Pierre, IN	•	•			•	•						
Canterbury Place — Valparaiso, IN	•	•	•	•	•			•				•
Pavilion Health Care Center — Valparaiso, IN	•	•	•	•	•	•	•	•	•	•		
Whispering Pines Health Care Center — Valparaiso, IN	•	•	•	•	•	•	•	•	•	•		
The Willow Rehabilitation Center — Valparaiso, IN	•	•	•	•	•	•	•	•	•	•	•	•
Hammond-Whiting Convalescent Center — Whiting, IN	•	•	•		•	•		•				

✔ In order to support future editions of this publication would you please mention *Elder Services* each time you contact any advertiser, facility, or service.

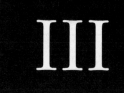

III

Nursing Homes

Facilities arranged by city.

Facilities	Dining Room	Physical Therapy Room	Activities Room	Chapel	Crafts Room	Laundry Room	Barber/Beauty Shop	Library	Greenhouse/Garden	Outdoor Patio/Yard	Enclosed Patio/Yard	Room	Lounge/Day Room	Ventilator Unit	Respiratory Unit
Americana Healthcare Center of Arlington Heights Arlington Heights, IL	•	•	•		•	•	•	•	•	•	•	•	•	•	
Lutheran Home & Services for the Aged Arlington Heights, IL	•	•	•	•	•	•	•	•	•	•	•	•	•		
Marriott Church Creek Health Care Center Arlington Heights, IL	•	•	•			•	•	•		•	•		•		
The Moorings Health Center Arlington Heights, IL	•		•		•		•	•	•	•	•	•	•		
Northwest Community Continuing Care Center Arlington Heights, IL	•	•		•			•	•	•	•			•	•	
Countryside Healthcare Centre Aurora, IL	•	•				•	•	•	•	•			•	•	
Elmwood Nursing Home Aurora, IL	•	•	•	•			•			•			•	•	
McAuley Manor Aurora, IL	•	•	•	•		•	•			•	•				
New York Manor Inc Aurora, IL	•	•	•	•	•	•	•	•							
Governor's Park Nursing & Rehabilitation Center Barrington, IL	•	•	•			•	•		•	•			•	•	•
Firwood Health Care Center Batavia, IL	•		•		•		•				•		•		
Michealsen Health Center Batavia, IL	•	•	•				•		•	•	•	•	•		
The Anchorage of Beecher Beecher, IL	•	•	•				•								
The Anchorage of Bensenville Bensenville, IL	•	•	•	•	•	•	•	•							

Facilities	Dining Room	Physical Therapy Room	Activities Room	Chapel	Crafts Room	Laundry Room	Barber/Beauty Shop	Library	Greenhouse/Garden	Outdoor Patio/Yard	Enclosed Patio/Yard	Room	Lounge/Day Room	Ventilator Unit	Respiratory Unit
Fairfax Health Care Center Berwyn, IL	•	•	•				•			•		•	•	•	
Alden Nursing Center—Valley Ridge Rehabilitation & Health Care Center Bloomingdale, IL	•	•	•		•	•	•			•		•	•		
Bridgeview Convalescent Center Bridgeview, IL	•	•	•		•	•	•								
Metropolitan Nursing Center Bridgeview, IL	•	•	•	•	•	•	•	•		•	•	•	•		•
The British Home Brookfield, IL	•		•		•		•	•							
Brentwood Nursing & Rehabilitation Center Burbank, IL	•	•	•		•	•	•								
Parkside Gardens Nursing Home Burbank, IL	•		•			•	•				•	•	•		
King Bruwaert House Burr Ridge, IL	•		•		•	•	•	•							
Windsor Park Manor Carol Stream, IL	•	•	•			•	•			•		•	•		
Alden Nursing Center—Lakeland Rehabilitation & Health Care Center Chicago, IL	•	•	•		•	•	•	•		•		•	•		
Alden Nursing Center—Morrow Rehabilitation & Health Care Center Chicago, IL	•	•	•		•	•	•	•							
Alden Nursing Center—Princeton Rehabilitation & Health Care Center Chicago, IL	•	•	•		•	•	•	•		•		•	•		
Alden Nursing Center—Wentworth Rehabilitation & Health Care Center Chicago, IL	•	•	•		•	•	•	•		•		•	•		
All American Nursing Home Chicago, IL		•	•	•	•	•	•	•							
Alshore House Chicago, IL	•	•	•			•	•			•	•				
Ambassador Nursing Center Inc Chicago, IL	•	•	•	•	•	•	•	•							
Arbour Health Care Center Ltd Chicago, IL	•	•	•		•		•	•							
Atrium Health Care Center Ltd Chicago, IL	•	•	•		•	•	•	•		•		•	•		
Avenue Care Center Inc Chicago, IL	•	•	•	•	•	•	•								

✔ In order to support future editions of this publication would you please mention *Elder Services* each time you contact any advertiser, facility, or service.

III

Facilities	Dining Room	Physical Therapy Room	Activities Room	Chapel	Crafts Room	Laundry Room	Barber/Beauty Shop	Library	Greenhouse/Garden	Outdoor Patio/Yard	Enclosed Patio/Yard	Room	Lounge/Day Room	Ventilator Unit	Respiratory Unit
Warren Barr Pavilion of Illinois Masonic Medical Center Chicago, IL	•	•	•	•	•	•	•	•	•	•		•	•		
Belmont Nursing Home Inc Chicago, IL	•		•			•			•	•		•	•		
Bethesda Home & Retirement Center Chicago, IL	•	•		•		•	•			•		•			
Birchwood Plaza Nursing Home Chicago, IL	•	•	•	•	•	•	•	•	•	•		•	•		
Bohemian Home for the Aged Chicago, IL	•	•	•		•	•	•	•							
Boulevard Care Center Inc Chicago, IL	•	•	•	•	•	•	•								
Brightview Care Center Inc Chicago, IL	•	•	•		•	•	•	•							
Buckingham Pavilion Nursing & Rehabilitation Center Chicago, IL	•	•	•	•	•	•	•	•	•	•	•	•	•		
California Gardens Nursing Center Chicago, IL	•	•	•		•	•	•	•							
Carlton House Nursing Center—CH Nursing Center Inc Chicago, IL	•	•	•		•					•		•	•		
Carmen Manor Nursing Home Chicago, IL	•		•		•	•			•	•		•	•		
Central Nursing Chicago, IL	•	•	•	•		•	•			•		•	•		
Central Plaza Residential Home Chicago, IL	•	•	•		•	•		•							
Chevy Chase Nursing Center Chicago, IL	•	•	•	•	•	•	•								
Clark Manor Convalescent Center Chicago, IL	•	•			•	•	•	•							
Clayton Residential Home Chicago, IL	•	•	•		•	•									
Cojeunaze Nursing Center Chicago, IL	•		•		•	•	•	•							
Columbus Manor Residential Care Home Chicago, IL	•		•		•	•		•		•					
Community Care Center Inc Chicago, IL	•	•	•	•	•	•	•	•							
Congress Care Center Chicago, IL	•	•	•		•	•	•	•							

Facilities	Dining Room	Physical Therapy Room	Activities Room	Chapel	Crafts Room	Laundry Room	Barber/Beauty Shop	Library	Greenhouse/Garden	Outdoor Patio/Yard	Enclosed Patio/Yard	Room	Lounge/Day Room	Ventilator Unit	Respiratory Unit
Continental Care Center Inc — Chicago, IL	•	•	•		•		•	•	•				•		
Covenant Home of Chicago — Chicago, IL	•		•	•	•		•	•				•	•		
Deauville Healthcare Center — Chicago, IL	•	•	•	•	•	•	•	•							
Edgewater Nursing & Geriatric Center — Chicago, IL	•	•	•	•	•		•	•		•	•	•	•		•
Elston Home Inc — Chicago, IL	•	•	•		•	•	•								
Garden View Home Inc — Chicago, IL	•	•	•												
Glencrest Nursing Rehabilitation Center Ltd — Chicago, IL	•	•	•		•	•	•	•							
Grasmere Resident Home Inc — Chicago, IL	•		•		•	•	•	•							
Halsted Terrace Nursing Center — Chicago, IL	•	•	•		•	•	•								
Heritage Healthcare Centre — Chicago, IL	•	•	•		•	•	•								
The Imperial Convalescent & Geriatric Center Inc — Chicago, IL	•	•	•		•		•			•	•	•	•		
Johnson Rehabilitation Nursing Home — Chicago, IL	•	•	•			•									
Lake Front Healthcare Center Inc — Chicago, IL	•	•	•		•	•	•	•							
Lake Shore Nursing Centre Ltd — Chicago, IL	•	•	•		•	•	•			•		•	•		
Lakeview Nursing & Geriatric Center Inc — Chicago, IL	•	•	•		•		•	•							
Lincoln Park Terrace Inc — Chicago, IL	•	•	•		•	•	•								
Little Sisters of the Poor Center for the Aging — Chicago, IL	•	•	•	•	•	•	•	•							
Margaret Manor — Chicago, IL	•		•	•	•	•									
Margaret Manor—North Branch — Chicago, IL	•	•	•		•	•		•							
Maxwell Manor — Chicago, IL	•		•		•	•				•	•		•	•	

✓ In order to support future editions of this publication would you please mention *Elder Services* each time you contact any advertiser, facility, or service.

Facilities	Dining Room	Physical Therapy Room	Activities Room	Chapel	Crafts Room	Laundry Room	Barber/Beauty Shop	Library	Greenhouse/Garden	Outdoor Patio/Yard	Enclosed Patio/Yard	Room	Lounge/Day Room	Ventilator Unit	Respiratory Unit
The Methodist Home Chicago, IL	•	•	•	•	•	•	•	•	•	•	•	•	•	•	•
Mid-America Convalescent Centers Inc Chicago, IL	•	•	•		•	•	•	•							
Monroe Pavilion Health Center Inc Chicago, IL	•	•	•		•	•	•								
Montgomery Place Chicago, IL	•	•	•			•	•		•	•	•	•	•		
Northwest Home for the Aged Chicago, IL	•	•	•	•	•	•	•	•							
Norwood Park Home Chicago, IL	•	•	•	•	•	•	•	•							
Our Lady of the Resurrection—Extended Care Unit Chicago, IL	•	•	•	•								•	•		
Park House Ltd Chicago, IL	•	•	•		•	•									
Peterson Park Health Care Center Chicago, IL	•	•	•			•	•								
Rainbow Beach Nursing Center Inc Chicago, IL	•		•												
St Joseph Home of Chicago Inc Chicago, IL	•	•	•	•	•	•	•			•		•	•		
St Joseph Hospital & Health Care Center—Skilled Nursing Unit Chicago, IL	•	•	•	•	•		•	•							
St Martha Manor Chicago, IL	•	•	•		•	•	•								
St Paul's House & Health Care Center Chicago, IL	•	•	•	•	•	•	•	•	•	•		•	•		
Selfhelp Home for the Aged Chicago, IL	•	•	•	•	•	•	•	•							
Washington & Jane Smith Home Chicago, IL	•	•	•	•	•	•	•	•	•	•		•	•		
Society for Danish Old People's Home Chicago, IL	•		•			•	•	•							
Somerset House Chicago, IL	•	•	•		•	•	•	•							
Warren Park Nursing Pavilion Chicago, IL	•	•	•		•	•	•			•	•	•	•		
Waterfront Terrace Chicago, IL	•	•	•	•	•	•				•		•	•		

Facilities	Dining Room	Physical Therapy Room	Activities Room	Chapel	Crafts Room	Laundry Room	Barber/Beauty Shop	Library	Greenhouse/Garden	Outdoor Patio/Yard	Enclosed Patio/Yard	Room	Lounge/Day Room	Ventilator Unit	Respiratory Unit
Wellington Plaza Nursing & Therapy Center Chicago, IL	•	•	•	•	•	•	•	•							
The Westwood Manor Inc Chicago, IL	•	•	•		•										
The Whitehall Convalescent and Nursing Home Chicago, IL	•	•	•			•	•			•	•	•			
Wincrest Nursing Center Chicago, IL	•		•			•	•								
Woodbridge Nursing Pavilion Chicago, IL	•	•	•		•	•	•								
Prairie Manor Health Care Center Chicago Heights, IL	•	•	•	•	•	•	•	•		•	•		•		
Riviera Manor Inc Chicago Heights, IL	•	•	•	•	•	•	•	•	•	•	•	•	•		
Thornton Heights Terrace Ltd Chicago Heights, IL	•		•	•	•	•	•								
Chicago Ridge Nursing Center Chicago Ridge, IL	•	•	•	•			•			•	•	•			•
Lexington Health Care Center of Chicago Ridge Chicago Ridge, IL	•	•	•	•	•	•	•	•		•	•	•			
Alden Nursing Center—Town Manor Rehabilitation & Health Care Center Cicero, IL	•	•	•	•	•	•	•	•		•		•			
Westshire Retirement & Healthcare Centre Cicero, IL	•	•	•		•	•	•			•		•	•		
Crestwood Heights Nursing Centre Crestwood, IL	•	•	•	•	•	•	•			•	•	•	•		
St James Manor Crete, IL	•	•	•	•	•		•			•		•	•		
Canterbury Care Center Crystal Lake, IL	•	•	•	•	•	•	•	•		•	•	•	•		
Crystal Pines Health Care Center Crystal Lake, IL	•	•	•			•	•								
Fair Oaks Health Care Center Crystal Lake, IL	•	•	•			•	•			•	•	•	•		
De Kalb County Nursing Home De Kalb, IL	•	•	•		•	•	•	•	•	•		•	•		
Oak Crest—De Kalb Area Retirement Center De Kalb, IL	•	•	•	•	•	•	•	•							
Pine Acres Care Center De Kalb, IL	•	•				•									

✓ In order to support future editions of this publication would you please mention *Elder Services* each time you contact any advertiser, facility, or service.

Facilities	Dining Room	Physical Therapy Room	Activities Room	Chapel	Crafts Room	Laundry Room	Barber/Beauty Shop	Library	Greenhouse/Garden	Outdoor Patio/Yard	Enclosed Patio/Yard	Room	Lounge/Day Room	Ventilator Unit	Respiratory Unit
The Whitehall North Deerfield, IL	•	•	•	•	•	•	•	•		•		•	•		
Ballard Nursing Center Inc Des Plaines, IL	•	•	•			•	•	•	•	•	•	•	•	•	
Holy Family Health Center Des Plaines, IL	•	•	•	•			•			•		•	•	•	
Lee Manor Health Care Residence Des Plaines, IL	•	•	•			•	•	•		•		•	•		
Nazarethville Des Plaines, IL	•	•	•	•	•	•	•	•		•		•			
Oakton Pavilion Healthcare Facility Inc Des Plaines, IL	•	•	•	•	•	•	•	•							
Dolton Healthcare Center Inc Dolton, IL	•	•	•			•	•								
Fairview Baptist Home Downers Grove, IL	•	•	•	•	•	•	•	•	•	•		•	•		
Rest Haven West Skilled Nursing Center Downers Grove, IL	•	•	•		•		•		•	•	•	•	•		
Fernwood Health Care Center Dwight, IL	•	•	•	•	•	•									
Americana Healthcare Center of Elgin Elgin, IL	•	•	•		•	•	•	•	•	•	•	•	•		
Apostolic Christian Resthaven Elgin, IL	•	•	•		•	•									
Heritage Manor of Elgin Elgin, IL	•	•	•	•	•		•	•							
Metropolitan Nursing Center of Elgin Elgin, IL	•	•	•	•		•				•	•	•	•		•
Sherman West Court Elgin, IL	•	•	•		•	•	•	•	•	•		•	•		
Americana Healthcare Center of Elk Grove Elk Grove Village, IL	•	•	•		•	•	•	•	•	•	•	•	•		
Elmhurst Extended Care Center Inc Elmhurst, IL	•	•	•	•	•	•	•	•							
York Convalescent Center Elmhurst, IL	•	•	•		•		•	•			•	•	•		
Royal Elm Convalescent & Geriatric Center Inc Elmwood Park, IL	•	•	•	•	•		•	•		•		•	•		•
Dobson Plaza Evanston, IL	•	•	•		•		•	•		•		•	•		

Facilities	Dining Room	Physical Therapy Room	Activities Room	Chapel	Crafts Room	Laundry Room	Barber/Beauty Shop	Library	Greenhouse/Garden	Outdoor Patio/Yard	Enclosed Patio/Yard	Room	Lounge/Day Room	Ventilator Unit	Respiratory Unit
The King Home Evanston, IL	•	•	•		•		•	•							
McGaw Health Care Center Evanston, IL	•	•	•	•	•	•	•	•	•	•	•		•		
Oakwood Terrace Nursing Home Evanston, IL	•	•	•		•	•	•	•							
St Francis Extended Care Center Evanston, IL	•	•	•	•	•		•	•							
Swedish Retirement Association Evanston, IL	•	•	•	•	•	•	•	•							
Park Lane Nursing Center Association Evergreen Park, IL	•	•	•				•								
Peace Memorial Home Evergreen Park, IL	•	•	•	•			•								
Altenheim Forest Park, IL	•	•	•			•	•			•			•		
Westlake Pavilion Franklin Park, IL	•	•	•		•	•	•		•	•	•	•	•		
Geneva Care Center Geneva, IL	•	•	•	•		•	•	•	•			•	•		
The Abington of Glenview Glenview, IL	•	•	•	•	•	•	•	•	•	•		•	•		
Glenview Terrace Nursing Center Glenview, IL	•	•	•	•	•	•	•	•	•	•	•	•	•		
Maryhaven Inc Glenview, IL	•	•	•	•	•	•	•			•	•	•	•		
Glenwood Terrace Nursing Center Glenwood, IL	•	•	•		•		•		•	•		•	•		
Alden Nursing Center—Heather Rehabilitation & Health Care Center Harvey, IL	•	•	•		•	•	•			•		•	•		
Imperial Nursing Center of Hazel Crest Hazel Crest, IL	•	•	•	•	•	•	•	•		•	•	•			•
Hickory Nursing Pavilion Inc Hickory Hills, IL	•	•	•			•	•								
Abbott House Highland Park, IL	•		•		•	•	•			•	•	•	•		
Villa St Cyril Highland Park, IL	•		•	•		•	•			•		•	•		
Highland Park Health Care Center Inc Highwood, IL	•	•	•		•	•	•								
Americana-Monticello Healthcare Center of Hinsdale Hinsdale, IL	•	•	•		•	•	•		•	•	•		•		

✔ In order to support future editions of this publication would you please mention *Elder Services* each time you contact any advertiser, facility, or service.

Facilities	Dining Room	Physical Therapy Room	Activities Room	Chapel	Crafts Room	Laundry Room	Barber/Beauty Shop	Library	Greenhouse/Garden	Outdoor Patio/Yard	Enclosed Patio/Yard	Room	Lounge/Day Room	Ventilator Unit	Respiratory Unit
Alden—Poplar Creek Rehabilitation & Health Care Center Hoffman Estates, IL	•	•	•	•	•	•	•	•		•	•	•	•		
Mercy Health Care & Rehabilitation Center Homewood, IL	•	•	•	•		•	•	•	•	•		•	•		
Briar Place Ltd Indian Head Park, IL	•	•	•	•	•	•	•								
The Arbor Itasca, IL	•		•	•	•	•	•	•							
Deerbrook Nursing Centre Joliet, IL	•	•	•		•	•	•		•	•		•	•		
Draper Plaza Joliet, IL	•	•		•			•	•							
Metropolitan Nursing Center of Joliet Joliet, IL	•	•	•	•	•		•	•		•		•	•		•
Our Lady of Angels Retirement Home Joliet, IL	•	•	•	•	•	•	•		•	•		•	•		
Salem Village Joliet, IL	•	•	•	•	•	•	•	•							
Sunny Hill Nursing Home Joliet, IL	•	•	•	•	•	•	•								
Villa Franciscan Joliet, IL	•	•	•	•	•	•	•								
Rosary Hill Home Justice, IL	•		•	•	•	•	•			•	•	•	•		
Colonial Manor Healthcare Center La Grange, IL	•	•	•	•	•	•	•	•							
Fairview Health Care Center La Grange, IL	•	•	•		•		•								
Plymouth Place La Grange Park, IL	•	•	•	•	•	•	•	•							
Hill Top Sanitorium Lake Bluff, IL	•		•	•		•		•		•		•	•		
Lake Bluff Healthcare Centre Lake Bluff, IL	•	•	•	•	•					•		•	•		•
Holy Family Villa Lemont, IL	•	•	•	•		•	•			•	•	•	•		
Mother Theresa Home Lemont, IL	•	•	•	•	•		•			•	•	•			
Americana Healthcare Center of Libertyville Libertyville, IL	•	•	•			•	•	•							

Facilities	Dining Room	Physical Therapy Room	Activities Room	Chapel	Crafts Room	Laundry Room	Barber/Beauty Shop	Library	Greenhouse/Garden	Outdoor Patio/Yard	Enclosed Patio/Yard	Room	Lounge/Day Room	Ventilator Unit	Respiratory Unit
Libertyville Manor Extended Care Facility Libertyville, IL	•	•	•	•	•	•	•	•		•		•	•		
Winchester House Libertyville, IL	•	•	•	•	•	•	•	•							
Regency Park Manor Lincolnwood, IL	•	•	•	•	•	•	•	•	•	•	•	•	•		
Victory Lakes Continuing Care Center Lindenhurst, IL	•	•	•	•	•	•	•	•	•	•	•	•	•		
Snow Valley Living Center Lisle, IL	•	•	•			•				•		•	•		
Beacon Hill Lombard, IL	•	•	•		•		•			•	•	•			
Bloomingdale Pavilion Lombard, IL	•	•	•		•	•			•	•	•	•			
Maple Hill Nursing Home Ltd Long Grove, IL	•	•	•	•	•	•	•	•	•	•	•	•			
Florence Nursing Home Marengo, IL	•		•		•					•		•	•		
Applewood Living Center Matteson, IL	•	•	•		•	•	•	•		•		•	•		•
Baptist Retirement Home Maywood, IL	•	•	•	•	•	•	•	•							
Royal Terrace McHenry, IL	•	•	•	•	•	•	•								
Bowman Nursing Home Midlothian, IL	•		•		•	•				•		•	•		
Crestwood Terrace Midlothian, IL	•	•	•		•	•	•	•							
Grundy County Home Morris, IL	•	•	•	•	•	•	•								
Morris Lincoln Nursing Home Morris, IL	•					•	•								
Bethany Terrace Nursing Centre Morton Grove, IL	•	•	•	•	•	•	•	•		•	•	•	•		
Alden Nursing Center—Naperville Rehabilitation & Health Care Center Naperville, IL	•	•	•		•	•	•			•		•	•		
Americana Healthcare Center of Naperville Naperville, IL	•	•	•		•	•	•		•	•		•	•		
Community Convalescent Center of Naperville Naperville, IL	•	•	•	•	•	•	•			•	•	•	•		

✓ In order to support future editions of this publication would you please mention *Elder Services* each time you contact any advertiser, facility, or service.

Facilities	Dining Room	Physical Therapy Room	Activities Room	Chapel	Crafts Room	Laundry Room	Barber/Beauty Shop	Library	Greenhouse/Garden	Outdoor Patio/Yard	Enclosed Patio/Yard	Room	Lounge/Day Room	Ventilator Unit	Respiratory Unit
St Patrick's Residence Naperville, IL	•	•	•	•	•	•	•	•	•	•		•	•		
Forest Villa Nursing Center Niles, IL	•	•	•	•			•	•	•	•	•	•	•		
Glen Bridge Nursing & Rehabilitation Center Niles, IL	•	•	•	•	•	•	•								
George J Goldman Memorial Home for the Aged Niles, IL	•	•	•	•		•	•	•		•		•	•		
Hampton Plaza Niles, IL	•	•	•		•	•	•	•							
Regency Nursing Centre Niles, IL	•	•	•	•		•	•			•		•	•		
St Benedict Home for Aged Niles, IL	•		•	•		•	•								
Central Baptist Home for the Aged Norridge, IL	•	•	•	•	•	•	•			•	•	•	•		
Norridge Nursing Centre Inc Norridge, IL	•	•	•		•	•	•	•	•	•	•	•	•		
Maplewood Health Care Center North Aurora, IL	•	•	•		•	•	•		•	•	•	•	•		
The Scottish Home North Riverside, IL	•	•	•		•	•	•	•		•		•			
Brandel Care Center Northbrook, IL	•	•	•	•		•	•			•	•	•	•		
GAF/Lake Cook Terrace Northbrook, IL	•	•	•		•	•	•	•							
Glen Oaks Nursing Home Inc Northbrook, IL	•	•	•		•	•	•	•							
Villa Scalabrini Northlake, IL	•	•	•	•		•				•		•	•		
Oak Brook Healthcare Centre Oak Brook, IL	•	•				•	•				•	•	•		
Americana Healthcare Center of Oak Lawn Oak Lawn, IL	•	•	•			•	•	•							
Americana-Monticello Healthcare Center of Oak Lawn Oak Lawn, IL	•	•	•		•	•	•	•	•	•	•	•	•		
Concord Extended Care Oak Lawn, IL		•	•	•	•	•	•								
Oak Lawn Convalescent Home Oak Lawn, IL	•	•	•			•	•								

Facilities	Dining Room	Physical Therapy Room	Activities Room	Chapel	Crafts Room	Laundry Room	Barber/Beauty Shop	Library	Greenhouse/Garden	Outdoor Patio/Yard	Enclosed Patio/Yard	Room	Lounge/Day Room	Ventilator Unit	Respiratory Unit
Metropolitan Nursing Center of Oak Park Oak Park, IL	•	•	•	•		•	•	•		•	•	•	•		•
The Woodbine Convalescent Home Oak Park, IL	•	•	•			•	•			•	•	•	•		
The Tillers Nursing Home Oswego, IL	•	•	•	•	•	•	•	•	•	•	•	•	•		
Little Sisters of the Poor Palatine, IL	•	•	•	•	•	•	•	•		•	•	•	•		
Plum Grove Nursing Home Palatine, IL	•	•	•		•	•	•								
Americana Healthcare Center of Palos Heights Palos Heights, IL	•	•	•		•	•	•	•	•	•	•	•	•		
Rest Haven Central Nursing Home Palos Heights, IL	•	•	•	•	•	•	•	•	•	•	•	•	•		
Ridgeland Living Center Palos Heights, IL	•	•					•			•		•	•		
Windsor Manor Nursing & Rehabilitation Center Palos Hills, IL	•	•	•				•			•		•	•		
Park Ridge Healthcare Center Park Ridge, IL	•		•		•										
Resurrection Nursing Pavilion Park Ridge, IL	•	•	•	•	•		•			•	•	•	•		
St Matthew Lutheran Home Park Ridge, IL	•	•	•	•	•	•	•								
Lakewood Living Center Plainfield, IL	•		•	•	•		•								
Richton Crossing Convalescent Center Richton Park, IL	•	•	•				•	•							
Brentwood North Nursing & Rehabilitation Center Riverwoods, IL	•	•	•	•	•	•	•	•	•	•	•	•	•		
Lydia Healthcare Robbins, IL	•	•	•	•	•	•	•	•	•	•		•	•		
Americana Healthcare Center of Rolling Meadows Rolling Meadows, IL	•	•	•		•	•	•	•	•	•	•	•	•		
Abbington House Roselle, IL	•		•		•	•	•	•							
Hillcrest Nursing Center Round Lake Beach, IL	•		•		•	•	•			•		•	•		
Pine View Care Center Saint Charles, IL	•	•			•		•	•							

✔ In order to support future editions of this publication would you please mention *Elder Services* each time you contact any advertiser, facility, or service.

Facilities	Dining Room	Physical Therapy Room	Activities Room	Chapel	Crafts Room	Laundry Room	Barber/Beauty Shop	Library	Greenhouse/Garden	Outdoor Patio/Yard	Enclosed Patio/Yard	Room	Lounge/Day Room	Ventilator Unit	Respiratory Unit
Dogwood Health Care Center Sandwich, IL	•		•		•	•	•								
Willow Crest Nursing Pavilion Sandwich, IL	•	•	•			•	•		•	•		•	•		
Friendship Village of Schaumburg Schaumburg, IL	•	•	•		•	•	•	•							
Shabbona Health Care Center Inc Shabbona, IL	•		•		•	•	•								
Lieberman Geriatric Health Centre Skokie, IL	•	•	•		•	•	•	•	•	•			•		
Old Orchard Manor Skokie, IL	•	•	•	•	•	•	•		•	•		•			
Skokie Meadows Nursing Center 1 Skokie, IL	•	•	•		•	•	•	•							
Fox Valley Healthcare Inc South Elgin, IL	•	•	•	•	•										
Americana Healthcare Center of South Holland South Holland, IL	•	•	•		•	•	•	•	•	•	•	•	•		
Rest Haven South South Holland, IL	•	•	•	•	•	•	•	•	•	•	•	•	•		
Windmill Nursing Pavilion Ltd South Holland, IL	•	•	•	•	•	•	•	•							
Pershing Convalescent Home Inc Stickney, IL	•	•	•			•									
The McAllister Nursing Home Inc Tinley Park, IL	•	•	•	•	•	•	•	•							
Town Hall Estates—Wauconda Inc Wauconda, IL	•		•	•	•	•				•		•	•		
Bayside Terrace Waukegan, IL	•		•		•	•	•			•		•	•		
Lake Park Center Waukegan, IL	•	•	•				•				•		•		
Northshore Terrace Waukegan, IL	•	•	•	•	•	•	•	•							
The Terrace Nursing Home Inc Waukegan, IL	•	•	•		•	•	•	•							
Arbor Terrace Health Care Center West Chicago, IL	•	•	•	•	•	•	•	•	•			•	•		
West Chicago Terrace West Chicago, IL	•	•	•			•	•		•	•		•	•		
Americana Healthcare Center of Westmont Westmont, IL	•	•	•		•	•									

Facilities	Dining Room	Physical Therapy Room	Activities Room	Chapel	Crafts Room	Laundry Room	Barber/Beauty Shop	Library	Greenhouse/Garden	Outdoor Patio/Yard	Enclosed Patio/Yard	Room	Lounge/Day Room	Ventilator Unit	Respiratory Unit
Burgess Square Healthcare Centre Westmont, IL	•	•	•		•	•	•								
Westmont Convalescent Center Westmont, IL	•	•	•			•	•								
Du Page Convalescent Center Wheaton, IL	•	•	•		•	•	•	•							
Parkway Healthcare Center Wheaton, IL	•	•	•				•			•	•	•	•		
Sandalwood Healthcare Centre Wheaton, IL	•	•	•			•	•								
Addolorata Villa Wheeling, IL	•	•	•	•	•	•	•	•		•		•	•		
Chateau Village Living Center Willowbrook, IL	•	•	•	•	•		•			•		•	•		
Normandy House Wilmette, IL	•		•		•		•	•	•	•		•	•		
Royal Willow Nursing Care Center Wilmington, IL	•	•	•			•	•								
Liberty Hill Healthcare Center Winfield, IL	•	•	•	•	•	•	•								
Sunset Manor Woodstock, IL	•	•	•	•		•	•			•	•	•	•		
Valley Hi Nursing Home Woodstock, IL	•	•	•	•		•	•								
The Woodstock Residence Woodstock, IL	•	•	•	•	•	•	•	•							
Hillside Health Care Center Yorkville, IL	•		•			•	•			•		•	•		
Crown Manor Healthcare Center Zion, IL	•	•	•	•	•	•	•	•		•	•	•	•	•	•
Rolling Hills Manor Zion, IL	•	•	•		•	•	•								
Sheridan Health Care Center Zion, IL	•	•	•			•	•	•							
Colonial Nursing Home Crown Point, IN	•		•			•	•			•		•	•		
Lake County Convalescent Home Crown Point, IN	•	•	•	•	•		•	•							
Lutheran Home of Northwest Indiana Inc Crown Point, IN	•	•	•	•	•	•	•	•			•	•	•		
St Anthony Home Crown Point, IN	•		•	•			•			•			•		
Lake Holiday Manor Demotte, IN	•		•	•	•	•	•								

✔ In order to support future editions of this publication would you please mention *Elder Services* each time you contact any advertiser, facility, or service.

Facilities	Dining Room	Physical Therapy Room	Activities Room	Chapel	Crafts Room	Laundry Room	Barber/Beauty Shop	Library	Greenhouse/Garden	Outdoor Patio/Yard	Enclosed Patio/Yard	Room	Lounge/Day Room	Ventilator Unit	Respiratory Unit
Meridian Nursing Center—Dyer Dyer, IN	•	•	•		•	•	•			•	•	•	•		
Lake County Rehabilitation Center Inc East Chicago, IN	•		•		•	•	•								
Green's Geriatric Health Center Gary, IN	•		•			•									
West Side Health Care Center Gary, IN	•	•	•	•	•	•	•		•	•	•	•	•		
Wildwood Manor—Clark Gary, IN	•	•	•	•	•	•									
Wildwood Manor—Mount Gary, IN	•		•		•	•	•								
Highland Nursing Home Highland, IN	•		•			•						•	•		
Miller's Merry Manor Hobart, IN	•	•	•		•	•	•								
Sebo's Heritage Manor Hobart, IN	•		•			•	•		•	•	•	•	•		
Fountainview Terrace La Porte, IN	•	•	•	•	•	•	•	•							
Lowell Health Care Center Lowell, IN	•		•		•	•	•								
Towne Centre Merrillville, IN	•	•	•		•	•	•			•		•	•		
Michigan City Health Care Michigan City, IN	•	•	•	•	•	•	•	•							
Red Oaks Healthcare Center Michigan City, IN	•	•	•	•		•	•								
Munster Med-Inn Munster, IN	•	•	•			•	•	•							
Fountainview Place Portage, IN	•	•	•		•	•	•								
Miller's Merry Manor Portage, IN	•	•	•		•	•	•								
Little Company of Mary Health Facility Inc San Pierre, IN	•		•	•	•	•	•								
Canterbury Place Valparaiso, IN	•	•	•		•	•	•	•		•		•	•		
Pavilion Health Care Center Valparaiso, IN	◦	•	•												
Whispering Pines Health Care Center Valparaiso, IN	•	•	•	•	•	•	•	•							
The Willow Rehabilitation Center Valparaiso, IN	•	•				•	•			•			•		

Facilities	Dining Room	Physical Therapy Room	Activities Room	Chapel	Crafts Room	Laundry Room	Barber/Beauty Shop	Library	Greenhouse/Garden	Outdoor Patio/Yard	Enclosed Patio/Yard	Room	Lounge/Day Room	Ventilator Unit	Respiratory Unit
Hammond-Whiting Convalescent Center Whiting, IN	●		●			●	●								

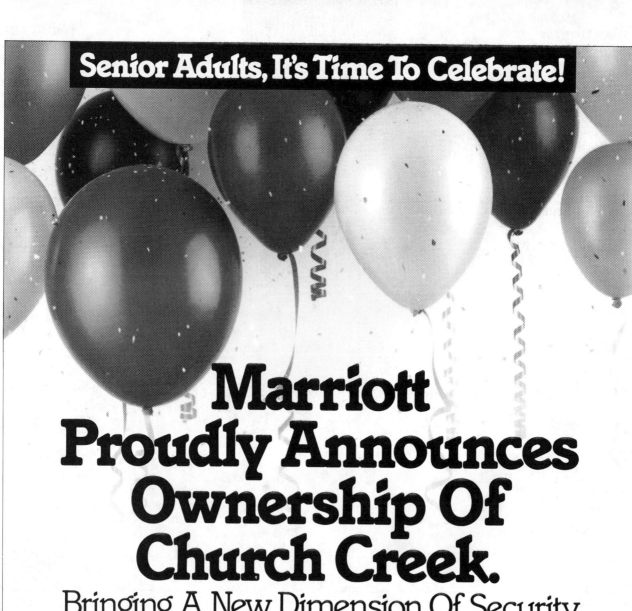

Sheltered and Congregate Care

ILLINOIS

Alsip

Windsor Place of Alsip
5450 W 127th St, Alsip, IL 60658
(708) 385-5200
CONGREGATE LIVING: Room for rent; Entrance fee $300;
Residents 30; Max. no. residents 52; Units 32
Facility Profile
ENTRANCE AGE REQUIREMENT: (min) 60
See ad page 283

Arlington Heights

Lutheran Home & Services for the Aged
800 W Oakton St, Arlington Heights, IL 60004
(708) 253-3710
SHELTERED CARE: Private room; Entrance fee is monthly
rate in advance; Residents 167; Max. no. residents
167; Units 167; Occupancy level 97%
Facility Profile
SERVICES: Central dining; Housekeeping; Transportation; Social and recreational; Financial
management/counseling; Social worker/Mental
health; Physical therapy and rehabilitation; Alzheimer's day, respite, residential care; Medical care;
Security; Library; Chapel
See ads pages 69, 202

The Moorings of Arlington Heights
811 E Central Rd, Arlington Heights, IL 60005
(708) 437-6700
SHELTERED CARE: Private room; Semiprivate room; Private bath; Residents 66; Max. no. residents 69;
Units 69; Occupancy level 97%
Facility Profile
SERVICES: Central dining; Housekeeping; Transportation; Social and recreational; Financial
management/counseling; Social worker/Mental
health; Physical therapy and rehabilitation; Medical
care; Library; Long-term care insurance; 24-hour
security; Laundry facilities; Personal storage areas;
Indoor swimming pool; Walking path; Fitness center; Woodworking shop; Convenience mart;
Beauty/barber shop; Arts/crafts room; Heated underground parking; Billiards room; Individual garden plots; Meditation room; Chaplain
ENTRANCE AGE REQUIREMENT: (min) 62
See ads pages 140, 202, 301

Aurora

Fox Knoll Retirement Community
412 N Lake St, Aurora, IL 60506
(708) 844-0380
SHELTERED CARE: Private room; Semiprivate room; Private bath; Entrance fee $0; Units 80
Facility Profile
AVERAGE MONTHLY FEES: $0-$1000
SERVICES: Central dining; Housekeeping; Transportation; Social and recreational; Financial
management/counseling; Social worker/Mental
health; Security; Library; Religious services
ENTRANCE AGE REQUIREMENT: (min) 62

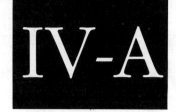

Jennings Terrace
275 S Lasalle, Aurora, IL 60505
(708) 897-6946
SHELTERED CARE: Private room; Semiprivate room; Residents 104

Sunnymere Inc
925 6th Ave, Aurora, IL 60505
(708) 898-7844
SHELTERED CARE: Private room; Entrance fee $0; Residents 43; Max. no. residents 48; Units 48; Occupancy level 100%
Facility Profile
AVERAGE MONTHLY FEES: $0-$1000
SERVICES: Central dining; Housekeeping; Social and recreational; Social worker/Mental health; Library
ENTRANCE AGE REQUIREMENT: (min) 65

Batavia

Colonial House at The Holmstad
831 N Batavia Ave, Batavia, IL 60510
(708) 879-4300, 879-1153 FAX
SHELTERED CARE: Private room; Units 26
See ads pages iv, 300

Bridgeview

Moraine Court Senior Apartments
8080 S Harlem Ave, Bridgeview, IL 60455
(708) 594-2700
CONGREGATE LIVING: Suite/Apt for rent; Room for rent; Entrance fee $0; Residents 150; Max. no. residents 165; Units 155
Facility Profile
AVERAGE MONTHLY FEES: $0-$1000; $1001-$2000
SERVICES: Central dining; Housekeeping; Social and recreational; Security; Library; Country store; Beauty/Barber shop; Chapel; Billiard room

Brookfield

The British Home
31st & McCormick, Brookfield, IL 60513
(708) 485-0135
SHELTERED CARE: Private room; Entrance fee $0; Residents 59; Max. no. residents 64; Units 64; Occupancy level 93%
Facility Profile
AVERAGE MONTHLY FEES: $1001-$2000
SERVICES: Central dining; Housekeeping; Transportation; Social and recreational; Social worker/Mental health; Physical therapy and rehabilitation; Medical care; Security; Library
ENTRANCE AGE REQUIREMENT: (min) 65

The Wye Valley Apartments
2940 S McCormick Ave, Brookfield, IL 60513
(708) 387-7799
SHELTERED CARE: Private room; Private bath; Residents 60; Max. no. residents 64; Units 64; Occupancy level 90%
Facility Profile
AVERAGE MONTHLY FEES: $0-$1000
SERVICES: Central dining; Housekeeping; Transportation; Social and recreational; Security; Library
ENTRANCE AGE REQUIREMENT: (min) 65

Burr Ridge

King Bruwaert House
6101 County Line Rd, Burr Ridge, IL 60521
(708) 323-2250
SHELTERED CARE: Private room; Residents 76; Max. no. residents 80; Units 83; Occupancy level 95%
Facility Profile
AVERAGE MONTHLY FEES: $1001-$2000
SERVICES: Central dining; Housekeeping; Transportation; Social and recreational; Social worker/Mental health; Physical therapy and rehabilitation; Medical care; Security; Library
ENTRANCE AGE REQUIREMENT: (min) 60

Carol Stream

Windsor Park Manor
124 Windsor Park Dr, Carol Stream, IL 60188
(708) 682-4377
SHELTERED CARE: Private room; Residents 22; Units 23
Facility Profile
AVERAGE MONTHLY FEES: $1001-$2000
SERVICES: Central dining; Housekeeping; Transportation; Social and recreational; Social worker/Mental health; Physical therapy and rehabilitation; Medical care; Security; Library; Rock shop; Photography/darkroom
ENTRANCE AGE REQUIREMENT: (min) 60

Chicago

2960 North Lake Shore Dr, A Classic Residence by Hyatt
2960 N Lake Shore Dr, Chicago, IL 60657
(800) 882-2960; (312) 882-2960
CONGREGATE LIVING: Suite/Apt for rent; Entrance fee $11,000-$35,000; Units 340

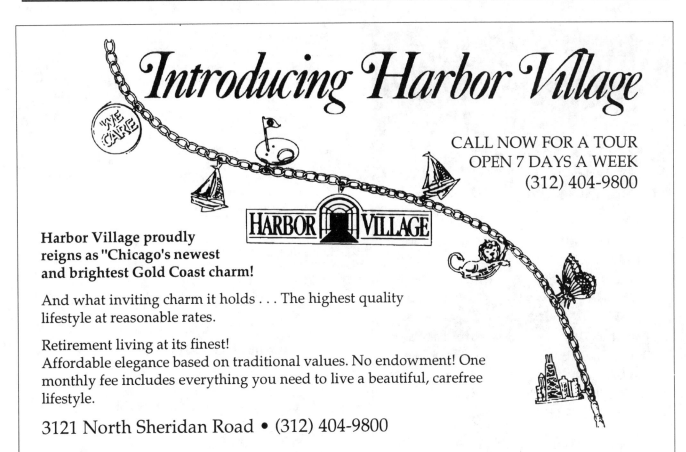
Facility Profile

AVERAGE MONTHLY FEES: $2001-$3000

SERVICES: Central dining; Housekeeping; Transportation; Social and recreational; Security; Library; Fitness center

ENTRANCE AGE REQUIREMENT: (min) 62

Bethany Retirement Home

4950 N Ashland Ave, Chicago, IL 60640

(312) 989-1501

SHELTERED CARE: Private room; Private bath; Entrance fee $7,500; Residents 24; Max. no. residents 26; Units 26; Occupancy level 92%

Facility Profile

AVERAGE MONTHLY FEES: $0-$1000

SERVICES: Central dining; Housekeeping; Transportation; Social and recreational; Social worker/Mental health; Physical therapy and rehabilitation; Medical care; Security; Library

ENTRANCE AGE REQUIREMENT: (min) 60

Bethesda Home & Retirement Center

2833 N Nordica Ave, Chicago, IL 60634

(312) 622-6144

SHELTERED CARE: Private room; Semiprivate room; Private bath; Residents 45; Max. no. residents 67; Occupancy level 67%

Facility Profile

AVERAGE MONTHLY FEES: $1001-$2000

SERVICES: Central dining; Housekeeping; Transporta-

tion; Social and recreational; Social worker/Mental health; Physical therapy and rehabilitation; Medical care; Security

ENTRANCE AGE REQUIREMENT: (min) 62

Buckingham Pavilion Nursing & Rehabilitation Center

2625 W Touhy Ave, Chicago, IL 60645

(312) 764-6850

SHELTERED CARE: Private room; Semiprivate room; Residents 80; Max. no. residents 80; Units 34; Occupancy level 100%

Facility Profile

AVERAGE MONTHLY FEES: $2001-$3000

ENTRANCE AGE REQUIREMENT: (min) 65

Cortland Manor Retirement Home

1900 N Karlov, Chicago, IL 60639

(312) 235-3670

CONGREGATE LIVING: Room for rent; Residents 53; Max. no. residents 56; Occupancy level 95%

Facility Profile

AVERAGE MONTHLY FEES: $0-$1000

SERVICES: Central dining; Housekeeping; Medical care; Security

Covenant Home of Chicago

2725 W Foster, Chicago, IL 60625

(312) 878-8200, 334-7516 FAX

SHELTERED CARE: Private room; Entrance fee $11,000-$13,500; Units 70

✓ In order to support future editions of this publication would you please mention *Elder Services* each time you contact any advertiser, facility, or service.

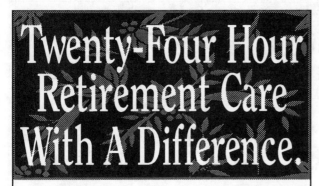

Facility Profile
SERVICES: Central dining; Housekeeping; Social and recreational; Medical care; Security; Library; Pastoral care
See ads pages iv, 300

Harbor Village
3121 N Sheridan Rd, Chicago, IL 60657
(312) 404-9800
CONGREGATE LIVING: Suite/Apt for rent; Entrance fee $0; Units 144
Facility Profile
AVERAGE MONTHLY FEES: $0-$1000; $1001-$2000
SERVICES: Central dining; Housekeeping; Social and recreational; Medical care; Library; Store; Private dining room; TV room; Game room; Prayer room; Cafe; Laundry facility; Activity room; Billard room
ENTRANCE AGE REQUIREMENT: (min) 65
See ad page 285

Kagan Home for the Blind
3525 W Foster Ave, Chicago, IL 60625
(312) 478-7040
SHELTERED CARE: Private room; Residents 31; Max. no. residents 53
Facility Profile
AVERAGE MONTHLY FEES: $0-$1000
SERVICES: Central dining; Housekeeping; Transportation; Social and recreational; Physical therapy and rehabilitation; Security; Library

Kraus Home
1620 W Chase, Chicago, IL 60626
(312) 973-2100
SHELTERED CARE: Private room; Semiprivate room; Residents 61; Max. no. residents 62; Occupancy level 99%
Facility Profile
AVERAGE MONTHLY FEES: $1001-$2000
SERVICES: Central dining; Housekeeping; Transportation; Social and recreational; Financial management/counseling; Social worker/Mental health; Medical care; Security; Library
ENTRANCE AGE REQUIREMENT: (min) 60
See ad page 286

Lakeside Boarding Home
6330 N Sheridan Rd, Chicago, IL 60660
(312) 338-2811
SHELTERED CARE: Private room; Semiprivate room; Ward; Residents 30; Max. no. residents 34; Units 19; Occupancy level 95%
Facility Profile
AVERAGE MONTHLY FEES: $0-$1000
SERVICES: Central dining; Housekeeping; Transportation; Social and recreational; Financial management/counseling; Social worker/Mental health; Physical therapy and rehabilitation; Medical care; Security; Library
ENTRANCE AGE REQUIREMENT: (min) 18

Lincoln Park Retirement Apartments
2437 N Southport, Chicago, IL 60614
(312) 248-9300
CONGREGATE LIVING: Suite/Apt for rent; Room for rent; Entrance fee $0; Residents 110; Max. no. residents 119; Units 119
Facility Profile
AVERAGE MONTHLY FEES: $1001-$2000
SERVICES: Central dining; Housekeeping; Transportation; Social and recreational; Security; Library; Store; TV room; Laundry room; Storage room
ENTRANCE AGE REQUIREMENT: (min) 55

The Methodist Home
1415 W Foster Ave, Chicago, IL 60640
(312) 769-5500, (312) 769-6287 FAX
SHELTERED CARE: Private room; Residents 9; Max. no. residents 11; Units 11
Facility Profile
AVERAGE MONTHLY FEES: $1001-$2000
SERVICES: Central dining; Housekeeping; Transportation; Social and recreational; Social worker/Mental health; Physical therapy and rehabilitation; Alzheimer's day, respite, residential care; Medical care; Security; Library
ENTRANCE AGE REQUIREMENT: (min) 60

Park Plaza Retirement Center
6840 N Sacramento, Chicago, IL 60645
(312) 465-6700

CONGREGATE LIVING: Suite/Apt for rent; Residents 205; Max. no. residents 205; Units 164; Occupancy level 100%

Facility Profile

AVERAGE MONTHLY FEES: $1001-$2000

SERVICES: Central dining; Housekeeping; Transportation; Social and recreational; Financial management/counseling; Social worker/Mental health; Medical care; Security; Library

Plaza on the Lake

7301 N Sheridan Rd, Chicago, IL 60626

(312) 743-7600

SHELTERED CARE: Private room; Semiprivate room; Private bath

CONGREGATE LIVING: Suite/Apt for rent; Units 98; Occupancy level 80%

Facility Profile

AVERAGE MONTHLY FEES: $1001-$2000

SERVICES: Central dining; Housekeeping; Transportation; Social and recreational; Alzheimer's day, respite, residential care; Security; Library

ENTRANCE AGE REQUIREMENT: (min) 62

St Joseph Home of Chicago Inc

2650 N Ridgeway Ave, Chicago, IL 60647

(312) 235-8600

SHELTERED CARE: Private room

CONGREGATE LIVING: Suite/Apt; Residents 177

Facility Profile

AVERAGE MONTHLY FEES: $2001-$3000

SERVICES: Medical care; Physical therapy and rehabilitation; Spiritual; Central dining; Security

ENTRANCE AGE REQUIREMENT: (min) 65

St Paul's House

3831 N Mozart St, Chicago, IL 60618

(312) 478-4222

SHELTERED CARE: Private room; Private bath; Entrance fee $0; Residents 60; Units 74; Occupancy level 79

Facility Profile

AVERAGE MONTHLY FEES: $0-$1000

SERVICES: Central dining; Housekeeping; Transportation; Social and recreational; Financial management/counseling; Social worker/Mental health; Physical therapy and rehabilitation; Alzheimer's day, respite, residential care; Medical care; Security; Library; Chapel

ENTRANCE AGE REQUIREMENT: (min) 65

See ad page 9

Selfhelp Home for the Aged

908 W Argyle St, Chicago, IL 60640

(312) 271-0300

SHELTERED CARE: Private room

CONGREGATE LIVING: Suite/Apt; Residents 46

Washington & Jane Smith Home

2340 W 113th Pl, Chicago, IL 60643

(312) 779-8010

SHELTERED CARE: Private room; Residents 234

Society for Danish Old People's Home

5656 N Newcastle Ave, Chicago, IL 60631

(312) 775-7383

SHELTERED CARE: Semiprivate room; Residents 59

Squire's Sheltered Care Home

2601 N California, Chicago, IL 60647

(312) 278-5300

SHELTERED CARE: Private room; Semiprivate room; Private bath; Entrance fee $535; Residents 37

Facility Profile

AVERAGE MONTHLY FEES: $0-$1000

SERVICES: Physical therapy and rehabilitation; Housekeeping; Social and recreational; Financial management/counseling; Central dining; Classes; Shopping; Laundry

ENTRANCE AGE REQUIREMENT: (min) 18

Uptown Shelter Care Home

4646 N Beacon, Chicago, IL 60640

(312) 561-7707

SHELTERED CARE: Private room; Semiprivate room; Entrance fee $678; Residents 52; Units 19; Occupancy level 95%

Facility Profile

AVERAGE MONTHLY FEES: $0-$1000

SERVICES: Central dining; Housekeeping; Social and recreational; Financial management/counseling; Social worker/Mental health; Medical care; Library

ENTRANCE AGE REQUIREMENT: (min) 21

Crete

Rest Haven Village Woods

2681 S Rte 394, Crete, IL 60417

(708) 672-6111, 672-8914 FAX

CONGREGATE LIVING: Room for rent; Units 128

Facility Profile

AVERAGE MONTHLY FEES: $0-$1000

SERVICES: Central dining; Housekeeping; Transportation; Social and recreational; Financial management/counseling; Security; Library; Beauty shop; Laundry facility; Catered living option

See ad on page i

Crystal Lake

Canterbury Place Retirement Community

965 N Brighton Cir W, Crystal Lake, IL 60012

(815) 455-8400

CONGREGATE LIVING: Suite/Apt for rent; Entrance fee $0; Residents 100; Max. no. residents 240; Units 200; Occupancy level 50%

Facility Profile

AVERAGE MONTHLY FEES: $1001-$2000

SERVICES: Central dining; Housekeeping; Transportation; Social and recreational; Security; Library; Beauty shop; Convenience store; Game room; Arts & crafts room; Fitness area; Linen service; TV

Lounge; Private dining areas; Free health screening; Seminars; Gardening area; Multi-denominational religious service

Darien

Carmelite Carefree Village

8419 Bailey Rd, Darien, IL 60559
(708) 960-4060
CONGREGATE LIVING: Room for rent; Entrance fee $0; Residents 103; Max. no. residents 103-105; Units 96; Occupancy level 100%

Des Plaines

The Breakers at Golf Mill

8975 Golf Rd, Des Plaines, IL 60016
(708) 296-0333
CONGREGATE LIVING: Suite/Apt for rent; Residents 325; Units 282; Occupancy level 98%
Facility Profile
AVERAGE MONTHLY FEES: $1001-$2000
SERVICES: Central dining; Housekeeping; Transportation; Social and recreational; Security; Library; Pool; Fitness center; Craft studio
ENTRANCE AGE REQUIREMENT: (min) 62
See ad page 305

The Heritage of Des Plaines

800 S River Rd, Des Plaines, IL 60016
(708) 699-8600
SHELTERED CARE: Private room; Private bath; Entrance fee $0; Units 50
CONGREGATE LIVING: Suite/Apt for rent; Entrance fee $0; Units 206
Facility Profile
AVERAGE MONTHLY FEES: $0-$1000; $1001-$2000
SERVICES: Central dining; Housekeeping; Transportation; Social and recreational; Security; Library; Staff available 24 hours a day; Comprehensive emergency response system; Life enrichment program; General store; Ice cream parlor; Full-service bank; Health and fitness center including indoor swimming pool and whirlpool; Woodworking shop; Beauty/barber shop; Clubroom/billiards; Covered parking; Pet and smoking wings; Travel & save program
See ad page 288, 292

Oakton Arms

1665 Oakton Pl, Des Plaines, IL 60018
(708) 827-4200
CONGREGATE LIVING: Suite/Apt for rent; Residents 106; Units 102; Occupancy level 100%

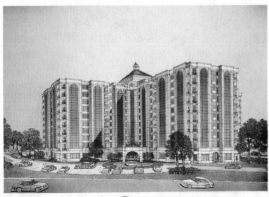 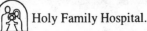

Facility Profile

AVERAGE MONTHLY FEES: $1001-$2000

SERVICES: Central dining; Housekeeping; Transportation; Social and recreational; Social worker/Mental health; Medical care; Security; Library

Downers Grove

Fairview Village

7 S 241 Fairview Ave, Downers Grove, IL 60516

(708) 852-0426

CONGREGATE LIVING: Suite/Apt

Facility Profile

AVERAGE MONTHLY FEES: $0-$1000

SERVICES: Central dining; Housekeeping; Transportation; Social and recreational; Security; Library

ENTRANCE AGE REQUIREMENT: (min) 55

See ads pages 136, 219

Saratoga Grove Christian Retirement Center

3460 Saratoga Ave, Downers Grove, IL 60515

(708) 971-1995

SHELTERED CARE: Private room; Entrance fee $0; Max. no. residents 96

CONGREGATE LIVING: Suite/Apt for rent; Entrance fee $0; Max. no. residents 96; Units 96; Occupancy level 100%

Facility Profile

AVERAGE MONTHLY FEES: $1001-$2000

SERVICES: Central dining; Housekeeping; Transportation; Social and recreational; Financial management/counseling; Social worker/Mental health; Physical therapy and rehabilitation; Security; Library

ENTRANCE AGE REQUIREMENT: (min) 62

See ad on page i

Elgin

Countryside Manor

971 Bode Rd, Elgin, IL 60120

(708) 695-9600

SHELTERED CARE: Semiprivate room; Entrance fee $1,425; Residents 39; Max. no. residents 39; Units 22; Occupancy level 39

Facility Profile

AVERAGE MONTHLY FEES: $1001-$2000

SERVICES: Central dining; Housekeeping; Transportation; Social and recreational; Social worker/Mental health; Physical therapy and rehabilitation; Library

ENTRANCE AGE REQUIREMENT: (min) 55

Oak Crest Residence

204 S State St, Elgin, IL 60123

(708) 742-2255

SHELTERED CARE: Private room; Entrance fee $0; Residents 31; Max. no. residents 39; Units 39; Occupancy level 39

Facility Profile

AVERAGE MONTHLY FEES: $1001-$2000

SERVICES: Central dining; Housekeeping; Social and recreational; Alzheimer's day, respite, residential care; Library; Day care; Respite care

ENTRANCE AGE REQUIREMENT: (min) 60

Sherman West Court

1950 Larkin Ave, Elgin, IL 60123

(708) 742-7070

SHELTERED CARE: Semiprivate room; Residents 10; Max. no. residents 28

Facility Profile

AVERAGE MONTHLY FEES: $2001-$3000

SERVICES: Central dining; Housekeeping; Social and recreational; Financial management/counseling; Social worker/Mental health; Physical therapy and rehabilitation; Alzheimer's day, respite, residential care; Medical care; Security

ENTRANCE AGE REQUIREMENT: (min) 62

Evanston

Homecrest Foundation

1430 Chicago Ave, Evanston, IL 60201

(708) 869-2162

SHELTERED CARE: Private room; Semiprivate room; Residents 110

Normandy Hall

2601 Central St, Evanston, IL 60201

(708) 869-6065

CONGREGATE LIVING: Room for rent; Entrance fee $0; Residents 22; Max. no. residents 25; Units 25

Facility Profile

AVERAGE MONTHLY FEES: $1001-$2000

SERVICES: Central dining; Housekeeping; Transportation; Social and recreational; Social worker/Mental health; Security; Library

ENTRANCE AGE REQUIREMENT: (min) 55

North Shore Retirement Hotel

1611 Chicago Ave, Evanston, IL 60201

(708) 864-6400, 570-7880 FAX

CONGREGATE LIVING: Suite/Apt for rent; Entrance fee is a security deposit; Residents 238; Max. no. residents 245; Units 239; Occupancy level 99%

Facility Profile

AVERAGE MONTHLY FEES: $0-$1000

SERVICES: Central dining; Housekeeping; Transportation; Social and recreational; Security; Library; Movie theater; Private garden; Swimming pool; Ballroom; Billiard room; Card room; Laundry room

ENTRANCE AGE REQUIREMENT: (min) 60

Wilson/Sidwell Apartments

3200 Grant St, Evanston, IL 60201

(708) 570-3422

SHELTERED CARE: Private room; Entrance fee; Max. no. residents 39; Units 34

✔ In order to support future editions of this publication would you please mention *Elder Services* each time you contact any advertiser, facility, or service.

Facility Profile

AVERAGE MONTHLY FEES: $1001-$2000

SERVICES: Central dining; Housekeeping; Transportation; Social and recreational; Social worker/Mental health; Physical therapy and rehabilitation; Medical care; Security; Library; Pharmacy; Dental exams; Eye exams; Chapel; Lounges; Convenience store; Recreation; Flat linen service

ENTRANCE AGE REQUIREMENT: (min) 65

Forest Park

Altenheim

7824 W Madison St, Forest Park, IL 60130

(708) 366-2206

SHELTERED CARE: Private room; Entrance fee $0; Units 50

Facility Profile

AVERAGE MONTHLY FEES: $2001-$3000

SERVICES: Central dining; Housekeeping; Transportation; Social and recreational; Physical therapy and rehabilitation; Alzheimer's day, respite, residential care; Medical care; Security

ENTRANCE AGE REQUIREMENT: (min) 65

Harvey

Dixie Manor Sheltered Care

15535 Dixie Hwy, Harvey, IL 60426

(708) 339-6438

SHELTERED CARE: Private room; Semiprivate room; Residents 23

Halsted Manor

16044 S Halsted St, Harvey, IL 60426

(708) 339-5311

SHELTERED CARE: Private room; Semiprivate room; Residents 42

Kenniebrew Home

14812 S Marshfield Ave, Harvey, IL 60426

(708) 339-9345

SHELTERED CARE: Private room; Semiprivate room; Residents 21

Hinsdale

West Suburban Shelter Care Center

Rte 83 and 91st St, Hinsdale, IL 60521

(708) 323-0198

SHELTERED CARE: Private room; Semiprivate room; Residents 46

Joliet

Broadway Residence

PO Box 2757, 216 N Broadway, Joliet, IL 60434

(815) 727-7672

CONGREGATE LIVING: Room for rent; Entrance fee $0; Residents 10; Max. no. residents 24; Units 15; Occupancy level 45%

Facility Profile

ENTRANCE AGE REQUIREMENT: (min) 50

Our Lady of Angels Retirement Home

1201 Wyoming Ave, Joliet, IL 60435

(815) 725-6631

SHELTERED CARE: Private room; Semiprivate room; Residents 46

Facility Profile

AVERAGE MONTHLY FEES: $1001-$2000

SERVICES: Central dining; Housekeeping; Transportation; Social and recreational; Social worker/Mental health; Medical care; Security; Library; Religious services

ENTRANCE AGE REQUIREMENT: (min) 65

Justice

Rosary Hill Home

9000 W 81st St, Justice, IL 60458

(708) 458-3040

SHELTERED CARE: Private room; Max. no. residents 50

La Grange

Windsor Place

42 S Ashland Ave, La Grange, IL 60525

(708) 354-6670

CONGREGATE LIVING: Room for rent; Entrance fee $300; Residents 36; Max. no. residents 42; Units 38

Facility Profile

AVERAGE MONTHLY FEES: $0-$1000

SERVICES: Central dining; Housekeeping; Transportation; Social and recreational; Financial management/counseling; Alzheimer's day, respite, residential care; Chapel

ENTRANCE AGE REQUIREMENT: (min) 60

See ad page 283

Lemont

Alvernia Manor Retirement Home

1598 Main St, Lemont, IL 60439

(708) 257-7721

SHELTERED CARE: Private room; Entrance fee $1000; Residents 48; Max. no. residents 50; Units 50; Occupancy level 96%

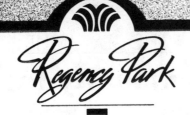
Facility Profile
AVERAGE MONTHLY FEES: $0-$1000
SERVICES: Central dining; Housekeeping; Transportation; Social and recreational; Library
ENTRANCE AGE REQUIREMENT: (min) 65

Franciscan Village
1270 Village Dr, Lemont, IL 60439
(708) 257-3377
SHELTERED CARE: Private room; Entrance fee $0
Facility Profile
AVERAGE MONTHLY FEES: $0-$1000; $1001-$2000
SERVICES: Central dining; Housekeeping; Transportation; Social and recreational; Security; Library
ENTRANCE AGE REQUIREMENT: (min) 55

Mother Theresa Home
1270 Franciscan Dr, Lemont, IL 60439
(708) 257-5801, 257-8615 FAX
SHELTERED CARE: Private room; Units 30

Libertyville

Americana Healthcare Center of Libertyville
1500 S Milwaukee Ave, Libertyville, IL 60048
(708) 816-3200
SHELTERED CARE: Private room; Semiprivate room; Private bath; Max. no. residents 25
See ad page 200

Lincolnwood

Regency Park
7000 N McCormick Blvd, Lincolnwood, IL 60645
(708) 673-7166
SHELTERED CARE: Private room; Private bath
CONGREGATE LIVING: Suite/Apt for rent
Facility Profile
SERVICES: Central dining; Housekeeping; Transportation; Social and recreational; Financial management/counseling; Social worker/Mental health; Physical therapy and rehabilitation; Medical care; Security; Library
See ad page 291

Lisle

The Devonshire
1700 Robin Ln, Lisle, IL 60532
(708) 963-1600
SHELTERED CARE: Private room; Private bath; Entrance fee $0; Residents 60; Max. no. residents 60; Units 60
CONGREGATE LIVING: Suite/Apt for rent; Entrance fee $0; Residents 250; Units 324; Occupancy level 75%

✔ In order to support future editions of this publication would you please mention *Elder Services* each time you contact any advertiser, facility, or service.

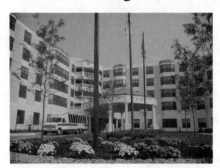
Facility Profile
AVERAGE MONTHLY FEES: $1001-$2000
SERVICES: Central dining; Housekeeping; Transportation; Social and recreational; Security; Library; Comprehensive emergency response system; General store; Full-service bank; Fine arts & crafts room; Beauty/barber shop; Woodworking shop; Health and fitness center with pool, sauna, whirlpool, and exercise equipment; Pet wing; Club room with pub; Gardening areas; Guest suites; Community room with large screen TV; Outdoor patio; Concierge services; Garage parking; Billiards
ENTRANCE AGE REQUIREMENT: (min) 62
See ads pages 288, 292

Queen of Peace Retirement Center
1910 Maple Ave, Lisle, IL 60532
(708) 852-5360
SHELTERED CARE: Private room
Facility Profile
AVERAGE MONTHLY FEES: $0-$1000
SERVICES: Central dining; Housekeeping; Social and recreational; Security; Wellness exercise
ENTRANCE AGE REQUIREMENT: (min) 62

Maywood

Baptist Retirement Home
316 W Randolph, Maywood, IL 60153
(708) 344-1541
SHELTERED CARE: Semiprivate room; Ward
Facility Profile
AVERAGE MONTHLY FEES: $1001-$2000
SERVICES: Central dining; Housekeeping; Transportation; Social and recreational; Social worker/Mental health; Physical therapy and rehabilitation; Alzheimer's day, respite, residential care; Medical care; Security; Library
ENTRANCE AGE REQUIREMENT: (min) 70

McHenry

McHenry Villa
3516 W Waukegan Rd, McHenry, IL 60050
(815) 344-0246
CONGREGATE LIVING: Suite/Apt for rent; Units 112
Facility Profile
AVERAGE MONTHLY FEES: $0-$1000; $1001-$2000
SERVICES: Central dining; Housekeeping; Transportation; Social and recreational; Security; Library; Beauty/barber shop; Card & game room; Lounge;

Outdoor patio & gardens; Linen service; Laundry rooms; Sunday van service to local churches; Low-income units
ENTRANCE AGE REQUIREMENT: (min) Retired adults
See ad page 293

Midlothian

Golfview Retirement Manor
14500 S Long Ave, Midlothian, IL 60445
(708) 385-6080
CONGREGATE LIVING: Room for rent; Residents 26
Facility Profile
AVERAGE MONTHLY FEES: $0-$1000
SERVICES: Central dining; Housekeeping; Transportation; Social and recreational; Library
ENTRANCE AGE REQUIREMENT: (min) 45

Morris

Morris Lincoln Nursing Home
916 Fremont, Morris, IL 60450
(815) 942-1202
SHELTERED CARE: Private room; Semiprivate room; Units 34

Naperville

St Patrick's Residence
1400 Brookdale Rd, Naperville, IL 60563-2126
(708) 416-6565
SHELTERED CARE: Private room; Semiprivate room; Residents 61
Facility Profile
AVERAGE MONTHLY FEES: $1001-$2000; $2001-$3000
SERVICES: Central dining; Housekeeping; Social and recreational; Physical therapy and rehabilitation; Medical care; Security; Spiritual services; Coffee shop; Resident lift-bus; Beauty/barber shop
ENTRANCE AGE REQUIREMENT: (min) 65

Niles

St Andrew Home for the Aged
7000 N Newark Ave, Niles, IL 60648
(708) 647-8332
SHELTERED CARE: Private room; Semiprivate room; Private bath; Residents 57
CONGREGATE LIVING: Room, units 143, for rent; Residents 137

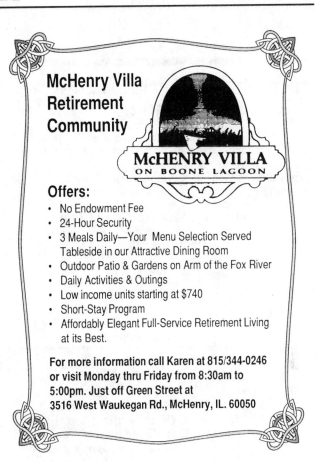
Facility Profile
AVERAGE MONTHLY FEES: $0-$1000
SERVICES: Medical care; Housekeeping; Shopping; Spiritual; Social and recreational; Financial management/counseling; Central dining; Security
ENTRANCE AGE REQUIREMENT: (min) 65; (max) 85

Norridge

Central Baptist Home for the Aged
4750 N Orange, Norridge, IL 60656
(708) 452-3700
SHELTERED CARE: Private room
CONGREGATE LIVING: Suite/Apt; Residents 136

North Aurora

Asbury Court
210 Airport Rd, North Aurora, IL 60542
(708) 896-7778
SHELTERED CARE: Private room; Private bath
CONGREGATE LIVING: Suite/Apt, for rent; Entrance fee $0; Residents 150; Units 193

✔ In order to support future editions of this publication would you please mention *Elder Services* each time you contact any advertiser, facility, or service.

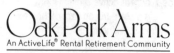

Facility Profile
AVERAGE MONTHLY FEES: $1001-$2000
SERVICES: Central dining; Housekeeping; Social and recreational; Library; Chapel; Medical office; Beauty shop; Billiard room; TV room; Activity room; Store

North Riverside

The Scottish Home
2800 S Des Plaines Ave, North Riverside, IL 60546
(708) 447-5092
SHELTERED CARE: Private room
CONGREGATE LIVING: Suite/Apt; Residents 63

Northbrook

Axelson Manor
2195 Foxglove Dr, Northbrook, IL 60062
(708) 480-7110
SHELTERED CARE: Private room; Private bath; Residents 50; Max. no. residents 52; Units 52; Occupancy level 100%
Facility Profile
AVERAGE MONTHLY FEES: $1001-$2000; $2001-$3000
SERVICES: Central dining; Housekeeping; Transportation; Social and recreational; Financial management/counseling; Social worker/Mental health; Physical therapy and rehabilitation; Security
ENTRANCE AGE REQUIREMENT: (min) 62
See ads pages iv, 300

Northlake

Villa Scalabrini
480 N Wolf Rd, Northlake, IL 60164
(708) 562-0040
SHELTERED CARE: Private room; Semiprivate room; Entrance fee $100; Residents 265
Facility Profile
AVERAGE MONTHLY FEES: $0-$1000
SERVICES: Physical therapy and rehabilitation; Housekeeping; Spiritual; Social and recreational; Central dining; Security

Oak Park

The Oak Park Arms
408 S Oak Park Ave, Oak Park, IL 60302
(708) 386-4040
CONGREGATE LIVING: Suite/Apt for rent; Room for rent; Entrance fee $1000; Residents 185; Max. no. residents 200; Units 194; Occupancy level 90%
Facility Profile
AVERAGE MONTHLY FEES: $0-$1000
SERVICES: Central dining; Housekeeping; Transportation; Social and recreational; Medical care; Security; Library
ENTRANCE AGE REQUIREMENT: (min) 62
See ads pages xiv, xix, 122, 294

Olympia Fields

Mercy Residence at Tolentine Center
20300 Governors Hwy, Olympia Fields, IL 60461
(708) 748-9500
CONGREGATE LIVING: Suite/Apt for rent; Room for rent; Entrance fee is a security deposit; Residents 50; Max. no. residents 52; Units 49; Occupancy level 50
Facility Profile
AVERAGE MONTHLY FEES: $0-$1000; $1001-$2000
SERVICES: Central dining; Housekeeping; Transportation; Social and recreational; Financial management/counseling; Social worker/Mental health; Security; Library; Medical care; Massage therapy; Tai chi exercises; Crafts; Beauty shop
ENTRANCE AGE REQUIREMENT: (min) 60

Palatine

St Joseph's Home
80 W Northwest Hwy, Palatine, IL 60067
(708) 358-5700
SHELTERED CARE: Private room; Semiprivate room; Residents 130

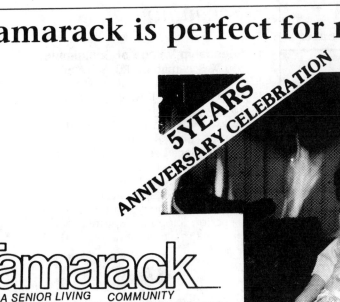

Tamarack
55 S Greeley St, Palatine, IL 60067
(708) 991-4700
CONGREGATE LIVING: Suite/Apt for rent; Entrance fee $1500; Residents 129; Max. no. residents 150; Units 133; Occupancy level 92%
Facility Profile
ENTRANCE AGE REQUIREMENT: (min) 62
See ad page 295

Palos Heights

Americana Healthcare Center of Palos Heights
7850 W College Dr, Palos Heights, IL 60463
(708) 361-6990
SHELTERED CARE: Private room; Semiprivate room; Private bath; Max. no. residents 29
See ad page 200

Park Ridge

St Matthew Lutheran Home
1601 N Western Ave, Park Ridge, IL 60068
(708) 825-5531
SHELTERED CARE: Private room
CONGREGATE LIVING: Suite/Apt; Residents 176

Summit Square Retirement Hotel
10 N Summit, Park Ridge, IL 60068
(708) 825-1161
CONGREGATE LIVING: Suite/Apt for rent; Room for purchase; Entrance fee $0; Residents 225; Max. no. residents 225; Units 223; Occupancy level 100%
Facility Profile
SERVICES: Central dining; Housekeeping; Transportation; Social and recreational; Security
ENTRANCE AGE REQUIREMENT: (min) 62

Peotone

Peotone Bensenville Home
104 S West St, Peotone, IL 60468
(708) 258-6879
SHELTERED CARE: Private room; Private bath; Entrance fee $0; Residents 27; Max. no. residents 28; Units 28; Occupancy level 96%
Facility Profile
AVERAGE MONTHLY FEES: $1001-$2000
SERVICES: Central dining; Housekeeping; Transportation; Social and recreational; Security
ENTRANCE AGE REQUIREMENT: None

IV-A

Hotel Baker Living Center

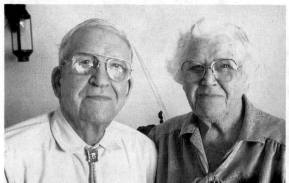

We're All Family

Hotel Baker Living Center
100 W. Main St.
St. Charles
Illinois
60174
708/584-2100

Bringing a parent to a retirement home is extremely stressful—for both the new resident and family members. But it can be the best and wisest move. At Hotel Baker Living Center, we can help you decide if it's the right step. If it is, we help everyone in your family adjust to ours.

Come talk with us.

A program of Lutheran Social Services of Illinois

Saint Charles

Hotel Baker Living Center—Lutheran Social Services of Illinois
100 W Main St, Saint Charles, IL 60174
(708) 584-2100
CONGREGATE LIVING: Suite/Apt for rent; Room for rent; Entrance fee $846-$1600; Units 52
Facility Profile
AVERAGE MONTHLY FEES: $0-$1000
SERVICES: Central dining; Housekeeping; Social and recreational; Social worker/Mental health; Security; Library; Church services
See ad page 296

Sandwich

Dogwood Health Care Center
902 E Arnold Ave, Sandwich, IL 60548
(815) 786-8409
CONGREGATE LIVING: Suite/Apt, units 20, for rent
Facility Profile
AVERAGE MONTHLY FEES: $0-$1000
SERVICES: Medical care; Spiritual; Social and recreational; Central dining; Security
ENTRANCE AGE REQUIREMENT: (min) 55

Schaumburg

Friendship Village of Schaumburg
350 W Schaumburg Rd, Schaumburg, IL 60194
(708) 884-5000, 884-5053 FAX
SHELTERED CARE: Private room; Units 76
Facility Profile
AVERAGE MONTHLY FEES: $1001-$2000
SERVICES: Central dining; Housekeeping; Transportation; Social and recreational; Financial management/counseling; Social worker/Mental health; Physical therapy and rehabilitation; Alzheimer's day, respite, residential care; Medical care; Security; Library; Gardens; Garages; Bank; Beauty parlor; Shopping; Spiritual
ENTRANCE AGE REQUIREMENT: (min) 62
See ad page 317

Skokie

Robineau Group Living Residence
7550 N Kostner, Skokie, IL 60076
(312) 508-1000
CONGREGATE LIVING: Room for rent; Residents 24; Max. no. residents 24; Units 24
Facility Profile
ENTRANCE AGE REQUIREMENT: (min) 60

South Holland

Holland Home
16300 Louis Ave, South Holland, IL 60473
(708) 596-3050, 596-3067 FAX
SHELTERED CARE: Private room; Entrance fee $0; Residents 305; Max. no. residents 312; Units 312; Occupancy level 98%
Facility Profile
AVERAGE MONTHLY FEES: $0-$1000
SERVICES: Central dining; Housekeeping; Transportation; Social and recreational; Financial management/counseling; Social worker/Mental health; Physical therapy and rehabilitation; Medical care; Security; Library; Chaplain
ENTRANCE AGE REQUIREMENT: (min) 65
See ad on page i

Tinley Park

Royal Acres Retirement Village
16301 S Brementowne Dr, Tinley Park, IL 60477
(708) 532-7800
CONGREGATE LIVING: Suite/Apt for rent; Entrance fee $400 refundable; Units 108

✔ In order to support future editions of this publication would you please mention *Elder Services* each time you contact any advertiser, facility, or service.

Facility Profile

AVERAGE MONTHLY FEES: $0-$1000; $1001-$2000

SERVICES: Central dining; Housekeeping; Transportation; Social and recreational; Security; Library; Exercise equipment; Beauty/Barber shops; Card room; Billiard room; Craft room; Church services

ENTRANCE AGE REQUIREMENT: (min) 62

Vernon Hills

Hawthorn Lakes of Lake County

10 E Hawthorn Pkwy, Vernon Hills, IL 60061

(708) 367-2516

CONGREGATE LIVING: Suite/Apt for rent; Entrance fee $0

Facility Profile

AVERAGE MONTHLY FEES: $1001-$2000

SERVICES: Central dining; Housekeeping; Transportation; Social and recreational; Security; Library

ENTRANCE AGE REQUIREMENT: (min) 62

See ads pages xiv, xix, 122, 294

West Chicago

Arbor Terrace Health Care Center

30 W 300 North Ave, West Chicago, IL 60185

(708) 231-4050

SHELTERED CARE: Private room; Entrance fee $0; Units 70

CONGREGATE LIVING: Room for rent; Entrance fee $0; Units 178

Facility Profile

AVERAGE MONTHLY FEES: $1001-$2000

SERVICES: Central dining; Housekeeping; Transportation; Social and recreational; Financial management/counseling; Social worker/Mental health; Physical therapy and rehabilitation; Alzheimer's day, respite, residential care; Medical care; Security; Library; Chapel

ENTRANCE AGE REQUIREMENT: (min) 18

Wheeling

Addolorata Villa

555 McHenry Rd, Wheeling, IL 60090

(708) 537-2900

SHELTERED CARE: Private room; Private bath; Residents 43; Max. no. residents 45; Units 45; Occupancy level 95%

Facility Profile

AVERAGE MONTHLY FEES: $1001-$2000

SERVICES: Central dining; Housekeeping; Transportation; Social and recreational; Financial

management/counseling; Social worker/Mental health; Physical therapy and rehabilitation; Alzheimer's day, respite, residential care; Medical care; Security; Library

ENTRANCE AGE REQUIREMENT: (min) 62

Wilmette

Baha'i Home

401 Greenleaf Ave, Wilmette, IL 60091

(708) 251-7000

SHELTERED CARE: Private room; Residents 20; Max. no. residents 20; Units 20

Facility Profile

AVERAGE MONTHLY FEES: $1001-$2000

SERVICES: Central dining; Housekeeping; Social and recreational; Social worker/Mental health; Security; Library

ENTRANCE AGE REQUIREMENT: (min) 65

Klafter Residence

615 Ridge Rd, Wilmette, IL 60091

(708) 251-7799

CONGREGATE LIVING: Suite/Apt for rent; Residents 29; Max. no. residents 29

Facility Profile

AVERAGE MONTHLY FEES: $1001-$2000

SERVICES: Central dining; Housekeeping; Transportation; Social and recreational; Social worker/Mental health; Security

ENTRANCE AGE REQUIREMENT: (min) 62

Woodstock

Carefree Village

840 N Seminary Ave, Woodstock, IL 60098

(800) 339-CARE; (815) 338-2110

CONGREGATE LIVING: Suite/Apt for purchase, for rent; Entrance fee $41,500-$89,500; Residents 65; Max. no. residents 80; Units 71; Occupancy level 85%

Facility Profile

AVERAGE MONTHLY FEES: $1001-$2000

SERVICES: Central dining; Housekeeping; Transportation; Social and recreational; Financial management/counseling; Security; Library; Country store; Beauty/barber shop; Private dining room; Exercise room; Garages

ENTRANCE AGE REQUIREMENT: (min) 60

Sunset Manor

PO Box 520, 920 N Seminary Ave, Woodstock, IL 60098

(815) 338-1749, 338-0062 FAX

SHELTERED CARE: Private room; Units 63

✔ In order to support future editions of this publication would you please mention *Elder Services* each time you contact any advertiser, facility, or service.

INDIANA

Demotte

Lake Holiday Manor
10325 County Line Rd, Demotte, IN 46310
(219) 345-5211
SHELTERED CARE: Private room
CONGREGATE LIVING: Suite/Apt; Units 16

Dyer

Regency Place
2300 Great Lakes Dr, Dyer, IN 46311
(219) 322-3555
SHELTERED CARE: Private room; Semiprivate room; Residents 150

Hammond

Albertine Home
1501 Hoffman St, Hammond, IN 46327
(219) 937-0575
CONGREGATE LIVING: Suite/Apt for rent; Residents 37

La Porte

Fountainview Terrace
1900 Andrew Ave, La Porte, IN 46350
(219) 362-7014
SHELTERED CARE: Private room; Semiprivate room; Residents 194
Facility Profile
AVERAGE MONTHLY FEES: $2001-$3000
SERVICES: Medical care; Physical therapy and rehabilitation; Housekeeping; Spiritual; Social and recreational; Central dining; Transportation
ENTRANCE AGE REQUIREMENT: (min) 21

Merrillville

Southlake Care Center
8800 Virginia Pl, Merrillville, IN 46410
(219) 736-1310
SHELTERED CARE: Private room; Semiprivate room; Private bath
Facility Profile
SERVICES: Central dining; Housekeeping; Social and recreational; Financial management/counseling; Social worker/Mental health; Physical therapy and rehabilitation; Medical care; Library

Towne Centre
7250 Arthur Blvd, Merrillville, IN 46410
(219) 736-2900
SHELTERED CARE: Private room; Entrance fee $56.00 per day; Residents 34; Max. no. residents 34; Units 34; Occupancy level 100%
CONGREGATE LIVING: Suite/Apt for rent; Entrance fee $995-$1800; Residents 137; Max. no. residents 162; Units 148; Occupancy level 93%
Facility Profile
SERVICES: Central dining; Housekeeping; Transportation; Social and recreational; Physical therapy and rehabilitation; Alzheimer's day, respite, residential care; Security; Library; Resident services
ENTRANCE AGE REQUIREMENT: (min) 55

Michigan City

Wedow Private Home Care
602 Spring St, Michigan City, IN 46360
(219) 879-0140
SHELTERED CARE: Private room; Semiprivate room; Residents 17

Portage

Fountainview Place
3175 Lancer St, Portage, IN 46368
(219) 762-9571
SHELTERED CARE: Semiprivate room; Units 226

WHY BE BOTHERED?

Wrong numbers. Unsolicited solicitations. Pranksters. Nosy neighbors. How do you separate these little annoyances from the phone calls you really care about? Like calls from your favorite friends and family?

The solution is Caller ID, new from Illinois Bell. Caller ID clearly shows the caller's number on a display screen that's attached to your phone. It's incredibly easy to use. And affordable, too.

When the phone rings and you're not sure how to answer, the answer is Caller ID.

CALLER ID.
For information and availability, call
1-800-428-2111
Dept. 89.

During its introduction, Caller ID will give you numbers of calls placed within your local Illinois Bell calling area. Both you and the caller must be in specially-equipped calling areas for numbers to appear on your display screen. Display equipment is purchased separately. If you want to block the appearance of your number when you place a call, dial *67 on your touchtone phone, or 1167 on rotary dials. The activation of your blocking is confirmed with a stutter, followed by a dial tone.

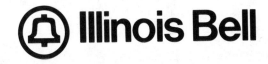

Illinois Bell

AMERITECH

In the Chicago area...

Your new retirement life is waiting at

A Covenant Retirement Community ®

with the active lifestyle you want now and the loving care you may need later.

The full, rich, active life you've planned for your retirement years can now be yours at Covenant Village of Northbrook and The Holmstad of Batavia, both Covenant Continuing Care Retirement Communities. Beautiful apartments, beautiful grounds, caring staff and more ... fellowship, friendship, companionship and loving care later, if you need it, are here. Owned by the Evangelical Covenant Church, both Northbrook and The Holmstad as well as the Covenant's other 10 not-for-profit retirement communities reflect a 100 year tradition of caring and financial stability...

strengths rarely found elsewhere. It's your assurance that your retirement years will be rich, rewarding and independent ... with personal freedom to pursue any interest or activity you desire. Here you'll share those retirement years with others who have your interests, faith and heritage in a beautiful environment of meaningful Christian fellowship ... with the added assurance, if care is ever needed it is close at hand. To obtain information about Covenant Village of Northbrook or The Holmstad please call or fill out and mail the coupon below to the appropriate address.

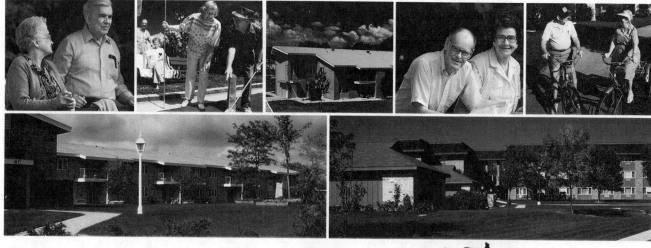

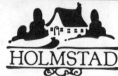

Independent Living

ILLINOIS

Addison

Indian Trail Apartments
601 Meadows Blvd, Addison, IL 60101
(708) 627-5332
INDEPENDENT LIVING: Apt, for rent; Entrance fee $480-
$700; Units 200

Arlington Heights

Greencastle of Arlington Heights
320 W Campbell, Arlington Heights, IL 60005
(708) 506-1010

INDEPENDENT LIVING: Apt; Units 80
Facility Profile
AVERAGE MONTHLY FEES: Govt-subsidized

Luther Village
1280 Village Dr, Arlington Heights, IL 60004
(708) 506-1919
CONTINUING CARE: Apt units; Private home units; Nursing on-site; Purchase price as a cooperative with
full equity
Facility Profile
AVERAGE MONTHLY FEES: $0-$1000
SERVICES: Central dining; Housekeeping; Transportation; Social and recreational; Medical care; Security; Library; Health club; Indoor swimming pool
ENTRANCE AGE REQUIREMENT: (min) 55
See ad page 302

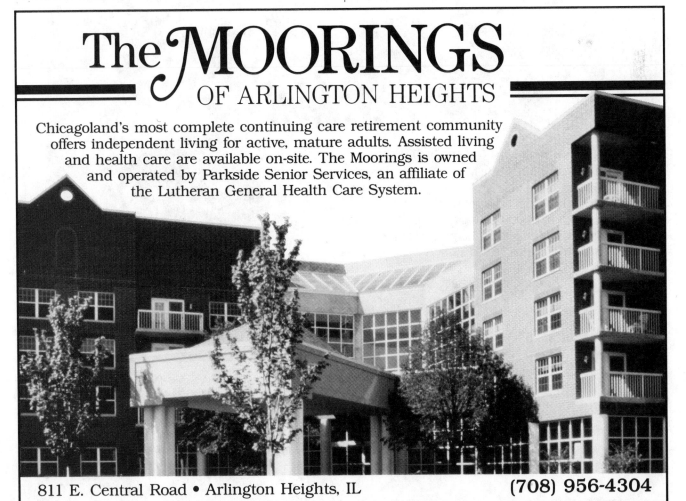

Profiles in Retirement Living

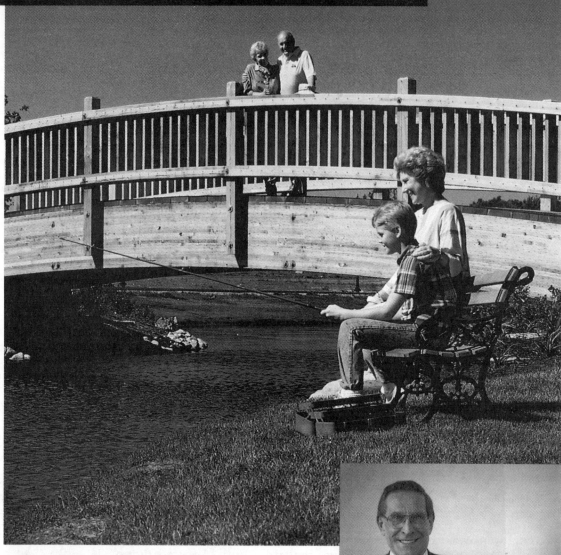

"This is ideal...it's a wonderfully planned community.
We were impressed with the quality of home construction, the beautiful lake and campus-like landscaping. No lawn maintenance or snow shoveling. We're still active in business and after raising our family we decided to semi-retire. We have the freedom to come and go as we please."

Luther Village has the quality and independence Don & Nancy Huebner were looking for.

Luther Village is the retirement lifestyle you're looking for.

LUTHER VILLAGE

1280 Village Drive, #147 • Arlington Heights, IL 60004
For more information please call (708) 506-1919.

A nondenominational development of The Charles H. Shaw Company in affiliation with The Lutheran Home healthcare services.

Don & Nancy Huebner
Luther Village Residents

Marriott Church Creek Retirement Center

1250 W Central Rd, Arlington Heights, IL 60005
(708) 506-3200
CONTINUING CARE: Apt units; Residents 216; Max. no. residents 246; Units 246; Occupancy level 88%; Rental program; Nursing on-site
Facility Profile
AVERAGE MONTHLY FEES: $1001-$2000
SERVICES: Central dining; Housekeeping; Transportation; Social and recreational; Financial management/counseling; Social worker/Mental health; Physical therapy and rehabilitation; Medical care; Security; Library
ENTRANCE AGE REQUIREMENT: (min) 60
See ad page 282

The Moorings of Arlington Heights

811 E Central Rd, Arlington Heights, IL 60005
(708) 437-6700
CONTINUING CARE: Apt units; Private home units; Entrance fee $43,000-$262,000; Residents 315; Max. no. residents 547; Units 291; Occupancy level 91%; Endowment program; Nursing on-site
Facility Profile
SERVICES: Central dining; Housekeeping; Transportation; Social and recreational; Financial management/counseling; Social worker/Mental health; Physical therapy and rehabilitation; Medical care; Library; Long-term care insurance; 24-hour security; Laundry facilities; Personal storage areas; Indoor swimming pool; Walking path; Fitness center; Woodworking shop; Convenience mart; Beauty/barber shop; Arts/crafts room; Heated underground parking; Billiards room; Individual garden plots; Meditation room; Chaplain
ENTRANCE AGE REQUIREMENT: (min) 62
See ads pages 140, 202, 301

Aurora

Aurora Housing Authority—Centennial House

1630 W Plum St, Aurora, IL 60506
(708) 859-7210
INDEPENDENT LIVING: Apt for rent; Residents 131; Units 126; Occupancy level 125
Facility Profile
AVERAGE MONTHLY FEES: Govt-subsidized
ENTRANCE AGE REQUIREMENT: (min) 62

Aurora Housing Authority—Maple Terrace Apartments

905 2nd Ave, Aurora, IL 60505
(708) 859-7362
INDEPENDENT LIVING: Apt for rent; Residents 189; Units 208
Facility Profile
AVERAGE MONTHLY FEES: Govt-subsidized

Fox Knoll Retirement Community

412 N Lake St, Aurora, IL 60506
(708) 844-0380
INDEPENDENT LIVING: Apt for rent; Entrance fee $0; Units 90
Facility Profile
AVERAGE MONTHLY FEES: $0-$1000
SERVICES: Central dining; Housekeeping; Transportation; Social and recreational; Financial management/counseling; Social worker/Mental health; Security; Library; Religious services
ENTRANCE AGE REQUIREMENT: (min) 62

Plum Landing

495 N Lake St, Aurora, IL 60506
(708) 896-5031
INDEPENDENT LIVING: Apt for rent; Entrance fee $0; Residents 68; Max. no. residents 70; Units 70; Occupancy level 97%
Facility Profile
AVERAGE MONTHLY FEES: $0-$1000
SERVICES: Central dining; Housekeeping; Transportation; Social and recreational; Security; Library; Commissary; Beauty/Barber shop; Activity rooms; Laundry

Batavia

Green Meadows

1187 W Wilson St, Batavia, IL 60510
(708) 879-8300
INDEPENDENT LIVING: Apt for rent; Entrance fee $0; Units 150; Occupancy level 100%
Facility Profile
AVERAGE MONTHLY FEES: Govt-subsidized
SERVICES: Social and recreational

The Holmstad

700 W Fabyan Pkwy, Batavia, IL 60510
(708) 879-4000, 879-1153 FAX
CONTINUING CARE: Apt units; Entrance fee $47,000-$99,500; Units 370; Nursing on-site
Facility Profile
SERVICES: Central dining; Housekeeping; Transportation; Social and recreational; Medical care; Library; Linen service; Spiritual activities; Indoor/outdoor parking; Beauty/Barber shop; Convenience store; Access banking; Woodshop; Gardening; Exercise equipment; Health services; 24-hour security
ENTRANCE AGE REQUIREMENT: (min) 62
See ads pages iv, 300

✔ In order to support future editions of this publication would you please mention *Elder Services* each time you contact any advertiser, facility, or service.

Bensenville

Bridgeway of Bensenville
113 E Memorial, Bensenville, IL 60106
(708) 766-0605
CONTINUING CARE: Apt units; Entrance fee $40,000-
$57,000; Max. no. residents 240; Units 172; Nursing
on-site
Facility Profile
AVERAGE MONTHLY FEES: $1001-$2000
SERVICES: Central dining; Housekeeping; Transportation; Social and recreational; Physical therapy and
rehabilitation; Alzheimer's day, respite, residential
care; Security; Library
ENTRANCE AGE REQUIREMENT: (min) 62

Castle Towers & Meadow Crest
325 S York Rd, Bensenville, IL 60106
(708) 766-5800
INDEPENDENT LIVING: Apt, units 160, for rent
Facility Profile
SERVICES: Social and recreational; Transportation
ENTRANCE AGE REQUIREMENT: (min) 62

Bridgeview

Moraine Court Senior Apartments
8080 S Harlem Ave, Bridgeview, IL 60455
(708) 594-2700
INDEPENDENT LIVING: Apt for rent; Entrance fee $0;
Residents 150; Max. no. residents 165; Units 155
Facility Profile
AVERAGE MONTHLY FEES: $0-$1000; $1001-$2000
SERVICES: Central dining; Housekeeping; Social and re-
creational; Security; Library; Country store; Beauty/
Barber shop; Chapel; Billiard room

Brookfield

The Wye Valley Apartments
2940 S McCormick Ave, Brookfield, IL 60513
(708) 387-7799
INDEPENDENT LIVING: Apt for rent; Residents 74;
Units 66; Occupancy level 100%
Facility Profile
AVERAGE MONTHLY FEES: $0-$1000
SERVICES: Central dining; Housekeeping; Transporta-
tion; Social and recreational; Security; Library
ENTRANCE AGE REQUIREMENT: (min) 65

Burr Ridge

King Bruwaert House
6101 County Line Rd, Burr Ridge, IL 60521
(708) 323-2250
INDEPENDENT LIVING: Private home for rent;
Residents 48; Units 31; Occupancy level 98%
CONTINUING CARE: Rental program; Nursing on-site
Facility Profile
AVERAGE MONTHLY FEES: $1001-$2000
SERVICES: Central dining; Housekeeping; Transporta-
tion; Social and recreational; Social worker/Mental
health; Physical therapy and rehabilitation; Medical
care; Security; Library
ENTRANCE AGE REQUIREMENT: (min) 60

Carol Stream

Windsor Park Manor
124 Windsor Park Dr, Carol Stream, IL 60188
(708) 682-4377
INDEPENDENT LIVING: Apt for purchase
CONTINUING CARE: Apt units; Occupancy level 91%;
Nursing on-site
Facility Profile
AVERAGE MONTHLY FEES: $1001-$2000
SERVICES: Central dining; Housekeeping; Transporta-
tion; Social and recreational; Social worker/Mental
health; Physical therapy and rehabilitation; Medical
care; Security; Library; Rock shop; Photography/
darkroom
ENTRANCE AGE REQUIREMENT: (min) 60

Chicago

The Admiral
909 W Foster Ave, Chicago, IL 60640-2515
(312) 561-2900
INDEPENDENT LIVING: Apt for rent; Entrance fee $22,000-
$63,000; Residents 108; Units 120
CONTINUING CARE: Apt units; Entrance fee $22,000-
$55,000; Residents 150; Units 120 apts; Endowment
program; Nursing on-site
Facility Profile
AVERAGE MONTHLY FEES: $1001-$2000
SERVICES: Central dining; Housekeeping; Social and re-
creational; Social worker/Mental health; Physical
therapy and rehabilitation; Medical care; Security;
Library
ENTRANCE AGE REQUIREMENT: (min) 65

Adorn Pavilion Inc
2201 N Sacramento, Chicago, IL 60647
(312) 235-8200
INDEPENDENT LIVING: Apt for rent; Entrance fee $500;
Residents 32; Max. no. residents 50; Units 36; Occupancy level 65%

Facility Profile
AVERAGE MONTHLY FEES: $0-$1000
SERVICES: Housekeeping; Shopping; Spiritual; Social and recreational; Transportation
ENTRANCE AGE REQUIREMENT: (min) 50

Arlington House Retirement Club
616 W Arlington Pl, Chicago, IL 60614
(312) 929-5380
INDEPENDENT LIVING: Apt, units 130

Bethany Retirement Home
4950 N Ashland Ave, Chicago, IL 60640
(312) 989-1501
INDEPENDENT LIVING: Apt for rent; Entrance fee; Residents 166; Max. no. residents 269; Units 176; Occupancy level 94%
Facility Profile
AVERAGE MONTHLY FEES: $0-$1000
SERVICES: Central dining; Housekeeping; Transportation; Social and recreational; Social worker/Mental health; Physical therapy and rehabilitation; Medical care; Security; Library
ENTRANCE AGE REQUIREMENT: (min) 60

Bethesda Home & Retirement Center
2833 N Nordica Ave, Chicago, IL 60634
(312) 622-6144
INDEPENDENT LIVING: Apt; Residents 13; Max. no. residents 19; Occupancy level 68
CONTINUING CARE: Apt units; Entrance fee approx $40,000; Residents 13; Max. no. residents 19; Units 19
Facility Profile
AVERAGE MONTHLY FEES: $1001-$2000
SERVICES: Central dining; Housekeeping; Transportation; Social and recreational; Social worker/Mental health; Physical therapy and rehabilitation; Medical care; Security
ENTRANCE AGE REQUIREMENT: (min) 62

Johnston R Bowman Residential Apartments
710 S Paulina, Chicago, IL 60612
(312) 942-7049
INDEPENDENT LIVING: Apt for rent; Entrance fee $0; Residents 30; Max. no. residents 40; Units 29; Occupancy level 100%
Facility Profile
AVERAGE MONTHLY FEES: $0-$1000
SERVICES: Housekeeping; Transportation; Social and recreational; Financial management/counseling; Social worker/Mental health; Physical therapy and rehabilitation; Medical care; Security; Library; Meal delivery; Home response unit

The Breakers at Edgewater Beach
5333 N Sheridan Rd, Chicago, IL 60640
(312) 878-5333
INDEPENDENT LIVING: Apt for rent; Entrance fee is one month's rent; Residents 449; Units 476; Occupancy level 88%

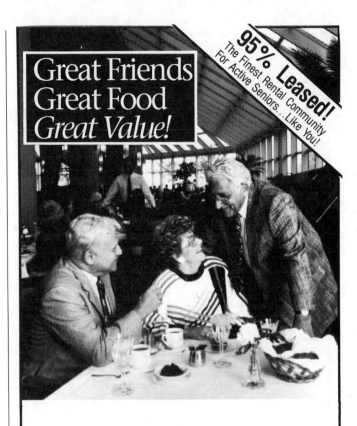
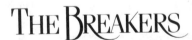

✔ In order to support future editions of this publication would you please mention *Elder Services* each time you contact any advertiser, facility, or service.

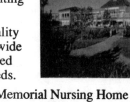
Facility Profile
AVERAGE MONTHLY FEES: $1001-$2000
SERVICES: Central dining; Housekeeping; Transportation; Social and recreational; Security; Library; Pool; Exercise facilities; Arts & crafts
ENTRANCE AGE REQUIREMENT: (min) 62
See ad page 305

Campbell Terrace
2061 N Campbell, Chicago, IL 60647
(312) 486-3666
INDEPENDENT LIVING: Apt, units 248
Facility Profile
AVERAGE MONTHLY FEES: Govt-subsidized
SERVICES: Social and recreational; Laundry
ENTRANCE AGE REQUIREMENT: (min) 62; Handicapped

Chatham Park South Cooperative
660 E 85th St, Chicago, IL 60619
(312) 873-9480
INDEPENDENT LIVING: Apt; Units 112
Facility Profile
AVERAGE MONTHLY FEES: Govt-subsidized

Drexel Square Apartments
810 Hyde Park, Chicago, IL 60615
(312) 268-2120
INDEPENDENT LIVING: Apt; Residents 156

Edgewater Shores Retirement Apartments
5326 N Winthrop, Chicago, IL 60640
(312) 275-9779
INDEPENDENT LIVING: Apt, for rent; Units 70
Facility Profile
AVERAGE MONTHLY FEES: $0-$1000
SERVICES: Central dining; Housekeeping; Social and recreational; Security
ENTRANCE AGE REQUIREMENT: (min) 55

Evergreen Tower Apartments
425 W Evergreen, Chicago, IL 60610
(312) 787-5741
INDEPENDENT LIVING: Apt; Units 122
Facility Profile
AVERAGE MONTHLY FEES: Govt-subsidized

Farwell Avenue
1420 W Farwell Ave, Chicago, IL 60626
(312) 262-1361
INDEPENDENT LIVING: Apt; Max. no. residents 45
Facility Profile
AVERAGE MONTHLY FEES: $0-$1000
SERVICES: Social and recreational; Security

Friendly Towers
920 W Wilson Ave, Chicago, IL 60640
(312) 989-6323
INDEPENDENT LIVING: Apt for rent; Residents 60; Max. no. residents 100; Units 100

Facility Profile

AVERAGE MONTHLY FEES: $0-$1000

SERVICES: Central dining; Housekeeping; Transportation; Social and recreational; Financial management/counseling; Social worker/Mental health; Security; Library; Visiting doctor & podiatrist

ENTRANCE AGE REQUIREMENT: (min) 55

Good Shepherd Tower

55 E Garfield Blvd, Chicago, IL 60637

(312) 643-5555

INDEPENDENT LIVING: Apt; Units 60

Facility Profile

AVERAGE MONTHLY FEES: Govt-subsidized

Greencastle Morgan Park/Beverly

10860 S Vincennes, Chicago, IL 60628

(312) 238-8380

INDEPENDENT LIVING: Apt; Units 60

Facility Profile

AVERAGE MONTHLY FEES: Govt-subsidized

Greencastle of Englewood

6344 S Peoria, Chicago, IL 60621

(312) 488-4999

INDEPENDENT LIVING: Apt; Units 60

Facility Profile

AVERAGE MONTHLY FEES: Govt-subsidized

Harper Square Cooperatives

4800 S Lake Park Blvd, Chicago, IL 60615

(312) 285-8600

INDEPENDENT LIVING: Apt; Units 591; Occupancy level 100%

Facility Profile

AVERAGE MONTHLY FEES: $0-$1000; Govt-subsidized

SERVICES: Social and recreational; Laundry

Hiewa Terrace

920 W Lawrence, Chicago, IL 60640

(312) 989-7333

INDEPENDENT LIVING: Apt; Units 201

Facility Profile

AVERAGE MONTHLY FEES: Govt-subsidized

Hollywood House & Club

5700 N Sheridan Rd, Chicago, IL 60660

(312) 728-2600

INDEPENDENT LIVING: Apt, units 198

Jarvis Avenue

1345 W Jarvis Ave, Chicago, IL 60626

(312) 262-3113

INDEPENDENT LIVING: Apt for rent; Max. no. residents 39; Units 39

Facility Profile

AVERAGE MONTHLY FEES: $0-$1000

SERVICES: Social and recreational

ENTRANCE AGE REQUIREMENT: (max) 62

Jugan Terrace

2300 N Racine Ave, Chicago, IL 60614

(312) 935-9600

INDEPENDENT LIVING: Apt, units 50

Lawrence House

1020 W Lawrence, Chicago, IL 60640

(312) 561-2100

INDEPENDENT LIVING: Apt for rent; Entrance fee is a security deposit; Residents 372; Max. no. residents 386; Units 372; Occupancy level 97%

Facility Profile

AVERAGE MONTHLY FEES: $0-$1000

SERVICES: Central dining; Housekeeping; Transportation; Medical care; Security; Library; Private park; Theater; Billiard room

ENTRANCE AGE REQUIREMENT: (min) 55

Levy House

1221 W Sherwin Ave, Chicago, IL 60626

(312) 262-3113

INDEPENDENT LIVING: Apt for rent; Residents 61; Max. no. residents 61; Units 61

Facility Profile

AVERAGE MONTHLY FEES: $0-$1000

SERVICES: Social and recreational; Security

ENTRANCE AGE REQUIREMENT: (max) 62

The Lorali

1039 W Lawrence, Chicago, IL 60640

(312) 561-1133

INDEPENDENT LIVING: Apt for rent; Residents 72; Max. no. residents 143; Units 143; Occupancy level 50%

Facility Profile

AVERAGE MONTHLY FEES: $0-$1000

SERVICES: Central dining; Housekeeping; Social and recreational; Financial management/counseling; Social worker/Mental health; Medical care; Security; Library

ENTRANCE AGE REQUIREMENT: (min) 50

Meds Apartments

60 E 36th Pl, Chicago, IL 60653

(312) 268-4811

INDEPENDENT LIVING: Apt; Units 111

Facility Profile

AVERAGE MONTHLY FEES: Govt-subsidized

Montgomery Place

5550 S Shore Dr, Chicago, IL 60637

(312) 753-4100

INDEPENDENT LIVING: Apt for rent; Residents 70; Max. no. residents 200; Units 165; Occupancy level 35%

Facility Profile

AVERAGE MONTHLY FEES: $1001-$2000

SERVICES: Central dining; Housekeeping; Transportation; Social and recreational; Social worker/Mental health; Security; Library

ENTRANCE AGE REQUIREMENT: (min) 60

Norwood Park Home

6016 N Nina Ave, Chicago, IL 60631

(312) 631-4856

✔ In order to support future editions of this publication would you please mention *Elder Services* each time you contact any advertiser, facility, or service.

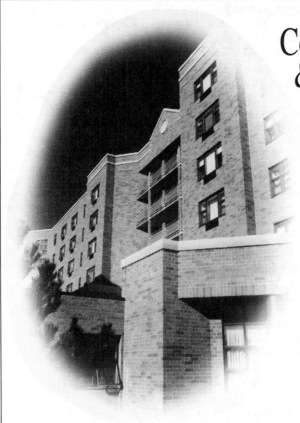
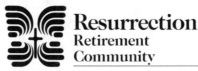
CONTINUING CARE: Apt units; Residents 186; Max. no. residents 261; Units 148; Occupancy level 80%; Nursing on-site
Facility Profile
AVERAGE MONTHLY FEES: $1001-$2000
SERVICES: Central dining; Housekeeping; Transportation; Social and recreational; Social worker/Mental health; Physical therapy and rehabilitation; Medical care; Security; Library
ENTRANCE AGE REQUIREMENT: (min) 65

Plaza on the Lake
7301 N Sheridan Rd, Chicago, IL 60626
(312) 743-7600
INDEPENDENT LIVING: Apt for rent
CONTINUING CARE: Apt units; Occupancy level 10%
Facility Profile
AVERAGE MONTHLY FEES: $1001-$2000
SERVICES: Central dining; Housekeeping; Transportation; Social and recreational; Alzheimer's day, respite, residential care; Security; Library
ENTRANCE AGE REQUIREMENT: (min) 62

Resurrection Retirement Community
7262 W Peterson Ave, Chicago, IL 60631
(312) 792-7930
INDEPENDENT LIVING: Apt; Entrance fee $28,000-$68,000; Residents 486; Max. no. residents 500; Units 473; Occupancy level 98%

Facility Profile
AVERAGE MONTHLY FEES: $0-$1000
SERVICES: Central dining; Transportation; Social and recreational; Security; Library; In-house banking; Chapel services
ENTRANCE AGE REQUIREMENT: (min) 62
See ads pages 163, 308

St Joseph Home of Chicago Inc
2650 N Ridgeway Ave, Chicago, IL 60647
(312) 235-8600
INDEPENDENT LIVING: Apt
Facility Profile
AVERAGE MONTHLY FEES: $2001-$3000
SERVICES: Medical care; Physical therapy and rehabilitation; Spiritual; Central dining; Security
ENTRANCE AGE REQUIREMENT: (min) 65

Selfhelp Home for the Aged
908 W Argyle St, Chicago, IL 60640
(312) 271-0300
INDEPENDENT LIVING: Apt; Units 46

South Chicago YMCA
3039 E 91st St, Chicago, IL 60642
(312) 721-9100
INDEPENDENT LIVING: Apt; Units 101

Facility Profile
AVERAGE MONTHLY FEES: Govt-subsidized

Swartzberg House
3001 Touhy, Chicago, IL 60645
(312) 262-3113
INDEPENDENT LIVING: Apt for rent; Residents 99; Max.
no. residents 99; Units 99
Facility Profile
AVERAGE MONTHLY FEES: $0-$1000
SERVICES: Social and recreational; Security; Access to
other CJE services

Woodlawn Residences II
6033 S Cottage Grove, Chicago, IL 60637
(312) 643-8100
INDEPENDENT LIVING: Apt; Units 60
Facility Profile
AVERAGE MONTHLY FEES: Govt-subsidized

Crete

The Fairways
2681 S Rte 394, Crete, IL 60417
(708) 672-3181
INDEPENDENT LIVING: Condo for purchase; Units 20
See ad on page i

De Kalb

**Golden Years Plaza—Dekalb County Housing
Authority**
507 E Taylor, De Kalb, IL 60115
(815) 758-4396
INDEPENDENT LIVING: Apt; Units 16
Facility Profile
AVERAGE MONTHLY FEES: Govt-subsidized

Oak Crest—De Kalb Area Retirement Center
2944 Greenwood Acres Dr, De Kalb, IL 60115
(815) 756-8461
CONTINUING CARE: Apt units; Private home units; Entrance fee $17,000-$53,000; Residents 173; Max. no.
residents 173; Units 112; Occupancy level 100%
Facility Profile
AVERAGE MONTHLY FEES: $1001-$2000; $2001-$3000
SERVICES: Central dining; Housekeeping; Transportation; Social and recreational; Financial
management/counseling; Social worker/Mental
health; Physical therapy and rehabilitation; Alzheimer's day, respite, residential care; Medical care;
Security; Library; Shop; Beauty salon
ENTRANCE AGE REQUIREMENT: (min) 62

Des Plaines

Nazarethville
300 N River Rd, Des Plaines, IL 60016
(708) 297-5900
CONTINUING CARE: Apt units
Facility Profile
AVERAGE MONTHLY FEES: $2001-$3000
SERVICES: Central dining; Housekeeping; Transportation; Social and recreational; Physical therapy and
rehabilitation; Alzheimer's day, respite, residential
care; Medical care; Library
ENTRANCE AGE REQUIREMENT: (min) 60

Downers Grove

Fairview Village
7 S 241 Fairview Ave, Downers Grove, IL 60516
(708) 852-0426
INDEPENDENT LIVING: Private home; Units 56; Entrance
fee $170,000 to $200,000
CONTINUING CARE: Apt units; Condo units; Private home
units
Facility Profile
AVERAGE MONTHLY FEES: $0-$1000
SERVICES: Central dining; Housekeeping; Transporta-
tion; Social and recreational; Security; Library
ENTRANCE AGE REQUIREMENT: (min) 55
See ads pages 136, 219

Peace Memorial Manor
3737 Highland Ave, Downers Grove, IL 60515
(708) 960-5770
INDEPENDENT LIVING: Apt; Units 150
Facility Profile
AVERAGE MONTHLY FEES: Govt-subsidized

Elgin

Westwind Towers
104 S State St, Elgin, IL 60123
(708) 697-6600
INDEPENDENT LIVING: Apt, units 149, for rent
Facility Profile
SERVICES: Shopping; Spiritual; Social and recreational;
Financial management/counseling; Security
ENTRANCE AGE REQUIREMENT: (min) 62

Elk Grove Village

Village Grove Apartments
1130 Cheekwood Ct, Elk Grove Village, IL 60007
(708) 593-4280
INDEPENDENT LIVING: Apt, units 300

Facility Profile
AVERAGE MONTHLY FEES: Govt-subsidized
SERVICES: Social and recreational; Laundry
ENTRANCE AGE REQUIREMENT: (min) 62

Elmhurst

Greencastle of Elmhurst
190 Michigan, Elmhurst, IL 60126
(708) 941-8894
INDEPENDENT LIVING: Apt; Units 80
Facility Profile
AVERAGE MONTHLY FEES: Govt-subsidized

Lexington Square of Elmhurst
400 Butterfield Rd, Elmhurst, IL 60126
(708) 832-9922
CONTINUING CARE: Condo units; Entrance fee $79,900-$179,900; Units 320; Occupancy level 78%; Nursing on-site
Facility Profile
AVERAGE MONTHLY FEES: $0-$1000; $1001-$2000
SERVICES: Central dining; Housekeeping; Transportation; Social and recreational; Financial management/counseling; Social worker/Mental health; Physical therapy and rehabilitation; Alzheimer's day, respite, residential care; Medical care; Security; Library; Swimming pool; Garage
ENTRANCE AGE REQUIREMENT: (min) 62

Evanston

Ebenezer Prime Towers
1001 Emerson, Evanston, IL 60201
(708) 864-0052
INDEPENDENT LIVING: Apt; Units 107

Geneva Place at the Presbyterian Home
3200 Grant St, Evanston, IL 60201
(708) 570-3422
CONTINUING CARE: Apt units; Entrance fee $0; Max. no. residents 96; Units 92; Endowment program; Nursing on-site
Facility Profile
AVERAGE MONTHLY FEES: $2001-$3000
SERVICES: Central dining; Housekeeping; Transportation; Social and recreational; Social worker/Mental health; Physical therapy and rehabilitation; Medical care; Security; Library; Beauty/barber shop; Dental exams; Eye exams; Chapel; Greenhouse; Lounges/meeting rooms; Pharmacy; Hobby shop; Convenience store
ENTRANCE AGE REQUIREMENT: (min) 65

The Georgian
422 Davis St, Evanston, IL 60201
(708) 475-4100

CONTINUING CARE: Apt units; Residents 156; Units 131; Nursing on-site
Facility Profile
AVERAGE MONTHLY FEES: $1001-$2000
SERVICES: Central dining; Housekeeping; Transportation; Social and recreational; Financial management/counseling; Social worker/Mental health; Physical therapy and rehabilitation; Medical care; Security; Library; Chapel; Linen service
ENTRANCE AGE REQUIREMENT: (min) 65

The King Home
1555 Oak Ave, Evanston, IL 60201
(708) 864-5460
CONTINUING CARE: Apt units; Entrance fee $0; Max. no. residents 76; Units 56; Endowment program; Nursing on-site
Facility Profile
AVERAGE MONTHLY FEES: $1001-$2000
SERVICES: Central dining; Housekeeping; Transportation; Social and recreational; Social worker/Mental health; Physical therapy and rehabilitation; Alzheimer's day, respite, residential care; Medical care; Security; Library; Barber shop; Dental exams; Eye exams; Woodworking shop; Indoor gardening; Lounge/Meeting rooms; Pharmacy; Laundry service
ENTRANCE AGE REQUIREMENT: (min) 60

The Mather Home
1615 N Hinman Ave, Evanston, IL 60201
(708) 492-7600
CONTINUING CARE: Apt units; Entrance fee $60,000; Residents 119; Max. no. residents 139; Units 123; Occupancy level 85%; Endowment program; Nursing on-site
Facility Profile
AVERAGE MONTHLY FEES: $2001-$3000
SERVICES: Central dining; Housekeeping; Transportation; Social and recreational; Financial management/counseling; Social worker/Mental health; Physical therapy and rehabilitation; Medical care; Security; Library; Beauty shop
ENTRANCE AGE REQUIREMENT: (min) 65

Swedish Retirement Association
2320 Pioneer Rd, Evanston, IL 60201
(708) 998-9406
CONTINUING CARE: Apt units; Entrance fee is variable; Max. no. residents 115; Units 80; Endowment program; Nursing on-site
Facility Profile
AVERAGE MONTHLY FEES: $0-$1000
SERVICES: Central dining; Housekeeping; Transportation; Social and recreational; Financial management/counseling; Social worker/Mental health; Physical therapy and rehabilitation; Alzheimer's day, respite, residential care; Medical care; Security; Library
ENTRANCE AGE REQUIREMENT: (min) 65

Ten Twenty Grove
1020 Grove St, Evanston, IL 60201
(708) 864-5451

INDEPENDENT LIVING: Apt; Entrance fee $35,000-$120,000; Max. no. residents 88; Units 48
Facility Profile
AVERAGE MONTHLY FEES: $1001-$2000
SERVICES: Central dining; Housekeeping; Transportation; Social and recreational; Social worker/Mental health; Security; Library; Pharmacy; Free laundry room; Lounges
ENTRANCE AGE REQUIREMENT: (min) 60

Westminster Place at the Presbyterian Home
3200 Grant St, Evanston, IL 60201
(708) 492-2800, 570-3422
CONTINUING CARE: Apt units; Private home units; Entrance fee $25,000-$295,000; Max. no. residents 371; Units 255; Nursing on-site
Facility Profile
AVERAGE MONTHLY FEES: $1001-$2000; $2001-$3000
SERVICES: Central dining; Housekeeping; Transportation; Social and recreational; Social worker/Mental health; Physical therapy and rehabilitation; Alzheimer's day, respite, residential care; Medical care; Security; Library; Beauty shop; Pharmacy; Dental exams; Eye exams; Craft room & woodworking shop; Convenience store
ENTRANCE AGE REQUIREMENT: (min) 65

Wilson/Sidwell Apartments
3200 Grant St, Evanston, IL 60201
(708) 570-3422
CONTINUING CARE: Apt units; Units 39; Endowment program; Rental program; Nursing on-site
Facility Profile
AVERAGE MONTHLY FEES: $1001-$2000
SERVICES: Central dining; Housekeeping; Transportation; Social and recreational; Social worker/Mental health; Physical therapy and rehabilitation; Medical care; Security; Library; Pharmacy; Dental exams; Eye exams; Chapel; Lounges; Convenience store; Recreation; Flat linen service
ENTRANCE AGE REQUIREMENT: (min) 65

Forest Park

Altenheim
7824 W Madison St, Forest Park, IL 60130
(708) 366-2206
INDEPENDENT LIVING: Private home for purchase; Apt for rent; Residents 35; Max. no. residents 35; Units 35; Occupancy level 100%
Facility Profile
AVERAGE MONTHLY FEES: $2001-$3000
SERVICES: Central dining; Housekeeping; Transportation; Social and recreational; Physical therapy and rehabilitation; Alzheimer's day, respite, residential care; Medical care; Security
ENTRANCE AGE REQUIREMENT: (min) 65

Fox Lake

Leisure Village
7313 E Leisure Ave, Fox Lake, IL 60020
(708) 587-6795
INDEPENDENT LIVING: Private home; Apt; Condo; Residents 360

Glenview

Glenview Elderly Housing
939 Harlem, Glenview, IL 60025
(708) 724-6308
INDEPENDENT LIVING: Apt for rent; Residents 85; Units 80; Occupancy level 100%
Facility Profile
AVERAGE MONTHLY FEES: Govt-subsidized
SERVICES: Transportation; Social and recreational; Social worker/Mental health; Security; Library
ENTRANCE AGE REQUIREMENT: (min) 62

Harvard

Harvard Retirement Home
210 E Front, Harvard, IL 60033
(815) 943-3350
INDEPENDENT LIVING: Apt; Units 20

Highland Park

Walnut Place
654 Walnut Ave, Highland Park, IL 60035
(708) 433-7694
INDEPENDENT LIVING: Apt, units 67, for rent
Facility Profile
ENTRANCE AGE REQUIREMENT: (min) 62

Hinsdale

Washington Square Retirement Community
10 N Washington St, Hinsdale, IL 60521
(708) 986-5625
INDEPENDENT LIVING: Apt for purchase; Entrance fee $26,950-$95,920; Residents 65; Max. no. residents 137; Units 71
Facility Profile
AVERAGE MONTHLY FEES: $0-$1000
SERVICES: Central dining; Transportation; Social and recreational; Security; Library
ENTRANCE AGE REQUIREMENT: (min) 60

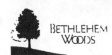
Hoffman Estates

The Benchmark of Hoffman Estates
1515 Barrington Rd, Hoffman Estates, IL 60194
(708) 490-5800
INDEPENDENT LIVING: Apt for rent; Residents 284; Max. no. residents 300; Units 251; Occupancy level 98
Facility Profile
AVERAGE MONTHLY FEES: $1001-$2000
SERVICES: Central dining; Housekeeping; Transportation; Social and recreational; Financial management/counseling; Social worker/Mental health; Physical therapy and rehabilitation; Medical care; Security; Library; Home health care
ENTRANCE AGE REQUIREMENT: (min) 62
See ad on inside back cover

Joliet

Salem Village
1314 Rowell Ave, Joliet, IL 60433
(815) 727-5451
INDEPENDENT LIVING: Apt; Condo; Units 248

La Grange Park

Bethlehem Woods Retirement Living Center
1571 W Ogden Ave, La Grange Park, IL 60525
(708) 579-3663
CONTINUING CARE: Apt units; Entrance fee $34,000-$73,000; Residents 243; Max. no. residents 350; Units 268; Occupancy level 76%; Endowment program
Facility Profile
AVERAGE MONTHLY FEES: $0-$1000; $1001-$2000
SERVICES: Central dining; Housekeeping; Transportation; Social and recreational; Financial management/counseling; Social worker/Mental health; Physical therapy and rehabilitation; Medical care; Security; Library; Barber/beauty shops; Chaplain; Bank; Travel agency
ENTRANCE AGE REQUIREMENT: (min) 62
See ad page 312

Plymouth Place
315 N La Grange Rd, La Grange Park, IL 60525
(708) 354-0340
CONTINUING CARE: Apt units; Private home units; Entrance fee $33,000-$150,000; Residents 302; Max. no. residents 305; Units 300; Occupancy level 99%; Endowment program; Nursing on-site
Facility Profile
AVERAGE MONTHLY FEES: $0-$1000
SERVICES: Central dining; Housekeeping; Transportation; Social and recreational; Financial management/counseling; Social worker/Mental health; Physical therapy and rehabilitation; Medical care; Security; Library; Gift shops; Beauty/barber shop; Music room; Banking services; Guest rooms
ENTRANCE AGE REQUIREMENT: (min) 60

Lemont

Franciscan Village
1270 Village Dr, Lemont, IL 60439
(708) 257-3377
INDEPENDENT LIVING: Private home for rent; Apt for rent; Entrance fee Apts $0; Homes $77,000; Residents 160; Max. no. residents 300; Units 128; Occupancy level 85%
Facility Profile
AVERAGE MONTHLY FEES: $0-$1000; $1001-$2000
SERVICES: Central dining; Housekeeping; Transportation; Social and recreational; Security; Library
ENTRANCE AGE REQUIREMENT: (min) 55

Libertyville

Liberty Towers
130 E Cook St, Libertyville, IL 60048
(708) 367-5503
INDEPENDENT LIVING: Apt, units 120

Lisle

Queen of Peace Retirement Center
1910 Maple Ave, Lisle, IL 60532
(708) 852-5360
INDEPENDENT LIVING: Apt for rent; Entrance fee $45,000-
$60,000; Residents 30; Max. no. residents 40;
Units 32
Facility Profile
AVERAGE MONTHLY FEES: $0-$1000
SERVICES: Central dining; Housekeeping; Social and re-
creational; Security; Wellness exercise
ENTRANCE AGE REQUIREMENT: (min) 62

Lombard

Beacon Hill
2400 S Finley Rd, Lombard, IL 60148
(708) 620-5850
INDEPENDENT LIVING: Apt; Units 200
CONTINUING CARE: Apt units 300; Entrance fee $77,000;
Residents 350
Facility Profile
AVERAGE MONTHLY FEES: $0-$1000
SERVICES: Medical care; Physical therapy and rehabilita-
tion; Housekeeping; Shopping; Spiritual; Social
and recreational; Central dining; Security; Trans-
portation

Lexington Square of Lombard
555 Foxworth Blvd, Lombard, IL 60148
(708) 832-9922, 620-0099
CONTINUING CARE: Condo units; Entrance fee $69,900-
$159,900; Units 230; Occupancy level 98%; Nursing
on-site
Facility Profile
AVERAGE MONTHLY FEES: $0-$1000; $1001-$2000
SERVICES: Central dining; Housekeeping; Transportation; Social and recreational; Financial
management/counseling; Social worker/Mental
health; Physical therapy and rehabilitation; Alzheimer's day, respite, residential care; Medical care;
Security; Library; Pool; Garage
ENTRANCE AGE REQUIREMENT: (min) 60

Lyons

Golden Age Retirement Home
7848 W Ogden Ave, Lyons, IL 60534
(708) 442-1515
INDEPENDENT LIVING: Apt; Units 60

Maywood

Baptist Retirement Home
316 W Randolph, Maywood, IL 60153
(708) 344-1541
INDEPENDENT LIVING: Private home for rent; Apt for rent
CONTINUING CARE: Rental program; Nursing on-site
Facility Profile
AVERAGE MONTHLY FEES: $1001-$2000
SERVICES: Central dining; Housekeeping; Transporta-
tion; Social and recreational; Social worker/Mental
health; Physical therapy and rehabilitation; Alzhei-
mer's day, respite, residential care; Medical care;
Security; Library
ENTRANCE AGE REQUIREMENT: (min) 70

Garden House of Maywood
515 S 2nd Ave, Maywood, IL 60153
(708) 343-4511
INDEPENDENT LIVING: Apt, units 144
Facility Profile
AVERAGE MONTHLY FEES: Govt-subsidized
SERVICES: Social and recreational; Community room;
Laundry
ENTRANCE AGE REQUIREMENT: (min) 62; Handicapped

Naperville

Martin Manor Apartments
310 W Martin Ave, Naperville, IL 60540
(708) 357-0909
INDEPENDENT LIVING: Apt; Residents 121
Facility Profile
SERVICES: Social and recreational; Central dining;
Transportation; Shopping; Spiritual; Store; Barber/
Beauty Shop
ENTRANCE AGE REQUIREMENT: (min) 62

North Riverside

The Scottish Home
2800 S Des Plaines Ave, North Riverside, IL 60546
(708) 447-5092
INDEPENDENT LIVING: Apt

Northbrook

Covenant Village of Northbrook
2625 Techny Rd, Northbrook, IL 60062
(708) 480-6380
CONTINUING CARE: Apt units; Entrance fee $44,900-
$126,000; Units 310; Nursing on-site

✔ In order to support future editions of this publication would you please mention *Elder Services* each time you contact
any advertiser, facility, or service.

Facility Profile

AVERAGE MONTHLY FEES: $0-$1000; $1001-$2000

SERVICES: Central dining; Housekeeping; Transportation; Social and recreational; Financial management/counseling; Library; Spiritual activities; Woodshop; Creative art center; Gardening; Health services; 24-hour security

ENTRANCE AGE REQUIREMENT: (min) 62

See ads pages iv, 300

Northlake

Casa San Carlo Retirement Community

420 N Wolf Rd, Northlake, IL 60164

(708) 562-4300

INDEPENDENT LIVING: Apt; Entrance fee $50,000; Residents 195; Units 183; Occupancy level 92%

Facility Profile

AVERAGE MONTHLY FEES: $0-$1000

SERVICES: Central dining; Housekeeping; Transportation; Social and recreational; Financial management/counseling; Medical care; Security; Library; Spa; Fitness center

ENTRANCE AGE REQUIREMENT: (min) 62

Concord Plaza Retirement Community

401 W Lake St, Northlake, IL 60164

(708) 562-9000

INDEPENDENT LIVING: Apt; Units 400

Facility Profile

AVERAGE MONTHLY FEES: $0-$1000

SERVICES: Central dining; Housekeeping; Social and recreational; Financial management/counseling; Social worker/Mental health; Physical therapy and rehabilitation; Medical care; Security; Library; Indoor heated swimming pool; Chapel; Penthouse greenhouse; Exercise class; Gift shop; Wood shop; Laundry; Penthouse party room with live entertainment; Bakery; Beauty salon; Barber shop

ENTRANCE AGE REQUIREMENT: (min) 62

Oak Brook

Mayslake Village

1801 35th St, Oak Brook, IL 60521

(708) 654-3280

INDEPENDENT LIVING: Apt for rent; Residents 750; Max. no. residents 825; Units 630; Occupancy level 100%

Facility Profile

AVERAGE MONTHLY FEES: Govt-subsidized

SERVICES: Central dining; Transportation; Social and recreational; Financial management/counseling; Social worker/Mental health; Security; Library; Chapel

ENTRANCE AGE REQUIREMENT: (min) 62

Oak Park

Holley Court Terrace

1111 Ontario St, Oak Park, IL 60302

(708) 383-1111

INDEPENDENT LIVING: Apt for rent; Entrance fee $2500 deposit; Units 180

Facility Profile

AVERAGE MONTHLY FEES: $1001-$2000; $2001-$3000

SERVICES: Central dining; Housekeeping; Transportation; Social and recreational; Medical care; Security; Library; Laundry service; Beauty/Barber shop; Convenience store; Guest apartments; Exercise room

ENTRANCE AGE REQUIREMENT: (min) 55

See ad page 315

Palos Park

Peace Memorial Village

10300 Village Circle Dr, Palos Park, IL 60464

(708) 361-3683

INDEPENDENT LIVING: Apt for purchase; Entrance fee $64,429-$121,650 (90% refundable); Units 240; Occupancy level 85%

Facility Profile

AVERAGE MONTHLY FEES: $0-$1000; $1001-$2000

SERVICES: Central dining; Housekeeping; Transportation; Social and recreational; Security; Library; Beauty shop, Bank

ENTRANCE AGE REQUIREMENT: (min) 62

See ad page 306

Park Ridge

St Matthew Lutheran Home

1601 N Western Ave, Park Ridge, IL 60068

(708) 825-5531

INDEPENDENT LIVING: Apt

Summit Square Retirement Hotel

10 N Summit, Park Ridge, IL 60068

(708) 825-1161

INDEPENDENT LIVING: Apt, units 240, for rent

Facility Profile

SERVICES: Central dining; Housekeeping; Transportation; Social and recreational; Security

ENTRANCE AGE REQUIREMENT: (min) 62

Saint Charles

Cumberland Green Cooperative

1796 Cumberland Green Dr Rm 456, Saint Charles, IL 60174

(708) 584-5150

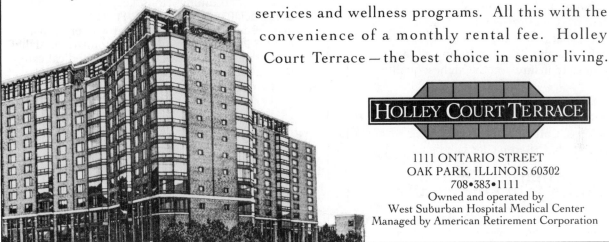
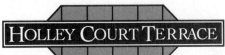
INDEPENDENT LIVING: Apt, units 204
Facility Profile
AVERAGE MONTHLY FEES: Govt-subsidized
SERVICES: Social and recreational; Laundry; Community room

Schaumburg

Friendship Village of Schaumburg
350 W Schaumburg Rd, Schaumburg, IL 60194
(708) 884-5000, 884-5053 FAX
CONTINUING CARE: Apt units; Entrance fee $59,000-$129,000; Residents 800; Units 546; Occupancy level 95%; Rental program; Nursing on-site; Nursing off-site
Facility Profile
AVERAGE MONTHLY FEES: $1001-$2000
SERVICES: Central dining; Housekeeping; Transportation; Social and recreational; Financial management/counseling; Social worker/Mental health; Physical therapy and rehabilitation; Alzheimer's day, respite, residential care; Medical care; Security; Library; Gardens; Garages; Bank; Beauty parlor; Shopping; Spiritual
ENTRANCE AGE REQUIREMENT: (min) 62
See ad page 317

Greencastle of Schaumberg
1335 S Mercury Dr, Schaumburg, IL 60193
(708) 980-3252
INDEPENDENT LIVING: Apt, units 90; Units 72
Facility Profile
AVERAGE MONTHLY FEES: Govt-subsidized

Skokie

Krasnow Residence
8901 Gross Point Rd, Skokie, IL 60076
(312) 262-3113
INDEPENDENT LIVING: Apt for rent; Residents 48; Max. no. residents 48; Units 48
Facility Profile
AVERAGE MONTHLY FEES: $0-$1000
SERVICES: Social and recreational; Security
ENTRANCE AGE REQUIREMENT: (max) 62

Tinley Park

Brementowne Manor
16130 S Oak Park Ave, Tinley Park, IL 60477
(708) 429-4088
INDEPENDENT LIVING: Apt, units 106, for rent; Residents 106

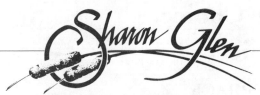
Facility Profile
AVERAGE MONTHLY FEES: $0-$1000
SERVICES: Social and recreational; Security; Transportation
ENTRANCE AGE REQUIREMENT: (min) 62

Vernon Hills

Hawthorn Lakes of Lake County
10 E Hawthorn Pkwy, Vernon Hills, IL 60061
(708) 367-2516
INDEPENDENT LIVING: Apt for rent; Entrance fee $0; Residents 240; Units 202; Occupancy level 95%
Facility Profile
AVERAGE MONTHLY FEES: $1001-$2000
SERVICES: Central dining; Housekeeping; Transportation; Social and recreational; Security; Library
ENTRANCE AGE REQUIREMENT: (min) 62
See ads pages xiv, xix, 122, 294

West Chicago

Arbor Terrace Health Care Center
30 W 300 North Ave, West Chicago, IL 60185
(708) 231-4050
INDEPENDENT LIVING: Apt for rent; Entrance fee $0; Units 178
CONTINUING CARE: Apt units; Entrance fee $0; Units 150; Rental program; Nursing on-site
Facility Profile
AVERAGE MONTHLY FEES: $1001-$2000
SERVICES: Central dining; Housekeeping; Transportation; Social and recreational; Financial management/counseling; Social worker/Mental health; Physical therapy and rehabilitation; Alzheimer's day, respite, residential care; Medical care; Security; Library; Chapel
ENTRANCE AGE REQUIREMENT: (min) 18

Wheaton

Marian Park
2126 W Roosevelt Rd, Wheaton, IL 60187
(708) 665-9100
INDEPENDENT LIVING: Apt for rent; Residents 127; Units 117; Occupancy level 100%
Facility Profile
AVERAGE MONTHLY FEES: Govt-subsidized
ENTRANCE AGE REQUIREMENT: (min) 62

Sharon Glen Village
c/o PO Box 1388, Geneva Rd at Pleasant Hill, Wheaton, IL 60189-1388
(708) 752-0400
CONTINUING CARE: Apt units; Private home units; Entrance fee $59,000-$235,000
Facility Profile
AVERAGE MONTHLY FEES: $1001-$2000
SERVICES: Central dining; Housekeeping; Transportation; Social and recreational; Financial management/counseling; Social worker/Mental health; Physical therapy and rehabilitation; Medical care; Security; Library
See ad page 316

Wheeling

Addolorata Villa
555 McHenry Rd, Wheeling, IL 60090
(708) 537-2900
INDEPENDENT LIVING: Apt for rent; Entrance fee is one month's rent; Residents 112; Units 100; Occupancy level 95%
Facility Profile
AVERAGE MONTHLY FEES: $1001-$2000
SERVICES: Central dining; Housekeeping; Transportation; Social and recreational; Financial management/counseling; Social worker/Mental

The First Nationally Accredited Retirement Community...

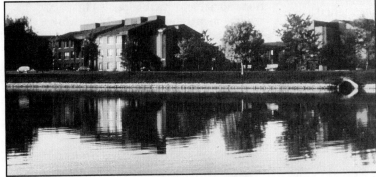

in all of Chicagoland.

health; Physical therapy and rehabilitation; Alzheimer's day, respite, residential care; Medical care; Security; Library
ENTRANCE AGE REQUIREMENT: (min) 62

Wilmette

Fairfield Court
2801 Old Glenview Rd, Wilmette, IL 60091
(708) 256-9300
CONTINUING CARE: Apt units; Residents 63; Max. no. residents 160; Units 143; Endowment program; Nursing on-site; Nursing off-site
Facility Profile
SERVICES: Central dining; Housekeeping; Transportation; Social and recreational; Financial management/counseling; Social worker/Mental health; Medical care; Security; Library
ENTRANCE AGE REQUIREMENT: (min) 65

Shore Line Place
324 Linden, Wilmette, IL 60091
(708) 251-6212
INDEPENDENT LIVING: Apt for rent; Residents 43; Max. no. residents 43; Units 43; Occupancy level 100%
Facility Profile
AVERAGE MONTHLY FEES: Govt-subsidized
SERVICES: Social and recreational; Social worker/Mental health

ENTRANCE AGE REQUIREMENT: (min) 62

Woodstock

Carefree Village Subdivision
840 N Seminary Ave, Woodstock, IL 60098
(800) 339-CARE; (815) 338-2110
INDEPENDENT LIVING: Private home for purchase, for rent; Entrance fee $33,000-$61,000; Residents 37; Max. no. residents 37; Units 31; Occupancy level 100%
Facility Profile
AVERAGE MONTHLY FEES: $0-$1000
SERVICES: Transportation; Social and recreational; Financial management/counseling; Library; Maintenance including lawn care and snow removal
ENTRANCE AGE REQUIREMENT: (min) 60

✔ In order to support future editions of this publication would you please mention *Elder Services* each time you contact any advertiser, facility, or service.

INDIANA

Crown Point

Lutheran Retirement Village
1200 E Luther Dr, Crown Point, IN 46307
(219) 663-3860, 662-3070 FAX
INDEPENDENT LIVING: Condo for rent; Units 40; Occupancy level 100%
Facility Profile
SERVICES: Central dining; Housekeeping; Transportation; Social and recreational; Social worker/Mental health; Physical therapy and rehabilitation; Alzheimer's day, respite, residential care; Medical care; Security
ENTRANCE AGE REQUIREMENT: (min) 60

Fort Wayne

Kingston Resident
7515 Winchester Rd, Fort Wayne, IN 46319
(219) 747-1523
INDEPENDENT LIVING: Apt; Units 45

Hammond

Mt Zion Pleasant View Plaza
940 Kenwood St, Hammond, IN 46320
(219) 931-3904
INDEPENDENT LIVING: Apt; Units 128
Facility Profile
AVERAGE MONTHLY FEES: Govt-subsidized

Merrillville

Towne Centre
7250 Arthur Blvd, Merrillville, IN 46410
(219) 736-2900
INDEPENDENT LIVING: Apt
Facility Profile
SERVICES: Central dining; Housekeeping; Transportation; Social and recreational; Physical therapy and rehabilitation; Alzheimer's day, respite, residential care; Security; Library; Resident services
ENTRANCE AGE REQUIREMENT: (min) 55

Valparaiso

Pines Village Retirement Community
3303 Pines Village Cir, Valparaiso, IN 46383
(219) 465-1591
CONTINUING CARE: Apt units; Residents 114; Max. no. residents 204; Units 111; Occupancy level 99%; Endowment program; Rental program; Nursing on-site
Facility Profile
AVERAGE MONTHLY FEES: $1001-$2000
SERVICES: Central dining; Housekeeping; Transportation; Social and recreational; Financial management/counseling; Social worker/Mental health; Security; Library; Laundry & free use of machines; Guest room
ENTRANCE AGE REQUIREMENT: (min) 60

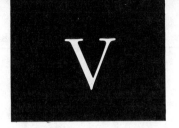

Alzheimer's Treatment Centers and Programs

ILLINOIS

Arlington Heights

Lutheran Home & Services for the Aged
800 W Oakton St, Arlington Heights, IL 60004
(708) 253-3710, 253-1427 FAX
Staff Profile
FULL-TIME STAFF: LPNs 15; Nurse's aides 76; Physical therapists 7; Physicians 1; RNs 19; Social workers 1.
PART-TIME STAFF: LPNs 7; Nurse's aides 41; Physical therapists 2; Physicians 5; Psychiatrists 2; RNs 25.
Program Profile
TYPE: Long-term residential program.
AFFILIATIONS: Lutheran Church.
ADMISSION: Physician's referral required.
INSURANCE PLANS ACCEPTED: Private group insurance; Medicaid; Medicare; Supplemental to Medicare.
CLIENT SERVICES: Sliding fee scale; Free initial interview; Evening hours; Weekend hours; Wheelchair access; Patient/client library; Educational workshops; Support groups; Information & referral; Hotline.
LANGUAGES SPOKEN: German, Spanish.
AGE REQUIREMENTS: Min 60.
See ads pages 69, 202

Berwyn

Fairfax Health Care Center
3601 S Harlem Ave, Berwyn, IL 60402
(708) 749-4160, 749-7696 FAX
Staff Profile
FULL-TIME STAFF: LPNs; Nurse's aides; Recreational therapists; RNs; Respiratory therapists; Social workers.
CONSULTING STAFF: Occupational therapists; Physical therapists; Physicians; Psychiatrists.
Program Profile
TYPE: Long-term residential program.
ACCREDITATIONS: JCAHO.
ADMISSION: Referral required.
INSURANCE PLANS ACCEPTED: Health maintenance organization (HMO); Private group insurance; Medicare.
CLIENT SERVICES: Free initial interview; Support groups.
AGE REQUIREMENTS: None.

MacNeal Outpatient Evaluation Program
3249 S Oak Park Ave, Berwyn, IL 60402
(708) 795-3600, 795-3518 FAX
Staff Profile
PART-TIME STAFF: RNs.
CONSULTING STAFF: Neurologists; Physicians; Social workers.
Program Profile
TYPE: Diagnostic and medical treatment; Family support group.
ADMISSION: Admission requirements include medical need for evaluation.
INSURANCE PLANS ACCEPTED: Preferred provider organization (PPO); Health maintenance organization (HMO); Private group insurance; Medicaid; Medicare.
CLIENT SERVICES: Evening hours; Wheelchair access; Support groups; Information & referral.
AGE REQUIREMENTS: None.
See ad page 174

Bloomingdale

Alden Nursing Center—Valley Ridge Rehabilitation & Health Care Center
275 Army Trail Rd, Bloomingdale, IL 60108
(708) 893-9616, 924-1059 FAX
Staff Profile
FULL-TIME STAFF: LPNs; Nurse's aides; Recreational therapists; RNs; Social workers.
PART-TIME STAFF: LPNs; Nurse's aides; RNs.
CONSULTING STAFF: Occupational therapists; Physical therapists; Physicians; Psychiatrists.
Program Profile
TYPE: Long-term residential program.
ADMISSION: Physician's referral required.
INSURANCE PLANS ACCEPTED: Medicaid; Medicare.
CLIENT SERVICES: Free initial interview; Wheelchair access; Information & referral.
LANGUAGES SPOKEN: Spanish, Tagalog, Polish, Italian.
AGE REQUIREMENTS: Min 18.

✔ In order to support future editions of this publication would you please mention *Elder Services* each time you contact any advertiser, facility, or service.

Bridgeview

Metropolitan Nursing Center
8540 S Harlem Ave, Bridgeview, IL 60455
(708) 598-2605, 598-5671 FAX
Program Profile
TYPE: Long-term residential program.

Burbank

Brentwood Nursing & Rehabilitation Center
5400 W 87th St, Burbank, IL 60459
(708) 423-1200
Staff Profile
FULL-TIME STAFF: LPNs; Nurse's aides; Occupational therapists; Physical therapists; Recreational therapists; RNs; Social workers.
CONSULTING STAFF: Neurologists; Psychiatrists; Psychologists; Respiratory therapists.
Program Profile
TYPE: Long-term residential program; Respite care program.

Chicago

Alden Nursing Center—Morrow Rehabilitation & Health Care Center
5001 S Michigan, Chicago, IL 60615
(312) 924-9292, 924-1308 FAX
Program Profile
TYPE: Long-term residential program.

Alzheimer's Disease Clinical Center
1725 W Harrison St, Chicago, IL 60612
(312) 942-4463
Program Profile
TYPE: Diagnostic and medical treatment.

Autumn Home Health & Case Management
1625 W Edgewater N-71, Chicago, IL 60660
(312) 769-9030
Staff Profile
FULL-TIME STAFF: LPNs 1.
PART-TIME STAFF: Nurse's aides 2.
CONSULTING STAFF: Physical therapists 1; Physicians 1; Psychiatrists 1; Psychologists 1; RNs 1; Social workers 1; Geriatricians 1.
Program Profile
TYPE: Home health care agency.
INSURANCE PLANS ACCEPTED: Preferred provider organization (PPO); Health maintenance organization (HMO); Private group insurance; Medicaid; Medicare; Veteran's insurance; Private pay.
CLIENT SERVICES: Evening hours; Weekend hours; Educational workshops; Support groups; Information & referral.
LANGUAGES SPOKEN: Spanish.

AGE REQUIREMENTS: Min 30; Max 100.

Birchwood Plaza Nursing Home
1426 W Birchwood Ave, Chicago, IL 60626
(312) 274-4405, 274-4763 FAX
Staff Profile
FULL-TIME STAFF: LPNs 7; Nurse's aides 42; RNs 8.
PART-TIME STAFF: LPNs 1; Nurse's aides 5; RNs 2.
CONSULTING STAFF: EEG technicians 1; Occupational therapists 1; Physical therapists 1; Physicians 50; Psychiatrists 2; Psychologists 2; Social workers 1.
Program Profile
TYPE: Long-term residential program.
ACCREDITATIONS: IDPH.
ADMISSION: No referral required.
INSURANCE PLANS ACCEPTED: Health maintenance organization (HMO); Private group insurance; Medicaid; Medicare; Humana Michael Reese Health Chicago.
CLIENT SERVICES: Wheelchair access; Support groups; Information & referral.
LANGUAGES SPOKEN: Russian, Yiddish.
AGE REQUIREMENTS: Min 62.

Buckingham Pavilion Nursing & Rehabilitation Center
2625 W Touhy Ave, Chicago, IL 60645
(312) 973-5333
Staff Profile
FULL-TIME STAFF: LPNs 8; Nurse's aides 25; Physical therapists 1; Physicians 1; Recreational therapists 1; RNs 12; Social workers 1.
PART-TIME STAFF: LPNs 4; Nurse's aides 10; RNs 2.
CONSULTING STAFF: EEG technicians; Neurologists; Occupational therapists; Physicians; Psychiatrists; Psychologists; Respiratory therapists.
Program Profile
TYPE: Diagnostic and medical treatment; Long-term residential program.
ADMISSION: Referral required; Referrals accepted from home, hospital.
INSURANCE PLANS ACCEPTED: Preferred provider organization (PPO); Health maintenance organization (HMO); Private group insurance; Medicaid; Medicare.
CLIENT SERVICES: Free initial interview; Evening hours; Weekend hours; Wheelchair access; Patient/client library; Educational workshops; Support groups; Information & referral.

Congress Care Center
901 S Austin Ave, Chicago, IL 60644
(312) 287-5959
Staff Profile
FULL-TIME STAFF: LPNs; Nurse's aides; Occupational therapists; Physical therapists; Physicians; Recreational therapists; RNs; Social workers.
PART-TIME STAFF: Neurologists; Psychiatrists; Psychologists; Respiratory therapists.

Program Profile

TYPE: Long-term residential program; Respite care program.

Glencrest Nursing Rehabilitation Center Ltd

2451 W Touhy Ave, Chicago, IL 60645
(312) 338-6800

Staff Profile

FULL-TIME STAFF: LPNs; Nurse's aides; Physicians; Psychologists; Recreational therapists; RNs; Social workers.

CONSULTING STAFF: Neurologists; Occupational therapists; Physical therapists; Psychiatrists; Respiratory therapists.

Program Profile

TYPE: Long-term residential program; Respite care program.

Kin Care Inc

3318 N Lincoln Ave, Chicago, IL 60657
(312) 975-7777

Staff Profile

FULL-TIME STAFF: RNs 2; Social workers 2.

CONSULTING STAFF: Physicians 1.

Program Profile

TYPE: Day care program; Home health care agency; Respite care program.

ADMISSION: Referrals accepted from anyone; Physician's referral not required.

INSURANCE PLANS ACCEPTED: Private group insurance; Private pay; Community Care/City of Chicago.

Kraus Home

1620 W Chase, Chicago, IL 60626
(312) 973-2100, 973-0480 FAX

Staff Profile

FULL-TIME STAFF: LPNs 6; Nurse's aides 5; Recreational therapists 1.

PART-TIME STAFF: RNs 1; Social workers 1.

CONSULTING STAFF: Neurologists 1; Occupational therapists 1; Physical therapists 1; Physicians 3; Psychiatrists 1; Psychologists 1.

Program Profile

TYPE: Long-term residential program.

ADMISSION: No referral required.

INSURANCE PLANS ACCEPTED: Private group insurance.

CLIENT SERVICES: Free initial interview; Evening hours; Weekend hours; Wheelchair access; Patient/client library; Educational workshops; Information & referral.

AGE REQUIREMENTS: None.

See ad page 286

Lakeview Nursing & Geriatric Center Inc

735 W Diversey Pkwy, Chicago, IL 60614
(312) 348-4055

Program Profile

TYPE: Diagnostic and medical treatment; Long-term residential program.

The Methodist Home

1415 W Foster Ave, Chicago, IL 60640
(312) 769-5500, 769-6287 FAX

Staff Profile

FULL-TIME STAFF: LPNs; Nurse's aides; RNs; Social workers.

PART-TIME STAFF: LPNs; Nurse's aides; Occupational therapists; Physical therapists; Physicians; RNs.

CONSULTING STAFF: Neurologists; Occupational therapists; Physical therapists; Psychiatrists; Psychologists; Recreational therapists; Respiratory therapists.

Program Profile

TYPE: Long-term residential program.

ADMISSION: Physician's referral required.

INSURANCE PLANS ACCEPTED: Health maintenance organization (HMO); Private group insurance; Medicaid; Medicare; Veteran's insurance.

CLIENT SERVICES: Free initial interview; Evening hours; Weekend hours; Wheelchair access; Patient/client library; Support groups.

AGE REQUIREMENTS: Min 60.

Rush Alzheimer's Disease Clinic

710 S Paulina 8 N, Chicago, IL 60612
(312) 942-4463

Staff Profile

FULL-TIME STAFF: LPNs 1; Neurologists 3; Psychologists 3; RNs 3; Social workers 3; Gerontologist 1.

PART-TIME STAFF: Social workers 1.

CONSULTING STAFF: Psychiatrists 1.

Program Profile

TYPE: Diagnostic and medical treatment.

ACCREDITATIONS: JCAHO; IDPH.

ADMISSION: Physician's referral not required.

INSURANCE PLANS ACCEPTED: Health maintenance organization (HMO); Private group insurance; Medicaid; Medicare.

CLIENT SERVICES: Wheelchair access; Educational workshops; Support groups; Information & referral; Alzheimer's related publications/periodicals.

Rush-Presbyterian-St Luke's Medical Center/ Alzheimer's Family Care Center

5522 N Milwaukee Ave, Chicago, IL 60630
(312) 763-1698, 763-8822 FAX

Staff Profile

FULL-TIME STAFF: Recreational therapists 4; RNs 1; Program coordinators; Program aides 2.

PART-TIME STAFF: Social workers 1.

Program Profile

TYPE: Day care program.

AFFILIATIONS: Chicago Chapter of Alzheimers Association.

ADMISSION: No referral required.

INSURANCE PLANS ACCEPTED: Veteran's insurance; CCP contract.

CLIENT SERVICES: Sliding fee scale; Free initial interview; Wheelchair access; Patient/client library; Educational workshops; Support groups; Information & referral.

AGE REQUIREMENTS: None.

See ad page 24

✔ In order to support future editions of this publication would you please mention *Elder Services* each time you contact any advertiser, facility, or service.

St Joseph Hospital & Health Care Center Alzheimer's Primary Provider Program
2900 N Lake Shore Dr Rm 730, Chicago, IL 60657-6274
(312) 975-3015 ext 6000, 975-3384 FAX
Staff Profile
PART-TIME STAFF: Physicians; RNs; Social workers; Chaplain.
CONSULTING STAFF: Neurologists; Occupational therapists; Physical therapists; Psychiatrists; Psychologists; Recreational therapists.
Program Profile
TYPE: Diagnostic and medical treatment.
AFFILIATIONS: Rush Alzheimer's Disease Center; Rush-Presbyterian-St Luke's Medical Center.
ADMISSION: Referral required; Referrals accepted from patients, family members, home health nurses, minister/priest/rabbi, social service agencies, law enforcement/police; Admission requirements include obvious suspected memory defects or other cognitive defects.
INSURANCE PLANS ACCEPTED: Medicare; Private insurance companies.
CLIENT SERVICES: Wheelchair access; Information & referral.
AGE REQUIREMENTS: None.
See ad page 11

University of Chicago Medical Center Alzheimer's Program
145 E 56th St, Windmere Health Center, Chicago, IL 60637
(312) 702-1000
Program Profile
TYPE: Diagnostic and medical treatment.

Waterfront Terrace
7750 S Shore Dr, Chicago, IL 60649
(312) 731-4200
Program Profile
TYPE: Long-term residential program.

Wellington Plaza Nursing & Therapy Center
504 W Wellington Ave, Chicago, IL 60657
(312) 281-6200
Staff Profile
FULL-TIME STAFF: LPNs 5; Nurse's aides 24; Recreational therapists 1; RNs 10.
PART-TIME STAFF: Physicians 3.
CONSULTING STAFF: Occupational therapists 1; Physical therapists 1; Psychiatrists 1; Social workers 1.
Program Profile
TYPE: Long-term residential program.
ADMISSION: Referrals accepted from hospital, family, social worker; Admission requirements include pre-admission screening; Physician's referral not required.
INSURANCE PLANS ACCEPTED: Medicare.
CLIENT SERVICES: Free initial interview; Wheelchair access; Patient/client library; Educational workshops; Support groups; Information & referral.

Woodbridge Nursing Pavilion
2242 N Kedzie Ave, Chicago, IL 60647
(312) 486-7700
Staff Profile
FULL-TIME STAFF: LPNs; Nurse's aides; Occupational therapists; Physical therapists; Physicians; Recreational therapists; RNs; Social workers.
PART-TIME STAFF: Psychiatrists; Psychologists.
CONSULTING STAFF: Neurologists; Respiratory therapists.
Program Profile
TYPE: Long-term residential program.

Cicero

Westshire Retirement & Healthcare Centre
5825 W Cermak Rd, Cicero, IL 60650
(708) 656-9120, 656-9128 FAX
Staff Profile
STAFF: LPNs; Nurse's aides; Physicians; Psychiatrists; RNs; Social workers.
Program Profile
TYPE: Family support group; Long-term residential program; Respite care program.
ACCREDITATIONS: University of Illinois at Chicago Teaching Affiliation.
ADMISSION: No referral required; Resident must have physical/history completed by physician if admitted from a non-medical setting.
INSURANCE PLANS ACCEPTED: Preferred provider organization (PPO); Health maintenance organization (HMO); Private group insurance; Medicaid.
CLIENT SERVICES: Free initial interview; Evening hours; Weekend hours; Wheelchair access; Support groups; Information & referral.
LANGUAGES SPOKEN: Spanish, Polish, Lithuanian, Czech, Italian.
AGE REQUIREMENTS: Min 18.
See ad on inside back cover

De Kalb

Pine Acres Care Center
1212 S 2nd St, De Kalb, IL 60115
(815) 758-8151, 758-6832 FAX
Staff Profile
FULL-TIME STAFF: LPNs 8; Nurse's aides 20; RNs 2; Social workers 1.
PART-TIME STAFF: LPNs 4; Nurse's aides 20; RNs 12.
CONSULTING STAFF: Occupational therapists 1; Physical therapists 1; Psychiatrists 1; Social workers 1.
Program Profile
TYPE: Long-term residential program.
AFFILIATIONS: United Church of Christ.
ADMISSION: Referrals accepted from anyone; Admission requirements include physician's orders.
CLIENT SERVICES: Free initial interview; Wheelchair access; Educational workshops; Support groups; Information & referral.

Des Plaines

Holy Family Health Center
2380 Dempster, Des Plaines, IL 60016
(708) 296-3335
Staff Profile
FULL-TIME STAFF: LPNs 5; Nurse's aides 96; Occupational therapists 1; Physical therapists 4; Physicians 3; RNs 30; Social workers 2.
PART-TIME STAFF: Nurse's aides 6; Occupational therapists 1; RNs 14.
CONSULTING STAFF: EEG technicians 1; Physical therapists 1; Psychiatrists 1; Respiratory therapists 2.
Program Profile
TYPE: Long-term residential program.
AFFILIATIONS: Rainbow Hospice; Share HMO.
ADMISSION: No referral required.
INSURANCE PLANS ACCEPTED: Preferred provider organization (PPO); Health maintenance organization (HMO); Private group insurance; Medicaid; Medicare; Private pay.
CLIENT SERVICES: Free initial interview; Evening hours; Weekend hours; Wheelchair access; Educational workshops.

Oakton Pavilion Healthcare Facility Inc
1660 Oakton Pl, Des Plaines, IL 60018
(708) 299-5588
Staff Profile
FULL-TIME STAFF: LPNs 8; Nurse's aides 125; Recreational therapists 8; RNs 28; Social workers 5.
PART-TIME STAFF: LPNs 1; Nurse's aides 6; Physicians 1; Recreational therapists 4; RNs 8.
CONSULTING STAFF: Occupational therapists 1; Physical therapists 1; Physicians 45; Psychiatrists 1; Psychologists 1; Respiratory therapists 1.
Program Profile
TYPE: Long-term residential program.
ACCREDITATIONS: JCAHO; IHCA.
ADMISSION: Physician's referral required.
INSURANCE PLANS ACCEPTED: Preferred provider organization (PPO); Health maintenance organization (HMO); Private group insurance; Medicare.
CLIENT SERVICES: Evening hours; Weekend hours; Wheelchair access; Patient/client library; Educational workshops; Information & referral.
LANGUAGES SPOKEN: German, Polish.
AGE REQUIREMENTS: Min 21.

Downers Grove

Rest Haven West
3450 Saratoga Ave, Downers Grove, IL 60515
(708) 969-2900, 241-0615 FAX
Staff Profile
FULL-TIME STAFF: LPNs 35; Nurse's aides 75; RNs 20.
PART-TIME STAFF: Occupational therapists 1; Physical therapists 1.
CONSULTING STAFF: Physicians; Psychiatrists 1; Psychologists 1; Recreational therapists 1; Social workers 1.

Program Profile
TYPE: Long-term residential program.
AFFILIATIONS: Christian Reformed & Reformed Churches.
ADMISSION: No referral required.
INSURANCE PLANS ACCEPTED: Medicaid; Medicare.
CLIENT SERVICES: Weekend hours; Wheelchair access; Support groups; Information & referral.
LANGUAGES SPOKEN: Spanish, Polish.
AGE REQUIREMENTS: Min 18.
See ad on page i

Elgin

Americana Healthcare Center of Elgin
180 S State St, Elgin, IL 60123
(708) 742-3310, 742-8112 FAX
Staff Profile
FULL-TIME STAFF: LPNs; Nurse's aides; Occupational therapists; Physical therapists; Physicians; Recreational therapists; RNs; Social workers.
PART-TIME STAFF: LPNs; Nurse's aides; RNs.
CONSULTING STAFF: EEG technicians; Neurologists; Psychiatrists; Psychologists; Respiratory therapists.
Program Profile
TYPE: Long-term residential program.
ADMISSION: Admission requirements include physician's orders.
INSURANCE PLANS ACCEPTED: Preferred provider organization (PPO); Health maintenance organization (HMO); Private group insurance; Medicare.
CLIENT SERVICES: Free initial interview; Evening hours; Weekend hours; Wheelchair access; Patient/client library; Educational workshops; Support groups; Information & referral; Alzheimer's related publications/periodicals.
LANGUAGES SPOKEN: Spanish, Italian, Polish.
AGE REQUIREMENTS: None.
See ad page 200

Oak Crest Residence
204 S State St, Elgin, IL 60123
(708) 742-2255
Staff Profile
FULL-TIME STAFF: LPNs 1; Nurse's aides 6.
PART-TIME STAFF: Nurse's aides 2.
Program Profile
TYPE: Long-term residential program.
ADMISSION: No referral required.
INSURANCE PLANS ACCEPTED: Private pay.
CLIENT SERVICES: Free initial interview.
AGE REQUIREMENTS: Min 60.

St Joseph Hospital—Alzheimer's Assessment Center
77 N Airlite, Elgin, IL 60123
(708) 695-3200

✔ In order to support future editions of this publication would you please mention *Elder Services* each time you contact any advertiser, facility, or service.

Program Profile

TYPE: Diagnostic and medical treatment.

ADMISSION: Physician's referral not required.

INSURANCE PLANS ACCEPTED: Preferred provider organization (PPO); Private group insurance; Medicare.

CLIENT SERVICES: Wheelchair access; Educational workshops; Information & referral.

See ads pages 18, 168

Elk Grove Village

Alexian Brothers Medical Center/Samaritan House

999A Leicester Rd, Elk Grove Village, IL 60007
(708) 437-5500 ext 5990

Staff Profile

PART-TIME STAFF: Neurologists; Psychologists; RNs; Social workers.

Program Profile

TYPE: Diagnostic and medical treatment.

ACCREDITATIONS: IDPH.

AFFILIATIONS: Rush-Presbyterian-St Luke's Alzheimer Center.

ADMISSION: Referrals accepted from self; Physician's referral not required.

INSURANCE PLANS ACCEPTED: Health maintenance organization (HMO); Private group insurance; Medicaid; Medicare.

CLIENT SERVICES: Information & referral.

Americana Healthcare Center of Elk Grove

1920 W Nerge Rd, Elk Grove Village, IL 60007
(708) 307-0550, 307-0735 FAX

Staff Profile

FULL-TIME STAFF: LPNs; Nurse's aides; Occupational therapists; Physical therapists; Physicians; Recreational therapists; RNs; Social workers.

PART-TIME STAFF: LPNs; Nurse's aides; RNs.

CONSULTING STAFF: EEG technicians; Neurologists; Psychiatrists; Psychologists; Respiratory therapists.

Program Profile

TYPE: Long-term residential program.

ADMISSION: Admission requirements include physician's orders.

INSURANCE PLANS ACCEPTED: Preferred provider organization (PPO); Health maintenance organization (HMO); Private group insurance; Medicare.

CLIENT SERVICES: Free initial interview; Evening hours; Weekend hours; Wheelchair access; Patient/client library; Educational workshops; Support groups; Information & referral; Alzheimer's related publications/periodicals.

LANGUAGES SPOKEN: Spanish, German, Polish.

AGE REQUIREMENTS: None.

See ad page 200

Elmhurst

Elmhurst Extended Care Center Inc

200 E Lake St, Elmhurst, IL 60126-2079
(708) 834-4337, 834-4122 FAX

Staff Profile

FULL-TIME STAFF: LPNs 9; Occupational therapists 1; Physical therapists 1; Recreational therapists 1; RNs 7.

PART-TIME STAFF: LPNs 3; Physicians 90; Recreational therapists 2; RNs 1; Respiratory therapists 1; Social workers 1.

CONSULTING STAFF: Occupational therapists 1; Physical therapists 2.

Program Profile

TYPE: Long-term residential program.

ACCREDITATIONS: IHCA; IDPH.

ADMISSION: Physician's referral required; Admission requirements include medical information.

INSURANCE PLANS ACCEPTED: Preferred provider organization (PPO); Health maintenance organization (HMO); Private group insurance; Medicare; Private pay.

CLIENT SERVICES: Free initial interview; Weekend hours; Wheelchair access; Patient/client library; Support groups; Information & referral.

LANGUAGES SPOKEN: Spanish, Italian.

AGE REQUIREMENTS: Min 18.

Elmhurst Memorial Hospital Senior Health Center at Concord Plaza

200 Berteau Ave, Elmhurst, IL 60126
(708) 833-1400

Program Profile

TYPE: Family support group.

Evanston

Council for Jewish Elderly Adult Day Care Center—Helen & Norman Asher Alzheimer's Care Program

1015 Howard St, Evanston, IL 60202
(708) 492-1400

Staff Profile

STAFF: Activity aides.

FULL-TIME STAFF: Nurse's aides 2; Recreational therapists 2; RNs 2.

PART-TIME STAFF: Social workers 1.

CONSULTING STAFF: Psychiatrists 2; Psychologists 1.

Program Profile

TYPE: Day care program; Family support group; Home health care agency.

ACCREDITATIONS: IDOA CCP.

ADMISSION: Admission requirements include ability to toilet oneself and feed oneself with assistance; No referral required.

CLIENT SERVICES: Sliding fee scale; Free initial interview; Wheelchair access; Support groups; Information & referral.

AGE REQUIREMENTS: Min 60.

Dobson Plaza

120 Dodge Ave, Evanston, IL 60202
(708) 869-7744, 869-2931 FAX

Staff Profile

FULL-TIME STAFF: LPNs 3; Nurse's aides 16; Occupational therapists 1; Recreational therapists 1; RNs 8; Social workers 1.

PART-TIME STAFF: Nurse's aides 4; RNs 3.

CONSULTING STAFF: EEG technicians; Neurologists; Occupational therapists; Physical therapists; Physicians; Psychiatrists; Psychologists; Recreational therapists; RNs; Respiratory therapists; Social workers; Opthalmologist; Podiatrist.

Program Profile

TYPE: Long-term residential program.

ACCREDITATIONS: IDPH.

AFFILIATIONS: Humana Michael Reese Health Plan; Chicagoland Hospice; Hospice North Shore.

ADMISSION: No referral required.

INSURANCE PLANS ACCEPTED: Health maintenance organization (HMO); Private group insurance; Medicaid; Medicare.

CLIENT SERVICES: Wheelchair access; Support groups; Information & referral.

LANGUAGES SPOKEN: Yiddish.

AGE REQUIREMENTS: Min 70.

The Evanston Hospital

2650 Ridge Ave, Evanston, IL 60201
(708) 570-2219

Staff Profile

FULL-TIME STAFF: EEG technicians; Neurologists; Occupational therapists; Physical therapists; Physicians; Psychiatrists; Psychologists; RNs; Respiratory therapists; Social workers.

Program Profile

TYPE: Diagnostic and medical treatment; Family support group.

ACCREDITATIONS: JCAHO.

ADMISSION: No referral required.

INSURANCE PLANS ACCEPTED: Preferred provider organization (PPO); Health maintenance organization (HMO); Private group insurance; Medicaid; Medicare; Veteran's insurance.

CLIENT SERVICES: Free initial interview; Wheelchair access; Educational workshops; Support groups; Information & referral.

AGE REQUIREMENTS: None.

The Oakwood Terrace Nursing Home

1300 Oak Ave, Evanston, IL 60201
(708) 869-1300, 869-1378 FAX

Staff Profile

FULL-TIME STAFF: LPNs 2; Nurse's aides 18; RNs 4.

PART-TIME STAFF: Nurse's aides 11; RNs 2.

CONSULTING STAFF: Occupational therapists 1; Physical therapists 1; Physicians 2; Psychiatrists 1; Social workers 1.

Program Profile

TYPE: Long-term residential program; Respite care program.

ADMISSION: No referral required.

LANGUAGES SPOKEN: Spanish, German, Hungarian.

AGE REQUIREMENTS: Min 21.

The Presbyterian Home

3200 Grant St, Evanston, IL 60201
(708) 492-4800

Staff Profile

FULL-TIME STAFF: LPNs 4; Nurse's aides 68; Occupational therapists 1; Physical therapists 1.

PART-TIME STAFF: LPNs 2; Nurse's aides 5; Occupational therapists 1; Physical therapists 1.

Program Profile

TYPE: Long-term residential program.

ACCREDITATIONS: CCAC.

AFFILIATIONS: Northwestern University Bueler Center on Aging.

INSURANCE PLANS ACCEPTED: Medicare.

CLIENT SERVICES: Wheelchair access; Patient/client library; Educational workshops; Support groups.

AGE REQUIREMENTS: Min 62.

Franklin Park

Westlake Pavilion

10500 W Grand Ave, Franklin Park, IL 60131
(708) 451-1520

Staff Profile

STAFF: EEG technicians; LPNs; Neurologists; Nurse's aides; Occupational therapists; Physical therapists; Physicians; Psychiatrists; Psychologists; Recreational therapists; RNs; Respiratory therapists; Social workers; Rehab therapists.

Program Profile

TYPE: Long-term residential program.

ACCREDITATIONS: IDPH.

ADMISSION: Physician's referral required.

INSURANCE PLANS ACCEPTED: Preferred provider organization (PPO); Health maintenance organization (HMO); Private group insurance; Medicaid; Medicare.

CLIENT SERVICES: Free initial interview; Evening hours; Weekend hours; Wheelchair access; Patient/client library; Educational workshops; Support groups; Information & referral; Hotline; Alzheimer's related publications/periodicals.

LANGUAGES SPOKEN: Spanish, Italian.

AGE REQUIREMENTS: Min 18.

Glenview

Glenview Terrace Nursing Center

1511 Greenwood Rd, Glenview, IL 60025
(708) 729-9090, 729-9135 FAX

Staff Profile

FULL-TIME STAFF: LPNs 5; Nurse's aides 84; Recreational therapists 1; RNs 28; Social workers 2.

CONSULTING STAFF: EEG technicians 1; Neurologists 1; Occupational therapists 1; Physical therapists 3; Physicians 3; Psychiatrists 2; Psychologists 4; Recreational therapists 1; Respiratory therapists 1.

✔ In order to support future editions of this publication would you please mention *Elder Services* each time you contact any advertiser, facility, or service.

Program Profile

TYPE: Long-term residential program.

ADMISSION: Referral required.

INSURANCE PLANS ACCEPTED: Medicaid; Medicare; Veteran's insurance.

CLIENT SERVICES: Free initial interview; Evening hours; Weekend hours; Wheelchair access; Patient/client library; Educational workshops; Support groups.

AGE REQUIREMENTS: Min 18.

See ad page 224

Harvey

Alden Nursing Center—Heather Rehabilitation & Health Care Center

15600 S Honore, Harvey, IL 60426

(708) 333-9550, 333-9554 FAX

Staff Profile

FULL-TIME STAFF: LPNs 14; Nurse's aides 35; Recreational therapists 5; Social workers 1.

PART-TIME STAFF: LPNs 6; Nurse's aides 15; Recreational therapists 1; Social workers 1.

CONSULTING STAFF: EEG technicians 1; Occupational therapists 2; Physical therapists 1; Physicians 12; Psychiatrists 1; Recreational therapists 1.

Program Profile

TYPE: Long-term residential program.

ADMISSION: Physician's referral required.

INSURANCE PLANS ACCEPTED: Health maintenance organization (HMO); Medicaid; Medicare; Veteran's insurance.

CLIENT SERVICES: Sliding fee scale; Free initial interview; Evening hours; Weekend hours; Wheelchair access; Patient/client library; Support groups; Information & referral.

AGE REQUIREMENTS: Min 18.

Hazel Crest

South Suburban Hospital—Alzheimer's Assessment Center

17800 S Kedzie Ave, Hazel Crest, IL 60429

(708) 799-8000, 799-8416 FAX

Staff Profile

FULL-TIME STAFF: Neurologists 1; RNs 1; Social workers 1.

PART-TIME STAFF: RNs 1.

Program Profile

TYPE: Diagnostic and medical treatment.

ACCREDITATIONS: IDPH.

ADMISSION: Referrals accepted from self, family members, health care providers.

INSURANCE PLANS ACCEPTED: Preferred provider organization (PPO); Health maintenance organization (HMO); Private group insurance; Medicare.

CLIENT SERVICES: Wheelchair access; Support groups; Information & referral; Alzheimer's related publications/periodicals.

AGE REQUIREMENTS: None.

Highland Park

Highland Park Hospital Alzheimer's Assessment Program

1936 Green Bay Rd, Highland Park, IL 60035

(708) 432-8000, 480-3974 FAX

Staff Profile

FULL-TIME STAFF: EEG technicians 5; LPNs 100; Neurologists 20; Nurse's aides 100; Occupational therapists 5; Physical therapists 30; Physicians 450; Psychiatrists 50; Recreational therapists 5; RNs 450; Respiratory therapists 20; Social workers 20.

Program Profile

TYPE: Diagnostic and medical treatment.

ACCREDITATIONS: JCAHO; Rush Primary Provider.

ADMISSION: No referral required.

INSURANCE PLANS ACCEPTED: Preferred provider organization (PPO); Health maintenance organization (HMO); Private group insurance; Medicare; Veteran's insurance.

CLIENT SERVICES: Evening hours; Wheelchair access; Educational workshops; Support groups; Information & referral.

AGE REQUIREMENTS: None.

Hinsdale

Americana-Monticello Healthcare Center of Hinsdale

600 W Ogden Ave, Hinsdale, IL 60521

(708) 325-9630, 325-9648 FAX

Staff Profile

FULL-TIME STAFF: LPNs; Nurse's aides; Occupational therapists; Physical therapists; Physicians; Recreational therapists; RNs; Social workers.

PART-TIME STAFF: LPNs; Nurse's aides; RNs.

CONSULTING STAFF: EEG technicians; Neurologists; Psychiatrists; Psychologists; Respiratory therapists.

Program Profile

TYPE: Long-term residential program.

ADMISSION: Admission requirements include physician's orders.

INSURANCE PLANS ACCEPTED: Preferred provider organization (PPO); Health maintenance organization (HMO); Private group insurance; Medicare.

CLIENT SERVICES: Free initial interview; Evening hours; Weekend hours; Wheelchair access; Patient/client library; Educational workshops; Support groups; Information & referral; Alzheimer's related publications/periodicals.

LANGUAGES SPOKEN: Italian, German.

AGE REQUIREMENTS: None.

See ad page 200

Suburban Hospital Alzheimer's Program

55th St & County Line Rd, Hinsdale, IL 60521

(708) 323-5800

Program Profile

TYPE: Family support group.

Hoffman Estates

Alden—Poplar Creek Rehabilitation & Health Care Center

1545 Barrington Rd, Hoffman Estates, IL 60194
(708) 884-0011, 884-0121 FAX

Staff Profile
FULL-TIME STAFF: LPNs; Nurse's aides; RNs; Social workers.
CONSULTING STAFF: Neurologists; Occupational therapists; Physical therapists; Physicians; Psychiatrists; Psychologists; Recreational therapists; Respiratory therapists.

Program Profile
TYPE: Day care program; Family support group; Long-term residential program; Respite care program.
ACCREDITATIONS: IHCA.
ADMISSION: No referral required.
INSURANCE PLANS ACCEPTED: Preferred provider organization (PPO); Health maintenance organization (HMO); Private group insurance; Medicaid; Medicare; Veteran's insurance; Hospice.
CLIENT SERVICES: Free initial interview; Evening hours; Weekend hours; Wheelchair access; Patient/client library; Educational workshops; Support groups; Information & referral.
AGE REQUIREMENTS: Min 18.

Joliet

Draper Plaza

777 Draper Ave, Joliet, IL 60432
(815) 727-4794

Program Profile
TYPE: Long-term residential program.

Salem Village

1314 Rowell Ave, Joliet, IL 60433
(815) 727-5451, 727-2220 FAX

Staff Profile
STAFF: LPNs; Nurse's aides.
FULL-TIME STAFF: Recreational therapists; RNs; Social workers.
PART-TIME STAFF: Physicians.
CONSULTING STAFF: Occupational therapists; Physical therapists.

Program Profile
TYPE: Long-term residential program.
ACCREDITATIONS: IDPH.
AFFILIATIONS: Lutheran Social Services of Illinois.
ADMISSION: Physician's referral required; Admission requirements include 1 year minimum private pay status.
CLIENT SERVICES: Free initial interview; Wheelchair access; Patient/client library; Support groups; Information & referral.
AGE REQUIREMENTS: Min 62.

Villa Franciscan

210 N Springfield, Joliet, IL 60435
(815) 725-3400

Program Profile
TYPE: Long-term residential program.

La Grange

Colonial Manor Healthcare Center

339 S 9th Ave, La Grange, IL 60525
(708) 354-4660

Staff Profile
FULL-TIME STAFF: LPNs; Nurse's aides; Occupational therapists; Physical therapists; Physicians; Recreational therapists; RNs; Social workers.
CONSULTING STAFF: Neurologists; Psychiatrists; Psychologists; Respiratory therapists.

Program Profile
TYPE: Long-term residential program.

La Grange Park

Plymouth Place

315 N La Grange Rd, La Grange Park, IL 60525
(708) 354-0340

Staff Profile
FULL-TIME STAFF: LPNs; Nurse's aides; RNs; Social workers.
PART-TIME STAFF: Occupational therapists; Physical therapists; Physicians.
CONSULTING STAFF: Psychiatrists; Psychologists; Recreational therapists; Respiratory therapists.

Program Profile
TYPE: Long-term residential program.
ACCREDITATIONS: JCAHO.
AFFILIATIONS: Lutheran.
ADMISSION: No referral required.
INSURANCE PLANS ACCEPTED: Health maintenance organization (HMO); Private pay.
CLIENT SERVICES: Free initial interview; Evening hours; Weekend hours; Wheelchair access; Patient/client library; Educational workshops; Support groups; Information & referral.
AGE REQUIREMENTS: Min 65.

Lake Bluff

Lake Bluff Healthcare Centre

700 Jenkisson Ave, Lake Bluff, IL 60044
(708) 295-3900

Staff Profile
FULL-TIME STAFF: LPNs; Nurse's aides; Recreational therapists; RNs; Social workers.
CONSULTING STAFF: Neurologists; Occupational therapists; Physical therapists; Physicians; Psychiatrists; Psychologists; Respiratory therapists.

Program Profile

TYPE: Diagnostic and medical treatment; Family support group; Long-term residential program; Respite care program.

Libertyville

Winchester House

1125 N Milwaukee Ave, Libertyville, IL 60048
(708) 362-4340

Staff Profile

FULL-TIME STAFF: LPNs 18; Nurse's aides 140; Occupational therapists 1; Physicians 1; RNs 25; Social workers 4.

PART-TIME STAFF: LPNs 4; Nurse's aides 20; Physicians 1; RNs 14.

CONSULTING STAFF: Physical therapists; Psychiatrists.

Program Profile

TYPE: Long-term residential program.

ADMISSION: Referral required; Referrals accepted from township supervisors in Lake County.

INSURANCE PLANS ACCEPTED: Medicaid; Medicare.

CLIENT SERVICES: Evening hours; Weekend hours; Wheelchair access; Patient/client library; Information & referral.

AGE REQUIREMENTS: Min 18.

Lindenhurst

Victory Lakes Continuing Care Center

1055 E Grand Ave, Lindenhurst, IL 60046
(708) 356-5900, 356-4570 FAX

Staff Profile

FULL-TIME STAFF: LPNs 1; Nurse's aides 12; RNs 1.

CONSULTING STAFF: EEG technicians; LPNs; Neurologists; Nurse's aides; Occupational therapists; Physical therapists; Physicians; Psychiatrists; Psychologists; Recreational therapists; RNs; Respiratory therapists; Social workers.

Program Profile

TYPE: Diagnostic and medical treatment; Long-term residential program.

ACCREDITATIONS: Alzheimer Disease Assistance Program of Illinois.

ADMISSION: Admission requirements include need for therapeutic environment; No referral required.

INSURANCE PLANS ACCEPTED: Private group insurance.

CLIENT SERVICES: Evening hours; Weekend hours; Wheelchair access; Educational workshops; Support groups; Information & referral.

AGE REQUIREMENTS: None.

See ad page 230

Lisle

Snow Valley Living Center

5000 Lincoln, Lisle, IL 60532
(708) 852-5100

Program Profile

TYPE: Long-term residential program.

Maywood

Loyola University Medical Center—Alzheimer Primary Provider Program

2160 S 1st Ave Room 2006, Maywood, IL 60153
(708) 216-3772

Staff Profile

FULL-TIME STAFF: EEG technicians; Neurologists; Nurse's aides; Occupational therapists; Physical therapists; Physicians; Psychiatrists; RNs; Respiratory therapists; Social workers.

PART-TIME STAFF: Psychologists.

Program Profile

TYPE: Diagnostic and medical treatment.

ACCREDITATIONS: JCAHO; State of Illinois Primary Provider.

ADMISSION: No referral required.

INSURANCE PLANS ACCEPTED: Preferred provider organization (PPO); Health maintenance organization (HMO); Private group insurance; Medicaid; Medicare.

CLIENT SERVICES: Evening hours; Wheelchair access; Patient/client library; Educational workshops; Support groups; Information & referral; Alzheimer's related publications/periodicals.

LANGUAGES SPOKEN: Spanish, Italian.

AGE REQUIREMENTS: None.

McHenry

Northern Illinois Medical Center

4201 Medical Center Dr, McHenry, IL 60050
(815) 344-6602

Staff Profile

FULL-TIME STAFF: Social workers 1.

PART-TIME STAFF: Neurologists 2; Occupational therapists 1; Physical therapists 1; Psychiatrists 1; Psychologists 1.

Program Profile

TYPE: Diagnostic and medical treatment.

ACCREDITATIONS: JCAHO; CARF.

ADMISSION: Referrals accepted from agencies, family; Admission requirements include possible diagnosis of dementia; Physician's referral not required.

INSURANCE PLANS ACCEPTED: Preferred provider organization (PPO); Health maintenance organization (HMO); Private group insurance; Medicaid; Medicare.

CLIENT SERVICES: Evening hours; Wheelchair access; Patient/client library; Information & referral; Alzheimer's related publications/periodicals.

Melrose Park

Gottlieb Memorial Hospital
701 W North Ave, Melrose Park, IL 60160
(708) 681-3200, 450-4526, 681-5412 FAX
Program Profile
TYPE: Diagnostic and medical treatment.
ACCREDITATIONS: JCAHO.
ADMISSION: No referral required.
INSURANCE PLANS ACCEPTED: Preferred provider organization (PPO); Health maintenance organization (HMO); Private group insurance; Medicare.
CLIENT SERVICES: Patient/client library; Educational workshops; Support groups; Information & referral to community resources; Hotline; Alzheimer's related publications/periodicals; Caregiver counseling; Clinical evaluation; Evening hours; Wheelchair access.
AGE REQUIREMENTS: None.
See ad page 127

Midlothian

Bowman Nursing Home
3249 W 147th St, Midlothian, IL 60445
(708) 389-3141
Program Profile
TYPE: Long-term residential program.

Morton Grove

Bethany Terrace Nursing Centre Alzheimer's Care Center
8425 N Waukegan, Morton Grove, IL 60053
(708) 965-8100, 965-8100 (ask to be connected) FAX
Staff Profile
FULL-TIME STAFF: LPNs 10; Nurse's aides 86; Physical therapists 1; Recreational therapists 7; RNs 13; Social workers 3.
PART-TIME STAFF: LPNs 11; Nurse's aides 43; Occupational therapists 1; Recreational therapists 6; RNs 18.
CONSULTING STAFF: Neurologists 1; Physicians; Psychiatrists 1; Dietician 1.
Program Profile
TYPE: Family support group; Long-term residential program; Respite care program.
ACCREDITATIONS: JCAHO.
AFFILIATIONS: United Methodist; Medicare/Medicaid; BCBS.
ADMISSION: No referral required; Admission requirements include completed application.

INSURANCE PLANS ACCEPTED: Health maintenance organization (HMO); Private group insurance; Medicaid; Medicare; Blue Cross-Blue Sheild.
CLIENT SERVICES: Free initial interview; Weekend hours; Wheelchair access; Patient/client library; Support groups; Information & referral.
AGE REQUIREMENTS: Min 18.
See ad page 233

Mount Prospect

Village of Mt Prospect Human Services Division
50 S Emerson, Mount Prospect, IL 60056
(708) 870-5680, 392-6022 FAX
Staff Profile
FULL-TIME STAFF: RNs 1; Social workers 3.
PART-TIME STAFF: RNs 1; Social workers 1.
Program Profile
TYPE: Family support group.
ADMISSION: No referral required.
INSURANCE PLANS ACCEPTED: Services are free.
CLIENT SERVICES: Free initial interview; Evening hours; Wheelchair access; Educational workshops; Support groups; Information & referral.
LANGUAGES SPOKEN: Spanish.
AGE REQUIREMENTS: None.

Naperville

Alden Nursing Center—Naperville Rehabilitation & Health Care Center
1525 S Oxford Ln, Naperville, IL 60565
(708) 983-0300
Staff Profile
FULL-TIME STAFF: LPNs; Nurse's aides; RNs; Social workers.
CONSULTING STAFF: Neurologists; Occupational therapists; Physical therapists; Physicians; Psychiatrists; Psychologists; Respiratory therapists.
Program Profile
TYPE: Day care program; Family support group; Long-term residential program; Respite care program.
ADMISSION: No referral required.
INSURANCE PLANS ACCEPTED: Preferred provider organization (PPO); Health maintenance organization (HMO); Private group insurance; Medicaid; Medicare; Veteran's insurance; Hospice.
CLIENT SERVICES: Free initial interview; Evening hours; Weekend hours; Wheelchair access; Patient/client library; Educational workshops; Support groups; Information & referral.
AGE REQUIREMENTS: Min 18.

Americana Healthcare Center of Naperville
200 Martin Ave, Naperville, IL 60540
(708) 355-4111, 355-1792 FAX

Staff Profile
FULL-TIME STAFF: LPNs; Nurse's aides; Occupational therapists; Physical therapists; Physicians; Recreational therapists; RNs; Social workers.
PART-TIME STAFF: LPNs; Nurse's aides; RNs.
CONSULTING STAFF: EEG technicians; Neurologists; Psychiatrists; Psychologists; Respiratory therapists.
Program Profile
TYPE: Long-term residential program.
ADMISSION: Admission requirements include physician's order.
INSURANCE PLANS ACCEPTED: Preferred provider organization (PPO); Health maintenance organization (HMO); Private group insurance; Medicaid; Medicare.
CLIENT SERVICES: Free initial interview; Evening hours; Weekend hours; Wheelchair access; Patient/client library; Educational workshops; Support groups; Information & referral; Alzheimer's related publications/periodicals.
LANGUAGES SPOKEN: German, Italian, Polish, Spanish.
AGE REQUIREMENTS: None.
See ad page 200

Community Convalescent Center of Naperville
1136 N Mill St, Naperville, IL 60563
(708) 355-3300, 355-1417 FAX
Staff Profile
FULL-TIME STAFF: LPNs; Nurse's aides; Recreational therapists; RNs; Social workers.
PART-TIME STAFF: LPNs; Nurse's aides; Occupational therapists; Physical therapists; Recreational therapists; RNs; Speech therapists.
CONSULTING STAFF: Physicians.
Program Profile
TYPE: Long-term residential program.
ACCREDITATIONS: JCAHO.
ADMISSION: Admission requirements include screening & assessment by Alzheimer's program coordinator, history & physical from physician.
INSURANCE PLANS ACCEPTED: Health maintenance organization (HMO); Private group insurance; Medicaid; Medicare.
CLIENT SERVICES: Free initial interview; Support groups; Information & referral.
AGE REQUIREMENTS: Min 18.
See ad page 138

St Patrick's Residence
1400 Brookdale Rd, Naperville, IL 60563-2126
(708) 416-6565
Program Profile
TYPE: Long-term residential program.

Niles

Regency Nursing Centre
6631 N Milwaukee Ave, Niles, IL 60648
(708) 647-7444, 647-6403 FAX

Program Profile
TYPE: Long-term residential program.
ACCREDITATIONS: JCAHO.
ADMISSION: Referrals accepted from hospital, day care, family, agencies; Admission requirements include a diagnosis of Alzheimer's disease; Physician's referral not required.
INSURANCE PLANS ACCEPTED: Health maintenance organization (HMO); Medicaid; Medicare; Private pay.
CLIENT SERVICES: Free initial interview; Evening hours; Weekend hours; Wheelchair access; Patient/client library; Educational workshops; Support groups.

Norridge

Norridge Nursing Centre Inc
7001 W Cullom Ave, Norridge, IL 60634
(708) 457-0700
Staff Profile
FULL-TIME STAFF: LPNs; Nurse's aides; Physical therapists; Physicians; RNs; Social workers.
CONSULTING STAFF: Neurologists; Occupational therapists; Psychiatrists; Psychologists; Recreational therapists; Respiratory therapists.
Program Profile
TYPE: Family support group; Long-term residential program; Respite care program.
ACCREDITATIONS: JCAHO.
CLIENT SERVICES: Hospice.
See ad on inside front cover

Northfield

North Shore Senior Center & House of Welcome
7 Happ Rd, Northfield, IL 60093
(708) 441-7775, 446-8762 FAX
Staff Profile
FULL-TIME STAFF: Social workers 1.
PART-TIME STAFF: Occupational therapists 1; RNs 3; Social workers 3; Program workers 2.
CONSULTING STAFF: Physicians 1; Psychiatrists 1; Music therapist 1.
Program Profile
TYPE: Day care program.
ADMISSION: Admission requirements include memory loss; Patients must be ambulatory; No referral required.
INSURANCE PLANS ACCEPTED: Private fee-for-service.
CLIENT SERVICES: Sliding fee scale; Educational workshops; Support groups; Information & referral.
AGE REQUIREMENTS: None.
See ad page 144

Northlake

Villa Scalabrini
480 N Wolf Rd, Northlake, IL 60164
(708) 562-0040, 562-3955 FAX
Staff Profile
FULL-TIME STAFF: LPNs; Nurse's aides; Recreational therapists; RNs; Social workers.
PART-TIME STAFF: EEG technicians; Physicians.
CONSULTING STAFF: Occupational therapists; Physical therapists; Psychiatrists; Psychologists.
Program Profile
TYPE: Long-term residential program.
ACCREDITATIONS: IDPH.
AFFILIATIONS: Catholic.
ADMISSION: Admission requirements include diagnosis of Alzheimer's or related disorders; No referral required.
INSURANCE PLANS ACCEPTED: Private group insurance; Medicaid; Medicare.
CLIENT SERVICES: Free initial interview; Wheelchair access; Support groups.
LANGUAGES SPOKEN: Italian.
AGE REQUIREMENTS: Min 60.

Oak Lawn

Americana-Monticello Healthcare Center of Oak Lawn
6300 W 95th St, Oak Lawn, IL 60453
(708) 599-8800, 598-7135 FAX
Staff Profile
FULL-TIME STAFF: LPNs; Nurse's aides; Occupational therapists; Physical therapists; Physicians; Recreational therapists; RNs; Social workers.
PART-TIME STAFF: LPNs; Nurse's aides; RNs.
CONSULTING STAFF: EEG technicians; Neurologists; Psychiatrists; Psychologists; Respiratory therapists.
Program Profile
TYPE: Long-term residential program.
ADMISSION: Admission requirements include physician's orders.
INSURANCE PLANS ACCEPTED: Preferred provider organization (PPO); Health maintenance organization (HMO); Private group insurance; Medicare.
CLIENT SERVICES: Free initial interview; Evening hours; Weekend hours; Wheelchair access; Patient/client library; Educational workshops; Support groups; Information & referral; Alzheimer's related publications/periodicals.
LANGUAGES SPOKEN: Spanish, German, Polish.
AGE REQUIREMENTS: None.
See ad page 200

Palatine

Palatine Township Senior Citizens Council
721 S Quentin Rd, Palatine, IL 60067
(708) 991-1112
Staff Profile
FULL-TIME STAFF: Social workers 2.
Program Profile
TYPE: Day care program; Family support group.
ADMISSION: Admission requirements include assessment; No referral required.
CLIENT SERVICES: Wheelchair access; Educational workshops; Support groups; Information & referral.
LANGUAGES SPOKEN: Polish.
AGE REQUIREMENTS: Min 55.

Plum Grove Nursing Home
24 S Plum Grove Rd, Palatine, IL 60067
(708) 358-0311, 358-8875 FAX
Program Profile
TYPE: Long-term residential program.

Palos Heights

Americana Healthcare Center of Palos Heights
7850 W College Dr, Palos Heights, IL 60463
(708) 361-6990, 361-9512 FAX
Staff Profile
FULL-TIME STAFF: LPNs; Nurse's aides; Occupational therapists; Physical therapists; Physicians; Recreational therapists; RNs; Social workers.
PART-TIME STAFF: LPNs; Nurse's aides; RNs.
CONSULTING STAFF: EEG technicians; Neurologists; Psychiatrists; Psychologists; Respiratory therapists.
Program Profile
TYPE: Long-term residential program.
ADMISSION: Admission requirements include physician's orders.
INSURANCE PLANS ACCEPTED: Preferred provider organization (PPO); Health maintenance organization (HMO); Private group insurance; Medicaid; Medicare.
CLIENT SERVICES: Free initial interview; Evening hours; Weekend hours; Wheelchair access; Patient/client library; Educational workshops; Support groups; Information & referral; Alzheimer's related publications/periodicals.
LANGUAGES SPOKEN: Spanish, German, Italian.
AGE REQUIREMENTS: None.
See ad page 200

Park Ridge

St Matthew Lutheran Home
1601 N Western Ave, Park Ridge, IL 60068
(708) 825-5531, 318-6659 FAX
Program Profile
TYPE: Long-term residential program.

✓ In order to support future editions of this publication would you please mention *Elder Services* each time you contact any advertiser, facility, or service.

Riverwoods

Brentwood North Nursing & Rehabilitation Center

3705 Deerfield Rd, Riverwoods, IL 60015
(708) 459-1200, 459-0113 FAX

Staff Profile
FULL-TIME STAFF: LPNs 3; Nurse's aides 44; Occupational therapists 3; Physical therapists 4; Recreational therapists 5; RNs 38; Social workers 1.
PART-TIME STAFF: LPNs 3; Nurse's aides 33; Occupational therapists 1; Recreational therapists 2; RNs 27.

Program Profile
TYPE: Long-term residential program.
ACCREDITATIONS: JCAHO.
ADMISSION: Referral required.
INSURANCE PLANS ACCEPTED: Health maintenance organization (HMO); Medicare.
CLIENT SERVICES: Free initial interview; Evening hours; Weekend hours; Wheelchair access; Patient/client library.
LANGUAGES SPOKEN: Spanish, German.
AGE REQUIREMENTS: Min 21.

Rolling Meadows

Americana Healthcare Center of Rolling Meadows

4225 W Kirchoff Rd, Rolling Meadows, IL 60008
(708) 397-2400, 397-2914 FAX

Staff Profile
FULL-TIME STAFF: LPNs; Nurse's aides; Occupational therapists; Physical therapists; Physicians; Recreational therapists; RNs; Social workers.
PART-TIME STAFF: LPNs; Nurse's aides; Occupational therapists; RNs.
CONSULTING STAFF: EEG technicians; Neurologists; Psychiatrists; Psychologists; Respiratory therapists.

Program Profile
TYPE: Long-term residential program.
ADMISSION: Admission requirements include physician's orders.
INSURANCE PLANS ACCEPTED: Preferred provider organization (PPO); Health maintenance organization (HMO); Private group insurance; Medicare.
CLIENT SERVICES: Free initial interview; Evening hours; Weekend hours; Wheelchair access; Patient/client library; Educational workshops; Support groups; Information & referral; Alzheimer's related publications/periodicals.
LANGUAGES SPOKEN: Spanish, Italian, Polish.
AGE REQUIREMENTS: None.
See ad page 200

Schaumburg

Friendship Village of Schaumburg

350 W Schaumburg Rd, Schaumburg, IL 60194
(708) 884-5000, 843-4271 FAX

Staff Profile
FULL-TIME STAFF: LPNs 1; Nurse's aides 11; Recreational therapists 1; RNs 4; Social workers 1.
CONSULTING STAFF: Neurologists; Occupational therapists; Physical therapists; Physicians; Psychiatrists; Psychologists; Respiratory therapists.

Program Profile
TYPE: Long-term residential program.
ACCREDITATIONS: CCAC.
AFFILIATIONS: ECFA.
ADMISSION: Physician's referral required.
INSURANCE PLANS ACCEPTED: Medicaid; Medicare.
AGE REQUIREMENTS: Min 62.
See ad page 317

Skokie

Alzheimer's Disease & Related Disorders Association

4709 Golf Rd Ste 1015, Skokie, IL 60076
(708) 864-0045

Lieberman Geriatric Health Centre

9700 Gross Point Rd, Skokie, IL 60076
(708) 674-7210, 674-6366 FAX

Staff Profile
STAFF: LPNs; Nurse's aides; Physicians; RNs.
FULL-TIME STAFF: Recreational therapists 7; Social workers 3.
PART-TIME STAFF: Psychiatrists 3; Psychologists 1; Recreational therapists 2; Social workers 3.
CONSULTING STAFF: Neurologists; Physical therapists.

Program Profile
TYPE: Long-term residential program.
ACCREDITATIONS: JCAHO.
AFFILIATIONS: Jewish.
ADMISSION: Admission requirements include need for long-term care—skilled or intermediate.
INSURANCE PLANS ACCEPTED: Medicaid; Private pay.
CLIENT SERVICES: Free initial interview; Educational workshops; Support groups; Information & referral.
LANGUAGES SPOKEN: Russian, Yiddish.

South Holland

Americana Healthcare Center of South Holland

2145 E 170th St, South Holland, IL 60473
(708) 895-3255, 895-3867 FAX

Staff Profile
FULL-TIME STAFF: LPNs; Nurse's aides; Occupational therapists; Physical therapists; Physicians; Recreational therapists; RNs; Social workers.
PART-TIME STAFF: LPNs; Nurse's aides; RNs.
CONSULTING STAFF: EEG technicians; Neurologists; Psychiatrists; Psychologists; Respiratory therapists.

Program Profile
TYPE: Long-term residential program.
ADMISSION: Admission requirements include physician's orders.

INSURANCE PLANS ACCEPTED: Preferred provider organization (PPO); Health maintenance organization (HMO); Private group insurance; Medicaid; Medicare.
CLIENT SERVICES: Free initial interview; Evening hours; Weekend hours; Wheelchair access; Patient/client library; Educational workshops; Support groups; Information & referral; Alzheimer's related publications/periodicals.
LANGUAGES SPOKEN: Spanish, German, Italian, Polish.
AGE REQUIREMENTS: None.
See ad page 200

Rest Haven South
16300 Wausau Ave, South Holland, IL 60473
(708) 596-5500, 596-6502 FAX
Staff Profile
FULL-TIME STAFF: LPNs; Nurse's aides; RNs; Social workers.
PART-TIME STAFF: Occupational therapists; Physical therapists.
CONSULTING STAFF: Neurologists; Physicians; Psychiatrists; Psychologists; Recreational therapists; Respiratory therapists.
Program Profile
TYPE: Long-term residential program.
ACCREDITATIONS: IDPH.
ADMISSION: No referral required.
INSURANCE PLANS ACCEPTED: Private group insurance.
CLIENT SERVICES: Free initial interview; Evening hours; Weekend hours; Wheelchair access; Patient/client library; Educational workshops; Support groups; Information & referral.
LANGUAGES SPOKEN: Spanish.
AGE REQUIREMENTS: None.
See ad on page i

Windmill Nursing Pavilion Ltd
16000 S Wabash Ave, South Holland, IL 60473
(708) 339-0600
Staff Profile
FULL-TIME STAFF: LPNs; Nurse's aides; Recreational therapists; RNs; Social workers.
CONSULTING STAFF: Neurologists; Occupational therapists; Physical therapists; Physicians; Psychiatrists; Psychologists.
Program Profile
TYPE: Diagnostic and medical treatment; Family support group; Long-term residential program.

Westmont

Americana Healthcare Center of Westmont
512 E Ogden Ave, Westmont, IL 60559
(708) 323-4400, 323-2083 FAX
Staff Profile
FULL-TIME STAFF: LPNs; Nurse's aides; Occupational therapists; Physical therapists; Physicians; Recreational therapists; RNs; Social workers.
PART-TIME STAFF: LPNs; Nurse's aides; RNs.

CONSULTING STAFF: EEG technicians; Neurologists; Psychiatrists; Psychologists; Respiratory therapists.
Program Profile
TYPE: Long-term residential program.
ADMISSION: Admission requirements include physician's orders.
INSURANCE PLANS ACCEPTED: Preferred provider organization (PPO); Health maintenance organization (HMO); Private group insurance.
CLIENT SERVICES: Free initial interview; Evening hours; Weekend hours; Wheelchair access; Educational workshops; Support groups; Information & referral; Hotline; Alzheimer's related publications/periodicals.
LANGUAGES SPOKEN: Spanish, Polish, German.
AGE REQUIREMENTS: None.
See ad page 200

Westmont Convalescent Center
6501 S Cass Ave, Westmont, IL 60559
(708) 960-2026
Program Profile
TYPE: Long-term residential program.

Wheaton

Sandalwood Healthcare Centre
2180 W Manchester Rd, Wheaton, IL 60187
(708) 665-4330, 665-4373 FAX
Staff Profile
FULL-TIME STAFF: LPNs; Nurse's aides.
PART-TIME STAFF: LPNs; Nurse's aides; Occupational therapists; Physical therapists; Physicians.
CONSULTING STAFF: Physicians.
Program Profile
TYPE: Long-term residential program.
ADMISSION: No referral required.
INSURANCE PLANS ACCEPTED: Medicaid; Medicare.
CLIENT SERVICES: Free initial interview; Weekend hours; Wheelchair access; Support groups; Alzheimer's related publications/periodicals.
LANGUAGES SPOKEN: Spanish, Polish, Tagalog.
AGE REQUIREMENTS: Min 65.

Wheeling

Addolorata Villa
555 McHenry Rd, Wheeling, IL 60090
(708) 537-2900
Program Profile
TYPE: Long-term residential program.

✔ In order to support future editions of this publication would you please mention *Elder Services* each time you contact any advertiser, facility, or service.

Wilmette

Normandy House
432 Poplar Dr, Wilmette, IL 60091
(708) 256-5000
Staff Profile
FULL-TIME STAFF: LPNs 2; Nurse's aides 22; Recreational therapists 1; RNs 10.
PART-TIME STAFF: Recreational therapists 3; RNs 8; Social workers 1.
CONSULTING STAFF: Physical therapists 1; Physicians 3; Psychiatrists 1.
Program Profile
TYPE: Long-term residential program.
ADMISSION: Physician's referral required.
INSURANCE PLANS ACCEPTED: Preferred provider organization (PPO); Health maintenance organization (HMO); Private group insurance.
CLIENT SERVICES: Free initial interview; Wheelchair access.
AGE REQUIREMENTS: Min 22.

Winfield

Central DuPage Hospital Alzheimer's Program
25 N Winfield Rd, Winfield, IL 60190
(708) 260-2685
Program Profile
CLIENT SERVICES: Diagnostic assessment; Medical referral; Support groups.
See ad page 138

Liberty Hill Healthcare Center
28 W 141 Liberty Rd, Winfield, IL 60190
(708) 668-2928
Staff Profile
STAFF: Physicians; Psychiatrists.
FULL-TIME STAFF: LPNs; Nurse's aides; RNs.
CONSULTING STAFF: Occupational therapists; Physical therapists; Psychologists; Social workers.
Program Profile
TYPE: Long-term residential program.
ADMISSION: No referral required.
INSURANCE PLANS ACCEPTED: Medicaid; Veteran's insurance; Private pay.
CLIENT SERVICES: Free initial interview; Wheelchair access; Information & referral.
AGE REQUIREMENTS: None.

Woodstock

Family Alliance Inc
670 S Eastwood Dr, Woodstock, IL 60098
(815) 338-3590, 337-4406 FAX
Staff Profile
FULL-TIME STAFF: LPNs; Nurse's aides; RNs; Social workers.
CONSULTING STAFF: Physicians; Psychiatrists.

Program Profile
TYPE: Day care program; Family support group.
CLIENT SERVICES: Sliding fee scale; Wheelchair access; Educational workshops; Support groups.
LANGUAGES SPOKEN: Spanish, Lithuanian.
AGE REQUIREMENTS: Min 55.

Sunset Manor
920 N Seminary Ave, Woodstock, IL 60098
(815) 338-1749
Program Profile
TYPE: Long-term residential program.

INDIANA

Crown Point

Lake County Convalescent Home
2900 W 93rd Ave, Crown Point, IN 46307
(219) 663-5118, 769-1708 FAX
Program Profile
TYPE: Long-term residential program.

Michigan City

Michigan City Health Care
1101 E Coolspring Ave, Michigan City, IN 46360
(219) 874-5211
Program Profile
TYPE: Diagnostic and medical treatment; Long-term residential program.

Portage

Fountainview Place
3175 Lancer St, Portage, IN 46368
(219) 762-9571
Program Profile
TYPE: Long-term residential program.

Valparaiso

Porter County Council on Aging & Aged
PO Box 246, 1005 Campbell, Valparaiso, IN 46384
(219) 464-9736
Program Profile
TYPE: Family support group.

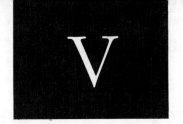

Alzheimer's Treatment Centers and Programs

Facilities arranged by city.

Services	Out-of-home Day Care	In-home Day Care	Out-of-home Respite Care	In-home Respite Care	Residential Facilities	Diagnostic and Treatment Programs
Lutheran Home & Services for the Aged Arlington Heights, IL			•	•	•	•
Fairfax Health Care Center Berwyn, IL					•	•
MacNeal Outpatient Evaluation Program Berwyn, IL						•
Alden Nursing Center—Valley Ridge Rehabilitation & Health Care Center Bloomingdale, IL			•		•	•
Brentwood Nursing & Rehabilitation Center Burbank, IL					•	
Autumn Home Health & Case Management Chicago, IL		•		•		•
Birchwood Plaza Nursing Home Chicago, IL					•	•
Buckingham Pavilion Nursing & Rehabilitation Center Chicago, IL	•		•		•	•
Congress Care Center Chicago, IL			•		•	
Glencrest Nursing Rehabilitation Center Ltd Chicago, IL			•		•	
Kin Care Inc Chicago, IL	•		•			

✔ In order to support future editions of this publication would you please mention *Elder Services* each time you contact any advertiser, facility, or service.

Services	Out-of-home Day Care	In-home Day Care	Out-of-home Respite Care	In-home Respite Care	Residential Facilities	Diagnostic and Treatment Programs
Kraus Home Chicago, IL					•	•
The Methodist Home Chicago, IL			•			•
Rush Alzheimer's Disease Clinic Chicago, IL						•
Rush-Presbyterian-St Luke's Medical Center/Alzheimer's Family Care Center Chicago, IL	•					
St Joseph Hospital & Health Care Center Alzheimer's Primary Provider Program Chicago, IL						•
Wellington Plaza Nursing & Therapy Center Chicago, IL			•			
Woodbridge Nursing Pavilion Chicago, IL					•	
Westshire Retirement & Healthcare Centre Cicero, IL				•	•	•
Pine Acres Care Center De Kalb, IL					•	
Holy Family Health Center Des Plaines, IL					•	•
Oakton Pavilion Healthcare Facility Inc Des Plaines, IL			•		•	•
Rest Haven West Downers Grove, IL	•				•	•
Americana Healthcare Center of Elgin Elgin, IL			•		•	•
Oak Crest Residence Elgin, IL	•		•			
St Joseph Hospital—Alzheimer's Assessment Center Elgin, IL						•
Alexian Brothers Medical Center/ Samaritan House Elk Grove Village, IL						•
Americana Healthcare Center of Elk Grove Elk Grove Village, IL			•		•	•

Services	Out-of-home Day Care	In-home Day Care	Out-of-home Respite Care	In-home Respite Care	Residential Facilities	Diagnostic and Treatment Programs
Elmhurst Extended Care Center Inc Elmhurst, IL			•		•	•
Council for Jewish Elderly Adult Day Care Center—Helen & Norman Asher Alzheimer's Care Program Evanston, IL	•	•			•	•
Dobson Plaza Evanston, IL	•				•	
The Evanston Hospital Evanston, IL						•
The Oakwood Terrace Nursing Home Evanston, IL			•			•
The Presbyterian Home Evanston, IL		•		•	•	•
Westlake Pavilion Franklin Park, IL			•			•
Glenview Terrace Nursing Center Glenview, IL					•	
Alden Nursing Center—Heather Rehabilitation & Health Care Center Harvey, IL					•	
South Suburban Hospital—Alzheimer's Assessment Center Hazel Crest, IL						•
Highland Park Hospital Alzheimer's Assessment Program Highland Park, IL		•				•
Americana-Monticello Healthcare Center of Hinsdale Hinsdale, IL			•		•	•
Alden—Poplar Creek Rehabilitation & Health Care Center Hoffman Estates, IL		•		•	•	•
Salem Village Joliet, IL			•		•	•
Colonial Manor Healthcare Center La Grange, IL					•	
Plymouth Place La Grange Park, IL		•			•	
Lake Bluff Healthcare Centre Lake Bluff, IL			•		•	•
Winchester House Libertyville, IL					•	•

✓ In order to support future editions of this publication would you please mention *Elder Services* each time you contact any advertiser, facility, or service.

338 / **ILLINOIS** / Lindenhurst

V ALZHEIMER'S TREATMENT CENTERS AND PROGRAMS

Services	Out-of-home Day Care	In-home Day Care	Out-of-home Respite Care	In-home Respite Care	Residential Facilities	Diagnostic and Treatment Programs
Victory Lakes Continuing Care Center Lindenhurst, IL	•		•		•	•
Loyola University Medical Center—Alzheimer Primary Provider Program Maywood, IL						•
Northern Illinois Medical Center McHenry, IL						•
Gottlieb Memorial Hospital Melrose Park, IL			•			•
Bethany Terrace Nursing Centre Alzheimer's Care Center Morton Grove, IL			•		•	•
Village of Mt Prospect Human Services Division Mount Prospect, IL		•		•		
Alden Nursing Center—Naperville Rehabilitation & Health Care Center Naperville, IL		•	•		•	•
Americana Healthcare Center of Naperville Naperville, IL			•		•	•
Community Convalescent Center of Naperville Naperville, IL			•		•	
St Patrick's Residence Naperville, IL					•	
Regency Nursing Centre Niles, IL					•	•
Norridge Nursing Centre Inc Norridge, IL			•		•	
North Shore Senior Center & House of Welcome Northfield, IL	•					
Villa Scalabrini Northlake, IL					•	
Americana-Monticello Healthcare Center of Oak Lawn Oak Lawn, IL			•		•	•
Palatine Township Senior Citizens Council Palatine, IL			•			
Americana Healthcare Center of Palos Heights Palos Heights, IL			•		•	•

Services	Out-of-home Day Care	In-home Day Care	Out-of-home Respite Care	In-home Respite Care	Residential Facilities	Diagnostic and Treatment Programs
Brentwood North Nursing & Rehabilitation Center Riverwoods, IL					•	
Americana Healthcare Center of Rolling Meadows Rolling Meadows, IL			•		•	•
Friendship Village of Schaumburg Schaumburg, IL					•	
Lieberman Geriatric Health Centre Skokie, IL					•	•
Americana Healthcare Center of South Holland South Holland, IL			•		•	•
Rest Haven South South Holland, IL		•			•	•
Windmill Nursing Pavilion Ltd South Holland, IL					•	
Americana Healthcare Center of Westmont Westmont, IL			•		•	•
Sandalwood Healthcare Centre Wheaton, IL					•	•
Normandy House Wilmette, IL					•	
Liberty Hill Healthcare Center Winfield, IL					•	
Family Alliance Inc Woodstock, IL	•					
Lake County Convalescent Home Crown Point, IN					•	

✔ In order to support future editions of this publication would you please mention *Elder Services* each time you contact any advertiser, facility, or service.

May we help you reach your rehabilitation goals?

Our team of expert rehabilitation specialists stands ready to work with you and your family in reaching your rehabilitation goals.

We believe that a comprehensive approach to rehabilitation starts with the patient and family telling us what they would like to achieve. We build each plan based on each patient's personal goals and needs.

Our special team of rehabilitation physicians, physical and occupational therapists, psychological staff, nutritional counselors, rehabilitation nurses and others will map out the best ways you can achieve your objectives. We will support you throughout every step.

Call today to learn more. Call **(312) 996-1087** to learn how we can become your rehabilitation team and help you achieve your very important rehabilitation goals.

Services offered
- **Rehabilitation physician specialists**
- **Physical therapy**
- **Occupational therapy**
- **Rehabilitation nursing**
- **Psychological services**
- **Speech therapy**
- **Nutritional counseling**
- **Social services**
- **Therapeutic recreation**

All these and other services are offered on an inpatient and outpatient basis.

The University of Illinois Hospital and Clinics
Specialty Care. Special Caring.

(312) 996-7210

UIC The University of Illinois at Chicago

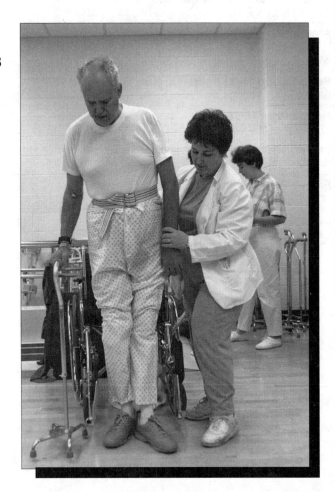

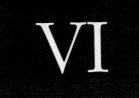

Medical Rehabilitation Facilities

ILLINOIS

Arlington Heights

Americana Healthcare Center of Arlington Heights
715 W Central Rd, Arlington Heights, IL 60005
(708) 392-2020, 392-3250 FAX
Program Profile
TYPE: Private medical rehabilitation facility.
INSURANCE PLANS ACCEPTED: Preferred provider organization (PPO); Health maintenance organization (HMO); Private group insurance; Medicare.
CLIENT SERVICES: Free initial interview; Evening hours; Weekend hours; Wheelchair access; Patient/Client library; Educational workshops; Support groups; Information and referral.

See ad page 200

Northwest Community Continuing Care Center
901 W Kirchoff Rd, Arlington Heights, IL 60005
(708) 259-5850, 577-4064 FAX
Staff Profile
FULL-TIME STAFF: Occupational therapists 2; Physical therapists 3; Physicians 1; Speech/Language therapists 1; Pharmacists 2.
PART-TIME STAFF: Occupational therapists 1; Pharmacists 2.
CONSULTING STAFF: Psychiatrists; Resident physicians; Respiratory therapists; Social workers; Physiatrists.
Program Profile
TYPE: Hospital-sponsored medical rehabilitation program.
ACCREDITATIONS: JCAHO.
INSURANCE PLANS ACCEPTED: Private group insurance; Medicare; Workers compensation.

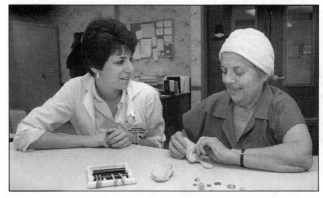

CLIENT SERVICES: Wheelchair access; Support groups; Information and referral.

See ads pages 203, 341

Aurora

Easter Seal Rehabilitation Center
1230 N Highland Ave, Aurora, IL 60506-1401
(708) 896-1961, 896-6257 FAX
Staff Profile
FULL-TIME STAFF: Occupational therapists 3; Physical therapists 2; Social workers 1; Special education instructors 2; Parent/Infant educators 8; Speech pathologists 4.
PART-TIME STAFF: Occupational therapists 2; Physical therapists 3.
CONSULTING STAFF: Physicians 1.
Program Profile
TYPE: Private medical rehabilitation facility.
ACCREDITATIONS: CARF.
AFFILIATIONS: National Easter Seal Society.
ADMISSION: Physician's referral required except some speech therapy referrals may be self-referred.
INSURANCE PLANS ACCEPTED: Preferred provider organization (PPO); Health maintenance organization (HMO); Private group insurance; Medicaid; Medicare; Veteran's insurance.
CLIENT SERVICES: Sliding fee scale; Free initial interview; Evening hours; Wheelchair access; Patient/Client library; Educational workshops; Support groups; Information and referral.

Fox Valley Rehabilitation Medicine Clinic
4050 Healthway Dr, Aurora, IL 60504
(708) 851-0008
Program Profile
TYPE: Hospital-sponsored medical rehabilitation program.

Mercy Center for Health Care Services Pain Treatment Center
1325 N Highland Ave, Aurora, IL 60506
(708) 859-2222
Program Profile
TYPE: Hospital-sponsored medical rehabilitation program.
ACCREDITATIONS: JCAHO.

Bolingbrook

Bolingbrook Medical Center
400 Medical Center Dr, Bolingbrook, IL 60440
(708) 759-0616, 759-0618 FAX
Staff Profile
STAFF: Occupational therapists; Physical therapists; Physicians.

Program Profile
TYPE: Out-patient medical rehabilitation component of private practice.
AFFILIATIONS: Seventh Day Adventist Church.
ADMISSION: Physician's referral required.
INSURANCE PLANS ACCEPTED: Preferred provider organization (PPO); Health maintenance organization (HMO); Private group insurance; Medicare.
CLIENT SERVICES: Evening hours; Wheelchair access; Educational workshops; Rehab-related publications/periodicals.

See ad page 73

Chicago

Allied Health Professionals
1871 N Maud Ave, Chicago, IL 60614
(312) 248-1676
Program Profile
TYPE: Private medical rehabilitation facility.

Baxter Work Center
6325 N Avondale Ave, Chicago, IL 60631
(312) 774-9398; (708) 605-1140
Program Profile
TYPE: Private medical rehabilitation facility.

Johnston R Bowman Health Center for the Elderly
710 S Paulina St, Chicago, IL 60612
(312) 942-7000
Program Profile
TYPE: Hospital-sponsored medical rehabilitation program.

The Center for Rehabilitation at Rush-Presbyterian-St Luke's Medical Center
1653 W Congress Pkwy, 710 S Paulina, Chicago, IL 60612
(312) 942-7161, 942-2323 FAX
Staff Profile
FULL-TIME STAFF: Occupational therapists; Physical therapists; Physicians 6; Psychiatrists; Psychologists; Recreational therapists; Rehabilitation nurses; Resident physicians 18; Social workers; Speech/Language therapists.
CONSULTING STAFF: Driver's education instructors; Orthotists/Prosthetists; Respiratory therapists; Vocational rehabilitation specialists; Pharmacists.
Program Profile
TYPE: Hospital-sponsored medical rehabilitation program.
ACCREDITATIONS: CARF; JCAHO.
ADMISSION: Referral required; Referrals accepted from discharge planner, case manager.
DIAGNOSTIC SERVICES: Physical; Psychological; Social.
INSURANCE PLANS ACCEPTED: Preferred provider organization (PPO); Health maintenance organization (HMO); Private group insurance; Medicaid; Medicare; Workers compensation.

CLIENT SERVICES: Free initial interview; Weekend hours; Wheelchair access; Patient/Client library; Educational workshops; Support groups; Information and referral.

Columbus Hospital Rehabilitation Program
2520 N Lakeview Ave, Chicago, IL 60614
(312) 883-7300
Staff Profile
FULL-TIME STAFF: Occupational therapists 6; Physical therapists 7; Physicians 1; Psychologists 1; Recreational therapists 1; Rehabilitation nurses 7; Social workers 1; Speech/Language therapists 2.
PART-TIME STAFF: Physicians 1.
CONSULTING STAFF: Orthotists/Prosthetists 4; Psychiatrists 2; Vocational rehabilitation specialists 1.
Program Profile
TYPE: Hospital-sponsored medical rehabilitation program.
ACCREDITATIONS: JCAHO.
AFFILIATIONS: Missionary Sisters of the Sacred Heart of Jesus.
DIAGNOSTIC SERVICES: Physical.
INSURANCE PLANS ACCEPTED: Preferred provider organization (PPO); Health maintenance organization (HMO); Private group insurance; Medicaid; Medicare.
CLIENT SERVICES: Wheelchair access; Patient/Client library; Information and referral.

Easter Seal Society of Metropolitan Chicago Inc
220 S State St 320, Chicago, IL 60604
(312) 939-5115
Staff Profile
FULL-TIME STAFF: Occupational therapists 2; Physical therapists 2; Social workers 2; Speech/Language therapists 4.
PART-TIME STAFF: Occupational therapists 1; Physical therapists 1; Social workers 1; Speech/Language therapists 1.
CONSULTING STAFF: Occupational therapists 1; Physical therapists 1; Psychologists 1.
Program Profile
TYPE: Private medical rehabilitation facility.
ACCREDITATIONS: CARF.
INSURANCE PLANS ACCEPTED: Preferred provider organization (PPO); Health maintenance organization (HMO); Private group insurance; Medicaid.
CLIENT SERVICES: Sliding fee scale; Wheelchair access; Support groups; Information and referral.

Foundation for Hearing & Speech Rehabilitation
18 S Michigan Ave, Chicago, IL 60603
(312) 704-1344
Program Profile
TYPE: Private medical rehabilitation facility.

Grant Hospital of Chicago
550 W Webster, Chicago, IL 60614
(312) 883-2000, 883-3883 FAX

Staff Profile

FULL-TIME STAFF: Occupational therapists 6; Physical therapists 7; Psychiatrists 1; Rehabilitation nurses 10; Resident physicians 1; Respiratory therapists; Social workers 1; Speech/Language therapists 2; Pharmacists.

PART-TIME STAFF: Occupational therapists 1; Psychiatrists 1; Recreational therapists 1.

CONSULTING STAFF: Orthotists/Prosthetists 2; Physicians; Psychologists 1.

Program Profile

TYPE: Hospital-sponsored medical rehabilitation program.

ACCREDITATIONS: JCAHO; IDPH.

ADMISSION: Physician's referral required; Admission requirements include need for comprehensive inpatient rehab, medically stable.

INSURANCE PLANS ACCEPTED: Preferred provider organization (PPO); Health maintenance organization (HMO); Private group insurance; Medicaid; Medicare; Veteran's insurance.

CLIENT SERVICES: Free initial interview; Evening hours; Weekend hours; Wheelchair access; Patient/Client library; Educational workshops; Support groups; Information and referral.

Hand Rehabilitation Services

1725 W Harrison, Chicago, IL 60612
(312) 243-6250

Program Profile

TYPE: Private medical rehabilitation facility.

Holy Cross Hospital Rehabilitation Unit

2701 W 68th St, Chicago, IL 60629
(312) 471-6700

Program Profile

TYPE: Hospital-sponsored medical rehabilitation program.

Humana Michael Reese Hospital & Medical Center

2929 S Ellis, Chicago, IL 60616
(312) 791-2000

Program Profile

TYPE: Hospital-sponsored medical rehabilitation program.

Loretto Hospital

645 S Central Ave, Chicago, IL 60644
(312) 626-4300

Staff Profile

FULL-TIME STAFF: Occupational therapists; Physical therapists; Physicians; Psychiatrists; Psychologists; Recreational therapists; Rehabilitation nurses; Respiratory therapists; Social workers.

PART-TIME STAFF: Physicians; Psychologists; Respiratory therapists.

Program Profile

TYPE: Hospital-sponsored medical rehabilitation program.

ACCREDITATIONS: JCAHO.

INSURANCE PLANS ACCEPTED: Preferred provider organization (PPO); Health maintenance organization (HMO); Medicaid; Medicare.

CLIENT SERVICES: Evening hours; Weekend hours; Wheelchair access.

Mercy Hospital & Medical Center

Stevenson Expwy at King Dr, Chicago, IL 60616-2477
(312) 567-2451, 567-7054 FAX

Staff Profile

FULL-TIME STAFF: Occupational therapists 2; Physical therapists 4; Physicians 2; Psychologists 1; Rehabilitation nurses 9; Resident physicians 2; Social workers 1; Speech/Language therapists 1.

PART-TIME STAFF: Orthotists/Prosthetists; Rehabilitation nurses 2; Chaplain; Dietician.

CONSULTING STAFF: Driver's education instructors; Orthotists/Prosthetists; Psychiatrists; Recreational therapists; Respiratory therapists; Vocational rehabilitation specialists; Pharmacists.

Program Profile

ADMISSION: Physician's referral required.

DIAGNOSTIC SERVICES: Physical; Psychological; Social.

INSURANCE PLANS ACCEPTED: Preferred provider organization (PPO); Health maintenance organization (HMO); Private group insurance; Medicaid; Medicare.

CLIENT SERVICES: Sliding fee scale; Wheelchair access; Educational workshops; Support groups; Information and referral.

See ads pages 116, 161, 351

The Methodist Home

1415 W Foster Ave, Chicago, IL 60640
(312) 769-5500

Staff Profile

FULL-TIME STAFF: Physicians 2; Recreational therapists 1; Rehabilitation nurses 1; Social workers 1.

PART-TIME STAFF: Physicians 1; Psychiatrists 1; Resident physicians 1.

CONSULTING STAFF: Occupational therapists 1; Orthotists/Prosthetists 1; Physical therapists 1; Physicians 5; Psychologists 2; Recreational therapists 1; Respiratory therapists 1; Speech/Language therapists 1.

Program Profile

TYPE: Private medical rehabilitation facility.

AFFILIATIONS: AAHA; IAHA.

DIAGNOSTIC SERVICES: Physical; Psychological; Social.

INSURANCE PLANS ACCEPTED: Medicare; Private resources.

CLIENT SERVICES: Evening hours; Weekend hours; Wheelchair access; Patient/Client library; Educational workshops; Support groups; Rehab-related publications/periodicals including "Courier" quarterly newsletter.

Pain Management Consultants

25 E Washington St 4th Floor, Chicago, IL 60602
(312) 726-9543

Staff Profile

CONSULTING STAFF: Occupational therapists; Physicians; Psychiatrists; Psychologists; Social workers.

STAFF: Occupational therapists; Physicians; Psychiatrists; Psychologists; Social workers.

Program Profile
TYPE: Hospital-sponsored medical rehabilitation program.
INSURANCE PLANS ACCEPTED: Preferred provider organization (PPO); Health maintenance organization (HMO); Private group insurance; Medicare.
CLIENT SERVICES: Sliding fee scale; Wheelchair access; Support groups; Information and referral.

Ravenswood Hospital Medical Center
4550 N Winchester St, Chicago, IL 60640
(312) 878-4300
Program Profile
TYPE: Hospital-sponsored medical rehabilitation program.

Rehabilitation Institute of Chicago
345 E Superior St, Chicago, IL 60611
(312) 908-6075, 908-6017, 908-4300 FAX
Staff Profile
FULL-TIME STAFF: Driver's education instructors 4; Occupational therapists 60; Orthotists/Prosthetists 7; Physical therapists 69; Physicians 26; Psychologists 16; Recreational therapists 9; Rehabilitation nurses 125; Resident physicians 40; Social workers 17; Speech/Language therapists 23; Vocational rehabilitation specialists 8; Pharmacists 5; Clinical rehabilitation engineers 3; Nursing assistants 136; Chaplains 2.
PART-TIME STAFF: Psychiatrists.
CONSULTING STAFF: Psychiatrists; Respiratory therapists 4; Special education instructors 2.
Program Profile
TYPE: Private medical rehabilitation facility.
ACCREDITATIONS: JCAHO; CARF.
ADMISSION: Referral required.
DIAGNOSTIC SERVICES: Physical; Psychological.
INSURANCE PLANS ACCEPTED: Preferred provider organization (PPO); Health maintenance organization (HMO); Private group insurance; Medicaid; Medicare.
CLIENT SERVICES: Weekend hours; Wheelchair access; Educational workshops; Support groups; Information and referral.

St Joseph Hospital & Health Care Center Physical Medicine & Rehabilitation Program (Inpatient)
2900 N Lake Shore Dr, Chicago, IL 60657
(312) 975-3000
Staff Profile
FULL-TIME STAFF: Occupational therapists 8; Physical therapists 16; Rehabilitation nurses 7; Speech/Language therapists 2; Audiologists 1.
Program Profile
TYPE: Hospital-sponsored medical rehabilitation program.
ACCREDITATIONS: JCAHO.
AFFILIATIONS: Catholic Church.
ADMISSION: Physician's referral required; Admission requirements include a need for both physical and occupational or speech therapy.
INSURANCE PLANS ACCEPTED: Health maintenance organization (HMO); Private group insurance; Medicaid; Medicare.

CLIENT SERVICES: Wheelchair access; Support groups; Information and referral.
See ad page 11

St Joseph Hospital Rehabilitation & Fitness Center (Outpatient)
2800 N Sheridan Rd Ste 150, Chicago, IL 60657
(312) 525-7868
Staff Profile
FULL-TIME STAFF: Physical therapists 6.
PART-TIME STAFF: Occupational therapists 1; Physical therapists 2; Speech/Language therapists 1.
Program Profile
TYPE: Out-patient medical rehabilitation component of private practice.
ACCREDITATIONS: JCAHO.
ADMISSION: Referral required; Referrals accepted from physician, dentists & podiatrists.
INSURANCE PLANS ACCEPTED: Preferred provider organization (PPO); Health maintenance organization (HMO); Private group insurance; Medicaid; Medicare.
CLIENT SERVICES: Sliding fee scale; Evening hours; Weekend hours; Wheelchair access; Educational workshops; Information and referral.
See ad page 11

St Mary of Nazareth Hospital Center
2233 W Division St, Chicago, IL 60622
(312) 770-2000
Program Profile
TYPE: Hospital-sponsored medical rehabilitation program.
ACCREDITATIONS: JCAHO.
See ad page 162

Schwab Rehabilitation Center
1401 S California Blvd, Chicago, IL 60608
(312) 522-2010, 522-4839 FAX
Staff Profile
CONSULTING STAFF: Orthotists/Prosthetists; Respiratory therapists; Pharmacists.
STAFF: Occupational therapists; Physical therapists; Physicians; Psychiatrists; Psychologists; Recreational therapists; Rehabilitation nurses; Resident physicians; Social workers; Speech/Language therapists; Vocational rehabilitation specialists; Physiatrists.
Program Profile
TYPE: Hospital-sponsored medical rehabilitation program.
ACCREDITATIONS: CARF; JCAHO.
AFFILIATIONS: Mount Sinai Hospital Medical Center, La Rabida Children's Hospital.
ADMISSION: Admission requirements include ability to benefit from rehabilitation; Referral required for inpatient but not for outpatient.
INSURANCE PLANS ACCEPTED: Preferred provider organization (PPO); Health maintenance organization (HMO); Private group insurance; Medicaid; Medicare.
CLIENT SERVICES: Free initial interview; Wheelchair access; Educational workshops; Support groups; Information and referral; Specialized outpatient programming.
See ad page 346

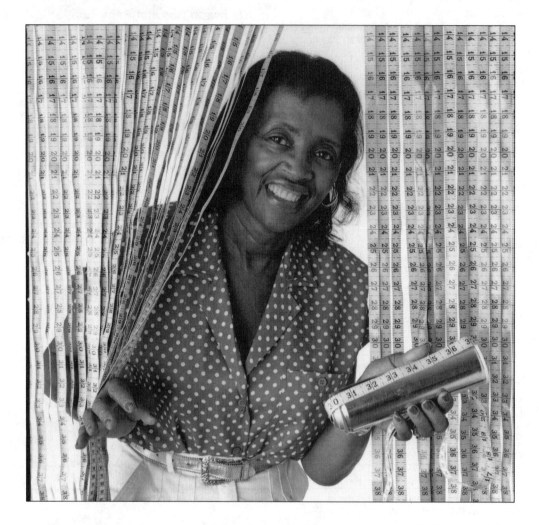
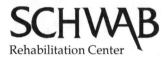

South Side Physical Medicine & Rehabilitation Center

3933 W Columbus Ave, Chicago, IL 60652
(312) 284-0022

Staff Profile

FULL-TIME STAFF: Physical therapists 2; Physicians 4.

PART-TIME STAFF: Psychologists 1.

CONSULTING STAFF: Orthotists/Prosthetists; Vocational rehabilitation specialists.

Program Profile

TYPE: Hospital-sponsored medical rehabilitation program.

ACCREDITATIONS: CARF.

INSURANCE PLANS ACCEPTED: Preferred provider organization (PPO); Health maintenance organization (HMO); Private group insurance; Medicaid; Medicare.

CLIENT SERVICES: Evening hours; Weekend hours; Wheelchair access; Educational workshops; Information and referral.

Swedish Covenant Hospital

5145 N California, Chicago, IL 60625
(312) 878-8200

Staff Profile

FULL-TIME STAFF: Occupational therapists 4; Physical therapists 7; Physicians 1; Psychiatrists 1; Rehabilitation nurses 5; Resident physicians 1; Social workers 2; Speech/Language therapists 3.

PART-TIME STAFF: Occupational therapists 1; Physical therapists 2; Physicians 1; Psychologists 2; Speech/Language therapists 1.

CONSULTING STAFF: Physical therapists 3.

Program Profile

TYPE: Hospital-sponsored medical rehabilitation program; Out-patient medical rehabilitation component of private practice.

ACCREDITATIONS: JCAHO.

ADMISSION: Referral required; Referrals accepted from social services, discharge planner, or utilization coordinators.

INSURANCE PLANS ACCEPTED: Preferred provider organization (PPO); Health maintenance organization (HMO); Private group insurance; Medicaid; Medicare.

CLIENT SERVICES: Wheelchair access; Educational workshops; Support groups.

The University of Illinois Hospital & Clinics

1740 W Taylor St Ste 1400 M/C 693, Chicago, IL 60612
(312) 996-7210, 996-7049 FAX

Staff Profile

FULL-TIME STAFF: Occupational therapists 5; Physical therapists 15; Psychiatrists 3; Psychologists 1; Recreational therapists 1; Rehabilitation nurses 10; Resident physicians 4; Social workers 1; Speech/Language therapists 3; Vocational rehabilitation specialists 1; Pharmacists 1.

PART-TIME STAFF: Occupational therapists 5; Physical therapists 2; Psychiatrists 1; Rehabilitation nurses 4; Vocational rehabilitation specialists 2.

CONSULTING STAFF: Orthotists/Prosthetists 2.

Program Profile

TYPE: Hospital-sponsored medical rehabilitation program.

ACCREDITATIONS: JCAHO.

ADMISSION: Physician's referral required; Admission requirements include transportation, medical records.

DIAGNOSTIC SERVICES: Economic.

INSURANCE PLANS ACCEPTED: Preferred provider organization (PPO); Health maintenance organization (HMO); Private group insurance; Medicaid; Medicare; Veteran's insurance.

CLIENT SERVICES: Weekend hours; Support groups.

See ad page 340

Veterans Affairs Lakeside Medical Center

333 E Huron St, Chicago, IL 60611
(312) 943-6600 ext 353, 943-6912 FAX

Staff Profile

FULL-TIME STAFF: Occupational therapists 5; Physical therapists 2; Physicians 2; Psychologists 1; Recreational therapists 1; Rehabilitation nurses 3; Resident physicians 3; Social workers 1; Speech/Language therapists 1.

PART-TIME STAFF: Physicians 2.

CONSULTING STAFF: Orthotists/Prosthetists 2; Vocational rehabilitation specialists 1.

Program Profile

TYPE: Hospital-sponsored medical rehabilitation program.

ACCREDITATIONS: JCAHO.

ADMISSION: Physician's referral required; Must be an eligible veteran.

DIAGNOSTIC SERVICES: Physical; Psychological; Social.

INSURANCE PLANS ACCEPTED: Veteran's insurance.

CLIENT SERVICES: Wheelchair access; Patient/Client library; Information and referral.

Veterans Affairs West Side Medical Center

820 S Damen Ave Ste B115, Rehab Medicine, Chicago, IL 60612
(312) 666-6500

Program Profile

TYPE: Hospital-sponsored medical rehabilitation program.

INSURANCE PLANS ACCEPTED: Veteran's insurance.

Des Plaines

Holy Family Health Center

2380 Dempster, Des Plaines, IL 60016
(708) 296-3335

Staff Profile

FULL-TIME STAFF: Occupational therapists 1; Physical therapists 4; Physicians 3; Rehabilitation nurses 1; Social workers 2; Special education instructors 1; Speech/Language therapists 1; Rehabilitation aides 4.

PART-TIME STAFF: Occupational therapists 1.

CONSULTING STAFF: Orthotists/Prosthetists 1; Physical therapists 1; Psychiatrists 1; Respiratory therapists 2; Pharmacists 1.

Program Profile

TYPE: Hospital-sponsored medical rehabilitation program.

ADMISSION: No referral required.

INSURANCE PLANS ACCEPTED: Preferred provider organization (PPO); Health maintenance organization (HMO); Private group insurance; Medicaid; Medicare; Private pay.

CLIENT SERVICES: Free initial interview; Evening hours; Weekend hours; Wheelchair access; Educational workshops.

Elgin

Americana Healthcare Center of Elgin

180 S State St, Elgin, IL 60123
(708) 742-3310, 742-8112 FAX

Program Profile

TYPE: Private medical rehabilitation facility.

INSURANCE PLANS ACCEPTED: Preferred provider organization (PPO); Health maintenance organization (HMO); Private group insurance; Medicare.

CLIENT SERVICES: Free initial interview; Evening hours; Weekend hours; Wheelchair access; Patient/Client library; Educational workshops; Support groups; Information and referral.

See ad page 200

Elgin Rehabilitation Center

1485 Davis Rd, Elgin, IL 60123
(708) 888-5540

Program Profile

TYPE: Private medical rehabilitation facility.

Jayne Shover Easter Seal Rehabilitation Center

799 S McLean Blvd, Elgin, IL 60123
(708) 742-3264, 742-9436 FAX

Staff Profile

FULL-TIME STAFF: Occupational therapists 3; Physical therapists 2; Rehabilitation nurses 1; Social workers 1; Speech/Language therapists 3; Audiologists 1.

PART-TIME STAFF: Physical therapists 2.

CONSULTING STAFF: Orthotists/Prosthetists 2; Physicians 1; Psychiatrists 1.

Program Profile

TYPE: Private medical rehabilitation facility.

ACCREDITATIONS: CARF; ASHA.

AFFILIATIONS: Local Easter Seal Affiliate.

ADMISSION: Referral required; Referrals accepted from hospitals, social service agencies, family, client, schools, Department of Rehabilitation Services (DORS); Admission requirements include residence in northern Kane County and Hanover Township, medical authorization for treatment, and immunization documentation 0-18 years.

DIAGNOSTIC SERVICES: Physical.

INSURANCE PLANS ACCEPTED: Preferred provider organization (PPO); Health maintenance organization (HMO); Private group insurance; Medicaid; Medicare; Veteran's insurance.

CLIENT SERVICES: Sliding fee scale; Wheelchair access; Patient/Client library; Support groups; Information and referral.

Elk Grove Village

Alexian Brothers Medical Center Physical Therapy

800 W Biesterfield Rd, Elk Grove Village, IL 60007
(708) 437-5500 ext 4563

Staff Profile

FULL-TIME STAFF: Occupational therapists 10; Physical therapists 6; Physicians; Psychiatrists 1; Psychologists 2; Recreational therapists 1; Rehabilitation nurses 31; Social workers 2; Speech/Language therapists 3.

PART-TIME STAFF: Physical therapists 15; Recreational therapists 1; Speech/Language therapists 25.

CONSULTING STAFF: Orthotists/Prosthetists; Psychiatrists 5; Respiratory therapists; Vocational rehabilitation specialists.

Program Profile

TYPE: Hospital-sponsored medical rehabilitation program.

ACCREDITATIONS: JCAHO; CARF.

INSURANCE PLANS ACCEPTED: Preferred provider organization (PPO); Health maintenance organization (HMO); Private group insurance; Medicaid; Medicare.

CLIENT SERVICES: Support groups.

Alexian Brothers Medical Center Rehabilitation Unit

955 Beisner Rd, Elk Grove Village, IL 60007
(708) 981-3592, 981-6554 FAX

Staff Profile

FULL-TIME STAFF: Occupational therapists 10; Physical therapists 7; Physicians 1; Psychologists 2; Recreational therapists 2; Rehabilitation nurses 30; Social workers 2; Speech/Language therapists 3.

CONSULTING STAFF: Orthotists/Prosthetists 2; Physicians 2; Psychiatrists 5; Respiratory therapists 4; Vocational rehabilitation specialists 2; Pharmacists 2.

Program Profile

TYPE: Hospital-sponsored medical rehabilitation program.

ACCREDITATIONS: JCAHO; CARF.

AFFILIATIONS: Alexian Brothers Health System.

ADMISSION: Physician's referral required.

DIAGNOSTIC SERVICES: Full service acute care hospital.

INSURANCE PLANS ACCEPTED: Preferred provider organization (PPO); Health maintenance organization (HMO); Private group insurance; Medicaid; Medicare; Workers compensation.

CLIENT SERVICES: Wheelchair access; Educational workshops; Support groups.

Americana Healthcare Center of Elk Grove
1920 W Nerge Rd, Elk Grove Village, IL 60007
(708) 307-0550, 307-0735 FAX
Program Profile
TYPE: Private medical rehabilitation facility.
INSURANCE PLANS ACCEPTED: Preferred provider organization (PPO); Health maintenance organization (HMO); Private group insurance; Medicare.
CLIENT SERVICES: Free initial interview; Evening hours; Weekend hours; Wheelchair access; Patient/Client library; Educational workshops; Support groups; Information and referral.
See ad page 200

Elmhurst

Lifeplan Center of Elmhurst Memorial Hospital
186 S West Ave, Elmhurst, IL 60126
(708) 543-3752
Program Profile
TYPE: Hospital-sponsored medical rehabilitation program.

Evanston

The Evanston Hospital Rehabilitation Unit
2650 Ridge Ave, Evanston, IL 60201
(708) 570-2061, 570-2901 FAX
Staff Profile
FULL-TIME STAFF: Occupational therapists 8; Physical therapists 36; Physicians 5; Physicians 4; Recreational therapists 1; Rehabilitation nurses 12; Resident physicians 3; Social workers 1; Speech/Language therapists 4.
PART-TIME STAFF: Occupational therapists 2; Physical therapists 15; Psychologists 1; Rehabilitation nurses 6; Special education instructors 1; Speech/Language therapists 2.
CONSULTING STAFF: Orthotists/Prosthetists 2.
STAFF: Respiratory therapists; Vocational rehabilitation specialists; Pharmacists.
Program Profile
TYPE: Hospital-sponsored medical rehabilitation program.
ACCREDITATIONS: JCAHO; CARF.
ADMISSION: Admission requirements include ability to fully participate in rehab program; No referral required.
INSURANCE PLANS ACCEPTED: Preferred provider organization (PPO); Health maintenance organization (HMO); Private group insurance; Medicaid; Medicare; Veteran's insurance.
CLIENT SERVICES: Evening hours; Weekend hours; Wheelchair access; Patient/Client library; Support groups; Information and referral.

St Francis Hospital of Evanston
355 Ridge Ave, Evanston, IL 60202
(708) 492-4000
Staff Profile
FULL-TIME STAFF: Occupational therapists 1; Physical therapists 8; Speech/Language therapists 2.
PART-TIME STAFF: Occupational therapists 2; Physical therapists 2.
Program Profile
TYPE: Hospital-sponsored medical rehabilitation program.
ACCREDITATIONS: JCAHO.
AFFILIATIONS: Sisters of St Francis of Perpetual Adoration.
INSURANCE PLANS ACCEPTED: Preferred provider organization (PPO); Health maintenance organization (HMO); Private group insurance; Medicaid; Medicare.
CLIENT SERVICES: Evening hours; Wheelchair access; Information and referral.

Glenview

Abington of Glenview
3901 Glenview Rd, Glenview, IL 60025
(708) 729-0000, 729-1552 FAX
Staff Profile
FULL-TIME STAFF: Occupational therapists; Physical therapists 2; Physicians 10; Psychiatrists 1; Recreational therapists 1; Rehabilitation nurses 1; Social workers 2; Speech/Language therapists 1; Pharmacists 1.
CONSULTING STAFF: Occupational therapists 2; Pharmacists 1.
STAFF: Physicians 20.
Program Profile
TYPE: Private medical rehabilitation facility.
ADMISSION: No referral required.
INSURANCE PLANS ACCEPTED: Preferred provider organization (PPO); Health maintenance organization (HMO); Private group insurance; Medicare.
CLIENT SERVICES: Free initial interview; Evening hours; Weekend hours; Wheelchair access; Patient/Client library; Educational workshops; Support groups; Information and referral.
See ad page 225

Harvey

Ingalls Memorial Hospital
One Ingalls Dr, Harvey, IL 60426
(708) 333-2300
Program Profile
TYPE: Hospital-sponsored medical rehabilitation program.
ACCREDITATIONS: JCAHO.

Highland Park

Highland Park Hospital

718 Glenview Ave, Highland Park, IL 60035
(708) 432-8000
Staff Profile
FULL-TIME STAFF: Occupational therapists 6; Physical therapists 11; Speech/Language therapists 2.
STAFF: Psychologists; Recreational therapists; Respiratory therapists; Social workers; Pharmacists.
Program Profile
TYPE: Hospital-sponsored medical rehabilitation program.
ACCREDITATIONS: JCAHO.
ADMISSION: Referral required.
INSURANCE PLANS ACCEPTED: Preferred provider organization (PPO); Health maintenance organization (HMO); Private group insurance; Medicaid; Medicare.
CLIENT SERVICES: Evening hours; Wheelchair access.

Hines

Edward Hines Jr Veterans Affairs Hospital

Roosevelt Rd & 5th Ave, Hines, IL 60141
(708) 343-7200
Program Profile
TYPE: Hospital-sponsored medical rehabilitation program.
INSURANCE PLANS ACCEPTED: Veteran's insurance.

Hinsdale

Americana-Monticello Healthcare Center of Hinsdale

600 W Ogden Ave, Hinsdale, IL 60521
(708) 325-9630, 325-9648 FAX
Program Profile
TYPE: Private medical rehabilitation facility.
ADMISSION: Admission requirements include physical exam.
INSURANCE PLANS ACCEPTED: Preferred provider organization (PPO); Health maintenance organization (HMO); Private group insurance; Medicare.
CLIENT SERVICES: Free initial interview; Evening hours; Weekend hours; Wheelchair access; Patient/Client library; Support groups; Information and referral.
See ad page 200

Paulson Rehab Network—Hinsdale Hospital

120 N Oak St, Hinsdale, IL 60521
(708) 887-2740, 887-2457 FAX
Staff Profile
STAFF: Driver's education instructors; Occupational therapists; Orthotists/Prosthetists; Physical therapists; Physicians; Psychiatrists; Psychologists; Recreational therapists; Rehabilitation nurses; Resident physicians; Respiratory therapists; Social

workers; Special education instructors; Speech/Language therapists; Vocational rehabilitation specialists.
Program Profile
TYPE: Hospital-sponsored medical rehabilitation program.
ACCREDITATIONS: JCAHO; CARF.
AFFILIATIONS: Seventh Day Adventist Church.
ADMISSION: Physician's referral required.
INSURANCE PLANS ACCEPTED: Preferred provider organization (PPO); Health maintenance organization (HMO); Private group insurance; Medicaid; Medicare.
CLIENT SERVICES: Evening hours; Wheelchair access; Educational workshops; Support groups; Information and referral; Hotline (708) 877-4100; Rehab-related publications/periodicals including "Network News".
See ad page 73

Hoffman Estates

Alden—Poplar Creek Hemodialysis Program

1545 Barrington Rd, Hoffman Estates, IL 60194
(708) 884-0011
Staff Profile
FULL-TIME STAFF: Physical therapists; Rehabilitation nurses; Social workers.
PART-TIME STAFF: Occupational therapists.
CONSULTING STAFF: Physicians; Hemodialysis technicians.
Program Profile
INSURANCE PLANS ACCEPTED: Preferred provider organization (PPO); Health maintenance organization (HMO); Private group insurance.
CLIENT SERVICES: Free initial interview; Evening hours; Weekend hours; Wheelchair access; Patient/Client library; Educational workshops; Support groups; Information and referral.

Homewood

Mercy Health Care & Rehabilitation Center

19000 S Halsted St, Homewood, IL 60430
(708) 957-9200, 799-4787 FAX
Staff Profile
FULL-TIME STAFF: Occupational therapists 3; Physical therapists 3; Recreational therapists 5; Rehabilitation nurses 4; Respiratory therapists 1; Social workers 2; Speech/Language therapists 1.
PART-TIME STAFF: Occupational therapists 1; Physicians 16.
CONSULTING STAFF: Physicians 4; Psychiatrists 1; Psychologists 1; Recreational therapists 1; Rehabilitation nurses 3; Pharmacists 1; Optometrists; Dentists; Podiatrists.

Program Profile
TYPE: Hospital-sponsored medical rehabilitation program.
ACCREDITATIONS: IDPH.
AFFILIATIONS: Sisters of Mercy.
ADMISSION: No referral required.
DIAGNOSTIC SERVICES: Physical; Psychological; Social.
INSURANCE PLANS ACCEPTED: Private group insurance; Medicaid; Medicare; Veteran's insurance.
CLIENT SERVICES: Free initial interview; Wheelchair access; Information and referral.
See ads pages 116, 161, 351

Joliet

Easter Seal Rehabilitation Center of Will-Grundy Counties Inc
257 Springfield Ave, Joliet, IL 60435
(815) 725-2194
Program Profile
TYPE: Out-patient medical rehabilitation component of private practice.

St Joseph Medical Center
333 N Madison St, Joliet, IL 60435
(815) 725-7133, 741-7376 FAX

Staff Profile
FULL-TIME STAFF: Occupational therapists 4; Physical therapists 4; Physicians 2; Recreational therapists 1; Rehabilitation nurses 8; Social workers 1; Speech/Language therapists 2.
PART-TIME STAFF: Rehabilitation nurses 10.
CONSULTING STAFF: Driver's education instructors 1; Orthotists/Prosthetists 5; Psychiatrists 10; Psychologists 1; Respiratory therapists 10; Vocational rehabilitation specialists 1; Pharmacists 9.
STAFF: Driver's education instructors; Occupational therapists; Orthotists/Prosthetists; Physical therapists; Physicians; Psychiatrists; Psychologists; Recreational therapists; Rehabilitation nurses; Respiratory therapists; Social workers; Speech/Language therapists; Vocational rehabilitation specialists; Pharmacists.
Program Profile
TYPE: Hospital-sponsored medical rehabilitation program.
ACCREDITATIONS: JCAHO; CARF.
ADMISSION: Physician's referral required; Admission requirements include medical stability, physical stamina, goals for functional improvement, motivation to participate in a rehabilitation program.
DIAGNOSTIC SERVICES: Physical; Psychological; Social; Economic.
INSURANCE PLANS ACCEPTED: Preferred provider organization (PPO); Health maintenance organization (HMO); Private group insurance; Medicaid; Medicare; Veteran's insurance; Workers compensation.

✔ In order to support future editions of this publication would you please mention *Elder Services* each time you contact any advertiser, facility, or service.

CLIENT SERVICES: Free initial interview; Evening hours; Weekend hours; Wheelchair access; Patient/Client library; Educational workshops; Support groups; Information and referral; Hotline (815) 725-7133; Rehab-related publications/periodicals including "Headlines" and "Stroke".

Silver Cross Hospital

1200 Maple Rd, Joliet, IL 60432
(815) 740-7119
Program Profile
TYPE: Hospital-sponsored medical rehabilitation program.

Lake Forest

Lake Forest Hospital Pain Treatment Center

660 N Westmoreland Rd, Lake Forest, IL 60045
(708) 234-6132, 234-9034 FAX
Staff Profile
FULL-TIME STAFF: Physical therapists 1; Rehabilitation nurses 2.
PART-TIME STAFF: Occupational therapists 1; Physical therapists 1; Physicians 2; Psychologists 2; Rehabilitation nurses 8; Biofeedback therapists.
CONSULTING STAFF: Psychiatrists 1; Social workers 1; Speech/Language therapists 1; Vocational rehabilitation specialists 1.
Program Profile
TYPE: Hospital-sponsored medical rehabilitation program.
ACCREDITATIONS: JCAHO; CARF.
ADMISSION: Referral required; Physician's referral not required.
DIAGNOSTIC SERVICES: Physical; Psychological.
INSURANCE PLANS ACCEPTED: Health maintenance organization (HMO); Private group insurance; Medicaid; Medicare.
CLIENT SERVICES: Wheelchair access; Support groups; Information and referral.

Libertyville

Americana Healthcare Center of Libertyville

1500 S Milwaukee Ave, Libertyville, IL 60048
(708) 816-3200, 816-6874 FAX
Program Profile
TYPE: Private medical rehabilitation facility.
ADMISSION: Admission requirements include history & physical.
INSURANCE PLANS ACCEPTED: Preferred provider organization (PPO); Health maintenance organization (HMO); Private group insurance; Medicaid; Medicare.
CLIENT SERVICES: Free initial interview; Evening hours; Weekend hours; Wheelchair access; Patient/Client library; Support groups; Information and referral.
See ad page 200

Lindenhurst

Victory Lakes Continuing Care Center

1055 E Grand, Lindenhurst, IL 60046
(708) 356-5900, 356-4570 FAX
Staff Profile
FULL-TIME STAFF: Rehabilitation nurses 6; Social workers 1.
PART-TIME STAFF: Occupational therapists 1; Physical therapists 1.
CONSULTING STAFF: Orthotists/Prosthetists; Physicians; Psychiatrists; Psychologists; Respiratory therapists; Speech/Language therapists; Pharmacists.
Program Profile
TYPE: Hospital-sponsored medical rehabilitation program.
ADMISSION: Physician's referral required; Admission requirements include Medicare SNF criteria.
INSURANCE PLANS ACCEPTED: Preferred provider organization (PPO); Health maintenance organization (HMO); Private group insurance; Medicare; Private pay.
CLIENT SERVICES: Evening hours; Weekend hours; Wheelchair access; Patient/Client library; Educational workshops; Information and referral.
See ad page 230

McHenry

Northern Illinois Medical Center

Rte 31 & Bull Valley Rd, McHenry, IL 60050
(815) 344-5000
Staff Profile
FULL-TIME STAFF: Occupational therapists 2; Physical therapists 2; Physicians 1; Rehabilitation nurses 3; Speech/Language therapists 1.
PART-TIME STAFF: Psychologists 1; Recreational therapists 1; Rehabilitation nurses 9; Respiratory therapists 1; Social workers 1.
CONSULTING STAFF: Physicians; Psychologists; Rehabilitation nurses 2; Social workers; Vocational rehabilitation specialists.
Program Profile
TYPE: Hospital-sponsored medical rehabilitation program.
ACCREDITATIONS: JCAHO; CARF.
DIAGNOSTIC SERVICES: Physical.
INSURANCE PLANS ACCEPTED: Preferred provider organization (PPO); Health maintenance organization (HMO); Private group insurance; Medicaid; Medicare.
CLIENT SERVICES: Wheelchair access; Support groups; Information and referral.

Melrose Park

Gottlieb Memorial Hospital
701 W North Ave, Melrose Park, IL 60160
(708) 450-4526, 681-5412 FAX
Staff Profile
STAFF: Occupational therapists; Physical therapists; Physicians; Psychiatrists; Recreational therapists; Rehabilitation nurses; Respiratory therapists; Social workers; Speech/Language therapists; Vocational rehabilitation specialists; Pharmacists; Exercise physiologists.
Program Profile
TYPE: Hospital-sponsored medical rehabilitation program.
ACCREDITATIONS: JCAHO.
AFFILIATIONS: Rehabilitation Institute of Chicago.
ADMISSION: Physician's referral required.
DIAGNOSTIC SERVICES: Physical; Psychological; Social.
INSURANCE PLANS ACCEPTED: Preferred provider organization (PPO); Health maintenance organization (HMO); Private group insurance; Medicaid; Medicare; Veteran's insurance; Workers compensation.
CLIENT SERVICES: Wheelchair access; Patient/Client library; Educational workshops; Support groups; Information and referral.
See ad page 127

Westlake Community Hospital Center for Rehabilitation
1225 Lake St, Melrose Park, IL 60160
(708) 681-3000, 681-0151 FAX
Staff Profile
FULL-TIME STAFF: Occupational therapists 15; Physical therapists 18; Psychiatrists 4; Psychologists 1; Recreational therapists 1; Rehabilitation nurses 22; Resident physicians 1; Respiratory therapists 2; Social workers 3; Speech/Language therapists 5; Pharmacists 2.
PART-TIME STAFF: Occupational therapists 10; Psychiatrists 1; Psychologists; Recreational therapists 2; Rehabilitation nurses 4; Social workers 1.
CONSULTING STAFF: Driver's education instructors; Orthotists/Prosthetists; Vocational rehabilitation specialists.
Program Profile
TYPE: Hospital-sponsored medical rehabilitation program.
ACCREDITATIONS: JCAHO; IDPH.
AFFILIATIONS: Syngeron.
ADMISSION: Referral required; Referrals accepted from family; assessors will contact attending physicians.
DIAGNOSTIC SERVICES: Physical.
INSURANCE PLANS ACCEPTED: Preferred provider organization (PPO); Health maintenance organization (HMO); Private group insurance; Medicaid; Medicare.
CLIENT SERVICES: Free initial interview; Weekend hours; Wheelchair access; Support groups; Information and referral.

Naperville

Americana Healthcare Center of Naperville
200 Martin Ave, Naperville, IL 60540
(708) 355-4111, 355-1792 FAX
Program Profile
TYPE: Private medical rehabilitation facility.
ADMISSION: No referral required.
INSURANCE PLANS ACCEPTED: Preferred provider organization (PPO); Health maintenance organization (HMO); Private group insurance; Medicaid; Medicare.
CLIENT SERVICES: Free initial interview; Evening hours; Weekend hours; Wheelchair access; Patient/Client library; Support groups; Information and referral.
See ad page 200

North Chicago

Veterans Affairs Medical Center—North Chicago
Rte 137 Buckley Rd, North Chicago, IL 60064
(708) 688-1900 ext 4211
Program Profile
TYPE: Hospital-sponsored medical rehabilitation program.
INSURANCE PLANS ACCEPTED: Veteran's insurance.

Oak Forest

Oak Forest Hospital
15900 S Cicero Ave, Oak Forest, IL 60452
(708) 687-7200, 687-7979 FAX
Staff Profile
FULL-TIME STAFF: Occupational therapists 5; Physical therapists 5; Physicians 3; Psychologists 3; Recreational therapists 3; Rehabilitation nurses 25; Social workers 3; Speech/Language therapists 3.
CONSULTING STAFF: Orthotists/Prosthetists 2.
STAFF: Vocational rehabilitation specialists.
Program Profile
TYPE: Hospital-sponsored medical rehabilitation program.
ACCREDITATIONS: JCAHO; CARF.
ADMISSION: Physician's referral required.
INSURANCE PLANS ACCEPTED: Health maintenance organization (HMO); Private group insurance; Medicaid; Medicare.
CLIENT SERVICES: Evening hours; Weekend hours; Wheelchair access; Patient/Client library; Educational workshops; Support groups; Rehab-related publications/periodicals including "Triumphs".

✔ In order to support future editions of this publication would you please mention *Elder Services* each time you contact any advertiser, facility, or service.

Oak Lawn

Americana Healthcare Center of Oak Lawn
9401 S Kostner Ave, Oak Lawn, IL 60453
(708) 423-7882, 423-5779 FAX
Program Profile
TYPE: Private medical rehabilitation facility.
ADMISSION: Admission requirements include history &
physical.
INSURANCE PLANS ACCEPTED: Preferred provider organiza-
tion (PPO); Health maintenance organization
(HMO); Private group insurance; Medicare.
CLIENT SERVICES: Free initial interview; Evening hours;
Weekend hours; Wheelchair access; Patient/Client
library; Educational workshops; Support groups;
Information and referral.
See ad page 200

**Americana-Monticello Healthcare Center of Oak
Lawn**
6300 W 95th St, Oak Lawn, IL 60453
(708) 599-8800, 598-7135 FAX
Program Profile
TYPE: Private medical rehabilitation facility.
ADMISSION: Admission requirements include physical
exam.
INSURANCE PLANS ACCEPTED: Preferred provider organiza-
tion (PPO); Health maintenance organization
(HMO); Private group insurance; Medicare.
CLIENT SERVICES: Free initial interview; Evening hours;
Weekend hours; Wheelchair access; Support
groups; Information and referral.
See ad page 200

Christ Hospital & Medical Center
4440 W 95th St, Oak Lawn, IL 60453
(708) 857-5431
Program Profile
TYPE: Hospital-sponsored medical rehabilitation program.

Olympia Fields

**Olympia Fields Osteopathic Hospital & Medical
Center**
20201 Crawford Ave, Olympia Fields, IL 60461
(708) 747-4000
Staff Profile
FULL-TIME STAFF: Occupational therapists 4; Physical
therapists 5; Rehabilitation nurses 7; Social workers
1; Speech/Language therapists 1.
PART-TIME STAFF: Physical therapists 2; Recreational
therapists 1; Rehabilitation nurses 6; Social workers
1.
CONSULTING STAFF: Orthotists/Prosthetists; Physicians;
Vocational rehabilitation specialists.
Program Profile
TYPE: Hospital-sponsored medical rehabilitation pro-
gram.
ACCREDITATIONS: AOA.

ADMISSION: Physician's referral required.
DIAGNOSTIC SERVICES: Physical; Psychological; Social.
INSURANCE PLANS ACCEPTED: Private group insurance;
Medicaid; Medicare.
CLIENT SERVICES: Wheelchair access.
See ad page xvii

Palos Heights

Americana Healthcare Center of Palos Heights
7850 W College Dr, Palos Heights, IL 60463
(708) 361-6990, 361-9512 FAX
Program Profile
TYPE: Private medical rehabilitation facility.
ADMISSION: Physician's referral required; Admission re-
quirements include history, physical, and physi-
cian's orders.
INSURANCE PLANS ACCEPTED: Preferred provider organiza-
tion (PPO); Health maintenance organization
(HMO); Private group insurance.
CLIENT SERVICES: Sliding fee scale; Free initial interview;
Evening hours; Weekend hours; Wheelchair access;
Patient/Client library; Educational workshops; Sup-
port groups; Information and referral.
See ad page 200

Park Ridge

Lutheran General Hospital
1775 Dempster St, Park Ridge, IL 60068
(708) 696-2210
Program Profile
TYPE: Hospital-sponsored medical rehabilitation program.
ACCREDITATIONS: CARF; JCAHO.

Prospect Heights

Excellcare Rehabilitation
664 N Milwaukee Ave, Prospect Heights, IL 60070
(708) 520-9850
Program Profile
TYPE: Private medical rehabilitation facility.

Riverwoods

Brentwood North Nursing & Rehabilitation Center
3705 Deerfield, Riverwoods, IL 60015
(708) 459-1200, 459-0113 FAX
Staff Profile
FULL-TIME STAFF: Occupational therapists 3; Physical
therapists 3; Recreational therapists 5; Social workers 1.

PART-TIME STAFF: Occupational therapists 1; Physical therapists 1; Recreational therapists 2.

CONSULTING STAFF: Speech/Language therapists 1; Pharmacists 1.

Program Profile

TYPE: Private medical rehabilitation facility.

ACCREDITATIONS: JCAHO.

ADMISSION: Physician's referral required.

INSURANCE PLANS ACCEPTED: Preferred provider organization (PPO); Health maintenance organization (HMO); Private group insurance; Medicare.

CLIENT SERVICES: Weekend hours; Wheelchair access; Patient/Client library; Information and referral.

Rolling Meadows

Americana Healthcare Center of Rolling Meadows

4225 W Kirchoff Rd, Rolling Meadows, IL 60008

(708) 397-2400, 397-2914 FAX

Program Profile

TYPE: Private medical rehabilitation facility.

INSURANCE PLANS ACCEPTED: Preferred provider organization (PPO); Health maintenance organization (HMO); Private group insurance; Medicaid; Medicare.

CLIENT SERVICES: Free initial interview; Evening hours; Weekend hours; Wheelchair access; Patient/Client library; Educational workshops; Support groups; Information and referral.

See ad page 200

South Holland

Americana Healthcare Center of South Holland

2145 E 170th St, South Holland, IL 60473

(708) 895-3255, 895-3867 FAX

Program Profile

TYPE: Private medical rehabilitation facility.

ADMISSION: Admission requirements include physical exam.

INSURANCE PLANS ACCEPTED: Preferred provider organization (PPO); Health maintenance organization (HMO); Private group insurance; Medicare.

CLIENT SERVICES: Free initial interview; Evening hours; Weekend hours; Wheelchair access; Patient/Client library; Support groups; Information and referral.

See ad page 200

Villa Park

Du Page Easter Seal Center

830 S Addison Ave, Villa Park, IL 60181

(708) 620-4433, 620-1148 FAX

Staff Profile

FULL-TIME STAFF: Occupational therapists 5; Physical therapists 4; Social workers 1; Speech/Language therapists 4; Audiologists 1.

PART-TIME STAFF: Occupational therapists 2; Physical therapists 6; Social workers 1; Speech/Language therapists 4; Audiologists 1.

CONSULTING STAFF: Orthotists/Prosthetists; Physicians; Psychiatrists; Psychologists.

Program Profile

TYPE: Private medical rehabilitation facility.

ACCREDITATIONS: CARF.

ADMISSION: Physician's referral required; Adult treatment limited to audiology.

DIAGNOSTIC SERVICES: Physical.

INSURANCE PLANS ACCEPTED: Preferred provider organization (PPO); Health maintenance organization (HMO); Private group insurance; Medicaid; Veteran's insurance.

CLIENT SERVICES: Sliding fee scale; Free initial interview; Wheelchair access; Patient/Client library; Educational workshops; Support groups; Information and referral.

Westmont

Americana Healthcare Center of Westmont

512 E Ogden Ave, Westmont, IL 60559

(708) 323-4400, 323-2083 FAX

Program Profile

TYPE: Private medical rehabilitation facility.

ADMISSION: Physician's referral required.

INSURANCE PLANS ACCEPTED: Preferred provider organization (PPO); Health maintenance organization (HMO); Private group insurance; Medicare; Veteran's insurance.

CLIENT SERVICES: Free initial interview; Evening hours; Weekend hours; Wheelchair access; Patient/Client library; Educational workshops; Support groups; Information and referral.

See ad page 200

Wheaton

Marianjoy Rehabilitation Hospital and Clinics

PO Box 795, 26 W 171 Roosevelt Rd, Wheaton, IL 60189

(708) 462-4000, 462-4442 FAX

Staff Profile

FULL-TIME STAFF: Occupational therapists 15; Physical therapists 24; Physicians 10; Psychologists 3; Recreational therapists 6; Rehabilitation nurses 68; Resident physicians 10; Social workers 7; Speech/Language therapists 6; Vocational rehabilitation specialists 2.

PART-TIME STAFF: Driver's education instructors 3; Occupational therapists 31; Physical therapists 15; Psychologists 2; Recreational therapists 1; Rehabilitation nurses 101; Social workers 2; Speech/Language therapists 16; Pharmacists 5.

CONSULTING STAFF: Orthotists/Prosthetists; Psychiatrists; Respiratory therapists.

✔ In order to support future editions of this publication would you please mention *Elder Services* each time you contact any advertiser, facility, or service.

Program Profile

TYPE: Hospital-sponsored medical rehabilitation program.

ACCREDITATIONS: JCAHO; CARF; CIRH.

ADMISSION: Physician's referral required.

DIAGNOSTIC SERVICES: Physical medicine; Rehabilitation.

INSURANCE PLANS ACCEPTED: Preferred provider organization (PPO); Health maintenance organization (HMO); Private group insurance; Medicaid; Medicare; Veteran's insurance; Workers compensation.

CLIENT SERVICES: Wheelchair access; Support groups; Information and referral; Rehab-related publications/periodicals include "Physicare" and "Marianjoy Matters".

See ad page 343

Willowbrook

Paulson Center for Rehabilitative Medicine

619 Plainfield Rd, Willowbrook, IL 60521-5381

(708) 323-5656, 323-5680 FAX

Staff Profile

FULL-TIME STAFF: Occupational therapists 3; Physical therapists 10; Rehabilitation nurses 1; Speech/Language therapists.

PART-TIME STAFF: Driver's education instructors; Occupational therapists 4; Physical therapists 8; Psychologists 1; Case managers.

CONSULTING STAFF: Orthotists/Prosthetists; Physicians; Psychologists 2; Recreational therapists 1; Social workers; Vocational rehabilitation specialists.

Program Profile

TYPE: Hospital-sponsored medical rehabilitation program.

ACCREDITATIONS: CORF.

AFFILIATIONS: Seventh Day Adventist Church.

ADMISSION: Physician's referral required.

INSURANCE PLANS ACCEPTED: Preferred provider organization (PPO); Health maintenance organization (HMO); Private group insurance; Medicare.

CLIENT SERVICES: Evening hours; Wheelchair access; Support groups.

See ad page 73

INDIANA

Crown Point

Rehabilitation Services of St Anthony Medical Center

Main & Franciscan Rd, Crown Point, IN 46307

(219) 663-8120

Staff Profile

FULL-TIME STAFF: Occupational therapists 6; Physical therapists 6; Physicians 1; Psychiatrists 3; Psychologists 1; Recreational therapists 1; Rehabilitation nurses 11; Social workers 1; Speech/Language therapists 6; Nurse liaison/Care manager 1.

PART-TIME STAFF: Occupational therapists 5; Rehabilitation nurses 4; Social workers 1.

Program Profile

TYPE: Hospital-sponsored medical rehabilitation program.

ACCREDITATIONS: JCAHO.

INSURANCE PLANS ACCEPTED: Preferred provider organization (PPO); Health maintenance organization (HMO); Private group insurance; Medicaid; Medicare.

CLIENT SERVICES: Free initial interview; Wheelchair access; Patient/Client library; Educational workshops; Support groups; Information and referral.

See ad page 245

Gary

Rehabilitation Institute of the Methodist Hospitals

600 Grant St, Gary, IN 46402

(219) 886-4566, 886-4107 FAX

Staff Profile

FULL-TIME STAFF: Occupational therapists 8; Physical therapists 18; Psychologists 1; Recreational therapists 2; Rehabilitation nurses 20; Social workers 2; Speech/Language therapists 4.

PART-TIME STAFF: Social workers 1.

CONSULTING STAFF: Driver's education instructors; Orthotists/Prosthetists; Physicians; Psychiatrists; Respiratory therapists; Vocational rehabilitation specialists; Pharmacists.

Program Profile

TYPE: Hospital-sponsored medical rehabilitation program.

ACCREDITATIONS: JCAHO; CARF.

ADMISSION: Physician's referral required.

INSURANCE PLANS ACCEPTED: Preferred provider organization (PPO); Health maintenance organization (HMO); Private group insurance; Medicaid; Medicare.

CLIENT SERVICES: Free initial interview; Wheelchair access; Support groups.

Hammond

St Margaret Hospital & Health Centers

5454 Hohman Ave, Hammond, IN 46320

(219) 932-2300

Staff Profile

FULL-TIME STAFF: Occupational therapists 5; Physical therapists 3; Recreational therapists 1; Rehabilitation nurses 17; Social workers 2; Speech/Language therapists 2.

PART-TIME STAFF: Physical therapists 1; Physicians 1; Speech/Language therapists 1.

CONSULTING STAFF: Orthotists/Prosthetists 1; Psychologists 1.

Program Profile

TYPE: Hospital-sponsored medical rehabilitation program.

ACCREDITATIONS: JCAHO.

INSURANCE PLANS ACCEPTED: Preferred provider organization (PPO); Health maintenance organization (HMO); Private group insurance; Medicaid; Medicare.

CLIENT SERVICES: Free initial interview; Evening hours; Weekend hours; Wheelchair access; Support groups; Information and referral.

La Porte

La Porte Hospital

100 Lincoln Way, La Porte, IN 46350

(219) 872-3331

Staff Profile

FULL-TIME STAFF: Occupational therapists 3; Physical therapists 4; Rehabilitation nurses 3; Speech/Language therapists 2.

PART-TIME STAFF: Physical therapists 1; Recreational therapists 1; Social workers 1.

CONSULTING STAFF: Orthotists/Prosthetists 1; Physicians 1; Psychiatrists 1; Psychologists 1.

Program Profile

TYPE: Hospital-sponsored medical rehabilitation program.

ACCREDITATIONS: JCAHO.

AFFILIATIONS: Veteran's Hospital Association.

INSURANCE PLANS ACCEPTED: Health maintenance organization (HMO); Private group insurance; Medicaid; Medicare.

CLIENT SERVICES: Weekend hours; Wheelchair access; Support groups.

Michigan City

St Anthony Hospital

301 Homer St, Michigan City, IN 46360

(219) 874-0586

Staff Profile

FULL-TIME STAFF: Occupational therapists 3; Physical therapists 4; Physicians 1; Rehabilitation nurses 1; Social workers 2; Speech/Language therapists 1.

PART-TIME STAFF: Orthotists/Prosthetists 1; Psychologists 1.

CONSULTING STAFF: Psychiatrists 1.

Program Profile

TYPE: Hospital-sponsored medical rehabilitation program.

ACCREDITATIONS: JCAHO.

AFFILIATIONS: Sisters of St Francis Health Services Inc.

DIAGNOSTIC SERVICES: Psychological.

INSURANCE PLANS ACCEPTED: Preferred provider organization (PPO); Health maintenance organization (HMO); Private group insurance; Medicaid; Medicare.

CLIENT SERVICES: Free initial interview; Wheelchair access; Patient/Client library; Support groups; Information and referral; Rehab-related publications/periodicals.

✔ In order to support future editions of this publication would you please mention *Elder Services* each time you contact any advertiser, facility, or service.

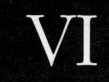

Medical Rehabilitation Facilities

Facilities arranged by city.

Programs	Paraplegia/Quadriplegia	Traumas	Stroke	Neurological/Neuromuscular Disorders	Language Disorders	Sensory Disorders	Musculoskeletal Disorders	Cardiovascular Disease	Pulmonary Diseases	Hematologic Diseases	Chronic Pain
Americana Healthcare Center of Arlington Heights Arlington Heights, IL	•	•	•	•	•	•	•	•	•		•
Northwest Community Continuing Care Center Arlington Heights, IL	•	•	•	•	•	•	•	•	•	•	•
Easter Seal Rehabilitation Center Aurora, IL	•	•	•	•	•	•	•				
Mercy Center for Health Care Services Pain Treatment Center Aurora, IL							•				•
Bolingbrook Medical Center Bolingbrook, IL	•	•	•	•	•		•				•
The Center for Rehabilitation at Rush-Presbyterian-St Luke's Medical Center Chicago, IL		•	•	•	•	•	•	•		•	
Columbus Hospital Rehabilitation Program Chicago, IL		•	•	•	•		•				
Easter Seal Society of Metropolitan Chicago Inc Chicago, IL				•	•	•	•		•		
Grant Hospital of Chicago Chicago, IL	•	•	•	•	•	•	•	•	•		•
Loretto Hospital Chicago, IL		•				•		•	•	•	
Mercy Hospital & Medical Center Chicago, IL	•	•	•	•		•	•	•			•
The Methodist Home Chicago, IL	•	•	•	•	•	•	•			•	

Programs	Paraplegia/Quadriplegia	Traumas	Stroke	Neurological/Neuromuscular Disorders	Language Disorders	Sensory Disorders	Musculoskeletal Disorders	Cardiovascular Disease	Pulmonary Diseases	Hematologic Diseases	Chronic Pain
Pain Management Consultants Chicago, IL											●
Rehabilitation Institute of Chicago Chicago, IL	●	●	●	●	●	●	●		●	●	●
St Joseph Hospital & Health Care Center Physical Medicine & Rehabilitation Program (Inpatient) Chicago, IL	●	●	●	●	●	●	●		●		
St Joseph Hospital Rehabilitation & Fitness Center (Outpatient) Chicago, IL	●	●	●	●	●	●					●
St Mary of Nazareth Hospital Center Chicago, IL	●	●	●	●	●	●	●				
Schwab Rehabilitation Center Chicago, IL	●	●	●	●	●	●	●	●		●	●
South Side Physical Medicine & Rehabilitation Center Chicago, IL	●	●	●	●			●				●
Swedish Covenant Hospital Chicago, IL	●	●	●	●	●	●	●				●
The University of Illinois Hospital & Clinics Chicago, IL	●	●	●	●	●	●	●	●	●	●	●
Veterans Affairs Lakeside Medical Center Chicago, IL		●	●	●			●				
Veterans Affairs West Side Medical Center Chicago, IL	●	●	●	●	●	●	●	●	●	●	●
Holy Family Health Center Des Plaines, IL	●										
Americana Healthcare Center of Elgin Elgin, IL	●	●	●	●	●	●	●	●	●		●
Jayne Shover Easter Seal Rehabilitation Center Elgin, IL	●	●	●	●	●	●					
Alexian Brothers Medical Center Physical Therapy Elk Grove Village, IL	●	●	●	●	●		●		●		
Alexian Brothers Medical Center Rehabilitation Unit Elk Grove Village, IL	●	●	●	●	●	●	●	●	●		●

✔ In order to support future editions of this publication would you please mention *Elder Services* each time you contact any advertiser, facility, or service.

Programs	Paraplegia/Quadriplegia	Traumas	Stroke	Neurological/Neuromuscular Disorders	Language Disorders	Sensory Disorders	Musculoskeletal Disorders	Cardiovascular Disease	Pulmonary Diseases	Hematologic Diseases	Chronic Pain
Americana Healthcare Center of Elk Grove Elk Grove Village, IL	•	•	•	•	•	•	•	•	•		•
The Evanston Hospital Rehabilitation Unit Evanston, IL	•	•	•	•	•		•	•	•		•
St Francis Hospital of Evanston Evanston, IL	•	•	•	•			•				
Abington of Glenview Glenview, IL	•	•	•	•		•	•		•	•	•
Ingalls Memorial Hospital Harvey, IL	•	•	•	•		•	•				
Edward Hines Jr Veterans Affairs Hospital Hines, IL	•	•	•	•	•	•	•	•	•	•	•
Americana-Monticello Healthcare Center of Hinsdale Hinsdale, IL				•							
Paulson Rehab Network—Hinsdale Hospital Hinsdale, IL	•	•	•	•	•	•	•	•	•	•	•
Mercy Health Care & Rehabilitation Center Homewood, IL	•	•	•	•	•	•	•	•	•		•
St Joseph Medical Center Joliet, IL	•	•	•	•		•	•	•	•	•	
Lake Forest Hospital Pain Treatment Center Lake Forest, IL		•		•			•				•
Americana Healthcare Center of Libertyville Libertyville, IL	•	•	•	•		•	•	•	•		•
Victory Lakes Continuing Care Center Lindenhurst, IL	•	•	•	•	•	•	•	•	•	•	•
Northern Illinois Medical Center McHenry, IL		•	•	•	•	•	•	•			
Gottlieb Memorial Hospital Melrose Park, IL		•	•	•	•	•	•	•	•		
Westlake Community Hospital Center for Rehabilitation Melrose Park, IL	•	•		•	•	•			•	•	
Americana Healthcare Center of Naperville Naperville, IL	•	•	•	•	•	•			•	•	

Programs	Paraplegia/Quadriplegia	Traumas	Stroke	Neurological/Neuromuscular Disorders	Language Disorders	Sensory Disorders	Musculoskeletal Disorders	Cardiovascular Disease	Pulmonary Diseases	Hematologic Diseases	Chronic Pain
Veterans Affairs Medical Center—North Chicago North Chicago, IL	●	●	●	●	●	●	●	●	●	●	●
Oak Forest Hospital Oak Forest, IL	●	●	●	●	●	●	●				
Americana Healthcare Center of Oak Lawn Oak Lawn, IL	●	●	●	●	●	●	●	●	●		●
Americana-Monticello Healthcare Center of Oak Lawn Oak Lawn, IL	●	●	●	●	●	●	●	●		●	●
Olympia Fields Osteopathic Hospital & Medical Center Olympia Fields, IL	●	●	●	●	●	●	●			●	
Americana Healthcare Center of Palos Heights Palos Heights, IL	●	●	●	●	●	●	●	●	●		●
Lutheran General Hospital Park Ridge, IL	●	●	●	●	●	●	●	●	●	●	
Brentwood North Nursing & Rehabilitation Center Riverwoods, IL	●	●	●	●	●	●	●	●	●		
Americana Healthcare Center of Rolling Meadows Rolling Meadows, IL	●	●	●	●	●	●	●	●	●		●
Americana Healthcare Center of South Holland South Holland, IL	●	●	●	●	●	●	●	●	●		●
Du Page Easter Seal Center Villa Park, IL				●	●	●	●				
Americana Healthcare Center of Westmont Westmont, IL	●	●	●	●	●	●	●	●	●		●
Marianjoy Rehabilitation Hospital and Clinics Wheaton, IL	●	●	●	●	●		●	●			●
Paulson Center for Rehabilitative Medicine Willowbrook, IL	●	●	●	●	●	●	●	●			●
Rehabilitation Services of St Anthony Medical Center Crown Point, IN	●	●	●	●	●	●	●				
Rehabilitation Institute of the Methodist Hospitals Gary, IN	●	●	●	●			●	●			

✔ In order to support future editions of this publication would you please mention *Elder Services* each time you contact any advertiser, facility, or service.

Programs	Paraplegia/Quadriplegia	Traumas	Stroke	Neurological/Neuromuscular Disorders	Language Disorders	Sensory Disorders	Musculoskeletal Disorders	Cardiovascular Disease	Pulmonary Diseases	Hematologic Diseases	Chronic Pain
St Margaret Hospital & Health Centers Hammond, IN	●	●	●	●	●		●				
La Porte Hospital La Porte, IN		●	●	●	●		●				
St Anthony Hospital Michigan City, IN	●	●	●	●	●	●	●				

INDEXES

Alphabetical Index

✔ In order to support future editions of this publication would you please mention *Elder Services* each time you contact any advertiser, facility, or service.

Americana Healthcare Center of Westmont, Westmont, IL, **III, V, VI**

Americana-Monticello Healthcare Center of Hinsdale, Hinsdale, IL, **III, V, VI**

Americana-Monticello Healthcare Center of Oak Lawn, Oak Lawn, IL, **III, V, VI**

Americanurse Ltd, Summit, IL, **II**

Amicare Home Health Services, Dyer, IN, **II**

The Anchorage of Beecher, Beecher, IL, **III**

The Anchorage of Bensenville, Bensenville, IL, **III**

Ancilla Home Health, East Chicago, IN, **II**

Ancilla Home Health, Oak Park, IL, **II**

Apostolic Christian Resthaven, Elgin, IL, **III**

Applewood Living Center, Matteson, IL, **I, III**

The Arbor, Itasca, IL, **III**

Arbor Terrace Health Care Center, West Chicago, IL, **III, IV-A, IV-B**

Arbour Health Care Center Ltd, Chicago, IL, **III**

Arlington House Retirement Club, Chicago, IL, **IV-B**

Around the Clock Nursing Registry Inc, Lake In The Hills, IL, **II**

Asbury Court, North Aurora, IL, **IV-A**

Ashwood Health Care Center, Elgin, IL, **III**

ASI Inc, Chicago, IL, **II**

At Home Health Inc, Oak Park, IL, **II**

Atrium Health Care Center Ltd, Chicago, IL, **III**

Aurora Housing Authority—Centennial House, Aurora, IL, **IV-B**

Aurora Housing Authority—Maple Terrace Apartments, Aurora, IL, **IV-B**

Aurora Manor, Aurora, IL, **III**

Autumn Country Club Adult Day Care, Frankfort, IL, **I**

Autumn Home Health & Case Management, Chicago, IL, **II, V**

Avenue Care Center Inc, Chicago, IL, **III**

Axelson Manor, Northbrook, IL, **IV-A**

Baha'i Home, Wilmette, IL, **IV-A**

Ballard Nursing Center Inc, Des Plaines, IL, **III**

Balmoral Nursing Centre Inc, Chicago, IL, **III**

Baptist Retirement Home, Maywood, IL, **III, IV-A, IV-B**

Warren Barr Pavilion of Illinois Masonic Medical Center, Chicago, IL, **I, III**

Baxter Work Center, Chicago, IL, **VI**

Bayside Terrace, Waukegan, IL, **III**

Beacon Hill, Lombard, IL, **III, IV-B**

Belhaven Inc, Chicago, IL, **III**

Belmont Nursing Home Inc, Chicago, IL, **III**

The Benchmark of Hoffman Estates, Hoffman Estates, IL, **IV-B**

Berwyn/Cicero Council on Aging, Cicero, IL, **II**

Bethany Retirement Home, Chicago, IL, **IV-A, IV-B**

Bethany Terrace Nursing Centre, Morton Grove, IL, **III**

Bethany Terrace Nursing Centre Alzheimer's Care Center, Morton Grove, IL, **V**

Bethel New Life, Chicago, IL, **I, II**

Bethesda Home & Retirement Center, Chicago, IL, **III, IV-A, IV-B**

Bethlehem Woods Retirement Living Center, La Grange Park, IL, **IV-B**

BHM Health Associates Inc, Merrillville, IN, **II**

Birchwood Plaza Nursing Home, Chicago, IL, **III, V**

Bloomingdale Pavilion, Lombard, IL, **III**

Blue Island Nursing Home Inc, Blue Island, IL, **III**

Bohemian Home for the Aged, Chicago, IL, **III**

Bolingbrook Medical Center, Bolingbrook, IL, **VI**

Boulevard Care Center Inc, Chicago, IL, **III**

Johnston R Bowman Health Center for the Elderly, Chicago, IL, **VI**

Johnston R Bowman Residential Apartments, Chicago, IL, **IV-B**

Bowman Nursing Home, Midlothian, IL, **III, V**

Brandel Care Center, Northbrook, IL, **III**

The Breakers at Edgewater Beach, Chicago, IL, **IV-B**

The Breakers at Golf Mill, Des Plaines, IL, **IV-A**

Brementowne Manor, Tinley Park, IL, **IV-B**

Brentwood North Nursing & Rehabilitation Center, Riverwoods, IL, **III, V, VI**

Brentwood Nursing & Rehabilitation Center, Burbank, IL, **III, V**

Briar Place Ltd, Indian Head Park, IL, **III**

Bridgeview Convalescent Center, Bridgeview, IL, **III**

Bridgeway of Bensenville, Bensenville, IL, **IV-B**

Brightview Care Center Inc, Chicago, IL, **III**

The British Home, Brookfield, IL, **III, IV-A**

Broadway Residence, Joliet, IL, **IV-A**

Bruce & Ken's Pharmacy, Chicago, IL, **II**

Bruce & Ken's Pharmacy, Oak Park, IL, **II**

Bryn Mawr Care Inc, Chicago, IL, **III**

Buckingham Pavilion Nursing & Rehabilitation Center, Chicago, IL, **III, IV-A, V**

Burgess Square Healthcare Centre, Westmont, IL, **III**

Burnham Terrace Ltd, Burnham, IL, **III**

California Gardens Nursing Center, Chicago, IL, **III**

Campbell Terrace, Chicago, IL, **IV-B**

Campbell's Personal Care, Chicago, IL, **II**

Canterbury Care Center, Crystal Lake, IL, **III**

Canterbury Place, Valparaiso, IN, **III**

Canterbury Place Retirement Community, Crystal Lake, IL, **IV-A**

Cardio Care Inc, Chicago, IL, **II**

Care Company Health Care Inc, Joliet, IL, **II**

Care Tech Inc, Elmhurst, IL, **II**

Carefree Village, Woodstock, IL, **IV-A**

Carefree Village Subdivision, Woodstock, IL, **IV-B**

Caregivers Home Health, Barrington, IL, **II**

Caregivers Home Health, Libertyville, IL, **II**

Caregivers Home Health, Woodstock, IL, **II**

Caremark Home Care Inc, Mount Prospect, IL, **II**

Caremark Inc, Homewood, IL, **II**

✔ In order to support future editions of this publication would you please mention *Elder Services* each time you contact any advertiser, facility, or service.

✔ In order to support future editions of this publication would you please mention *Elder Services* each time you contact any advertiser, facility, or service.

Nursefinders of Merrillville, Merrillville, IN, **II**
Nursefinders of Oak Lawn, Oak Lawn, IL, **II**
Nursefinders of Skokie, Skokie, IL, **II**
Nurses on Wheels, Chicago, IL, **II**
Nurses to You Ltd, Roselle, IL, **II**
Oak Brook Healthcare Centre, Oak Brook, IL, **III**
Oak Crest—De Kalb Area Retirement Center, De Kalb, IL, **III, IV-B**
Oak Crest Residence, Elgin, IL, **IV-A, V**
Oak Crest Residence Sharing Today, Elgin, IL, **I**
Oak Forest Hospital, Oak Forest, IL, **VI**
Oak Lawn Convalescent Home, Oak Lawn, IL, **III**
The Oak Park Arms, Oak Park, IL, **IV-A**
Oak Park Township Office, Oak Park, IL, **II**
Oakridge Convalescent Home Inc, Hillside, IL, **III**
Oakton Arms, Des Plaines, IL, **IV-A**
Oakton Pavilion Healthcare Facility Inc, Des Plaines, IL, **III, V**
Oakwood Terrace Nursing Home, Evanston, IL, **III, V**
Old Orchard Manor, Skokie, IL, **III**
Older Adult Rehabilitation Services (OARS) Adult Day Care, Cicero, IL, **I**
Older Adult Rehabilitation Service (OARS) Adult Day Care, Countryside, IL, **I**
Ollie's Adult Day Care, Hammond, IN, **I**
Olsten Healthcare, Lombard, IL, **II**
Olympia Fields Osteopathic Hospital & Medical Center, Olympia Fields, IL, **VI**
Omni Home Care, Park Ridge, IL, **II**
Operation Brotherhood, Chicago, IL, **II**
Option Care, Merrillville, IN, **II**
Orsini Nursing Agency Inc, Arlington Heights, IL, **II**
Osteopathic Home Health Service, Chicago, IL, **II**
Our Lady of Angels Retirement Home, Joliet, IL, **III, IV-A**
Our Lady of Mercy Hospital Transitional Care Center, Dyer, IN, **III**
Our Lady of the Resurrection—Extended Care Unit, Chicago, IL, **III**
Pain Management Consultants, Chicago, IL, **VI**
Palatine Township Senior Citizens Council, Palatine, IL, **V**
Park Forest Health Dept, Park Forest, IL, **II**
Park House Ltd, Chicago, IL, **III**
Park Lane Nursing Center Association, Evergreen Park, IL, **III**
Park Plaza Retirement Center, Chicago, IL, **IV-A**
Park Ridge Healthcare Center, Park Ridge, IL, **III**
Parkside Adult Day Health Center, Arlington Heights, IL, **I**
Parkside Adult Day Health Center, Des Plaines, IL, **I**
Parkside Adult Day Health Center, Northfield, IL, **I**
Parkside Gardens Nursing Home, Burbank, IL, **III**

Parkside—Trinity Adult Day Health Center, Roselle, IL, **I**
Parkway Healthcare Center, Wheaton, IL, **III**
Paulson Center Adult Care, Willowbrook, IL, **I**
Paulson Center for Rehabilitative Medicine, Willowbrook, IL, **VI**
Paulson Rehab Network—Hinsdale Hospital, Hinsdale, IL, **VI**
Pavilion Health Care Center, Valparaiso, IN, **III**
Pavilion of Waukegan Inc, Waukegan, IL, **III**
Peace Memorial Home, Evergreen Park, IL, **III**
Peace Memorial Home Health Service, Evergreen Park, IL, **II**
Peace Memorial Manor, Downers Grove, IL, **IV-B**
Peace Memorial Village, Palos Park, IL, **IV-B**
Peotone Bensenville Home, Peotone, IL, **IV-A**
Pershing Convalescent Home Inc, Stickney, IL, **III**
Peterson Park Health Care Center, Chicago, IL, **III**
Pine Acres Care Center, De Kalb, IL, **III, V**
Pine View Care Center, Saint Charles, IL, **III**
Pines Village Retirement Community, Valparaiso, IN, **IV-B**
Plaza on the Lake, Chicago, IL, **IV-A, IV-B**
Plows Council on Aging, Oak Lawn, IL, **II**
Plum Grove Nursing Home, Palatine, IL, **III, V**
Plum Landing, Aurora, IL, **IV-B**
Plymouth Place, La Grange Park, IL, **III, IV-B, V**
Polonia Home Health Care, Chicago, IL, **II**
Porter County Council on Aging & Aged, Valparaiso, IN, **V**
Prairie Manor Health Care Center, Chicago Heights, IL, **III**
The Presbyterian Home, Evanston, IL, **V**
Primary Health Care Services, Chicago, IL, **II**
Pro Tem Inc, Highland, IN, **II**
Professional Nurses Bureau, Chicago, IL, **II**
Professional Nursing Service—Division of L A Flowers Inc, Gary, IN, **II**
Promed Home Care of Northern Indiana Inc, Merrillville, IN, **II**
Proviso Council on Aging, Bellwood, IL, **II**
Proviso Council on Aging Adult Day Health Center, Bellwood, IL, **I**
Proviso Township Referral Office, Broadview, IL, **II**
Quality Home Health Care Inc, Arlington Heights, IL, **II**
Queen of Peace Retirement Center, Lisle, IL, **IV-A, IV-B**
Rainbow Beach Nursing Center Inc, Chicago, IL, **III**
Ravenswood Home Care, Chicago, IL, **II**
Ravenswood Hospital Medical Center, Chicago, IL, **VI**
Reach Out in Blue Island, Blue Island, IL, **II**
Red Oaks Healthcare Center, Michigan City, IN, **III**
Regency Home Health Care, Niles, IL, **II**
Regency Nursing Centre, Niles, IL, **III, V**

Sherman West Court, Elgin, IL, **III**, **IV-A**
Sherwin Manor Nursing Center, Chicago, IL, **III**
Shore Line Place, Wilmette, IL, **IV-B**
Jayne Shover Easter Seal Rehabilitation Center, Elgin, IL, **VI**
Silver Cross Hospital, Joliet, IL, **VI**
Simmons Loving Care Health Facility, Gary, IN, **III**
Skokie Health Dept, Skokie, IL, **II**
Skokie Meadows Nursing Center 1, Skokie, IL, **III**
Skokie Meadows Nursing Center 2, Skokie, IL, **III**
Washington & Jane Smith Home, Chicago, IL, **III**, **IV-A**
Snow Valley Living Center, Lisle, IL, **III**, **V**
Society for Danish Old People's Home, Chicago, IL, **III**, **IV-A**
Society of St Vincent De Paul of Chicago, Chicago, IL, **II**
Somerset House, Chicago, IL, **III**
South Chicago YMCA, Chicago, IL, **IV-B**
South Side Physical Medicine & Rehabilitation Center, Chicago, IL, **VI**
South Suburban Hospital—Alzheimer's Assessment Center, Hazel Crest, IL, **V**
South Suburban Senior Services of Catholic Charities, Harvey, IL, **II**
Southlake Care Center, Merrillville, IN, **III**, **IV-A**
The Sovereign Home, Chicago, IL, **III**
Squire's Sheltered Care Home, Chicago, IL, **IV-A**
Staff Builders Health Care Services, Crown Point, IN, **II**
Staff Builders Health Services, Chicago, IL, **II**
Staff Builders Services, Chicago, IL, **II**
Stickney Township Office on Aging, Burbank, IL, **II**
Stickney Township Office on Aging—North Stickney Medical Center, Stickney, IL, **I**
Suburban Adult Day Care Center, Oak Park, IL, **I**
Suburban Hospital Alzheimer's Program, Hinsdale, IL, **V**
Summit Home Health Inc, Chicago, IL, **II**
Summit Square Retirement Hotel, Park Ridge, IL, **IV-A**, **IV-B**
Sunny Hill Nursing Home, Joliet, IL, **III**
Sunnymere Inc, Aurora, IL, **IV-A**
Sunnyside Adult Day Center—Senior Services Associates Inc, Elgin, IL, **I**
Sunset Manor, Woodstock, IL, **III**, **IV-A**, **V**
Swartzberg House, Chicago, IL, **IV-B**
Swedish Covenant Hospital, Chicago, IL, **VI**
Swedish Retirement Association, Evanston, IL, **III**, **IV-B**
Tamarack, Palatine, IL, **IV-A**
Ten Twenty Grove, Evanston, IL, **IV-B**
The Terrace Nursing Home Inc, Waukegan, IL, **III**
Third Age Program, Chicago, IL, **II**
Thornton Heights Terrace Ltd, Chicago Heights, IL, **III**
The Tillers Nursing Home, Oswego, IL, **III**

Alice Toch Nurses Registry, Evanston, IL, **II**
Total Home Health Care of Chicago Inc, Chicago, IL, **II**
Town Hall Estates—Wauconda Inc, Wauconda, IL, **III**
Towne Centre, Merrillville, IN, **III**, **IV-A**, **IV-B**
Traycee Home Care, Highwood, IL, **II**
Tri State Manor Nursing Home, Lansing, IL, **III**
Ultra Care Home Medical, Chicago, IL, **II**
Umoja Care Inc, Chicago, IL, **I**, **II**
University of Chicago Medical Center Alzheimer's Program, Chicago, IL, **V**
The University of Illinois Hospital & Clinics, Chicago, IL, **VI**
Unlimited Home Care, Chicago, IL, **II**
Upjohn HealthCare Services, Chicago, IL, **II**
Upjohn HealthCare Services, Joliet, IL, **II**
Uptown Shelter Care Home, Chicago, IL, **IV-A**
Valley Hi Nursing Home, Woodstock, IL, **III**
Veterans Affairs Lakeside Medical Center, Chicago, IL, **VI**
Veterans Affairs Medical Center—North Chicago, North Chicago, IL, **VI**
Veterans Affairs Medical Center—North Chicago-Adult Day Health Care, North Chicago, IL, **I**
Veterans Affairs West Side Medical Center, Chicago, IL, **VI**
Victory Lakes Adult Day Care Center, Lindenhurst, IL, **I**
Victory Lakes Continuing Care Center, Lindenhurst, IL, **III**, **V**, **VI**
Victory Memorial Hospital Home Health Care, Waukegan, IL, **II**
Victory Memorial Hospital—Waukegan Adult Day Care Center, Waukegan, IL, **I**
Villa Franciscan, Joliet, IL, **III**, **V**
Villa St Cyril, Highland Park, IL, **III**
Villa Scalabrini, Northlake, IL, **III**, **IV-A**, **V**
Village Grove Apartments, Elk Grove Village, IL, **IV-B**
Village Nursing Home Inc, Skokie, IL, **III**
Village of Arlington Heights Health Services, Arlington Heights, IL, **II**
Village of Mt Prospect Human Services Division, Mount Prospect, IL, **II**, **V**
Visiting Nurse Association Home Care Services Inc, La Porte, IN, **II**
Visiting Nurse Association Hospice Home Care, Valparaiso, IN, **II**
Visiting Nurse Association North, Evanston, IL, **II**
Visiting Nurse Association of Chicago, Chicago, IL, **II**
Visiting Nurse Association of Fox Valley, Aurora, IL, **II**
Visiting Nurse Association of Fox Valley, Elgin, IL, **II**

✔ In order to support future editions of this publication would you please mention *Elder Services* each time you contact any advertiser, facility, or service.

Geographical Index

ILLINOIS

ADDISON

Indian Trail Apartments, Addison, IL, **IV-B**

ALSIP

Abbey Home Healthcare, Alsip, IL, **II**
Dyna Care Home Health Inc, Alsip, IL, **II**
Home Care Service South & West Inc, Alsip, IL, **II**
Windsor Place of Alsip, Alsip, IL, **IV-A**

ARGO

Des Plaines Valley Health Center, Argo, IL, **II**

ARLINGTON HEIGHTS

Alpha Home Health Care, Arlington Heights, IL, **II**
Americana Healthcare Center of Arlington Heights, Arlington Heights, IL, **III, VI**
Children's Memorial Home Health Inc, Arlington Heights, IL, **II**
Greencastle of Arlington Heights, Arlington Heights, IL, **IV-B**
Lifestyle Options Inc, Arlington Heights, IL, **II**
Luther Village, Arlington Heights, IL, **IV-B**
Lutheran Home & Services for the Aged, Arlington Heights, IL, **III, IV-A, V**
Marriott Church Creek Health Care Center, Arlington Heights, IL, **III**
Marriott Church Creek Retirement Center, Arlington Heights, IL, **IV-B**
The Moorings Health Center, Arlington Heights, IL, **III**
The Moorings of Arlington Heights, Arlington Heights, IL, **IV-A, IV-B**
Northwest Community Continuing Care Center, Arlington Heights, IL, **III, VI**
Northwest Community Health Services of Northwest Community Hospital, Arlington Heights, IL, **II**
Northwest Community Hospital Adult Day Care Center at Park Place Senior Center, Arlington Heights, IL, **I**
Nursefinders of Arlington Heights, Arlington Heights, IL, **II**
Orsini Nursing Agency Inc, Arlington Heights, IL, **II**
Parkside Adult Day Health Center, Arlington Heights, IL, **I**

Quality Home Health Care Inc, Arlington Heights, IL, **II**
Village of Arlington Heights Health Services, Arlington Heights, IL, **II**

AURORA

Alpha Home Health Care, Aurora, IL, **II**
Aurora Housing Authority—Centennial House, Aurora, IL, **IV-B**
Aurora Housing Authority—Maple Terrace Apartments, Aurora, IL, **IV-B**
Aurora Manor, Aurora, IL, **III**
Countryside Healthcare Centre, Aurora, IL, **III**
Easter Seal Rehabilitation Center, Aurora, IL, **VI**
Elmwood Nursing Home, Aurora, IL, **III**
Fox Knoll Retirement Community, Aurora, IL, **IV-A, IV-B**
Fox Valley Rehabilitation Medicine Clinic, Aurora, IL, **VI**
Hospitals Home Health Care Services Inc, Aurora, IL, **II**
Jennings Terrace, Aurora, IL, **III, IV-A**
McAuley Manor, Aurora, IL, **III**
Medical Personnel Pool, Aurora, IL, **II**
Mercy Center for Health Care Services Pain Treatment Center, Aurora, IL, **VI**
New Encounters Adult Day Care Centre, Aurora, IL, **I**
New York Manor Inc, Aurora, IL, **III**
Nursefinders of Aurora, Aurora, IL, **II**
Plum Landing, Aurora, IL, **IV-B**
Sunnymere Inc, Aurora, IL, **IV-A**
Visiting Nurse Association of Fox Valley, Aurora, IL, **II**

BARRINGTON

Caregivers Home Health, Barrington, IL, **II**
Farah Medical Group, Barrington, IL, **II**
Governor's Park Nursing & Rehabilitation Center, Barrington, IL, **III**

BATAVIA

Colonial House at The Holmstad, Batavia, IL, **IV-A**
Firwood Health Care Center, Batavia, IL, **III**
Fox Valley Hospice, Batavia, IL, **II**
Green Meadows, Batavia, IL, **IV-B**
The Holmstad, Batavia, IL, **IV-B**
Michealsen Health Center, Batavia, IL, **III**

✔ In order to support future editions of this publication would you please mention *Elder Services* each time you contact any advertiser, facility, or service.

✔ In order to support future editions of this publication would you please mention *Elder Services* each time you contact any advertiser, facility, or service.

Ravenswood Home Care, Chicago, IL, **II**
Ravenswood Hospital Medical Center, Chicago, IL,
  VI
Rehabilitation Institute of Chicago, Chicago, IL, **VI**
Resurrection Home Health Care Services, Chicago,
  IL, **II**
Resurrection Retirement Community, Chicago, IL,
  IV-B
Rush Alzheimer's Disease Clinic, Chicago, IL, **V**
Rush Home Health Service, Chicago, IL, **II**
Rush-Presbyterian-St Luke's Medical Center/
  Alzheimer's Family Care Center, Chicago, IL, **V**
Sacred Heart Home, Chicago, IL, **III**
St Agnes Health Care Center, Chicago, IL, **III**
St Gregory Socialcare, Chicago, IL, **II**
St James Place Ltd, Chicago, IL, **II**
St Joseph Home of Chicago Inc, Chicago, IL, **III,
  IV-A, IV-B**
St Joseph Hospital & Health Care Center
  Alzheimer's Primary Provider Program, Chicago,
  IL, **V**
St Joseph Hospital & Health Care Center Physical
  Medicine & Rehabilitation Program (Inpatient),
  Chicago, IL, **VI**
St Joseph Hospital & Health Care Center—Skilled
  Nursing Unit, Chicago, IL, **III**
St Joseph Hospital Rehabilitation & Fitness Center
  (Outpatient), Chicago, IL, **VI**
St Martha Manor, Chicago, IL, **III**
St Mary of Nazareth Hospital Center, Chicago, IL,
  VI
St Mary's Home Health Services, Chicago, IL, **II**
St Paul's House, Chicago, IL, **IV-A**
St Paul's House & Health Care Center, Chicago, IL,
  III
The Salvation Army—Family Service Division,
  Chicago, IL, **II**
The Salvation Army, Chicago, IL, **II**
Sargent—Water Tower Pharmacy, Chicago, IL, **II**
Sauganash Edgebrook Home Nursing Inc, Chicago,
  IL, **II**
SCH Home-Med North, Chicago, IL, **II**
Schwab Rehabilitation Center, Chicago, IL, **VI**
Selfhelp Home for the Aged, Chicago, IL, **III, IV-A,
  IV-B**
Senior Care Inc, Chicago, IL, **II**
Seniors Home Health Care Ltd, Chicago, IL, **II**
Sherwin Manor Nursing Center, Chicago, IL, **III**
Washington & Jane Smith Home, Chicago, IL, **III,
  IV-A**
Society for Danish Old People's Home, Chicago,
  IL, **III, IV-A**
Society of St Vincent De Paul of Chicago, Chicago,
  IL, **II**
Somerset House, Chicago, IL, **III**
South Chicago YMCA, Chicago, IL, **IV-B**

South Side Physical Medicine & Rehabilitation
  Center, Chicago, IL, **VI**
The Sovereign Home, Chicago, IL, **III**
Squire's Sheltered Care Home, Chicago, IL, **IV-A**
Staff Builders Health Services, Chicago, IL, **II**
Staff Builders Services, Chicago, IL, **II**
Summit Home Health Inc, Chicago, IL, **II**
Swartzberg House, Chicago, IL, **IV-B**
Swedish Covenant Hospital, Chicago, IL, **VI**
Third Age Program, Chicago, IL, **II**
Total Home Health Care of Chicago Inc, Chicago,
  IL, **II**
Ultra Care Home Medical, Chicago, IL, **II**
Umoja Care Inc, Chicago, IL, **I, II**
University of Chicago Medical Center Alzheimer's
  Program, Chicago, IL, **V**
The University of Illinois Hospital & Clinics,
  Chicago, IL, **VI**
Unlimited Home Care, Chicago, IL, **II**
Upjohn HealthCare Services, Chicago, IL, **II**
Uptown Shelter Care Home, Chicago, IL, **IV-A**
Veterans Affairs Lakeside Medical Center, Chicago,
  IL, **VI**
Veterans Affairs West Side Medical Center,
  Chicago, IL, **VI**
Visiting Nurse Association of Chicago, Chicago, IL,
  II
Vital Measurements Inc, Chicago, IL, **II**
Warren Park Nursing Pavilion, Chicago, IL, **III**
Waterfront Terrace, Chicago, IL, **III, V**
Wedgewood Nursing Pavilion Ltd, Chicago, IL, **III**
Wellington Plaza Nursing & Therapy Center,
  Chicago, IL, **III, V**
The Westwood Manor Inc, Chicago, IL, **III**
The Whitehall Convalescent and Nursing Home,
  Chicago, IL, **III**
Wilson Care Inc, Chicago, IL, **III**
Wincrest Nursing Center, Chicago, IL, **III**
Winston Manor Convalescent & Nursing Home,
  Chicago, IL, **III**
Wishing Well Health Services, Chicago, IL, **II**
Woodbridge Nursing Pavilion, Chicago, IL, **III, V**
Woodlawn Residences II, Chicago, IL, **IV-B**
YMCA of Metro Chicago, Chicago, IL, **I**
YWCA—Harriet M Harris Adult Day Care Center,
  Chicago, IL, **I**

CHICAGO HEIGHTS

Alpha Home Health Care, Chicago Heights, IL, **II**
Prairie Manor Health Care Center, Chicago
  Heights, IL, **III**
Riviera Manor Inc, Chicago Heights, IL, **III**
Thornton Heights Terrace Ltd, Chicago Heights, IL,
  III

Peace Memorial Home Health Service, Evergreen
   Park, IL, **II**
Wellspring Gerontological Services, Evergreen
   Park, IL, **I**

FLOSSMOOR

Home Health Plus, Flossmoor, IL, **II**

FOREST PARK

Altenheim, Forest Park, IL, **III, IV-A, IV-B**

FOX LAKE

Leisure Village, Fox Lake, IL, **IV-B**

FRANKFORT

Autumn Country Club Adult Day Care, Frankfort,
   IL, **I**
Frankfort Terrace, Frankfort, IL, **III**

FRANKLIN PARK

Leyden Adult Day Center, Franklin Park, IL, **I**
Leyden Family Service (Mental Health Center)
   Senior Citizen Program, Franklin Park, IL, **II**
Westlake Pavilion, Franklin Park, IL, **III, V**

GENEVA

Carlton Health Care, Geneva, IL, **II**
Community Contacts Inc, Geneva, IL, **II**
Geneva Care Center, Geneva, IL, **III**

GLEN ELLYN

Alpha Home Health Care, Glen Ellyn, IL, **II**
ESSE Adult Day Care—Ecumenical Support
   Services for the Elderly, Glen Ellyn, IL, **I**

GLENCOE

Chicagoland Therapy Associates, Glencoe, IL, **II**

GLENVIEW

The Abington of Glenview, Glenview, IL, **III, VI**
Glenview Elderly Housing, Glenview, IL, **IV-B**
Glenview Terrace Nursing Center, Glenview, IL,
   III, V
Maryhaven Inc, Glenview, IL, **III**

GLENWOOD

Glenwood Terrace Nursing Center, Glenwood, IL,
   III

HARVARD

Harvard Retirement Home, Harvard, IL, **IV-B**

HARVEY

Alden Nursing Center—Heather Rehabilitation &
   Health Care Center, Harvey, IL, **III, V**
Dixie Manor Sheltered Care, Harvey, IL, **IV-A**
Halsted Manor, Harvey, IL, **IV-A**
Ingalls Memorial Hospital, Harvey, IL, **VI**
Kenniebrew Home, Harvey, IL, **IV-A**
South Suburban Senior Services of Catholic
   Charities, Harvey, IL, **II**

HAZEL CREST

Home Health Services of South Suburban Hospital,
   Hazel Crest, IL, **II**
Imperial Nursing Center of Hazel Crest, Hazel
   Crest, IL, **III**
Lutheran Social Services—Home Helps for Seniors,
   Hazel Crest, IL, **I**
Nursefinders of Hazel Crest, Hazel Crest, IL, **II**
South Suburban Hospital—Alzheimer's Assessment
   Center, Hazel Crest, IL, **V**

HICKORY HILLS

Hickory Nursing Pavilion Inc, Hickory Hills, IL, **III**
Kimberly Quality Care—Hickory Hills, Hickory
   Hills, IL, **II**

HIGHLAND PARK

Abbott House, Highland Park, IL, **III**
Highland Park Hospital, Highland Park, IL, **VI**
Highland Park Hospital Alternative Adult Day
   Services, Highland Park, IL, **I**
Highland Park Hospital Alzheimer's Assessment
   Program, Highland Park, IL, **V**
Highland Park Hospital Home Health Services,
   Highland Park, IL, **II**
Villa St Cyril, Highland Park, IL, **III**
Walnut Place, Highland Park, IL, **IV-B**

HIGHWOOD

Highland Park Health Care Center Inc, Highwood,
   IL, **III**
Traycee Home Care, Highwood, IL, **II**

HILLSIDE

Oakridge Convalescent Home Inc, Hillside, IL, **III**

HINES

Edward Hines Jr Veterans Affairs Hospital, Hines,
   IL, **VI**

HINSDALE

Americana-Monticello Healthcare Center of
   Hinsdale, Hinsdale, IL, **III, V, VI**
Health Care at Home, Hinsdale, IL, **II**

Paulson Rehab Network—Hinsdale Hospital, Hinsdale, IL, **VI**

Suburban Hospital Alzheimer's Program, Hinsdale, IL, **V**

Washington Square Retirement Community, Hinsdale, IL, **IV-B**

West Suburban Shelter Care Center, Hinsdale, IL, **IV-A**

HOFFMAN ESTATES

Alden—Poplar Creek Hemodialysis Program, Hoffman Estates, IL, **VI**

Alden—Poplar Creek Rehabilitation & Health Care Center, Hoffman Estates, IL, **I, III, V**

The Benchmark of Hoffman Estates, Hoffman Estates, IL, **IV-B**

Kenneth W Young Center for Senior Services, Hoffman Estates, IL, **II**

HOMEWOOD

Caremark Inc, Homewood, IL, **II**

Concerned Care Inc, Homewood, IL, **II**

Heartland Health Care Center—Homewood, Homewood, IL, **III**

Ingalls Home Care, Homewood, IL, **II**

Mercy Health Care & Rehabilitation Center, Homewood, IL, **III, VI**

INDIAN HEAD PARK

Briar Place Ltd, Indian Head Park, IL, **III**

ISLAND LAKE

Sheltering Oak, Island Lake, IL, **III**

ITASCA

The Arbor, Itasca, IL, **III**

JOLIET

Broadway Residence, Joliet, IL, **IV-A**

Care Company Health Care Inc, Joliet, IL, **II**

Community Adult Day Care Systems Inc, Joliet, IL, **I**

Community Care System Inc, Joliet, IL, **II**

Deerbrook Nursing Centre, Joliet, IL, **III**

Draper Plaza, Joliet, IL, **III, V**

Easter Seal Rehabilitation Center of Will-Grundy Counties Inc, Joliet, IL, **VI**

Franciscan Home Health of St Joseph Medical Center, Joliet, IL, **II**

In Home Health Care Service—West Inc-Joliet Div, Joliet, IL, **II**

Joliet Terrace, Joliet, IL, **III**

Kimberly Quality Care—Joliet, Joliet, IL, **II**

Medical Personnel Pool, Joliet, IL, **II**

Metropolitan Nursing Center of Joliet, Joliet, IL, **III**

Nursefinders of Joliet, Joliet, IL, **II**

Our Lady of Angels Retirement Home, Joliet, IL, **III, IV-A**

Rosewood Care Center Inc—Joliet, Joliet, IL, **III**

St Joseph Medical Center, Joliet, IL, **VI**

Salem Village, Joliet, IL, **III, IV-B, V**

Silver Cross Hospital, Joliet, IL, **VI**

Sunny Hill Nursing Home, Joliet, IL, **III**

Upjohn HealthCare Services, Joliet, IL, **II**

Villa Franciscan, Joliet, IL, **III, V**

JUSTICE

Mercy Home Health Care, Justice, IL, **II**

Rosary Hill Home, Justice, IL, **III, IV-A**

LA GRANGE

Colonial Manor Healthcare Center, La Grange, IL, **III, V**

Fairview Health Care Center, La Grange, IL, **III**

La Grange Community Nurse & Service Association, La Grange, IL, **II**

Windsor Place, La Grange, IL, **IV-A**

LA GRANGE PARK

Bethlehem Woods Retirement Living Center, La Grange Park, IL, **IV-B**

Plymouth Place, La Grange Park, IL, **III, IV-B, V**

LAKE BLUFF

Hill Top Sanitorium, Lake Bluff, IL, **III**

Lake Bluff Healthcare Centre, Lake Bluff, IL, **III, V**

LAKE FOREST

Lake Forest Hospital Adult Day Care, Lake Forest, IL, **I**

Lake Forest Hospital Home Health, Lake Forest, IL, **II**

Lake Forest Hospital Pain Treatment Center, Lake Forest, IL, **VI**

LAKE IN THE HILLS

Around the Clock Nursing Registry Inc, Lake In The Hills, IL, **II**

LAKE VILLA

Family Care Services of Lake and McHenry Counties, Lake Villa, IL, **II**

Lake County Health Dept, Lake Villa, IL, **II**

LANSING

Tri State Manor Nursing Home, Lansing, IL, **III**

LEMONT

Alvernia Manor Retirement Home, Lemont, IL, **IV-A**

Franciscan Village, Lemont, IL, **IV-A, IV-B**

Holy Family Villa, Lemont, IL, **III**

✔ In order to support future editions of this publication would you please mention *Elder Services* each time you contact any advertiser, facility, or service.

Home Health Care Inc—Lemont, Lemont, IL, **II**
Mother Theresa Home, Lemont, IL, **III, IV-A**

LIBERTYVILLE

Americana Healthcare Center of Libertyville,
  Libertyville, IL, **III, IV-A, VI**
Caregivers Home Health, Libertyville, IL, **II**
Condell Day Center Intergenerational Care,
  Libertyville, IL, **I**
Liberty Towers, Libertyville, IL, **IV-B**
Libertyville Manor Extended Care Facility,
  Libertyville, IL, **III**
Medical Personnel Pool, Libertyville, IL, **II**
Nursefinders of Libertyville, Libertyville, IL, **II**
Winchester House, Libertyville, IL, **III, V**

LINCOLNWOOD

Regency Park, Lincolnwood, IL, **IV-A**
Regency Park Manor, Lincolnwood, IL, **III**

LINDENHURST

Victory Lakes Adult Day Care Center, Lindenhurst,
  IL, **I**
Victory Lakes Continuing Care Center, Lindenhurst,
  IL, **III, V, VI**

LISLE

The Devonshire, Lisle, IL, **IV-A**
Queen of Peace Retirement Center, Lisle, IL, **IV-A,
  IV-B**
Snow Valley Living Center, Lisle, IL, **III, V**

LOMBARD

Abbey Home Healthcare, Lombard, IL, **II**
Beacon Hill, Lombard, IL, **III, IV-B**
Bloomingdale Pavilion, Lombard, IL, **III**
Lexington Health Care Center of Lombard,
  Lombard, IL, **III**
Lexington Square of Lombard, Lombard, IL, **IV-B**
Olsten Healthcare, Lombard, IL, **II**

LONG GROVE

Maple Hill Nursing Home Ltd, Long Grove, IL, **III**

LYONS

Golden Age Retirement Home, Lyons, IL, **IV-B**
MacNeal Home Health Services, Lyons, IL, **II**

MARENGO

Florence Nursing Home, Marengo, IL, **III**

MATTESON

Applewood Living Center, Matteson, IL, **I, III**

MAYWOOD

Baptist Retirement Home, Maywood, IL, **III, IV-A,
  IV-B**
Garden House of Maywood, Maywood, IL, **IV-B**
Loyola University Medical Center—Alzheimer
  Primary Provider Program, Maywood, IL, **V**
NovaCare Inc, Maywood, IL, **II**

MCHENRY

McHenry Villa, McHenry, IL, **IV-A**
Northern Illinois Medical Center, McHenry, IL, **V,
  VI**
Northern Illinois Medical Center—Home Health
  Care, McHenry, IL, **II**
Royal Terrace, McHenry, IL, **III**

MELROSE PARK

Gottlieb Memorial Hospital, Melrose Park, IL, **II, V,
  VI**
Gottlieb Memorial Hospital Extended Care Unit,
  Melrose Park, IL, **III**
Westlake Community Hospital, Melrose Park, IL, **II**
Westlake Community Hospital Center for
  Rehabilitation, Melrose Park, IL, **VI**

MIDLOTHIAN

Bowman Nursing Home, Midlothian, IL, **III, V**
Crestwood Terrace, Midlothian, IL, **III**
Golfview Retirement Manor, Midlothian, IL, **IV-A**

MORRIS

Grundy County Home, Morris, IL, **III**
Morris Lincoln Nursing Home, Morris, IL, **III, IV-A**
Walnut Grove Village, Morris, IL, **III**

MORTON GROVE

Abbey Home Healthcare, Morton Grove, IL, **II**
Bethany Terrace Nursing Centre, Morton Grove, IL,
  III
Bethany Terrace Nursing Centre Alzheimer's Care
  Center, Morton Grove, IL, **V**
In Home Health Care—Suburban Chicago North,
  Morton Grove, IL, **II**
NMC Home Care, Morton Grove, IL, **II**

MOUNT PROSPECT

Caremark Home Care Inc, Mount Prospect, IL, **II**
Village of Mt Prospect Human Services Division,
  Mount Prospect, IL, **II, V**

NAPERVILLE

Alden Nursing Center—Naperville Rehabilitation &
  Health Care Center, Naperville, IL, **I, III, V**
Americana Healthcare Center of Naperville,
  Naperville, IL, **III, V, VI**

Community Convalescent Center of Naperville, Naperville, IL, **III, V**

Ecumenical Adult Care of Naperville, Naperville, IL, **I**

Health Force, Naperville, IL, **II**

Martin Manor Apartments, Naperville, IL, **IV-B**

St Patrick's Residence, Naperville, IL, **III, IV-A, V**

NILES

The Caring Touch, Niles, IL, **II**

Forest Villa Nursing Center, Niles, IL, **III**

Glen Bridge Nursing & Rehabilitation Center, Niles, IL, **III**

George J Goldman Memorial Home for the Aged, Niles, IL, **III**

Hampton Plaza, Niles, IL, **III**

Regency Home Health Care, Niles, IL, **II**

Regency Nursing Centre, Niles, IL, **III, V**

Roche Professional Services, Niles, IL, **II**

St Andrew Home for the Aged, Niles, IL, **III, IV-A**

St Benedict Home for Aged, Niles, IL, **III**

NORRIDGE

Central Baptist Home for the Aged, Norridge, IL, **III, IV-A**

Norridge Nursing Centre Inc, Norridge, IL, **III, V**

NORTH AURORA

Asbury Court, North Aurora, IL, **IV-A**

Maplewood Health Care Center, North Aurora, IL, **III**

NORTH CHICAGO

Veterans Affairs Medical Center—North Chicago, North Chicago, IL, **VI**

Veterans Affairs Medical Center—North Chicago-Adult Day Health Care, North Chicago, IL, **I**

NORTH RIVERSIDE

Kimberly Quality Care—North Riverside, North Riverside, IL, **II**

The Scottish Home, North Riverside, IL, **III, IV-A, IV-B**

NORTHBROOK

Axelson Manor, Northbrook, IL, **IV-A**

Brandel Care Center, Northbrook, IL, **III**

Caring Companions of the North Shore Inc, Northbrook, IL, **II**

Covenant Village of Northbrook, Northbrook, IL, **IV-B**

GAF/Lake Cook Terrace, Northbrook, IL, **III**

Glen Oaks Nursing Home Inc, Northbrook, IL, **III**

House of Welcome, Northbrook, IL, **I**

NORTHFIELD

North Shore Senior Center, Northfield, IL, **II**

North Shore Senior Center & House of Welcome, Northfield, IL, **V**

Parkside Adult Day Health Center, Northfield, IL, **I**

NORTHLAKE

The Caring Center—Casa San Carlo, Northlake, IL, **II**

Casa San Carlo Retirement Community, Northlake, IL, **IV-B**

Concord Plaza Retirement Community, Northlake, IL, **IV-B**

Villa Scalabrini, Northlake, IL, **III, IV-A, V**

OAK BROOK

EHS Home Health Care Service Inc, Oak Brook, IL, **II**

Mayslake Village, Oak Brook, IL, **IV-B**

Norrell Health Care, Oak Brook, IL, **II**

Oak Brook Healthcare Centre, Oak Brook, IL, **III**

OAK FOREST

Oak Forest Hospital, Oak Forest, IL, **VI**

OAK LAWN

Americana Healthcare Center of Oak Lawn, Oak Lawn, IL, **III, VI**

Americana-Monticello Healthcare Center of Oak Lawn, Oak Lawn, IL, **III, V, VI**

Christ Hospital & Medical Center, Oak Lawn, IL, **VI**

Concord Extended Care, Oak Lawn, IL, **III**

Medical Personnel Pool, Oak Lawn, IL, **II**

Nursefinders of Oak Lawn, Oak Lawn, IL, **II**

Oak Lawn Convalescent Home, Oak Lawn, IL, **III**

Plows Council on Aging, Oak Lawn, IL, **II**

OAK PARK

Ancilla Home Health, Oak Park, IL, **II**

At Home Health Inc, Oak Park, IL, **II**

Bruce & Ken's Pharmacy, Oak Park, IL, **II**

The Caring Center—Mills Tower, Oak Park, IL, **II**

The Caring Center—The Oaks, Oak Park, IL, **II**

Community Nursing Service West, Oak Park, IL, **II**

FirstChoice Home Health & Family Support Services, Oak Park, IL, **II**

Holley Court Terrace, Oak Park, IL, **IV-B**

Home Companion Service, Oak Park, IL, **II**

Home Medical Care Foundation, Oak Park, IL, **II**

HomeCare Resources—An Affiliate of West Suburban Hospital Medical Center, Oak Park, IL, **II**

Kimberly Quality Care—Oak Park, Oak Park, IL, **II**

Medical Personnel Pool, Oak Park, IL, **II**

✔ In order to support future editions of this publication would you please mention *Elder Services* each time you contact any advertiser, facility, or service.

Metropolitan Nursing Center of Oak Park, Oak Park, IL, **III**

The Oak Park Arms, Oak Park, IL, **IV-A**

Oak Park Township Office, Oak Park, IL, **II**

Suburban Adult Day Care Center, Oak Park, IL, **I**

The Woodbine Convalescent Home, Oak Park, IL, **III**

OLYMPIA FIELDS

Kimberly Quality Care—Olympia Fields, Olympia Fields, IL, **II**

Mercy Residence at Tolentine Center, Olympia Fields, IL, **IV-A**

Olympia Fields Osteopathic Hospital & Medical Center, Olympia Fields, IL, **VI**

OSWEGO

The Tillers Nursing Home, Oswego, IL, **III**

PALATINE

Little Sisters of the Poor, Palatine, IL, **I, III**

Palatine Township Senior Citizens Council, Palatine, IL, **V**

Plum Grove Nursing Home, Palatine, IL, **III, V**

St Joseph's Home, Palatine, IL, **IV-A**

Tamarack, Palatine, IL, **IV-A**

PALOS HEIGHTS

Americana Healthcare Center of Palos Heights, Palos Heights, IL, **III, IV-A, V, VI**

Rest Haven Central Nursing Home, Palos Heights, IL, **III**

Ridgeland Living Center, Palos Heights, IL, **III**

PALOS HILLS

Shay Health Care Services Inc, Palos Hills, IL, **II**

Windsor Manor Nursing & Rehabilitation Center, Palos Hills, IL, **III**

PALOS PARK

The Club Adult Day Care Centers Inc, Palos Park, IL, **I**

Peace Memorial Village, Palos Park, IL, **IV-B**

PARK FOREST

The Club Adult Day Care Centers Inc, Park Forest, IL, **I**

Park Forest Health Dept, Park Forest, IL, **II**

PARK RIDGE

A-Abiding Care Inc, Park Ridge, IL, **II**

The Center of Concern, Park Ridge, IL, **II**

Lutheran General Hospital, Park Ridge, IL, **VI**

Omni Home Care, Park Ridge, IL, **II**

Park Ridge Healthcare Center, Park Ridge, IL, **III**

Resurrection Nursing Pavilion, Park Ridge, IL, **III**

St Matthew Lutheran Home, Park Ridge, IL, **III, IV-A, IV-B, V**

Summit Square Retirement Hotel, Park Ridge, IL, **IV-A, IV-B**

PEOTONE

Peotone Bensenville Home, Peotone, IL, **IV-A**

PLAINFIELD

Lakewood Living Center, Plainfield, IL, **III**

PROSPECT HEIGHTS

Excellcare Rehabilitation, Prospect Heights, IL, **VI**

RICHTON PARK

Rich Township Senior Services, Richton Park, IL, **II**

Richton Crossing Convalescent Center, Richton Park, IL, **III**

RIVER FOREST

Home Infusion Therapy, River Forest, IL, **II**

RIVERWOODS

Brentwood North Nursing & Rehabilitation Center, Riverwoods, IL, **III, V, VI**

ROBBINS

Lydia Healthcare, Robbins, IL, **III**

Senior Citizens Services, Robbins, IL, **II**

ROLLING MEADOWS

Americana Healthcare Center of Rolling Meadows, Rolling Meadows, IL, **III, V, VI**

Home Health Plus, Rolling Meadows, IL, **II**

ROSELLE

Abbington House, Roselle, IL, **III**

Nurses to You Ltd, Roselle, IL, **II**

Parkside—Trinity Adult Day Health Center, Roselle, IL, **I**

ROUND LAKE BEACH

Hillcrest Nursing Center, Round Lake Beach, IL, **III**

SAINT CHARLES

Concerned Care Inc, Saint Charles, IL, **II**

Country Care Inc, Saint Charles, IL, **II**

Cumberland Green Cooperative, Saint Charles, IL, **IV-B**

Hotel Baker Living Center—Lutheran Social Services of Illinois, Saint Charles, IL, **IV-A**

Pine View Care Center, Saint Charles, IL, **III**

SANDWICH

Dogwood Health Care Center, Sandwich, IL, **III**, **IV-A**
Willow Crest Nursing Pavilion, Sandwich, IL, **III**

SCHAUMBURG

Alexian Home Health, Schaumburg, IL, **II**
Friendship Village of Schaumburg, Schaumburg, IL, **III**, **IV-A**, **IV-B**, **V**
Greencastle of Schaumberg, Schaumburg, IL, **IV-B**
In Home Health Care Service—West Inc, Schaumburg, IL, **II**
Lexington Health Care Center of Schaumburg, Schaumburg, IL, **III**
Medical Personnel Pool, Schaumburg, IL, **II**

SHABBONA

Shabbona Health Care Center Inc, Shabbona, IL, **III**

SKOKIE

Alzheimer's Disease & Related Disorders Association, Skokie, IL, **V**
Concerned Care Inc, Skokie, IL, **II**
Extended Health Services Inc, Skokie, IL, **II**
Great Opportunities Adult Day Care, Skokie, IL, **I**
Health Connections, Skokie, IL, **II**
Kelly Assisted Living, Skokie, IL, **II**
Kimberly Quality Care—Skokie, Skokie, IL, **II**
Krasnow Residence, Skokie, IL, **IV-B**
Lieberman Geriatric Health Centre, Skokie, IL, **III**, **V**
Nursefinders of Skokie, Skokie, IL, **II**
Old Orchard Manor, Skokie, IL, **III**
Robineau Group Living Residence, Skokie, IL, **IV-A**
Skokie Health Dept, Skokie, IL, **II**
Skokie Meadows Nursing Center 1, Skokie, IL, **III**
Skokie Meadows Nursing Center 2, Skokie, IL, **III**
Village Nursing Home Inc, Skokie, IL, **III**

SOUTH CHICAGO HEIGHTS

Woodside Manor, South Chicago Heights, IL, **III**

SOUTH ELGIN

Alderwood Health Care Center, South Elgin, IL, **III**
Fox Valley Healthcare Inc, South Elgin, IL, **III**

SOUTH HOLLAND

Americana Healthcare Center of South Holland, South Holland, IL, **III**, **V**, **VI**
Holland Home, South Holland, IL, **IV-A**
Lutheran Social Services of Illinois—Home Helps for Seniors, South Holland, IL, **II**
Rest Haven South, South Holland, IL, **I**, **III**, **V**

Windmill Nursing Pavilion Ltd, South Holland, IL, **III**, **V**

STICKNEY

Pershing Convalescent Home Inc, Stickney, IL, **III**
Stickney Township Office on Aging—North Stickney Medical Center, Stickney, IL, **I**

STREAMWOOD

Family Service—Hanover Township, Streamwood, IL, **II**

SUMMIT

Americanurse Ltd, Summit, IL, **II**

TINLEY PARK

Brementowne Manor, Tinley Park, IL, **IV-B**
The McAllister Nursing Home Inc, Tinley Park, IL, **III**
Royal Acres Retirement Village, Tinley Park, IL, **IV-A**

VERNON HILLS

Hawthorn Lakes of Lake County, Vernon Hills, IL, **IV-A**, **IV-B**
The Helping Hand Private Duty—DME, Vernon Hills, IL, **II**

VILLA PARK

Du Page Easter Seal Center, Villa Park, IL, **VI**
Elmhurst Memorial Home Health Care Services, Villa Park, IL, **II**

WAUCONDA

Town Hall Estates—Wauconda Inc, Wauconda, IL, **III**

WAUKEGAN

Bayside Terrace, Waukegan, IL, **III**
Franciscan Home Health, Waukegan, IL, **II**
Helping Care Inc, Waukegan, IL, **II**
Home Health Services of Lake County Health Dept, Waukegan, IL, **II**
Kimberly Quality Care—Waukegan, Waukegan, IL, **II**
Lake Park Center, Waukegan, IL, **III**
Northshore Terrace, Waukegan, IL, **III**
Pavilion of Waukegan Inc, Waukegan, IL, **III**
The Terrace Nursing Home Inc, Waukegan, IL, **III**
Victory Memorial Hospital Home Health Care, Waukegan, IL, **II**
Victory Memorial Hospital—Waukegan Adult Day Care Center, Waukegan, IL, **I**

✔ In order to support future editions of this publication would you please mention *Elder Services* each time you contact any advertiser, facility, or service.

WEST CHICAGO

Arbor Terrace Health Care Center, West Chicago, IL, **III, IV-A, IV-B**
Kimberly Quality Care—West Chicago, West Chicago, IL, **II**
West Chicago Terrace, West Chicago, IL, **III**

WESTCHESTER

Home Health Plus, Westchester, IL, **II**
In Home Health Care Service—West Inc, Westchester, IL, **II**
Westchester Manor, Westchester, IL, **III**

WESTMONT

Americana Healthcare Center of Westmont, Westmont, IL, **III, V, VI**
Burgess Square Healthcare Centre, Westmont, IL, **III**
Home Health Care Providers Inc, Westmont, IL, **II**
Westmont Convalescent Center, Westmont, IL, **III, V**

WHEATON

Denson Optioncare Pharmacy, Wheaton, IL, **II**
Denson Shops Inc, Wheaton, IL, **II**
Du Page Convalescent Center, Wheaton, IL, **III**
Marian Park, Wheaton, IL, **IV-B**
Marianjoy Rehabilitation Hospital and Clinics, Wheaton, IL, **VI**
Parkway Healthcare Center, Wheaton, IL, **III**
Sandalwood Healthcare Centre, Wheaton, IL, **III, V**
Sharon Glen Village, Wheaton, IL, **IV-B**
Wheaton Convalescent Center, Wheaton, IL, **III**

WHEELING

Addolorata Villa, Wheeling, IL, **III, IV-A, IV-B, V**

WILLOWBROOK

Chateau Village Living Center, Willowbrook, IL, **III**
Paulson Center Adult Care, Willowbrook, IL, **I**
Paulson Center for Rehabilitative Medicine, Willowbrook, IL, **VI**

WILMETTE

Altru Nurses Registry, Wilmette, IL, **II**
Baha'i Home, Wilmette, IL, **IV-A**
Fairfield Court, Wilmette, IL, **IV-B**
House of Welcome, Wilmette, IL, **I**
Klafter Residence, Wilmette, IL, **IV-A**
Normandy House, Wilmette, IL, **III, V**
North Shore Visiting Nurse Association, Wilmette, IL, **II**
Shore Line Place, Wilmette, IL, **IV-B**

WILMINGTON

Royal Willow Nursing Care Center, Wilmington, IL, **III**

WINFIELD

Central DuPage Hospital Alzheimer's Program, Winfield, IL, **V**
Liberty Hill Healthcare Center, Winfield, IL, **III, V**

WINNETKA

House of Welcome, Winnetka, IL, **I**

WOODSTOCK

Carefree Village, Woodstock, IL, **IV-A**
Carefree Village Subdivision, Woodstock, IL, **IV-B**
Caregivers Home Health, Woodstock, IL, **II**
Easter Seal Adult & Child Rehabilitation Center, Woodstock, IL, **II**
Family Alliance Inc, Woodstock, IL, **I, V**
Healthtrends Ltd, Woodstock, IL, **II**
McHenry County Dept of Health, Woodstock, IL, **II**
Sunset Manor, Woodstock, IL, **III, IV-A, V**
Valley Hi Nursing Home, Woodstock, IL, **III**
The Woodstock Residence, Woodstock, IL, **III**

YORKVILLE

Hillside Health Care Center, Yorkville, IL, **III**

ZION

Crown Manor Healthcare Center, Zion, IL, **III**
Rolling Hills Manor, Zion, IL, **III**
Sheridan Health Care Center, Zion, IL, **III**

INDIANA

CHESTERTON

Chesterton Health Care Facility, Chesterton, IN, **III**

CROWN POINT

The Caring Co Inc, Crown Point, IN, **II**
Caritas Center Adult Day Care, Crown Point, IN, **I**
Colonial Nursing Home, Crown Point, IN, **III**
ElderCare Services Inc, Crown Point, IN, **II**
Lake County Convalescent Home, Crown Point, IN, **III, V**
Lutheran Home of Northwest Indiana Inc, Crown Point, IN, **III**
Lutheran Retirement Village, Crown Point, IN, **IV-B**
Meals on Wheels—Northwest Indiana, Crown Point, IN, **II**
Rehabilitation Services of St Anthony Medical Center, Crown Point, IN, **VI**
St Anthony Home, Crown Point, IN, **III**
Staff Builders Health Care Services, Crown Point, IN, **II**

✔ In order to support future editions of this publication would you please mention *Elder Services* each time you contact any advertiser, facility, or service.

Index of Advertisers

✔ In order to support future editions of this publication would you please mention *Elder Services* each time you contact any advertiser, facility, or service.

✔ In order to support future editions of this publication would you please mention **Elder Services** each time you contact any advertiser, facility, or service.